Clinical Procedures in
OPTOMETRY

J. Boyd Eskridge, O.D., Ph.D.

School of Optometry / The Medical Center
University of Alabama at Birmingham
Birmingham, Alabama

John F. Amos, O.D., M.S.

School of Optometry / The Medical Center
University of Alabama at Birmingham
Birmingham, Alabama

Jimmy D. Bartlett, O.D., D.O.S.

School of Optometry / The Medical Center
University of Alabama at Birmingham
Birmingham, Alabama

With 41 additional contributors

J. B. Lippincott Company   Philadelphia
New York   London   Hagerstown

Library of Congress Cataloging-in-Publication Data

Eskridge, J. Boyd.
  Clinical procedures in optometry / J. Boyd Eskridge, John
Amos, Jimmy D. Bartlett, with 41 additional contributors.
    p.   cm.
  Includes bibliographical references and index.
  ISBN 0–397–50984–7
  1. Optometry.   I. Amos, John F.   II. Bartlett, Jimmy D.
III. Title.
  [DNLM: 1. Contact Lenses.   2. Eye Diseases—diagnosis.
3. Optometry—methods.   4. Vision Disorders—diagnosis.
WW 141 E75c]
RE951.E85   1991
617.7'5—dc20
DNLM/DLC
for Library of Congress   91–8590
                                                                    CIP

Acquisitions Editor: Nancy Mullins
Production Manager: Janet Greenwood
Production: P. M. Gordon Associates
Compositor: Bi-Comp, Inc.
Printer/Binder: Halliday Lithograph Corp.

1   3   5   6   4   2

The authors and publisher have exerted every effort to ensure that
drug selection and dosage set forth in this text are in accord with
current recommendations and practice at the time of publication.
However, in view of ongoing research, changes in government
regulations, and the constant flow of information relating to drug
therapy and drug reactions, the reader is urged to check the package insert for each drug for any change in indications and dosage
and for added warnings and precautions. This is particularly important when the recommended agent is a new or infrequently
employed drug.

We sincerely thank our dear wives and children for their understanding of the time commitment required to produce this book.

Contributors

John F. Amos, OD, MS
Professor of Optometry
Director, Residency Programs
School of Optometry/The
    Medical Center
University of Alabama at
    Birmingham
Birmingham, Alabama

**Ian L. Bailey, OD, MS,
    FBCO**
Professor of Optometry and
    Vision Science
Director of Low Vision Center
School of Optometry
University of California at
    Berkeley
Berkeley, California

James E. Bailey, OD, PhD
Professor and Chairman
Department of Basic and
    Visual Sciences
Southern California College
    of Optometry
Fullerton, California

Felix M. Barker, OD, MS
Associate Professor and
    Director
The Light and Laser Institute
Pennsylvania College of
    Optometry
Philadelphia, Pennsylvania

Jimmy D. Bartlett, OD
Associate Professor of
    Optometry
School of Optometry/The
    Medical Center
University of Alabama at
    Birmingham
Birmingham, Alabama

Linda J. Bass, OD
Adjunct Assistant Professor
University of Houston College
    of Optometry
Southern California College
    of Optometry
Chief of Optometry
Bay Pines Veterans Affairs
    Medical Center
Bay Pines, Florida

Sherry J. Bass, OD
Associate Professor
State University of New York
State College of Optometry
New York, New York

Clifford W. Brooks, OD
Associate Professor of
    Optometry
Indiana University School of
    Optometry
Bloomington, Indiana

**William L. Brown, OD,
    PhD**
Associate Professor of
    Optometry
Illinois College of Optometry
Director
Center for the Partially
    Sighted
Illinois Eye Institute
Chicago, Illinois

Linda Casser Locke, OD
Associate Professor of
    Optometry
Department of Clinical
    Sciences
Indiana University School of
    Optometry
Bloomington, Indiana
Director
Indianapolis Clinics
Indianapolis, Indiana

**Anthony A.
    Cavallerano, OD**
Associate Professor of
    Optometry
The New England College of
    Optometry
Eye Health Services
Weymouth, Massachusetts

**Jerry D. Cavallerano, OD,
    PhD**
Staff Optometrist
Joslin Diabetes Center
Boston, Massachusetts

Richard J. Clompus, OD
Adjunct Faculty Member
Pennsylvania College of
    Optometry
Philadelphia, Pennsylvania

**David M. Cockburn, DSc,
    MScOptom**
Senior Academic Associate
Department of Optometry
University of Melbourne
Victoria, Australia

Roy Gordon Cole, OD
Associate Professor
Department of Clinical
    Sciences
State University of New York
State College of Optometry
New York, New York

George W. Comer, OD
Associate Professor
Chief, Ocular Disease Service
Southern California College
    of Optometry
Fullerton, California

Jeffrey Cooper, OD
Associate Clinical Professor of
   Optometry
State University of New York
State College of Optometry
New York, New York

Kent M. Daum, OD, PhD
Associate Professor of
   Optometry
School of Optometry/The
   Medical Center
University of Alabama at
   Birmingham
Birmingham, Alabama

**David W. Davidson, OD,
MS**
Associate Dean
School of Optometry
University of Missouri-
   St. Louis
St. Louis, Missouri

**Pierrette Dayhaw-Barker,
PhD**
Assistant Dean for Basic
   Sciences and Associate
   Professor
Pennsylvania College of
   Optometry
Philadelphia, Pennsylvania

J. Boyd Eskridge, OD, PhD
Professor of Optometry
School of Optometry/The
   Medical Center
University of Alabama at
   Birmingham
Birmingham, Alabama

Troy E. Fannin, OD
Professor
University of Houston College
   of Optometry
Houston, Texas

Adam Gordon, OD, MPH
Clinical Associate Professor
School of Optometry/The
   Medical Center
University of Alabama at
   Birmingham
Birmingham, Alabama

David A. Goss, OD, PhD
Professor of Optometry
College of Optometry
Northeastern State University
Clinical Optometrist
W. W. Hastings Public Health
   Service—Indian Health
   Service Hospital
Tahlequah, Oklahoma

**Barbara J. Jennings, MA,
OD**
Chapman Professor of Vascu-
   lar Research and Director
Chapman Vascular Clinic
Southern College of
   Optometry
Memphis, Tennessee

Richard London, OD, MA
Oakland, California

William F. Long, PhD, OD
Associate Professor
School of Optometry
University of Missouri-St.
   Louis
St. Louis, Missouri

**Gerald E. Lowther, OD,
PhD**
Professor and Associate Dean
School of Optometry/The
   Medical Center
University of Alabama at
   Birmingham
Birmingham, Alabama

Michel Millodot, OD, PhD
Professor and Head
Department of Optometry
University of Wales
Cardiff, Wales
United Kingdom

Leonard J. Oshinskie, OD
Chief, Optometry Section
Department of Veteran's
   Affairs Medical Center
Newington, Connecticut
Clinical Professor of
   Optometry
New England College of
   Optometry
Boston, Massachusetts

Charles J. Patorgis, OD
Adjunct Clinical Professor of
   Optometry
New England College of
   Optometry
Director of Optometric
   Services
Center for Sight
Venice, Florida

Michael Polasky, OD
Assistant Professor
Assistant Dean for
   Professional Affairs
College of Optometry
The Ohio State University
Columbus, Ohio

Robert Rosenberg, MS, OD
Professor of Optometry and
   Vision Sciences
State University of New York
State College of Optometry
Associate Director of
   Optometry
Low Vision Clinic
The Lighthouse—New York
   Association for the Blind
New York, New York

Bruce P. Rosenthal, OD
Professor
Department of Clinical Sci-
   ences
State University of New York
State College of Optometry
New York, New York

Robert P. Rutstein, OD, MS
Associate Professor
Chief of Binocular Vision and
   Pediatric Clinic
School of Optometry/The
   Medical Center
University of Alabama at
   Birmingham
Birmingham, Alabama

Mitchell Scheiman, OD
Chief, Pediatric and
   Binocular Vision Service
Associate Professor
Pennsylvania College of
   Optometry
Philadelphia, Pennsylvania

Leo P. Semes, OD
Associate Professor
Chief, Primary Vision Care
   Services
School of Optometry/The
   Medical Center
University of Alabama at
   Birmingham
Birmingham, Alabama

Jerome Sherman, OD
Professor
State University of New York
State College of Optometry
Director of Professional
   Relations
Nassau Medical Eye Care
New York, New York

Vesna G. Sutija, PhD
Associate Professor
Department of Clinical
   Sciences
State University of New York
State College of Optometry
Member
Schnurmacher Institute for
   Vision Research
New York, New York

John C. Townsend, OD
Associate Professor
Southern California College
   of Optometry
Fullerton, California
Assistant Chief, Optometry
   Service
Department of Veterans
   Affairs Medical Center
Los Angeles, California

Norman J. Weiss, OD
Chief of Clinical Services and
   Executive Director
Western New York Center for
   the Visually Impaired
Buffalo, New York

Bruce Wick, OD
Associate Professor
College of Optometry
University of Houston
Houston, Texas

**T. David Williams, OD,
PhD**
Professor
School of Optometry
University of Waterloo
Waterloo, Ontario, Canada

Diane P. Yolton, OD, PhD
Associate Professor
College of Optometry
Pacific University
Forest Grove, Oregon

Foreword

Optometry has been greatly influenced by the fact that although its heritage resides in long-established optical and physical principles, its involvement as a health care delivery profession has placed it among the youngest of such disciplines. The history of early optometric development indicates that only a few of the founding practitioners had credible formal education in the basic sciences that underlay their applied endeavors. This early education consisted of rather elementary surveys of the basics in anatomy, physiology, and optics (upon which the tenets of refractive "testing" rested), with major emphasis upon subjective and some objective clinical processes aimed at determining the basic "refractive status" of the eye. Such routines exhibited some vague uniformity but essentially were derived from personal experience of the teachers. Almost no textbooks existed that dealt with the techniques of examination. The teachers developed their personal syllabi and compiled notes to serve the purpose. Perhaps one of the earliest texts was that written by Lionel Lawrence, in England, in the early part of the century. Although many concepts, and even instrumentation, varied between England and the United States, this volume remained the basic text in the field until it was replaced by *Clinical Refraction* in 1949.

As the scope and concern of optometry expanded beyond the elementary process of simple technical manipulation to the cognitive aspects of diagnosis and management, the priority turned to understanding and evaluating the inferences derived from the data accumulated by the clinical procedures. Accurate diagnosis and treatment depend on credible inferences that, in turn, depend on meaningful data. It obviously follows that the quality of the data is totally dependent on the procedures by which they are gathered. To present authentic data, procedures must fulfill several qualifications. They must be reliable—that is, they must be consistent in their determinations when used, so they do not present widely varying values for the same condition when repeated under comparable circumstances. They must be valid—that is, they test and evaluate the condition for which they are intended and not some other condition or a combination of both sought and unsought situations. They should also present respectably compatible findings when used on the same patient under similar circumstances by different examiners or upon the same patient at different times.

In addition, the expansion of the field of optometry into primary care has placed an added responsibility on the clinician. Because the examination must penetrate newly expanded realms of function and structure, new clinical test procedures become essential. Although many of these are detailed in scattered texts, descriptions and delineations of the soundest procedures for given purposes have not been compiled in a single textbook designed for the optometrist's use.

This volume was motivated by an attempt to compile a complete and comprehensive text of the clinical procedures involved in the performance of a thorough and embracing optometric examination and to indicate those procedures that lend themselves to efficient and facile clinical utilization and provide valid and reliable data from which a high level of diagnostic significance can be reached. Still another objective was that of enabling optometrists to accurately cooperate with each other, to have confidence in the progression of data from series of examinations performed either by themselves or by colleagues, and to arrive at maximum consistency of procedure, finer rapport in interpretation, and greater trust among themselves.

The aspiration of the editors and the contributors are that this volume may result in more consistency, harmony, and unity in the profession. The future of the profession may be reflected in that aspiration.

Irvin M. Borish, OD, DOS, LLD, DSc

Preface

The profession of optometry is relatively young, less than 100 years old. The teaching of clinical optometry has changed from correspondence courses taught by lens and frame manufacturers to the comprehensive postbaccalaureate professional education programs of today. The growth of clinical optometry has occurred because of the development of professional education programs, the involvement in vision and ocular research, the publication of scientific articles and textbooks, and the broadening of the legal definition of optometry. We believe there is currently a great need for a textbook that discusses the clinical procedures that need to be appreciated, understood, and utilized by contemporary optometrists. We feel that this information is the foundation of progressive clinical education and the comprehensive practice of optometry. Optometry, as a young profession, has developed divergent philosophies in some areas of clinical care, and even though this has some benefits, there is a substantial need for more clinical harmony so that optometry will provide better vision and ocular health care to patients and will have greater growth as a health care profession.

The main purpose of this book is to provide a clinical reference in the needed area of clinical procedures, and through its use to unify components of the optometric curriculum and thereby produce greater unity within the profession of optometry. We have placed more emphasis on those clinical procedures that will be used by the primary care practitioner.

We hope this book will be used by students, residents, faculty, and practitioners and thereby bring more consistency to the teaching and practice of optometry. It is our desire that this book will help students gain a greater understanding of the clinical procedures, how to obtain the needed patient care information, and how to use this information in patient care decisions. We hope this book will also broaden the perspective of students and practitioners with regard to the scope of the clinical practice of optometry. To help produce this effect, we have included nearly all the clinical procedures used in optometry that require the development of technical skills.

We have developed an outline, with major headings, that is used in most of the chapters, thus producing consistency and uniformity and making the contents easier to understand and use. Any shortcomings in the chapters produced by this outline are the responsibility of the editors, not the contributing authors. The outline begins with an Introduction section which defines the clinical procedure, includes a brief history, and indicates the general clinical use of the procedure. This is followed by a section on Instrumentation that discusses the theoretical basis of the involved instrument. The Commercially Available Instruments section is next and discusses most of the instruments that are available to perform the clinical procedure. We have attempted to be as current as possible, but because of ongoing changes in manufacturers there will be some errors in the sources and commercial names of the instruments. The next section, a Clinical Procedure section, is a step-by-step outline of how to perform the clinical procedure. Most chapters conclude with a section on Clinical Implications that discusses the clinical significance of the obtained information and how to interpret and use the information in the clinical care of the patient. The main thrust of each chapter is directed toward performing and understanding the clinical procedures, with less emphasis on the clinical management of disorders.

To facilitate the use of this book we have divided it into seven separate parts. The first part covers the clinical procedures used for general patient care. The next five parts cover the clinical procedures used in special areas of patient care: ocular disease, contact lenses, pediatrics, binocular vision, and low vision. The final part covers the clinical patient care decision making process and reimbursement. The clinical procedures discussed in the parts on general patient care are more routine and are performed on most general patients. The clinical procedures discussed in the parts on special patient care are more specialized procedures that are used for patients with special needs. The decisions of what clinical procedures to include in the book and then what procedures to place in the various parts were studied and made by the editors. The chapters in all of the parts are grouped into similar clinical testing areas and are not necessarily in a sequential order of testing.

Finally, a word is in order regarding the color of the cover. In the late 1800s, it was recommended that universities and colleges use a uniform color code on academic hoods to represent the various educational programs. Although the color has not been completely specified, seafoam green is the color generally used on academic hoods in schools of optometry. The cover of the book is green, symbolizing optometry.

Many people have assisted with the development and production of this book, and we sincerely appreciate their contributions. We are grateful for the outstanding work of the contributing au-

thors, for without their contributions, the book would still be a dream. We acknowledge the typing and preparation of the manuscripts by Affie Martin, Carolyn Rickels, and Ann Simpson; the assistance of Ann Richardson; the line drawings and graphics by Ken Norris; and the helpful advice offered by many people. We thank Bradford W. Wild, O.D., Ph.D., for his support of this project.

We also acknowledge all those people who, over the years, have significantly contributed to the evolution of clinical optometry. We salute them and hope that this textbook will be a contribution to the continuing growth and development of our beloved health care profession—optometry.

JBE
JFA
JDB

Contents

Clinical Procedures in
OPTOMETRY

PART 1

General Procedures

Binocular Subjective Refraction

John F. Amos

INTRODUCTION

Definition

Binocular refraction is a clinical procedure in which the subjective refraction is performed monocularly under binocular-viewing conditions. This situation may be achieved by several methods. These include positioning a septum, using polarized targets, or blurring vision in one eye such that each eye sees only its respective target.

History

Bannon[1] has provided a survey of many of the suggested procedures used for binocular refraction. The following is intended largely as a historical overview, since some of these procedures are no longer used with any frequency in contemporary clinical practice.

Cyclodamia was first reported in 1930 by Smith.[2] It represents one of the first attempts to measure the refractive error under binocular conditions. By having the patient view the letters through the retinoscopic findings, with the working distance dioptric equivalent in place, the patient was "fogged" and, thereby, encouraged to relax accommodation maximally. The power of the spherical lenses was gradually reduced and the cylindrical correction checked by cross cylinder under binocular conditions. In 1940, Copeland[3] proposed a method of binocular refraction that was a variation of that suggested by Smith. With this procedure a +2.00-D working lens was placed before the eye not undergoing refraction. This served to "fog" vision of one eye yet allow binocular fixation.

Sugar[4] in 1944, suggested using the cross cylinder on each eye following the monocular postcycloplegic examination under binocular-viewing conditions. According to his procedure the cross cylinder test for cylinder axis and power was performed on each eye in succession. He did not utilize any means to suspend or occlude vision in the eye not undergoing testing.

In 1946, Turville,[5] an English optometrist, introduced the procedure of binocular refraction that was modified by Morgan and others in subsequent years. The basic premise was to block or occlude a binocularly viewed target so that the right eye views the right side of the target and the left eye views the left side of the target. Turville accomplished this by placing a vertical septum over the patient's viewing mirror, thereby preventing the possibility of the right eye viewing the left target. This is the same procedure used in contemporary practice if one has access to an optically folded operatory or examination room.

Several investigators have used polarizing techniques that covered the entire chart or only the letters, or developed special instrumentation utilizing polarizing methods. A new approach to binocular refraction was introduced in 1966 by American Optical. The American Optical Vectographic slide was manufactured by depositing a dicroic dye on a stretched polyvinyl alcohol film.[6] In this manner, polarized or vectographic symbols and characters were formed. This allowed the projection of a target in which, with analyzers in place, the right eye sees only characters designed to be seen by the right eye and the left eye would see only characters designed to be seen by the left eye, yet both eyes remain open. This represented a unique method, not only in character design, but in chart or slide design as well. It allowed easy access to procedures that could be used in a 20-ft operatory or examination room.

In 1963, Humphriss[7] described the procedure of binocular refraction in which a low power plus lens (+0.75 D) was used to suspend foveal vision while refraction was performed on the eye

Table 19–1
Rationale for Binocular Refraction

Study	Difference Between Monocular and Binocular Refraction Results	Sphere Power Difference
Morgan[9]	0.25 D difference, 20%	0.50 D or more difference, 2%
Norman[10]	0.25 D difference, 35%	0.50 D or more difference, 12%
Spherical Balance		
Norman[10]	0.25-D difference between eyes, 28%	0.50-D or more difference between eyes, 5.6%
Campbell[8]	Fluctuations in accommodation up to 0.50 D with retinal image blur	
Fry, Reese,[8] and Flom	Found that adding plus lenses created varying amounts of visual acuity loss among individuals	
Flom and Goodwin[8]	Found an unequal decrease in visual acuity between the two eyes with the addition of plus lenses	
Cylindrical Axis		
Morgan[9]	Found over 2% of patients in his study had a 10° or greater change in cylinder axis with binocular viewing conditions	
Miles[8]	Found the cylinder axis differed an average of 8° under monocular and binocular conditions	
Rutstein and Eskridge[12]	Found that patients with paretic extraocular muscles producing 3° or more of cyclodeviation should have refractive status measured under binocular viewing conditions.	

not under fog. He called this immediate contrast refraction. Although not a procedure that is widely used, it is easily available and does not necessitate any extra or special equipment.

Clinical Use

As most patients have binocular vision, it seems reasonable that clinicians should use procedures that permit measurement of the refractive error under binocular viewing conditions. Several procedures have been proposed for this purpose, some simple in design, others more elaborate, yet binocular refraction remains relatively unused by most clinicians. Why is this so? Is it from a lack of knowledge of the procedure, a result of having to use different instrumentation, a result of not having the proper perspective about the procedure, or all of these? It is most likely a combination of all the foregoing factors. This chapter on subjective refraction will explore the rationale for binocular refraction as well as describe the more commonly used procedures.

Binocular refraction has a variety of advantages over the monocular subjective refractive procedure. Eskridge[8] has provided an excellent review of the clinical research supporting the rationale for binocular refraction (Table 19–1). Several investigators[9–12] have concluded that refractive differences may be measured in a substantial number of patients under monocular versus binocular viewing conditions. However, these differences are usually not significant for most patients. In certain conditions, however, the binocular refraction procedure may result in significantly different measurements, and it is clearly indicated as the refractive procedure of choice (Table 19–2). These conditions include hyperopic anisometropia, antimetropia, amblyopia, latent hyperopia, pseudo-myopia, cyclophoria, latent nystagmus, and paretic extraocular muscles, among others.

A principal advantage of binocular refraction is that it allows greater relaxation of accommodation than do traditional monocular procedures. This permits a more complete and accurate mea-

surement of such conditions as hyperopic anisometropia, antimetropia, latent hyperopia, or pseudymopia. In conditions such as cyclophoria or latent nystagmus, binocular refraction prevents the interruption of fusion and, therefore, the manifestation of these conditions. Without their manifestation, they are unable to influence the refractive condition or visual acuity.

INSTRUMENTATION

Theory

The theoretical principle involved in binocular refraction is that by some means each eye views its respective target, yet both eyes remain open. The right eye views only the right target, the left eye only the left target, and the single precept is represented cortically.

Table 19–2
Clinical Indications for Binocular Refraction

Refractive Considerations
  Hyperopic anisometropia
  Antimetropia
  Latent hyperopia (intermittent)
  Pseudomyopia

Visual Acuity Considerations
  Anisooxyopia (unequal acuity between the eyes)
    Unilateral amblyopia (physiologic or organic)
    Unilateral reduced acuity as a result of ocular disease
    Physiologic differences between best corrected acuities

Ocular Motility Considerations
  Significant horizontal-, vertical-, or cyclo-associated phoria
  Cyclophoria (physiologic or paretic)
  Latent nystagmus

This monocular viewing under binocular conditions may be achieved by several methods.

Use

Septum

A commonly used method for each eye viewing its respective target is to physically block or obstruct part of the target. The septum concept was originally described by Turville,[5] and its effect is illustrated diagrammatically in Figure 19–1. This technique is particularly effective when using an optically folded operatory or examination room because the septum may be quickly centered on the mirror. However, it may also be utilized in a 20-ft examination room.

Polarization

A variety of investigators have suggested the use of polarization as a means to achieve monocular viewing under binocular conditions. With this method, the analyzer and polarized target have the same axis of polarization, allowing the right eye to view the right half of the target, but blocking the left half of the target from view (Fig. 19–2). A variation of this technique is to polarize only the letters, leaving the background normal. This is the technique utilized in the Reichert (formerly American Optical) Vectographic slide (Fig. 19–3).

Fogging

A different approach to monocular refraction under binocular conditions is to slightly blur the central vision in the eye not under test. This slight blurring suspends foveal vision, such that each eye is refracted under conditions of binocular vision with peripheral fusion[13] (Fig. 19–4).

COMMERCIALLY AVAILABLE INSTRUMENTS

The American Optical Vectograph slide has been the only commercially available equipment made expressly for binocular refraction in the United States. This slide, originally introduced in 1966, is

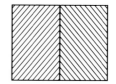
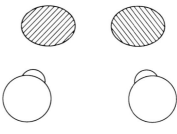

FIGURE 19–2. The polarizing method for producing monocular viewing under binocular conditions. The viewing analyzers have crossed axes and thus prevent the right eye from seeing the left target and vice versa.

now commercially available from Reichert Ophthalmic Instruments.* Slides are available for adults and children. Stereo Optical Company has introduced a similar slide for binocular refraction.†

When Turville[5] first introduced the infinity balance test, in 1946, his apparatus consisted of a double vertical column of test characters that were viewed in a mirror and to which a 3-cm wide opaque septum was attached. As a result of the almost exclusive use of 20-ft examination rooms in the United States at that time the procedure never gained popularity. The test cabinet was commercially available for many years in the United Kingdom, especially England.

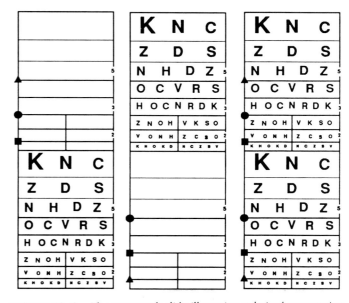

FIGURE 19–3. The vectograph slide illustrating polarized presentation of targets to the right, left, and both eyes.

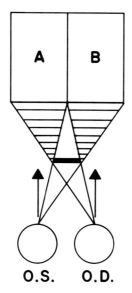

FIGURE 19–1. The effect of occluding the central portion of an acuity target by placing a septum midway between the patient and the target.

* Reichert Ophthalmic Instruments, a division of Cambridge Instruments, Inc., Buffalo, NY 14240.

† Available from Stereo Optical Company, 3539 North Kenton Ave., Chicago, IL 60641.

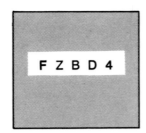

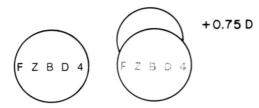

FIGURE 19–4. A low-power plus lens (+0.75-D sphere) fogs the right retinal image sufficiently to suspend foveal vision and allow monocular refraction of the left eye with both eyes open.

Morgan[9] first advocated the use of the American Optical Robinson Cohen Slide in 1949 because of its double vertical columns of characters and clear central area. Again, because almost all examination rooms were 20-ft in design, Morgan, in 1951, suggested an American Optical Project-O-Chart slide that could be used in the "straight-thru" examination room.[1] With this slide a free-standing septum must be positioned approximately halfway between the patient and the projected target.

In contemporary practice the only practical inexpensive and easy method for performing binocular refraction is to utilize the procedure in a folded examination room. In this setting a manila file folder or similar cardboard can be quickly cut and folded to act as a septum. Almost any projected chart may be used, although the septum reduces the numbers of characters by obstructing the central one or two letters in the line of characters (Fig. 19–5).

CLINICAL PROCEDURE

Septum Technique

1. Once the decision to perform binocular refraction has been reached the patient should be seated behind the phoroptor and the 20/40 or 20/50 line of Snellen characters projected on the screen. The septum should be placed

in the center of the patient's viewing mirror and the patient instructed to hold his or her head in an upright position and not to move the head from side to side. If, for example, the 20/50 line of letters of the American Optical Paraboline slide is used, the septum should be positioned such that with the right eye closed only the U and 5 are visible with the left eye. Conversely, with the left eye closed only the E and G are visible with the right eye. When both eyes are open and binocular overlap is present all four characters will be visible (two to each eye) and the center letter (in this case N) will be blocked by the septum. The edge of the mirror and frame will serve as peripheral fusion stimuli and stabilize binocular vision.

2. Once proper alignment is achieved the procedure for binocular refraction may begin. The patients attention is directed to the right side of the chart and, with the retinoscopic findings or present prescription in place, the appropriate-sized characters are projected on the screen.

3. If the letters are blurred, then a best-sphere determination should be made until approximately 20/25 or 20/20 characters are clear. If this level of visual acuity is not attainable, then retinoscopy should be repeated or other factors such as amblyopia or ocular disease considered.

4. Once the appropriate level of visual acuity is attained, the patient's attention should be directed to the right side of the chart, and the cross cylinder introduced parallel to the axis of the cylinder present. If cylinder is not present, then an arbitrary amount and position of the cylinder may be introduced (e.g., −0.50 × 180). In this manner, the presence, amount, and orientation of astigmatism may be measured in the right eye using the same procedure described in Chapter 18.

5. The next step after astigmatism determination is to blur or fog the characters to approximately the 20/40 level. This may be achieved by adding 0.75- or 1.00-D sphere more plus or less minus to the sphere power. From this point, power is decreased in 0.25-D steps until best or maximum visual acuity is attained.

6. Care should be taken to avoid overminusing the patient by questioning him or her as to the improvement in clarity of the letters with each step in decreased power. It is important to monitor the patient concerning character size and clarity, since any decrease in clarity or size is likely to indicate the sphere power has been decreased too much. This same end point may be monitored by red–green balance, as opposed to visual acuity.

7. The same procedure is repeated for the left eye. Next each eye is blurred or fogged by +0.75 D or 1.00 D, and this amount reduced binocularly until best visual acuity is attained. A separate step for balancing sphere power is not necessary because the best procedure to ensure equal stimulus to accommodation is best visual acuity in each eye.

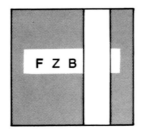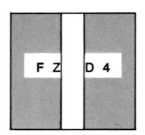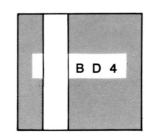

FIGURE 19–5. An example of a septum that can be hung over the upper edge of the viewing mirror to occlude the middle letter in a line of acuity letters. The figure on the left illustrates what the left eye sees, the middle figure shows what both eyes see, and the right figure illustrates what the right eye sees.

Vectographic Technique

The technique using the American Optical Vectographic slide involves changing the position of the slide.

1. With the slide in place, polarizing lenses must be placed in front of the patient's eyes, either by having them available in the lens well of the phoropter or by hanging analyzer lenses in front of the phoropter. Most contemporary phoropters have polarizing analyzers built in the phoropter.
2. The polarizing analyzers are oriented in a 45° to 135° axis orientation.* In this manner the 45° axis is placed over the right eye and the 135° axis is placed over the left eye. With this orientation, the right eye sees those characters composed of crystals that are oriented along the 45° axis, and the left eye sees those oriented along the 135° axis. Remembering that the characters are polarized also, the right eye sees only those characters with polarization axis 45° and the left eye sees only those characters with polarization axis 135°. Those characters intended to be viewed with both eyes are not polarized. Therefore, the right eye cannot see the letters viewed by the left eye and vice versa.
3. With a portion of the top chart (right eye), refraction is performed on the right eye in the usual manner of axis and power determination of the astigmatism and appropriate sphere power. The procedure is then repeated for the left eye.
4. The slide also has charts containing the clock dial, binocular balance, binocular function (suppression), monocular and binocular acuity, fixation disparity, and stereopsis. The monocular and binocular acuity charts may also be used for refraction.

Immediate Contrast Technique (Psychological Septum)

1. A +0.75-D sphere, such as that found in a trial set, is placed before one eye and serves to inhibit foveal vision by blurring central vision.
2. The fellow eye may then be refracted in the usual manner.

CLINICAL IMPLICATIONS

Clinical Significance

The value of binocular refraction lies not so much in its being a procedure for routine refraction, but in its use for specific conditions. Foremost among these is hyperopic anisometropia or antimetropia, in which monocular refraction under binocular conditions encourages greater relaxation of accommodation and, thereby, allows the correction of a greater amount of hyperopia.

Binocular refraction may also be the procedure of choice for determining the appropriate spectacle correction for the management of latent hyperopia. This is particularly true in cases of intermittent latent hyperopia, in which accommodation is more likely to relax its tonic position.

Binocular refraction frequently allows sufficient plus power to be prescribed to relieve the patient's symptoms in a manner that makes adaptation to the spectacles relatively easy for the patient. Plus power may then be gradually increased over time until the entire refractive error has been optically compensated. This results in a more agreeable approach than having the patient suffer decreased vision while they adapt to spectacles.

One of the best features of binocular refraction is that it does not require a separate step for the balancing technique. In cases of unilateral or unequal functional amblyopia, or physiological differences between best corrected visual acuity, or decreased vision as a result of ocular disease, balance is achieved when best visual acuity is measured in each eye. Possible errors are avoided by circumventing fogging procedures for biocular balancing, as conducted in monocular subjective refractive procedures.

Occasionally, the clinician encounters a patient with latent nystagmus in which, as one eye is covered, both eyes manifest a jerk-type nystagmus. As a result of the nystagmus, visual acuity is slightly decreased. Binocular refraction does not result in the occlusion of either eye and permits refraction without the annoyance and visual decrement induced by the nystagmus.

The same concept is involved in circumventing the effects of cyclodeviation on visual acuity in the presence of an astigmatic refractive error. In those rare cases for whom a physiologic cyclophoria significantly changes the cylinder axis, thereby decreasing visual acuity, its effect may be negated by employing binocular refraction. A change in cylinder axis, in the presence of significant cylinder power, may also occur in a paretic cyclovertical extraocular muscle that produces 3° or more cyclodeviation. In these cases, since this procedure does not interrupt fusion, the cyclodeviation is not manifested.

Clinical Interpretation

In general, interpretation of the measurement of refractive error using the procedure of binocular refraction is straightforward. The usual clinical interpretation, particularly in the conditions listed in Table 19–2 is to prescribe the dioptric values measured under manifest conditions. Modification of the prescription may be made based on such usual considerations as age of the patient, refractive amount, and occupation, among others.

REFERENCES

1. Bannon RE. Binocular refraction. A survey of various techniques. Optom Weekly 1965;56:25–31.
2. Smith D. The estimation of the total refractive error without a cycloplegia. Trans Am Acad Ophthalmol Otolarygol 1930;35:101–127.
3. Copeland JC. Locating the astigmatic axes under binocular fixation. Ten Years of Optical Developments. Chicago: Rigg's Optical Co, 1942: Nov.
4. Sugar SH. Binocular refraction with cross cylinder technique. Arch Ophthalmol 1944;31:34–42.
5. Turville AE. Outline of infinity balance. London: Raphael's Ltd, 1946.
6. Grolman B. Binocular refraction. A new system. N Engl J Optom 1966;17:118–129.
7. Humphriss D. Binocular vision technique. The psychological septum. Opt J Rev Optom 1962;99:19–21.
8. Eskridge JE. Rationale for binocular refraction. N Engl J Optom 1971; 123:160–166.
9. Morgan MW. The Turville infinity balance test. Am J Optom 1949; 26:231–239.
10. Norman SL. Plus acceptance in binocular refraction. Optom Weekly 1953;44:45–46.
11. Gentsch L, Goodwin H. A comparison of methods for the determination of binocular refractive balance. Am J Optom 1966;43:658.
12. Rutstein RP, Eskridge JB. The effect of cyclodeviations on the axis of astigmatism. Optom Vis Sci 1990;67:80–83.
13. Humphriss D. The psychological septum. An investigation into its function. Am J Optom Physiol Opt 1982;59:639–641.

---

* The polarizing analyzers must be oriented in the same axes as the targets are to be visible. In theory this could be any axis as long as the orientation of the analyzers over each eye are 90° apart.

Near Subjective Refraction

John F. Amos

INTRODUCTION

Definition

Near refraction refers to the measurement of the refractive state when the patient is fixating at the near point.

History

A review of many of the techniques and instruments used for near refraction has been provided by Borish.[1] The first clinicians to describe a procedure for near refraction were Esdaile and Turville in 1934.[2] Variations of these near targets and procedures have been described in the literature by many writers since then. The most contemporary review and description of the procedure has been presented by Bannon.[3] Basically, these devices can be divided into three groups (1) those utilizing a septum and existing near cards, (2) devices requiring polarizing filters, and (3) devices requiring bichrome or duochrome and polarizing filters.

Clinical Use

The primary use of the near subjective refraction procedure is to measure the refractive error with the patient fixating at a near distance. This procedure is utilized only when the patient's near symptoms cannot be explained by other findings.

There are a variety of clinical procedures that optometrists may use to assess vision at near. These include procedures to measure visual acuity, accommodation, ocular coordination, fusion ability, and stereopsis. One clinical procedure that is generally not used is subjective refraction with a near fixation distance. Clinicians devote a significant amount of time to the measurement of refractive errors and the optical correction of these errors with

accommodation relaxed, but seldom is the refractive state evaluated with accommodation stimulated. However, on occasion, changes may occur that significantly alter the refractive error when the patient fixates at near. This chapter addresses the etiologic factors responsible for producing a different near refraction and describes procedures for measuring the near subjective refraction.

Factors that May Be Responsible for a Different Near Refraction[3–6]

Possible Causes of a Different Cylinder Axis with Near Fixation

1. *Excyclotorsion.* When a patient fixates at a near distance, accommodation, convergence, pupillary constriction, and excyclotorsion occur. Although the effect of excyclophoria is generally nullified under conditions of binocularity, excyclotorsion may affect the cylinder axis position, even if sufficient encyclofusion is present to maintain binocular vision.
2. *Other possible factors that may affect the cylinder axis position include:*

   • Muscular contributions from the medial recti during convergence may produce unequal ciliary contraction and, therefore, astigmatic accommodation.
   • Lenticular contributions from such factors as aspheric surfaces, inhomogeneity of the ocular media, and tilting of the crystalline lens surfaces, similarly may change or produce astigmatism.
   • Corneal curvature changes may occur secondary to accommodation and convergence[6–8] or associated with eyelid pressure.[9,10]
   • Pupillary diameter changes with near fixation may result in different positions of the lens being exposed.

• Zonular weaknesses affecting one area of the ciliary body may affect the accommodative mechanism.

Possible Causes for a Different Cylinder Power with Near Fixation[11–14]

1. *Effectivity.* Effectivity is an optical phenomenon in which there is a change in the stimulus to accommodation from that which is theoretically necessary for a particular near distance. This change in stimulus is brought about by the patient fixating a near object while wearing a spectacle prescription. The greater the spherical or cylindrical power of the spectacle prescription, the greater the change in the stimulus to accommodation.

Possible Causes for a Different Sphere Power with Near Fixation

1. *Effectivity of the Spectacle Correction.* As previously mentioned, there is a change in the stimulus to accommodation from that theoretically necessary for a particular near point because the patient is fixating at near distance through a spectacle prescription. This effectivity is greatest when the sphere power is high. This is generally of clinical concern only if there is a significant anisometropia or astigmatism present.

2. *Anatomic and Physiologic Factors*

   • *Astigmatic Accommodation (Sectional or Asymmetric Astigmatism).* Although meridional lenticular astigmatism can possibly account for changes in astigmatism when the patient fixates at a near distance, there is no overwhelming clinical evidence that its affect is significant.[15–17]

   Possible suggested causes for meridional lenticular astigmatism include asymmetric contractions of the ciliary muscle or unequal distribution of the ciliary body around the crystalline lens.

   • *Corneal Contributions.* Near astigmatism may be induced by changes in corneal curvature with accommodation and convergence.[6–8] Most investigators have found that accommodation does not affect corneal curvature, but that corneal curvature does definitely flatten with convergence (i.e., there is a decrease in power of the horizontal meridian). This flattening during convergence could definitely be the result of the extraocular muscles exerting pressure on the globe.

   • *Lenticular Factors.* There are several possible lenticular factors that may contribute to a different near refraction. These include aspheric lenticular surfaces, inhomogeneity of the lenticular equator, and tilting of the crystalline lens.

   • *Pupillary Factors.* The pupil may cover a different area of the lens when the eyes converge than when fixating at distance. This may affect not only the cylinder axis, but power as well.

3. *Differential Accommodation.* Although accommodative effort may be the same for each eye, an unequal amount of accommodation does occur in a few patients and can create an anisometropia with near fixation.

INSTRUMENTATION

Theory

The theory of near subjective refraction is the same as that for distance subjective refraction. The goal of the procedure is to determine the lenses that will permit the near object to be focused on the retina. The primary difference is that with near refraction some degree of accommodation is usually being exerted, the eyes are being converged and undergoing excyclotorsion, and the pupils are miotic. Apart from the possible anatomic and physiologic changes that may influence a different near refraction, optical effectivity is likely to be a major cause in producing a near refraction that is different from the distance refraction. All near refraction procedures utilize binocular refraction, and the procedure used at near is, in theory, no different from that at distance.

COMMERCIALLY AVAILABLE INSTRUMENTS

Basic Design

The Borish card* is a near card in which the characters and targets are polarized for the purpose of binocular refraction (Fig. 20–1). Likewise, Stereo Optical Company has a vectographic near acuity card which may also be used.† Several instruments manufactured in England may also be used for near refraction. These instruments include the Turville near unit, the Freeman Bi-chromatic unit, and the Mallet unit, among others. However, unlike the Borish card, these targets were not designed to mount on the near-reading rod and must be hand-held. In addition to being polarized, these units also have duochrome filters for equalizing sphere power both monocularly and binocularly.

A simple and effective approach is to construct a near target using a near card and septum (Fig. 20–2). This approach has been described by Esdaile and Turville,[2] Jacques,[3] and, more recently, Bannon.[3] Any near card can be mounted on the reading rod and a septum (such as a PD ruler or other flat object) interposed midway between the card and the patient.

CLINICAL PROCEDURE

Although near refraction may be performed monocularly, the presence of a small amount of cyclodeviation will generally occur with near fixation and may result in a different cylinder axis. Therefore, it is best to perform a near binocular refraction. One can approach this procedure in one of two ways: (1) with a near card and a PD ruler held vertically as the septum and positioned midpoint between the phoropter and the target, or (2) with a polarized target, such as the Borish card or appropriate American Optical Near Vectograph cards. As in distance refraction, it is important to control accommodation.

Cylinder Determination

1. The polarized near card or the near card and septum are set at the appropriate working distance (usually 40 cm) on the reading rod. The distance cylindrical correction is left in place.
2. Plus power is added in +0.25-D steps alternately before each eye until the near target is first blurred.
3. Plus power is decreased alternately until the 20/20 line just becomes clear. This serves to place the circle of least confusion on the retina for the near working distance, while stabilizing accommodation. (The amount of plus power required to achieve the foregoing end point over the distance refraction usually ranges from +0.75 D to +2.00 D.)

---

* Available from Ophthalmic Research Institute, Suite 1149, 5530 Wisconsin Avenue, NW, Washington, DC 20815 ($50).
† Available from Stereo Optical Company, 3539 North Kenton Ave., Chicago, IL 60641.

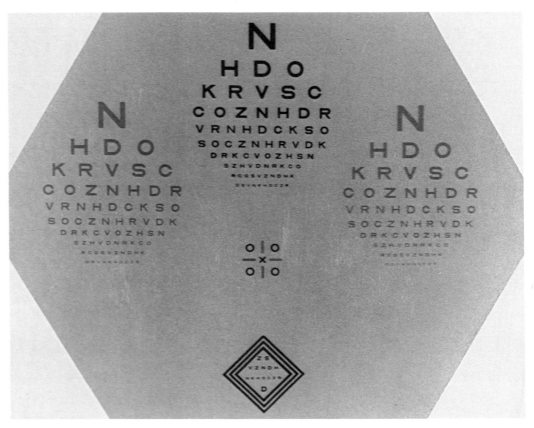

FIGURE 20–1. The Borish card for near binocular procedures.

4. The correcting cylinder axis and power are then determined for each eye by using the cross cylinder technique in the same manner discussed in the chapter on monocular subjective refraction.

Sphere Determination

Near sphere power is determined for each eye separately using the criteria of least plus power to achieve maximum or best visual acuity.

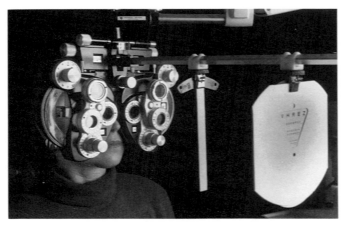

FIGURE 20–2. Septum and near card position for near binocular refraction.

CLINICAL IMPLICATIONS

Clinical Significance

The amount of demand on the visual system for near use has steadily increased during the past century. This is a result of the need for increased reading to cope in an increasing complex society, and to technological advances, such as the sewing machine, industrial machines, typewriter, and more recently, the word processor, computers, and their video display terminals.

The value of near refraction is greatest when patient symptoms such as discomfort, strain, or headache with near work, or persistent near blurred vision through the distance refraction, cannot be explained by other tests. This may be most obvious in patients whose spectacle prescription in sphere and/or cylinder power equals or exceeds 3.00 D. It may also be found in corrected anisometropic patients in which an unequal accommodative stimulus exists.

Clinical Interpretation

Regardless of the etiologic factors involved in the production of a different near refraction, prescribing is based on measurement of the near refraction.

When a difference between the refraction at distance and the refraction at near results, several options exist for prescribing a refractive correction. These include (1) prescribing the distance sphere with the near cylinder power and axis; (2) prescribing a separate pair of glasses for near work, including the appropriate near sphere, cylinder, and axis; or (3) changing from spectacle lenses to contact lenses, thereby greatly minimizing effectivity as a factor.

REFERENCES

1. Borish IM. Clinical refraction, 3rd ed. Chicago: Professional Press, 1975:777–782.
2. Turville AE. The common complaint. Dioptric Rev 1934;36:199–205.
3. Bannon RE. Near point binocular problems—astigmatism and cyclophoria. Ophthal Optician 1971;11:158–168.
4. Hughes W. Changes of axis of astigmatism on accommodation. Arch Ophthalmol 1941;26:742–749.
5. Rabbetts RB. A comparison of astigmatism and cyclophoria in distance and near vision. Br J Physiol Opt 1972;27:161–190.
6. Beau–Seigneur W. Changes in power and axis of cylindrical errors after convergence. Am J Optom 1946;23:111–121.
7. Fairmaid JA. The constancy of corneal curvature. Br J Physiol Opt 1959;16:2–23.
8. Lopping B, Weale RA. Changes in corneal curvature following ocular convergence. Vision Res 1965;5:207–215.
9. Miller E. Pressure of the lid on the eye. Arch Ophthalmol 1967;78:328–330.
10. Wilson G. The effect of lifting the lids on corneal astigmatism. Am J Optom Physiol Opt 1982;59:670–674.
11. Pascal JI. Intrinsic variability of astigmatic errors. Arch Ophthalmol 1944;32:123–124.
12. Hofstetter HW. The correction of astigmatic errors. Am J Optom 1945;22:121–131.
13. O'Brien JM, Bannon RE. Accommodative astigmatism. Am J Ophthalmol 1947;30:289–296.
14. Roth N. The problem of the undependable cylinder. Surv Ophthalmol 1969;14:112–115.
15. Erggelet H. The near glass for the accommodating astigmatic eye. J Optik 1925;13–14:146–147.
16. Bannon RE. A study of astigmatism at the near point with special reference to astigmatic accommodation. Am J Optom 1946;23:53–72.
17. Fletcher RJ. Astigmatic accommodation. Br J Physiol Opt 1952;9:8–32.

Presbyopic Addition

Troy E. Fannin

INTRODUCTION

Definition

The amplitude of accommodation diminishes gradually and uninterruptedly in the normal patient from early age to approximately age 60. When the amplitude of accommodation is insufficient to permit sustained, clear, comfortable vision at the customary near working distances, clinically the condition is classified as *presbyopia* (old sight). The *presbyopic addition* is the additional plus lens power prescribed to augment the available accommodation so near visual activity may be performed clearly and comfortably.

Presbyopia may also be defined and classified as incipient presbyopia, premature presbyopia, manifest presbyopia, and absolute presbyopia. *Incipient presbyopia* is the beginning stage of presbyopia when symptoms or difficulty are first encountered in near vision activities. The patient can still see clearly and comfortably most of the time at near-viewing distances. *Premature presbyopia* is the need of additional plus lens power for near-viewing distances at an earlier age than expected for the population. Premature presbyopia is usually associated with ocular or systemic disease, nutritional deficiencies, trauma, environmental factors, or the ingestion of certain drugs. *Manifest presbyopia* is presbyopia with some amplitude of accommodation present. *Absolute presbyopia* exists when the amplitude of accommodation is completely absent.

History

Presbyopia

Although refractive anomalies of the eye have been a matter of interest from ancient times, their clarification took centuries. Aristotle is reported to have appreciated presbyopia, the long sight of old age, and differentiated it from myopia.[1] Although myopia and presbyopia were thought to be antitheses, long sight (hyperopia) was considered to be identical with presbyopia. This conclusion, no doubt, seemed reasonable, for both hyperopia and presbyopia are corrected by convex lenses.

James Ware was the first person in the 19th century to understand that long sight was not necessarily associated with presbyopia.[2] His explanation was not immediately appreciated and confusion prevailed among writers of that period until Stellwag von Carion, in 1855, provided a relatively clear description with an optical explanation of the differences between hyperopia and presbyopia.[3]

In 1856, Hermann von Helmholtz published his standard work on vision, *Handbook of Physiological Optics,* which laid the scientific groundwork for future progress. In 1858, Frans Cornelius Donders began publishing his work on ametropia and its correction with an elegant simplicity. In 1864, he published his classic book *On the Anomalies of Accommodation and Refraction of the Eye.* The text, in clear and simple language, not only established fully the optical nature of hyperopia and its differentiation from presbyopia, but also placed the theory of refractive errors and their correction on a scientific basis. The diminution of the amplitude of accommodation with age was first assessed and recorded by Donders.

Optical Assistance In Presbyopia

Seneca's comment that writing, however small and distinct, appears larger and clearer through a bowl filled with water is the first reference indicating the appreciation and significance of the magnification of print.[4] In 1267, the Francescan monk, Roger Bacon of Oxford, in a monumental work, *Opus Majus,* provided a detailed description of magnification produced by a strong plano–convex lens when placed on a manuscript. Undoubtedly, Bacon understood the benefits of employing convex lenses as a near vision aid. Whether Bacon moved the lens to the eye or mounted the lenses in a framelike device is unknown. However, it is not likely that Bacon invented spectacles, but his research provided an impetus for further development.

In the period following Bacon's work, simple hand-held magnifying lenses, as reading aids, came widely into use. The first usage and place of origin of rudimentary eye-glasses for spectacles (two mounted magnifying lenses connected by a bridge or nose piece) are still unknown. In a erudite, exhausting historical analysis, Rosen[5] concluded that no single person could be declared to be the inventor of spectacles. Ronchi has summarized the dilemma by stating: "Much has been written ranging from the valuable to the worthless about the invention of eyeglasses; but when it is all summed up, the fact remains that the world has found lenses on its nose without knowing whom to thank.[5]

The earliest known lenses for near work were approximately +3.00 D sphere in power and made in plano–convex form. The surface quality was often poor and uneven.

Benjamin Franklin is usually credited with the invention of bifocals. Franklin, while a minister to France, wrote a letter dated August 21, 1784 to his friend George Whately in London describing his double spectacles: ". . . I cannot distinguish a Letter of even of Large Print; but am happy in the invention of Double Spectacles, which serving for distant objects as well as near ones, makes my eyes as ever they were: If all other defects and infirmities were as easily and cheaply remedied, it would be worth while for friends to live a deal longer. . . ."[6] Some evidence exists that crediting Franklin with being the sole inventor of bifocals is questionable.[7]

With greater certainty John Isaac Hawkins, a prolific and imaginative inventor, is recognized as the inventor of trifocals in 1826. Hawkins had previously coined the term "bifocal" and invented a pupillary distance (PD) gauge. The trifocals described by Hawkins were for his own use and consisted of three separate lenses of +1.50 D for distance, +3.25 D for 12 to 30 in., and +5.50 D for 8 to 12 in.

Clinical Use

The purpose for determining the presbyopic addition is to provide a correction that renders vision clear and comfortable at the desired near distance. The decrease in accommodative ability is generally agreed to be related to changes in the crystalline lens. Normally, when the ciliary muscle contracts, tension is released on the zonular fibers attached to the capsule containing the lens. The release of tension allows the highly elastic capsule to mold the lens into a more convex form (Helmholtz theory of relaxation). Thus, contraction of the ciliary body produces positive accommodation; relaxation of the ciliary body provides for relaxation of accommodation. The loss of accommodation with age that results in presby-

opia is thought to be due to decreases in the elasticity of the capsule and increasing rigidity of the lens itself.

Signs and Symptoms of Presbyopia

The finding common in all presbyopic patients is the recession of the near point of accommodation. Although the amplitude of accommodation decreases gradually and linearly with age, even among different individuals, the patient often reports a sudden and rapidly progressive loss of near vision. As long as the available amplitude exceeds the demand, the patient can see the target clearly. When sufficient accommodation is no longer available to meet the actual demand, further decline in the amplitude of accommodation rapidly decreases the visual acuity. Although the deterioration in the accommodative amplitude expressed in diopters is approximately linear, the regression of the near point in centimeters or inches will proceed at a progressively accelerated rate because the distance of the near point of accommodation is a reciprocal of the amplitude. The patient history, however, if carefully taken will determine the nature of the onset. If the onset is truly precipitous, the cause is not likely a result of the normal loss of amplitude of accommodation. A sudden loss of accommodative amplitude can occur with diseases such as glaucoma, diabetes, anemia, tuberculosis, focal infection, alcoholism, neurologic dysfunction, and the use of certain drugs.

Blurred vision at near is the most frequent symptom reported. Difficulty in threading a needle and the inability to read the telephone directory are common occurrences that initially direct the patient's attention to a beginning near point problem.

The patient may push near work away from the customary near position until clear vision is achieved. The patient may report this behavior by stating "there is nothing wrong with my eyes but my arms aren't long enough." More difficulty may be encountered late in the work day when fatigue is present. Conversely, some incipient presbyopic patients report difficulty upon arising in the morning when they attempt to read the morning paper. As the morning passes, their vision improves, as if their accommodative activity needed a "warming up period." Sluggishness in the velocity of accommodative change and the rate of relaxation may be reported.

The incipient presbyopic patient is likely to see better under bright than dim illumination due to the decrease in pupil size and improved contrast.

Presbyopic patients are more likely to complain of poor vision, such as blurring, smudging or smearing, print running together, and double vision, rather than visual fatigue or asthenopia. The eyes may tire quickly and letters of the print begin to blur after only a few minutes. If the near work continues, symptoms of eye strain, such as stinging, burning, tearing, aching, and headaches, may occur. The symptoms may be intermittent or constant, but are invariably associated with near work.

As the amplitude of accommodation decreases to the point that a patient encounters difficulty seeing clearly at the near point, the patient may resort to four different solutions to see clearly and comfortably.[8] The patient may

1. Avoid the problem by decreasing the amount of near work
2. Allow the print to blur slightly and take advantage of the depth of focus
3. Increase the reading distance by holding the work farther from the eye
4. Use all of the amplitude in spite of the tremendous effort required to obtain the last portion of the amplitude

Strategies 1 and 3 are often used, but the patient may use each strategy at different times. The last solution may result in asthenopia or micropsia, or both. On occasion the incipient presbyopic patient does not complain of indistinct vision, but of seeing the print smaller and farther away. Usually the micropsia occurs only after prolonged near work. This phenomenon in beginning presbyopia is probably associated with excess ciliary muscle activity, as it occurs in cases of paresis of the ciliary muscle as well.

INSTRUMENTATION

The instrumentation and devices required to determine the presbyopic addition include a phoropter or refractor; retinoscope; trial frame and trial lens set; tape measure, meter stick, or near point rod; and assorted near point cards (Fig. 21–1).

CLINICAL PROCEDURE

Determination of the Tentative Presbyopic Addition

A review of the ophthalmic literature reveals many procedures for ascertaining a suitable tentative near addition.[9–11] Most clinicians usually select only one or two procedures to use routinely, but since no single procedure works equally well for all patients, a clinician should be skillful in using several alternative procedures to select the test providing the greatest efficacy for a given patient.

Because many presbyopic patients will be unable to see the near card with their distance correction, the tentative correction provides clear vision at the near point such that heterophoria, vergences, relative accommodation tests, and other near tests may begin with clear vision. Typically, the tentative near addition is modified according to other test results, the patient's history, and clinical experience to arrive at the amount of the final addition.

Addition Based on the Amplitude of Accommodation

Many patients report difficulty at the near working distances long before the amplitude of accommodation has decreased to the dioptric value of the working distance. Donders[12] placed the commencement of presbyopia when the near point of accommodation exceeded 8 Parisian inches (22 cm). This denotes an amplitude of accommodation of about 4.50 D. Morgan[13] stated that presbyopia exists when the measured amplitude of accommodation is less than 5.00 D.

On the basis of these observations, various clinical "rules-of-thumb" have been advanced that state that the amount of a new addition should permit a certain percentage of the amplitude of

accommodation to remain in reserve. Lawrence[14] and Maxwell[15] have advocated leaving one-half of the amplitude in reserve, whereas Sheard[16] and Giles[17] suggest that only one-third be held in reserve. Although it is difficult to find an explanation for such practices in the physiology of the mechanism of accommodation, to the clinician they are justified merely because they satisfy the needs of the patient.

1. With this method it is imperative to establish the patient's working distance accurately. Once the working distance and amplitude are known, it is easy to calculate the tentative presbyopic addition. For example, if the working distance is 40 cm and the amplitude is 2.00 D, and the patient is to hold one-half (1.00 D) of the amplitude in reserve, the available accommodative amplitude is 1.00 D. Since the patient will need 2.50 D to see clearly at 40 cm, the near addition is determined by subtracting from the near accommodative demand (2.50 D) the available accommodation (1.00 D) or 2.50 − 1.00 = +1.50 D addition.
2. If the working distance is less than 40 cm, consideration should be given to holding only one-third the amplitude in reserve. The application of the one-third rule for very close distances minimizes the addition and provides longer distances of clear vision through the bifocal segment.

Cross Cylinder Method

Many practitioners prefer to use the cross cylinder to determine the presbyopic addition.

1. A target consisting of four to five vertical and horizontal lines is presented to the patient at their customary working distance (Fig. 21–2). It is important that the illumination on the target be diffuse and subdued, although sufficient to allow the patient to see the target satisfactorily. If too high, the illumination will decrease pupil size, thereby increasing the depth of focus to such an extent that it exceeds the amount of the artificially created astigmatism. The patient will then find it difficult to distinguish the difference in focus between the two sets of lines.
2. If the patient cannot see the lines initially, sufficient plus lens power is added until the lines are recognized. Before

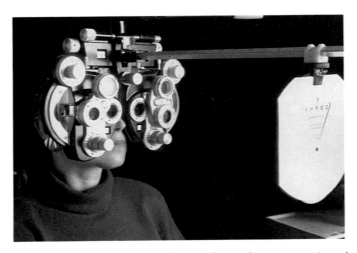

FIGURE 21–1. Phoroptor or refractor with a reading or near point rod and near card at the typical working distance of 40 cm.

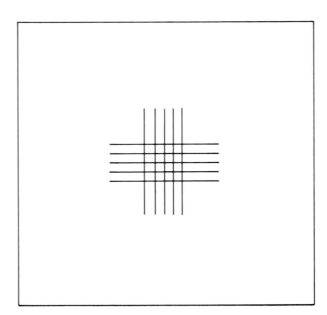

FIGURE 21–2. A typical near point cross target.

placing the cross cylinder lenses (± 0.50 DC) in front of the eyes, it is good practice to determine if the astigmatism at the near point is fully corrected by asking if the horizontal and vertical lines are equally black for each eye in turn. If one set of lines on the target appears blacker without the cross cylinder lenses before either eye, the cylindrical power should be altered until both sets of lines are equally clear for each eye. It is often necessary to alter the cylindrical correction to achieve equality between the lines. This may occur simply because of a difference in lens effectivity during near fixation, rather than because of an error in the astigmatic distance correction. Large cylindrical corrections for distance typically lose about 10% of their effectivity when used at near. However, the lenses that exactly correct the astigmatic error for near distance, overcorrect the astigmatic error at distance. Therefore, the temporary change in the cylindrical correction should be used only to achieve good results on the near point cross cylinder tests and not prescribed for the distance correction.

3. When the lines are equally clear for each eye, the cross cylinders with their minus axes vertical (+0.50 DS −1.00 DC × 090), are placed before the patient's eyes.

4. The test may be conducted initially monocularly and then binocularly. Although the presbyopic addition could be determined solely by the binocular (fused) cross cylinder test, the monocular cross cylinder test offers a check on the accuracy of the astigmatic correction and the binocular balance of the distance correction. If the monocular findings are different, the distance refraction or balance may be in error.

5. The monocular cross cylinder tests will usually result in a larger addition than the binocular cross cylinder, and the safer, more conservative approach is to use the binocular measurement as the tentative near addition.

6. The cross cylinder lenses create artificial astigmatism, with an interval of Sturm of 1 D (Fig. 21–3). The patient is asked to observe the target and report to the clinician *which set of lines,* the ones running across, or the ones running up and down, is clearer, blacker, or sharper. To prevent confusion, the terms *horizontal* and *vertical* should not be used because they may not be understood by all patients.

7. If the patient accommodates exactly for the target position, the two sets of lines should be equally clear, since the image of the horizontal lines is 0.50 D in front of the retina, and the vertical lines will lie 0.50 D behind the retina. If the patient is underaccommodated for the target,

as expected in the usual case of presbyopia, the horizontal lines will appear clearer.

8. The monocular cross cylinder test may be conducted by using alternate occlusion, dissociation with prisms, or by polarization (Borish Near Point Card). During monocular testing, sufficient plus power is added before each eye until the vertical lines are just barely clearer than the horizontal lines and retain their clearness upon changing from eye to eye.

9. As soon as the vertical lines, seen monocularly, are clearer than the horizontal, the patient is permitted fusion and now views the target binocularly. The patient is then asked which set of lines is clearer, and most patients are likely to respond that the vertical lines are clearer. The plus power is then reduced in 0.25-D steps until the lines are equally clear. If the patient seems uncertain about equality of the lines, plus power is reduced until the horizontal lines are clearer than the vertical. The amount of additional plus power remaining above that of the distance subjective correction represents the tentative binocular cross cylinder addition.

10. Some would argue that the end points of these tests should be equality of blackness or clarity of the horizontal and vertical lines. However, equality is usually not a point, but may extend over a range of 0.25 D to 0.75 D, and an equality finding may provide a measurement anywhere in this range. Establishing the end point at one end of the range of apparent equality yields a more consistent, precise measurement than accepting any value in the range.

For some patients the cross cylinder test may give more consistent results if the minus cylinder axes of the lenses are placed at 180°. When this is done, the end-point condition for the monocular cross cylinder test is slightly greater clarity or blackness of the horizontal lines, and for the binocular cross cylinder test the end point is when the vertical lines are slightly clearer or blacker.

Baxter[18] recommended that the lines forming the cross be segmented or made with dashes. The use of dashed lines in the cross cylinder test object gives the effect of solidity to the line most prominent, producing more sensitive and accurate results than the conventional grid test object.

Goldberg[19] suggested that a variable color near point grid consisting of a cross with multiple red horizontal and green vertical lines would minimize any tendency toward an overcorrection at near. However, Woo and Sivak[20] concluded that results obtained with a variable color near grid did not produce a statistically significant difference from a target composed of only black lines.

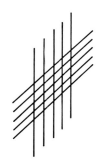
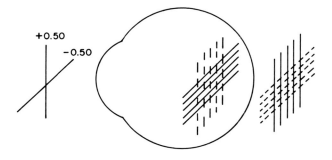

FIGURE 21–3. The optical representation of a typical near point cross cylinder target and a cross cylinder lens (+0.50 DS − 1.00 DC × 090) before an eye with no residual astigmatism. When the circle of least confusion in the astigmatic interval created by the cross cylinder is focused on the retina, by either accommodation or spherical lenses, the vertical and horizontal lines will appear equally distinct.

Balancing Positive and Negative Relative Accommodation

The procedure for balancing the positive and negative relative accommodation is based on the concept of placing the accommodative demand in the middle of the range of relative accommodation.

1. A target containing fine print is placed at the preferred near distance. If the print is blurred, sufficient plus lens power must be added to clear the target.
2. Plus sphere power is then added until a first sustained blur is reached (negative relative accommodation finding). This procedure is then repeated by adding minus sphere power (positive relative accommodation finding).
3. The optical range of clear vision can be determined from these two measurements. The power that results in equal negative relative and positive relative accommodation findings about the preferred working distance is the tentative presbyopic addition.

An example may illustrate how this method is used. Suppose a patient can read fine print with a +1.00-D addition. Blurring occurred when the addition was increased to +2.00 D and reduced to +0.50 D. The range of clear vision, therefore, extends from a +0.50-D addition to a +2.00-D addition or over a range of 1.50 D. The midpoint between +0.50 D and +2.00 D is +1.25 D, which is the tentative addition. The negative relative accommodation and positive relative accommodation findings with this tentative addition in place would be +0.75 D and -0.75 D, respectively.

If the negative relative accommodation finding (plus lens to blur) reduces the accommodation stimulus to zero at the preferred reading distance, the addition that balances the plus and minus lens to blur findings will be equal to the addition that leaves one-half of the amplitude in reserve. If the plus lens to blur does not reduce the accommodative stimulus to zero, the addition that balances the plus and minus lens blur points will be less than the addition that leaves one-half the amplitude of accommodation in reserve. In effect, the smaller addition will result in a smaller exophoria, reducing the demand on positive fusional convergence necessary to achieve single vision from that required had the one-half rule been used. Therefore, the amount of the addition determined by this method will always be equal to that produced by the one-half rule or less.

The Bichrome Method

The bichrome procedure provides a method for determining the presbyopic addition that is based on the natural chromatic aberration of the eye. The bichrome method enjoys wide use for determining the spherical component of the distant correction.

When an ametropic eye is out of focus for distance fixation, a red monochromatic target is seen clearer in myopia and a green target in hyperopia. The same principles apply at near distances. For presbyopic patients who are unable to accommodate adequately for near targets, both the red and green will focus behind the retina. Because the red light will focus farther behind the retina than the green, the uncorrected or undercorrected presbyopic patient will see the letters on the green background clearer in much the same manner as a hyperopic patient will for distant vision. Similarly, an overcorrection or an overaction of accommodation for a near target will cause the letters on the red background to appear clearer.

1. When the correct addition is placed before the eyes and a suitable bichromatic target is placed at near, the red and green foci are equally spaced dioptrically from the retina, the green in front, the red behind, and the letters will be equally distinct on both colors.

2. If the letters on the green side appear clearer, plus power is added until equality of the letters on the two colors is achieved. If the letters on the red side are clearer, the power of the addition is reduced.

The bichromatic test has a high degree of sensitivity for most patients. The primary problem with this test has been the scarcity of suitable near bichromatic targets. Targets that are translucent and transilluminated perform more efficiently than those printed on opaque backgrounds. The Freeman–Archer unit and the Mallett unit, both from England, provide excellent transilluminated targets.

Best Visual Acuity Subjective (Plus Buildup)

This procedure works best when the corrected visual acuity is normal at distance.

1. The power of the addition is increased binocularly in 0.25-D steps to the amount required for the patient to *first* read the smallest letters on the near point card at the customary working distance. The power of the addition is then increased in 0.25-D steps to the amount *preferred* by the patient. The result is usually about 0.50 D more plus than the lenses that provided minimum resolution of the smallest targets.
2. This procedure may also be conducted monocularly in the same manner as described in step 1. It usually results in a greater near addition, since less accommodation is available because of a lack of convergence accommodation. In addition, the results of this procedure may be used to indirectly confirm the accuracy of the balance of the distance refraction.

The method is fast and works rather well if the distance chosen for the test closely resembles the preferred working distance.

Addition Based on Age

Many investigators have reported on the manner in which the amplitude of accommodation decreases with age.[21] The basic assumption underlying this concept is that, for a given age, the amplitude of accommodation is a fixed value for all patients, and a near addition may be calculated using the values. Although this seems patently fallacious, the results from one study that used this procedure found that it fared as well as most other procedures.[22]

The mean amplitudes of accommodation for various age groups, as determined in major studies, are shown in Table 21–1. Hofstetter has derived formulas for calculating the maximum, probable, and minimum amplitudes of accommodation given the age of the patient to the nearest birthday (Table 21–2).[23] The power of the near addition required by the patient, given the calculated minimum expected amplitude of accommodation for patients whose ages range from 40 to 60, is illustrated in Table 21–3. The addition power is based on the assumption that one-half the accommodative amplitude is held in reserve and the working distance is 40 cm.

The association of chronologic age and near addition power quickly provides a tentative near addition. This may also be of great value to the clinician for comparison of the patient's present addition power to that expected by age.

Dynamic Retinoscopy

In this procedure a fixation distance is selected that represents the patient's preferred near working distance. The retinoscopic observation is made at the same position.

Table 21–1
The Mean Amplitude of Accommodation for Various Age Groups from Major Studies

Age	Donders (Monocular)	Duane (Monocular)	Jackson (Binocular)	Sheard (Monocular)	Turner (Monocular)
10	19.70	13.50	14.00		13.00
15	16.00	12.50	12.00	11.00	10.60
20	12.70	11.50	10.00	9.00	9.50
25	10.40	10.50	9.00	7.50	7.90
30	8.20	8.90	8.00	6.50	6.60
35	6.30	7.30	7.00	5.00	5.75
40	5.00	5.90	5.50	3.75	4.40
45	3.80	3.70	4.00		2.50
50	2.60	2.00	2.50		1.60
55	1.80	1.30	1.25		1.10
60	1.00	1.00	0.50		0.70

(Wold, RM. The spectacle amplitude of accommodation of children ages six to ten. Am J Optom 1967;44:642–664, © American Academy of Optometry 1967)

1. The patient is asked to fixate fine print (located in the plane of the retinoscope).
2. If the near point of accommodation is behind the peephole of the retinoscope, as usually expected, the examiner will observe a "with" motion when using a retinoscope in the plane mirror mode.
3. Convex lenses are then added until the with motion observed by the retinoscope first disappears. The amount of the additional convex lenses needed to first produce neutrality is the amount of the tentative presbyopic addition.

Determination of the Final Add

Hofstetter has reported that the distributions of additions at given age levels do not differ markedly with various clinicians.[24] Even though the stated criteria of the clinicians in the study were different, it is apparent that the individual optometrist takes into account many other criteria not usually described. However, it is apparent that the use of special criteria can usually be acquired quickly and easily, since the clinicians who were just entering practice had essentially the same dioptric averages as those with extensive experience.

Strict adherence to the use of any of the procedures previously described may avoid obvious errors and usually lead to success. Nevertheless, any method of presbyopic addition determination applied to all patients fails to take into account individual differences. No one procedure or set of data is sufficient unto itself.

The following factors should be considered when selecting the final presbyopic addition.

Table 21–2
Formulae for Calculating the Relationship of the Amplitude of Accommodation to Age

Maximum = 25.0 − 0.4 (age)
Probable = 18.5 − 0.3 (age)
Minimum = 15.0 − 0.25 (age)

(Hofstetter HW. A useful age–amplitude formula. Penn Optom 1947;7: 5–8)

Customary Near Working Distance

The identification of the customary working distance is essential in the selection of the final presbyopic addition. The patient's working distance becomes more critical as the amplitude becomes small. The clinician must know exactly this distance, and not accept a standard distance such as 40 cm. This is best accomplished by having the patient hold the appropriate reading material at their natural working distance when they are comfortable and relaxed. The patient is reminded to assume the position in which they would like to work and not the position that has been recently adapted to see clearly. It may be necessary for the patient to close his or her eyes and permit the kinesthetic sense to position the arms where they are most comfortable. Many patients may be required to perform various tasks at different distances from the eyes. Patients who use their eyes for visually demanding tasks in their work or spend considerable time with hobbies may need more than one pair of glasses. In any event, the use and limitation of any particular prescription should be explained and demonstrated to the patient. The near and far blur ranges should be demonstrated to the patient through the intended near prescription in a trial frame and the power of the addition changed to provide the most desirable range of clear vision.

Many advanced presbyopic patients may need trifocals to

Table 21–3
Calculated Near Addition Based on the Minimum Expected Amplitude of Accommodation

Age	Near Addition (D)
40	0
42	0.25
44	0.50
46	0.75
48	1.00
50	1.25
52	1.50
54	1.75
56	2.00
58	2.25
60	2.50

cover intermediate distances beyond 40 cm. With a declining amplitude of accommodation and an increasing near addition, the near point of accommodation through the distance portion moves farther from the patient, and the far point of accommodation through the near portion moves closer to the patient. When a physical range of blurred vision exists between the near point of accommodation through the distance portion and the far point of accommodation through the near portion, the patient is a candidate for a trifocal. This range begins when the near addition is +1.75 D or +2.00 D and increases as the near addition increases.

Before writing a final prescription the clinician should demonstrate the range of clear vision through the tentative distance and near corrections to acquaint the patient with this range or "gap" of indistinct vision and, furthermore, to demonstrate how the intermediate distance can be cleared with a trifocal. As a routine practice the clinician should demonstrate to any patient requiring a +1.75-D addition or greater that clear vision is available at distance, at 40 cm, and at intermediate ranges with appropriate lens powers.

Trifocals are usually available with the power of the intermediate portion being one-half the power of the near addition. Other percentages of the near addition may be available.

Nature of the Near Work

Many complex occupational tasks require prolonged, critical, clear vision at near distances: the accountant, proofreader, and oral surgeon are examples. The working distance must be measured precisely for these occupations, and the addition must be carefully determined. For patients whose near vision activities are casual and noncritical in their occupation or hobbies, the near distance needs not be identified as precisely.

Physical Nature of the Patient

In general, patients with long arms require slightly less power in their reading addition than patients with average arm lengths. Conversely, patients with short arms may require a slightly higher addition power. In addition, some patients are in good health, appear robust, and are physically active; these patients often require less power in their addition. However, other patients are asthenic, seem debilitated, for which near work is more difficult; a higher addition may be needed to relieve symptoms of eyestrain at near.

Illumination Levels

The illumination levels under which near work is performed may greatly affect the patient's visual acuity. Good illumination may greatly improve the ability to perform fine visual near tasks. This, in part, is due to the constriction of the pupil, but improvement in contrast also assists. When the lighting conditions are subdued, near vision efficiency is reduced. The patient should be questioned concerning the level of illumination under which their near work is performed, and appropriate recommendations provided. However, the level of illumination may not be under the control of the patient.

Status of the Accommodation–Convergence Relationship

The power of the addition may be modified to alleviate an existing convergence problem. In early presbyopia a patient with an overconvergence problem may be helped by prescribing a slightly higher addition than would otherwise be prescribed. Similarly, a patient manifesting an underconvergence problem may be given a slightly lower addition, but also may require positive fusional vergence therapy or base-in prism in the near prescription.

Change in the Amount of the Addition

Probably the single most important attitude the clinician should develop is to keep the presbyopic addition power *as weak as possible*. The range of clear vision is progressively longer as the power of the addition is reduced. If possible, keep any change under 0.50 D. If a patient is seen over an interval not exceeding 2 years, increments usually may be kept at 0.50 D or under.

Changes of 0.75 D or more materially affect the patients' customary near visual habits, most noticeably the decrease in the far point through the correction. If the changes are small and gradual, the patient is less likely to notice them.

Rarely are presbyopic additions prescribed under +0.75 D. Generally it is better to correct presbyopia when the addition is small (not more than +1.00 D). When a small addition is made, the adaptation will be quicker and easier than if the patient delays until the addition needed is +1.50 D or more.

In summary, the adaptation occurs more quickly and easily if the addition is prescribed early, when the amount is small, then gradually increased in increments not exceeding 0.50 D until the maximum addition is reached. Unless providing for low-vision assistance, an addition should always be less than the dioptric value of the working distance.

CLINICAL IMPLICATIONS

Clinical Significance

The percentage of the American population composed of presbyopic patients is increasing dramatically. Numerous people today live long enough to encounter problems of presbyopia long before their careers are completed. In addition, patients in the work force today are far more dependent on good near vision for adequate performance than ever before.

With the increasing prevalence of a specific and predictable visual disability affecting so many people in the population, optometrists must become more sensitive to the visual needs of this group and develop diagnostic procedures and visual aids that better serve these patients. Some aspects of the clinical care of the presbyopic patient are sufficiently different from the nonpresbyopic patient to warrant special attention.

The management of the presbyopic patient is one of the most challenging and satisfying aspects of optometric care. The success of the treatment program may have profound consequences for the patient. Often a small improvement in visual ability and patient education produce significant changes in the degree of function and the quality of life.

Clinical Interpretation

The onset of presbyopia typically begins in the early 40s and continues until absolute presbyopia is reached, generally in the late 50s but sometimes in the early 60s.[25] It is usual to expect small, but significant, changes in the near addition approximately every 2 years during the period of decreasing amplitude. The power of the first near addition is usually +0.75 D or +1.00 D, but may be greater if the patient has delayed correction. For a near working distance of 40 cm, the patient usually does not require a near addition greater than +2.25 D if the visual acuity is normal. Higher addition powers may be used for patients with a vocation or avocation requiring a nearer than 40-cm working distance or for patients requiring the magnification effects of low-vision aids.

Clinicians should provide advanced presbyopic patients with education and demonstrate the efficacy of progressive addition lenses or trifocals so that patients may make informed decisions that affect their visual performance at intermediate distances.

Other factors are involved in the interpretation of presbyopia. Uncorrected low or moderate myopic patients may avoid the need for a near addition. If their distance vision is corrected, they may remove their spectacles for near visual tasks. Lens effectivity varies with the amount and type of ametropia, and this factor will often influence when incipient presbyopia begins. The accommodative demand is greater for patients with high amounts of corrected hyperopia than for emmetropic patients; conversely the accommodative demand is smaller for patients with high amounts of corrected myopia. Consequently, corrected hyperopic patients are likely to need additional plus power for near distances sooner than corrected myopic patients.

The only presenting symptom of many presbyopic patients is indistinct near vision, with no complaint of their distance vision. The clinician should determine the distance power and the near power of the old lenses, the difference being the near addition. For many patients the cause of the indistinct near vision may be solely due to a change in their distance prescription. If additional plus power is added to the distance correction, the near addition may actually remain the same as the prior correction. The total change in power through the near portion is the sum of the additional plus power at distance plus any change in the power of the near addition. The concept of total plus power must be kept in mind when contemplating any power change, particularly changes in distance plus power.

REFERENCES

1. Levene JR. Clinical refraction and visual science. London: Butterworths, 1977:35.
2. Levene JR. Clinical refraction and visual science. London: Butterworths, 1977:39–41.
3. Duke–Elder WS, Abram D. Ophthalmic optics and refraction. In: Duke–Elder WS, ed. System of ophthalmology. London: Henry Kimpton, 1970:208.
4. Levene, JR. Clinical refraction and visual science. London: Butterworths, 1977:54.
5. Rosen E. The invention of eyeglasses. J Hist Med Allied Sci 1956;11:13–46, 183–218.
6. Smyth AH, ed. The writings of Benjamin Franklin. New York: Macmillan, 1905:246–266.
7. Levene JR. Clinical refraction and visual science. London: Butterworths, 1977:141.
8. Morgan MW. Accommodative changes in presbyopia and their correction. In: Hirsch M, Wick R, eds. Vision of the aging patient. Philadelphia: Chilton Book Co, 1960:93.
9. Patorgis CJ. Presbyopia. In: Amos J, ed. Diagnosis and management in vision care. Boston: Butterworths, 1987:203–238.
10. Grosvenor TP. Primary care optometry: a clinical manual, 2nd ed. Professional Press, 1989:334–336.
11. Borish IM. Clinical refraction, 3rd ed. Chicago: Professional Press, 1975:178–184.
12. Donders FC; Moore WD, trans. On the anomalies of accommodation and refraction of the eye. London: New Syndenham Society, 1864:212.
13. Morgan MW. Accommodative changes in presbyopia and their correction. In: Hirsch M, Wick R, eds. Vision of the aging patient. Philadelphia: Chilton Book Co, 1960:84.
14. Lawrence L. Visual optics and sight testing. London: School of Optics, 1920:216.
15. Maxwell JT. Outline of ocular refraction. Omaha: Medical Publishing Co, 1937:169.
16. Sheard C. Physiological optics. Chicago: Cleveland Press, 1918:98–99.
17. Giles GH. The principles and practice of refraction and its allied subjects, 2nd ed. London: Hammond, Hammond Co, 1965:161.
18. Baxter RC. A new cross cylinder test object for the determination of near point corrections. J Am Optom Assoc 1939;11:123–124.
19. Goldberg HB. New variable color-cross grid test card. Refraction Lett 1976;37:4.
20. Woo GC, Sivak JG. A comparison of three methods of determining the reading addition. Am J Optom Physiol Opt 1979;56:75–77.
21. Borish IM. Clinic refraction, 3rd ed. Chicago: Professional Press, 1975: 165–174.
22. Hanlon SD, Nakabayashi J, Shigezawa G. A critical view of presbyopic add determination. J Am Optom Assoc 1987;58:468–472.
23. Hofstetter HW. A useful age–amplitude formula. Penn Optom 1947; 7:5–8.
24. Hofstetter HW. Survey of practices in prescribing presbyopia adds. Am J Optom 1947;26:144–160.
25. Hamasaki D, Ong J, Marg E. The amplitude of accommodation in presbyopia. Am J Optom 1956;33:3–14.

Slit Lamp

Jimmy D. Bartlett

INTRODUCTION

Definition

Of all the procedures and techniques used by the primary care optometrist, slit lamp biomicroscopy represents one of the most important techniques for the physical assessment of the eye and adnexa. Careful slit lamp examination is performed during all comprehensive ocular examinations, and the procedure is usually employed for contact lens fitting and patient follow-up evaluations. Because of its clinical importance in the evaluation of ocular disease, the slit lamp biomicroscope is an essential component of the ophthalmic diagnostic and treatment armamentarium. The relative simplicity of the instrument—a microscope coupled with an illumination system—belies its use in clinical practice, for it requires many hours of practice and experience to gain even a minimal level of competency with the technique. It is essential that all optometrists become proficient in use of the slit lamp biomicroscope so it can be used with ease and without hesitation in the care of both routine patients and patients presenting with suspected ocular disease.

History

Alivar Gullstrand of Stockholm received the Nobel prize in medicine and physiology, in 1911, for his contributions to the dioptrics of the eye and for the development of the slit lamp biomicroscope.[1] By today's standards the Gullstrand instrument was quite crude and mechanically cumbersome, and modern instruments represent a considerable refinement of the illumination systems and mechanical convenience compared with the earlier designs. Even today, however, most models of slit lamps are still based on the principles of the original Gullstrand device.

One such modification in slit lamp technique was contributed in 1919 by Vogt.[2] Vogt was the first to describe the use of specular microscopy of the corneal endothelium, and, in recent years, use of specular illumination techniques and the evaluation potential they provide have become of considerable clinical importance. These procedures have gained popularity and widespread use in connection with the development of more sophisticated anterior segment surgical techniques.

Clinical Use

Slit lamp biomicroscopy is one of the most frequently employed clinical procedures in the practice of optometry. It is used for both diagnostic and treatment purposes to aid visualization of the anterior ocular structures, giving variable magnification, while maintaining a stereoscopic view. The combination of variable magnification with stereopsis is critically important when evaluating the presence and location of anterior segment lesions. The information provided by careful slit lamp examination generally cannot be obtained using any other procedure. Thus, slit lamp biomicroscopy represents a unique procedure that contributes vitally important information for the care of most optometric patients.

Patients presenting for routine, comprehensive eye examinations must receive a careful slit lamp examination to exclude the presence of disease or abnormality of the anterior ocular structures. Slit lamp examination is also indicated in contact lens-fitting procedures to evaluate proper fitting relationships between the lens and contiguous structures, such as the cornea, conjunctiva, and lids. Any anterior segment compromise induced by lens wear is usually best evaluated using the slit lamp instrument.

Beyond the "routine," asymptomatic patient, the slit lamp is regularly used to assist in the differential diagnosis of patients presenting with "red eyes." Conjunctival inflammations, eyelid disease, keratitis, anterior uveitis, ocular trauma, and diseases of the lacrimal system cannot be properly evaluated without the aid of the slit lamp. The slit lamp is often utilized in conjunction with ancillary procedures. These include the administration of diagnostic dyes such as sodium fluorescein and rose bengal. These tests are discussed in Chapter 38. Moreover, stereoscopic examination of the vitreous and retina is frequently accomplished in conjunction with the slit lamp; slit lamp biomicroscopy of the fundus utilizes ancillary diagnostic lenses and is discussed in detail in Chapter 47.

The slit lamp is often used therapeutically when highly magnified, stereoscopic observation of the anterior ocular structures is required. Examples include foreign body removal from the cornea, conjunctiva, or eyelids; insertion of punctal plugs; and corneal epithelial debridement in cases of herpetic keratitis.

INSTRUMENTATION

Theory

The operational components of the slit lamp biomicroscope consist of a binocular microscope, an illumination system, and joystick to provide movement of the microscope and illumination system (Fig. 22–1). The instrument is called a *slit lamp* because the illumination system (the lamp) is designed to provide broad-beam illumination or, more commonly, a tall but narrow "slit" of light, often referred to as an *optic section* or *parallelepiped,* depending on the beam width. Optic sections are extremely thin (less than 0.25 mm wide), whereas parallelepipeds are wider (1 to 2 mm wide). Although many variations are used in clinical practice, the most common configuration for the illumination system is to use a beam of moderate width (0.5 to 1.0 mm). This allows the incident light to "slice" through tissues of the anterior ocular structures to reveal the anatomic structures in their normal relationships and to allow the practitioner to ascertain departures from normal. The microscope merely allows maintenance of a stereoscopic view, with variable magnification according to the capabilities of the slit lamp instrument. The critical feature of the slit lamp biomicroscope that must be mastered by the practitioner is the utilization of various illumination techniques wherein the incident light from the illumination system is cast on the eye in a way such that it maximally exposes existing abnormalities when viewed through the binocular microscope. Although each of these illumination techniques will be discussed separately, it must be emphasized that, in practice, the clinician will usually use more than one of the techniques simultaneously and will, quite subconsciously, change illumination techniques to enable the best view of the structure under examination. This proficiency requires considerable practice on the part of the clinician, but it must be gained if effective slit lamp examination procedures are to be mastered.

The illumination techniques most often used are direct, indirect, sclerotic scatter, retroillumination, and specular reflection. Of these, direct illumination is most often used, but other types of illumination techniques may be chosen by the practitioner when direct observation seems inadequate to properly visualize the tissue or abnormality examined.

Direct Illumination

Direct focal illumination involves placing the light source at an angular separation of about 40° to 50° from the microscope, and both should be placed in coincident focus. This arrangement permits both the light beam and microscope to be sharply focused on the ocular tissue being observed. Several variations of direct illumination can be used, and each employs a variation of beam size and microscope magnification.[3]

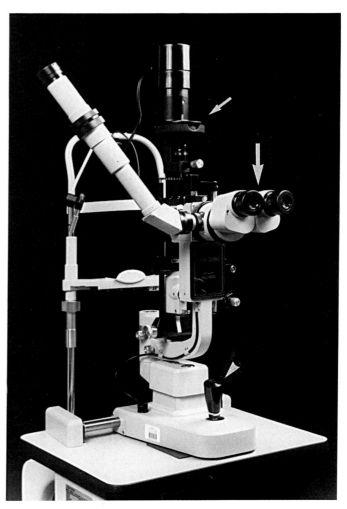

FIGURE 22–1. General features of a slit-lamp biomicroscope. Binocular microscope (*large arrow*), illumination system (*small arrow*), and joystick (*arrowhead*).

1. Wide-beam direct illumination is commonly used as a preliminary technique to evaluate a large area (Fig. 22–2).
2. A parallelepiped may be constructed by narrowing the beam to 1 to 2 mm in width to illuminate a rectangular area of the cornea (Fig. 22–3). This provides a layered view of the cornea and lens. Higher magnification than that used with wide-beam illumination is preferred to evaluate both the depth and extent of corneal abrasions, scarring, or foreign bodies. Such an illumination procedure is probably the most commonly used of all the illumination techniques.
3. An optic section is produced when the width of the parallelepiped is further reduced to an extremely thin slit beam (Fig. 22–4). Such an illumination technique is used primarily to evaluate structural layers of the cornea and lens, and it is quite useful when estimating the depth of an abnormality such as a corneal foreign body or position of cataract.
4. A conical beam may be produced by narrowing the vertical height of a parallelepiped to produce a small circular or square spot of light. This illumination technique is most useful when examining the transparency of the anterior

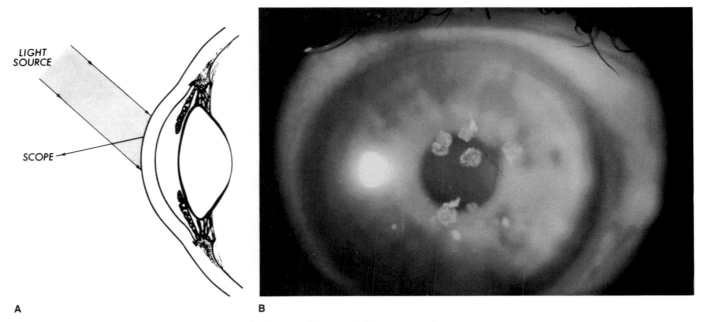

FIGURE 22–2. Wide-beam direct illumination. (*A*) Schematic drawing of illumination and microscope positions. (*B*) Clinical example showing general features of corneal stromal dystrophy. (Adapted from Eskridge JB, Schoessler J, Lowther G. A specific biomicroscopy procedure. J Am Optom Assoc 1973;45:400.)

chamber for evidence of floating cells and flare, as seen in anterior uveitis.

Indirect (Proximal) Illumination

Indirect illumination is formed by narrowing the slit beam to 1 to 2 mm in width. The beam is then focused on an area adjacent to the ocular tissue observed. The foci of the light source and microscope are not coincident (Fig. 22–5). The purpose of indirect illumination is to provide somewhat "softer" illumination to give better definition of the structural components of the iris, epithelial corneal edema, pigment spots, and corneal foreign bodies.

A dynamic source of illumination can be adapted from this technique by moving the light beam in and out of its "click" position while holding the microscope steady. Light will be alternately

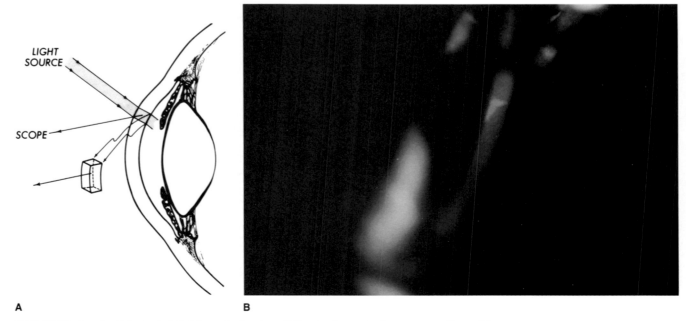

FIGURE 22–3. Parallelepiped. (*A*) Schematic drawing of illumination and microscope positions. (*B*) Clinical example showing epithelial basement membrane dystrophy. (Adapted from Eskridge JB, Schoessler J, Lowther G. A specific biomicroscopy procedure. J Am Optom Assoc 1973;45:400.)

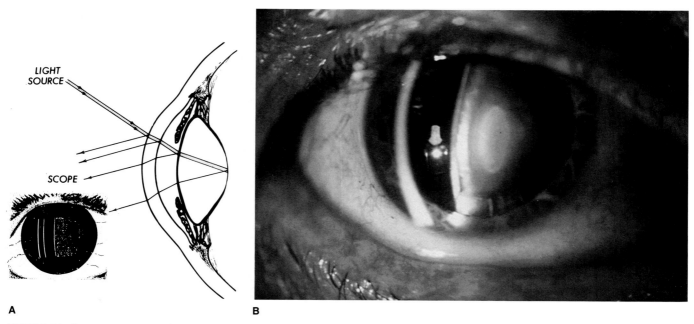

A **B**

FIGURE 22–4. Optic section. (*A*) Schematic drawing of illumination and microscope positions. (*B*) Clinical example showing zones of discontinuity of crystalline lens. (Adapted from Eskridge JB, Schoessler J, Lowther G. A specific biomicroscopy procedure. J Am Optom Assoc 1973;45:400.)

reflected and transmitted by the structure observed and, thereby, will enhance its three-dimensional appearance.

Retroillumination

Retroillumination is formed by reflecting light of the slit beam from a structure more posterior than the structure under observation. Some clinicians prefer to move the slit beam out of its click position, but this is not a necessary prerequisite for successful retroillumination. A vertical slit beam 1- to 4-mm wide can be used (Fig. 22–6).

The purpose of retroillumination is to place the object of regard against a bright background, allowing the object to appear dark or black. This technique is used most often in searching for keratic precipitates and other debris on the corneal endothelium. The crystalline lens can also be retroilluminated for viewing of

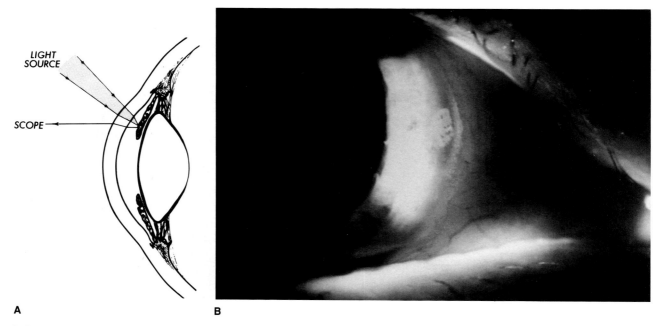

A **B**

FIGURE 22–5. Indirect (proximal) illumination. (*A*) Schematic drawing of illumination and microscope positions. (*B*) Clinical example showing Vogt's girdle and early band keratopathy. (Adapted from Eskridge JB, Schoessler J, Lowther G. A specific biomicroscopy procedure. J Am Optom Assoc 1973;45:400.)

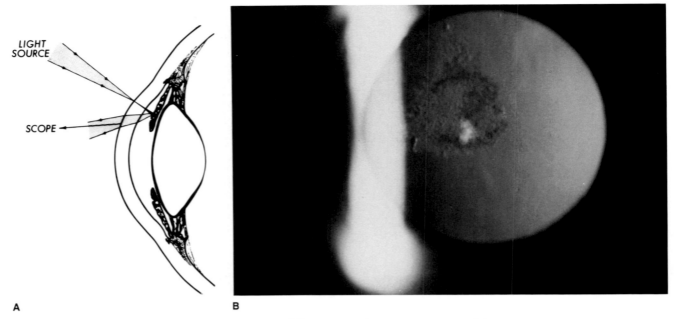

FIGURE 22–6.   Retroillumination. (*A*) Schematic drawing of illumination and microscope positions. (*B*) Clinical example showing posterior subcapsular cataract. (Adapted from Eskridge JB, Schoessler J, Lowther G. A specific biomicroscopy procedure. J Am Optom Assoc 1973;45:400.)

water clefts and vacuoles of the anterior lens and of posterior subcapsular cataract.

Specular Reflection

Specular reflection is established by separating the microscope and slit beam by equal angles from the normal to the cornea. The separation that seems to produce the best specular reflection is about 50°[4] (Fig. 22–7). The area of high reflectance is termed the *zone of specular reflection,* and only a small portion of the cornea can be viewed in this zone at any given time. The patient must be instructed to move his or her gaze in many directions to observe the specular reflection over most of the cornea.

Under specular reflection, the anterior corneal surface appears as a white, uniform surface, and the corneal endothelium takes on a golden mosaic pattern. Irregularities, deposits, or exca-

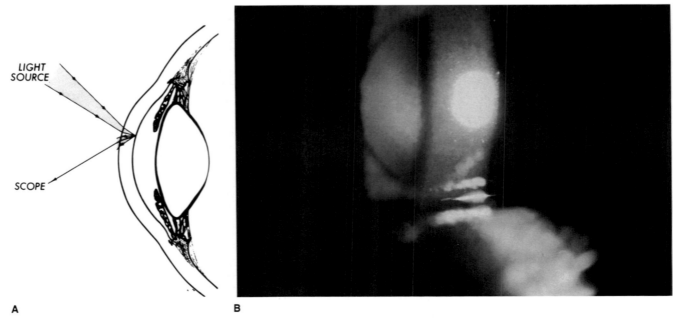

FIGURE 22–7.   Specular reflection. (*A*) Schematic drawing of illumination and microscope positions. (*B*) Clinical example showing irregular anterior corneal surface. (Adapted from Eskridge JB, Schoessler J, Lowther G. A specific biomicroscopy procedure. J Am Optom Assoc 1973;45:400.)

LIGHT SOURCE

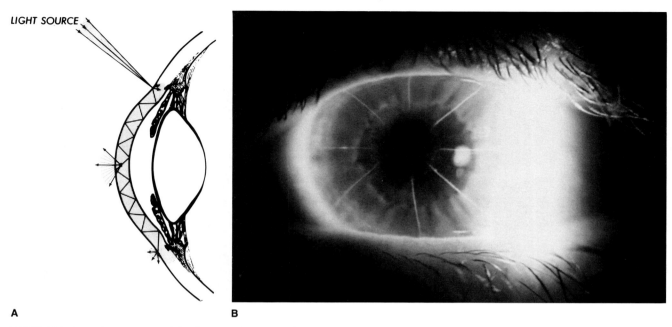

A   B

FIGURE 22–8. Sclerotic scatter. (A) Schematic drawing of illumination and microscope positions. (B) Clinical example showing radial keratotomy incisions. (Adapted from Eskridge JB, Schoessler J, Lowther G. A specific biomicroscopy procedure. J Am Optom Assoc 1973;45:400.)

vations in these smooth surfaces will fail to reflect light and thus will appear darker than the surroundings.

Sclerotic Scatter

The sclerotic scatter illumination technique is formed by focusing a bright, but narrow (1 mm), slit beam on the limbus and using the microscope on low magnification. Such an illumination technique causes the cornea to take on total internal reflection (Fig. 22–8). The slit beam should be placed approximately 40° to 60° from the microscope and out of its click position. The central corneal area can be viewed with the microscope without disturbing the slit beam focus at the limbus. When properly positioned, this technique will produce a halo glow of light around the limbus as the light is transmitted throughout the cornea. Because the light is internally reflected, no light will emerge toward the examiner, and, consequently, the cornea will appear black. An area of reduced light transmission within the cornea, however, will appear gray because light will be reflected toward the microscope. Although the slit beam must not necessarily be focused on the limbus to produce sclerotic scatter, it is generally necessary to rotate the beam out of its click position so that the beam is incident on the limbal area. Moreover, many practitioners prefer to observe the cornea during sclerotic scatter without aid of the slit lamp microscope. Central corneal epithelial edema can be easily observed using sclerotic scatter, even without the benefit of magnification afforded by the microscope. Other conditions that lend themselves to observation using sclerotic scatter include corneal abrasions as well as corneal nebulae and maculae.

Use

Routine biomicroscopy of the ophthalmic patient involves examining the patient in a seated position. Some clinical situations, however, may require a supine position. For example, patients under anesthesia, patients who have difficulty positioning the face or

head within the instrument, or those who are unable to cooperate properly may require examination in the supine position. A simple L-shaped device has been described for use with the Zeiss 100/16 slit lamp to enable examination of the supine patient.[5]

The basic design of the slit lamp can be incorporated into a videotape-recording system to enable recording and playback of dynamic anterior segment phenomena. Perhaps the most useful indication for such a system is contact lens research applications and clinical situations in which the practitioner wishes to demonstrate to the patient abnormal contact lens–eye dynamics. Such video recording of contact lens–eye relationships can be useful in the diagnosis of lens-fitting relationships.[6] The editing feature permits time-lapse documentation of adverse ocular responses.

COMMERCIALLY AVAILABLE INSTRUMENTS

Basic Design

The typical slit lamp biomicroscope (see Fig. 22–1) will accommodate most patients and allow comfortable examination. All slit lamps have a patient chin rest and forehead rest for correct patient positioning. The chin rest (Fig. 22–9) can be adjusted vertically to accommodate various facial features and head sizes. A fixation light or mirror (Fig. 22–10) is provided to help maintain steady patient fixation in the desired position of gaze to facilitate viewing of various ocular structures or lesions. A binocular microscopic system allows a stereoscopic view of anterior ocular structures and permits variable magnification, which is controlled by a rotatable lever or knob (Fig. 22–11). The interpupillary distance of the microscope eyepieces is continuously variable and is adjusted to the examiner's requirements.

The illumination system is mounted on the same axis as the microscope and has appropriate controls for the slit beam height, width, and rotation (Fig. 22–12). In addition, various filters can be inserted into the beam path and usually include neutral density, cobalt blue, and red-free filters. The entire illumination system

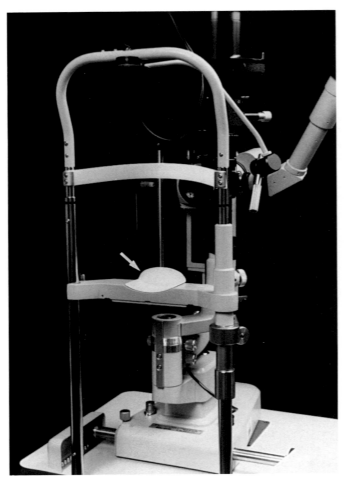

FIGURE 22–9. Chin rest (*arrow*).

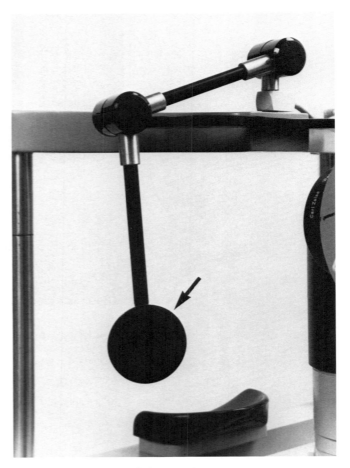

FIGURE 22–10. Fixation light (*arrow*).

usually swings freely from left to right for adequate examination of each eye from various angles.

Both the microscope and illumination system are moved as a single unit by use of a joystick (Fig. 22–13). Most joysticks allow easy maneuverability of the slit lamp and, by use of one or more controls, provide three-dimensional movement of the slit lamp (i.e., forward–backward, left–right, and up–down). In addition, most slit lamps are securely mounted on an examination table that is attached to the basic ophthalmic examination unit. The various controls allowing positioning of the table give the examiner even greater flexibility in making sure both the patient and practitioner are comfortable during slit lamp examination.

Although numerous models of slit lamps are commercially available, the following section describes the most commonly used slit lamp biomicroscopes. The basic features of each are described, but the reader is encouraged to consult current product information for specific details and commercial availability.

Haag–Streit Universal Slit Lamp Model 900 BM (Fig. 22–14)

The Haag–Streit slit lamp features a three-dimensional joystick control lever and has a slit beam that is continuously adjustable from hairline to a width or height of 8 mm. A tilting mechanism for the slit image permits examination in vertical, oblique, and horizontal sections. There are built-in heat-absorbing red-free and gray

filters, as well as aperture disks containing apertures of 0.2, 1, 2, 3, 5, and 8 mm. A fixation device allows a nondazzling annular fixation target to be set to remain within the patient's field of view. Standard magnifications are 10×, 16×, or 25×, but additional eyepieces are available for magnifications up to 40×. Many optional accessories are available, including a teaching microscope, depth-measuring attachment, and tonometer.

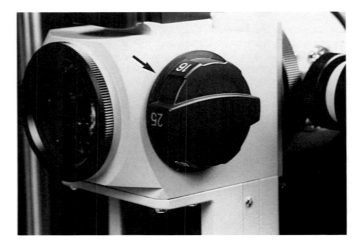

FIGURE 22–11. Magnification control (*arrow*).

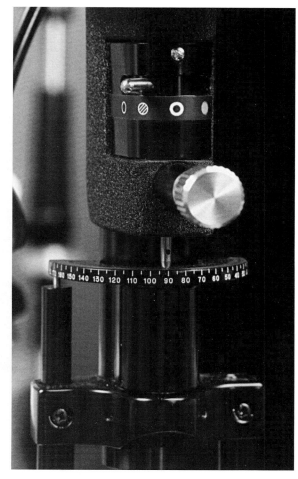

FIGURE 22–12. Illumination controls.

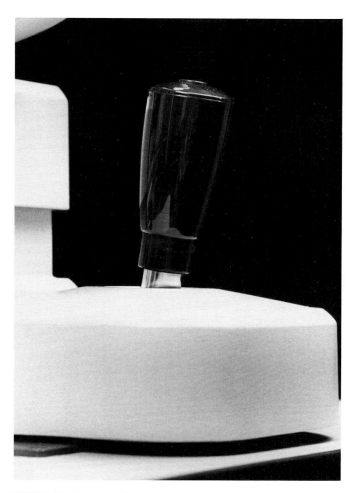

FIGURE 22–13. Joystick.

Marco IV Slit Lamp (Fig. 22–15)

The Marco IV instrument features a slit beam length that can be changed from 1 to 8 mm, and the slit lamp elevation can be controlled with a single hand on the joystick. This instrument contains a tilting mechanism that can be used during gonioscopy or fundus biomicroscopy.

The microscope is of the Galilean type and consists of a manual rotary objective changing system to produce five different magnifications ($6\times$, $10\times$, $16\times$, $25\times$, and $40\times$).

The slit beam width is continuously variable from 0 to 14 mm, and the slit length is continuously variable from 0.2 to 14 mm. Aperture diaphragms allow illumination in 0.2-, 1-, 2-, 3-, 5-, 9-, and 14-mm diameters. Built-in filters include cobalt blue, red-free, 13% neutral density, and heat absorbing.

Mentor Slit Lamp Model SH-12 (Fig. 22–16)

The Mentor model SH-12 provides a joystick to permit control in any direction on the horizontal and vertical plane. The instrument also provides for variable slit beam length and width. Six aperture diaphragms are selected by lever action and allow variable slit lengths from 0.2 to 10.0 mm. Slit width is adjustable from fully open to fully closed. A built-in slit aperture scale measures lesion size on a vernier slit length. Five built-in filters are selectable by lever action: cobalt, normal light, heat absorption, 50% neutral density, and blue-green.

The slit rotates 180° with an adjusting knob, and slit illumination can be displaced from the center of the field for indirect illumination.

The fixation light offers a choice of a bull's eye with dioptric adjustments or an annular target for patients with high myopia.

A rheostat permits variable brightness control, and a booster button projects brilliant slit illumination.

Eyepieces are available in $10\times$ and $16\times$ power, and a pivot point on the light column permits tilting the slit illumination system during gonioscopy.

Nikon NS-1 Zoom Slit Lamp (Fig. 22–17)

The Nikon NS-1 slit lamp allows continuously variable magnification from $7.5\times$ to $32\times$. The total magnification ranges from $5\times$ to $71\times$ with optional eyepieces.

The slit beam width is continuously variable from 0 to 14 mm, and the slit length is variable from 0.2 to 14 mm in preset steps. The slit length is also continuously variable from 1 to 12 mm.

A single joystick permits movement of the instrument in any direction.

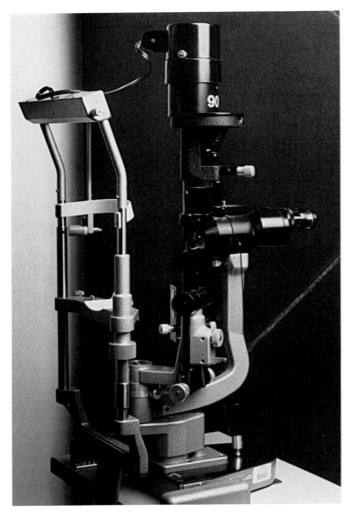

FIGURE 22–14. Haag-Streit Universal Slit Lamp Model 900 BM.

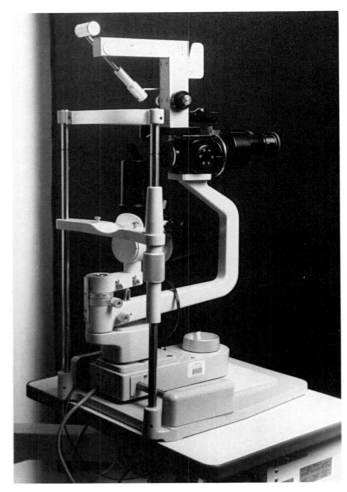

FIGURE 22–15. Marco IV Slit Lamp, No. 1040.

Topcon Model SL-4E Slit Lamp (Fig. 22–18)

The Topcon SL-4E slit lamp combines a converging binocular with a Galilean telescope with magnifications of 10×, 16×, and 25.6×. A halogen illumination system provides adjustable slit heights from 0 to 12 mm, as well as rotation, scanning controls, red-free and cobalt blue filters. The joystick control allows movement in all directions. Various accessories are available, including tonometers and photographic attachments.

Zeiss Slit Lamp 100/16 (Fig. 22–19)

The Zeiss 100/16 slit lamp includes a high-resolution stereoscopic corneal microscope with a manually-controlled magnification changing system for magnifications of 6×, 10×, 16×, 25×, and 40×. Eyepieces are 12.5× with ±8 Diopter correction range. Head and chin rest have screw-action height adjustment. A rotatable slit illuminator system has 6 repeatable slit heights and continuously-variable slit widths as well as red-free and cobalt blue filters. Various accessories are available, including Hruby lens and tonometers.

CLINICAL PROCEDURE

Special care must be taken to assure that the patient is comfortable during the slit lamp examination. This is particularly important for elderly patients, children, and others who cannot tolerate a prolonged procedure. Although most individuals can physically lean forward onto the chin rest, obese patients or those with large chests can be more appropriately accommodated by the instrument by lowering the instrument table and allowing the patient to take an excessive forward position onto the chin rest. Infants and small children can often be held in the parent's lap and the child's head can be gently placed in the chin rest. Hand rests are usually provided, and these serve to increase the patient's comfort and balance at the slit lamp. With the patient's chin in the chin rest, the slit lamp table should be lowered until the patient can place his or her forehead on the forehead rest.

Although the specific procedure varies greatly among practitioners, slit lamp examination can be simplified by following a routine, systematic procedure for most patients.[3] The following procedures, including illumination techniques, are recommended as serving to optimize and maximize the information obtained from slit-lamp biomicroscopy.

1. *Eyelids and lashes.* It is usually appropriate to begin the slit-lamp examination by evaluating the eyelids and

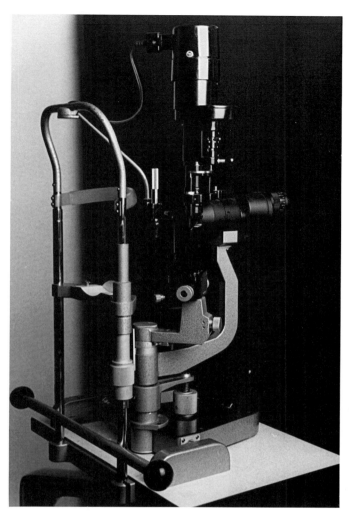

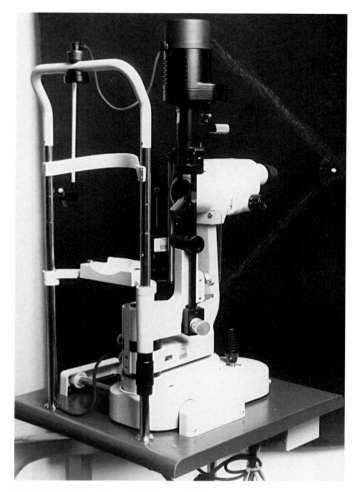

FIGURE 22–17. Nikon NS-1 Zoom Slit Lamp.

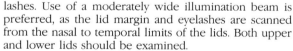

FIGURE 22–16. Mentor Slit Lamp Model SH-12.

lashes. Use of a moderately wide illumination beam is preferred, as the lid margin and eyelashes are scanned from the nasal to temporal limits of the lids. Both upper and lower lids should be examined.

2. *Palpebral conjunctiva.* The lower lid can be everted with the thumb or forefinger and, with low magnification, the inferior palpebral conjunctiva and inferior punctum should be examined. Following eversion of the upper lid (see Chap. 3), the upper palpebral conjunctiva can be examined in a similar fashion. Low magnification is usually sufficient, even when lesions such as follicles or papillae are observed.

3. *Bulbar conjunctiva.* The bulbar conjunctiva is most easily examined using direct illumination with a vertical slit.[3] The horizontal meridians of the conjunctiva can be examined with the patient in primary gaze, and the superior and inferior portions of the bulbar conjunctiva can be examined with the patient alternately gazing up and down or, alternatively, with the patient's eyelids retracted by the examiner. As the conjunctiva is scanned with the slit lamp, use of a medium-beam width about 5 mm in length should be sufficient to uncover any abnormality present.[4]

4. *Sclera.* Detection of inflammatory lesions of the episclera

or sclera is facilitated by the stereoscopic view afforded by the slit lamp. Differentiation between conjunctival and episcleral or scleral inflammation is usually straightforward, since involvement of the former is associated with superficial inflammatory signs, whereas inflammation of the latter is accompanied by deeply engorged episcleral or scleral vessels. The examiner can manually oscillate the eyelids over the inflamed region during slit lamp examination to ascertain whether the inflamed vessels move (conjunctiva) or whether they are stationary (episclera or sclera). A moderately wide slit lamp beam with low to medium magnification is usually sufficient to enable recognition of episcleral or scleral inflammation.

5. *Limbus.* A slit lamp beam of medium width and length is appropriate for examination of the limbus. Evaluation of the superior limbus requires that the patient gaze downward and the upper lid be retracted. Similarly, the inferior limbus can be evaluated with the patient gazing upward and with the lower lid retracted, if necessary.

6. *Cornea.* Because of its transparency, the cornea can be extremely difficult to examine. Consequently, it is often appropriate to use a variety of illumination techniques and variable magnification to maximize the ability to detect corneal abnormalities. The experienced examiner will often use a variety of illumination procedures, with-

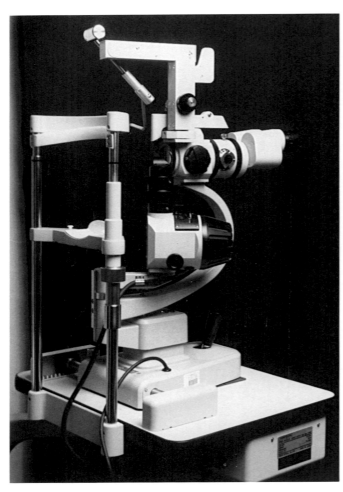

FIGURE 22–18. Topcon Model SL-4E Slit Lamp.

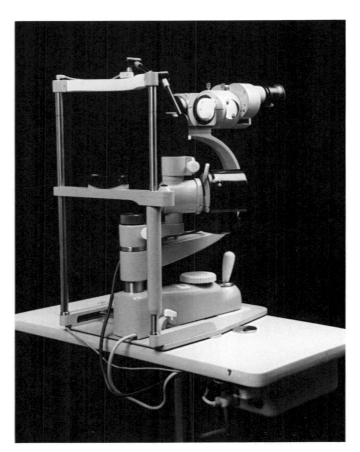

FIGURE 22–19. Zeiss Slit Lamp 100/16.

out realizing that the illumination technique has changed. When using direct illumination, including its various subtypes, the clinician should often look to the side of the illuminated area to view the corneal structures indirectly. If this is done successfully, numerous subtle corneal changes can be detected. Specular reflection, sclerotic scatter, and retroillumination should frequently be used to aid in the detection of specific corneal abnormalities. For example, sclerotic scatter is an illumination technique of choice to detect stromal or epithelial edema associated with contact lens wear or herpetic infection. Retroillumination from the iris can greatly assist in the detection of microcystic lesions or minute foreign bodies.

7. *Anterior chamber*. A simple and rapid estimation of the anterior chamber depth can be made during routine slit-lamp examination. This rapid assessment is usually sufficient to permit safe pupillary dilatation without the need for gonioscopy.[7] A vertical slit lamp beam is placed at the temporal limbus just inside the corneoscleral junction. The beam should be as narrow as possible and should be directed toward the eye at an angle of about 60° from the direction of the microscope (Fig. 22–20). The depth of the anterior chamber at the temporal limbus is compared with the thickness of the cornea through which the beam

travels.[7] Following estimation of the anterior chamber depth, the optical quality of the aqueous should be assessed. In its normal state, the aqueous is optically empty, and the slit-lamp beam will be invisible as it travels through the anterior chamber. Examination of the aqueous is most appropriately performed with a small square or circular beam directed through the anterior chamber into the pupil. High magnification is generally desired to enable detection of cells moving within the beam. The presence of cells indicates the existence of anterior uveal inflammation. This condition is also commonly associated with "flare," in which the aqueous takes on the appearance of smoke or fog, indicating elevated protein content of the aqueous. It is especially important during this examination to have minimal or no ambient illumination in the examination room.

8. *Iris*. The iris should be examined using direct illumination with a medium-width (1.5-mm) slit beam.[3] In some patients, especially those with light irides, the iris sphincter muscle can be best viewed by using indirect illumination combined with an oscillatory beam.[8]

9. *Crystalline lens*. It is often helpful to reduce the vertical height of the slit beam to control light intensity so that the pupil does not become excessively constricted during examination of the crystalline lens. Although specular reflection can be used to evaluate the anterior epithelial surface and lens capsule, direct illumination is sufficient to reveal pigment deposits on the anterior lens surface. Examination of the middle and posterior lenticular areas

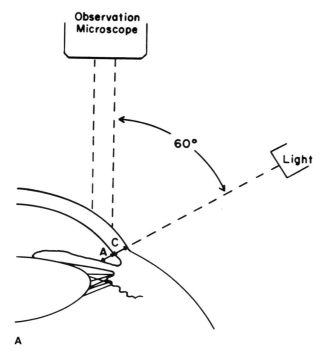

A

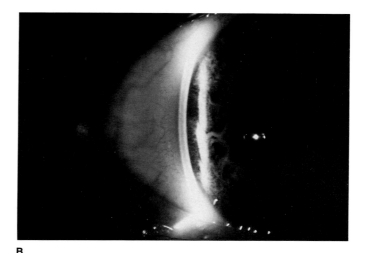

B

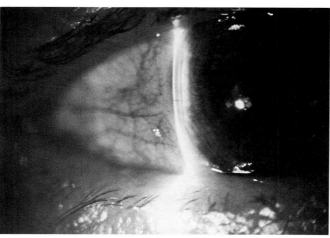

C

FIGURE 22–20. Slit lamp method for anterior angle evaluation. (*A*) The slit lamp beam should be as narrow as possible and should be directed toward the eye at an angle of approximately 60° from the direction of the microscope. The depth of the anterior chamber (*A*) is compared with the thickness of the cornea (*C*) through which the beam travels. (*B*) Slit lamp view of a wide-open (grade 4) angle in which the depth of the anterior chamber is greater than the thickness of the cornea. (*C*) Slit lamp view of a grade 2 angle in which the depth of the anterior chamber is one-fourth the thickness of the cornea. (Published with permission from Bartlett JD. Dilation of the pupil. In: Bartlett JD, Jaanus SD, eds. Clinical ocular pharmacology. Boston: Butterworth, 1989:393–419.)

is facilitated by retroillumination from the retina. This is especially helpful in the detection of early or subtle posterior subcapsular cataract. It may be helpful to narrow the slit beam to enable an optic section of the entire lens thickness. This may help localize any opacity in relation to the surrounding structural lenticular zones.

Retroillumination of the anterior layers of the lens may reveal vacuoles, water clefts, and anterior opacities. The use of wide-beam direct illumination should generally be discouraged because there is often intense reflection and diffusion from the anterior lens capsule, which may serve to mask the deeper structures of the lens and hinder localization of lenticular detail.[3] Narrow-beam direct illumination, coupled with retroillumination, are usually the best techniques to maximize examination of the crystalline lens. The detection and differentiation of cataracts and other lenticular abnormalities warrants wide

pupillary dilatation.[9] Hence, many clinicians often perform a cursory examination of the crystalline lens before routine pupillary dilation, followed by a more detailed examination after the pupil has reached its maximum diameter.

10. *Anterior vitreous.* Routine slit lamp examination encompasses evaluation of the anterior vitreous. Midvitreal and posterior vitreal abnormalities are generally best examined using auxilliary procedures, as discussed in Chapter 47. For routine examination purposes, it is usually sufficient to use a narrow beam that is focused through the pupil and lens, with the angle of separation of the microscope and slit beam kept small. The patient can be instructed to gaze alternately upward and downward to enable observation of the ascension phenomenon. Occasionally, asteroid bodies can be observed within the anterior vitreous.

CLINICAL IMPLICATIONS

Clinical Significance

Information derived from a careful slit lamp examination can be of vital importance in the care of the patient. Knowledge of the health of the anterior ocular structures is important to enable the clinician to make informed decisions about the source of the patient's complaint. Differentiation between refractive and pathologic causes of presenting signs and symptoms will often rest on the slit lamp examination. Thus, a careful slit lamp procedure performed during every comprehensive ocular examination is essential and, likewise, is necessary whenever the patient's complaint increases the suspicion of anterior segment abnormalities. Such complaints include symptoms of itching, tearing, scratchiness, pain, photophobia, or ocular discharge. A history of ocular foreign bodies will also necessitate careful evaluation with the slit lamp. It is important, both clinically and medicolegally, to document carefully the health and integrity of all anterior ocular structures.

Clinical Interpretation

A conscientious slit lamp examination should, with practice and experience, require only a few minutes of examination time, but it will yield invaluable information that will be used to document the health and integrity of the anterior ocular structures and, thereby, facilitate proper patient management. A discussion of abnormal findings is beyond the scope of this chapter, but the clinician can be guided by the following observations that define the "normal" slit lamp examination.[10]

Eyelids and Lashes

As the eyelid margins are examined, the practitioner should observe for signs of erythema and swelling as an indication of inflammation. No discharge should be observed, and the eyelashes should be free of debris, crusting, or eyelid matting. Eyelid crusting or scaling are signs of blepharitis and may warrant appropriate treatment.

Both the external lid tissues as well as internal tissues should be free of localized or diffuse areas of swelling, an indication of external or internal hordeola, respectively. These lesions must be differentiated from chalazia by the presence of tenderness on palpation in the former.

Several rows of lashes will be seen to emerge from their respective follicles along the lid margin. Abnormal lash architecture includes inturning lashes (trichiasis) and an auxilliary row of lashes emerging from the meibomian gland orifices (distichiasis).

The meibomian gland orifices should be inspected for signs of inspissation (clogging) with white or yellow caps overlying the orifices. This abnormal finding is indicative of meibomianitis.

The position of the lower and upper lids in relationship to the globe should be ascertained. Inward rolling of the lower eyelid is an abnormal finding (entropion), and an outward eversion of the eyelid can lead to serious ocular sequelae, a condition termed ectropion. In the presence of either condition the cornea should be carefully examined for signs of exposure keratitis or lash-induced trauma.

Finally, both the lower and upper puncta should be examined. A pointing, inflamed punctum suggests the diagnosis of canaliculitis. Discharge from the punctum may be noted when pressure is exerted over the lacrimal sac. The normal punctum should be open; a stenotic punctum can contribute to complaints of ocular tearing and may be a manifestation of an active infectious process or normal aging.

Palpebral Conjunctiva

Examination of the inferior palpebral conjunctiva should reveal a satinlike tissue generally free of follicles or papillae. Many patients, however, will be observed to have several follicles scattered throughout the palpebral conjunctiva, especially near the outer canthus. Moreover, many children may be seen to have many follicles, a normal finding known as folliculosis. The presence of abundant follicles in the symptomatic patient may be an indication of viral or toxic conjunctivitis.

Many patients will be observed to have lithiasis, creamy white calcium deposits located more commonly in the inferior palpebral conjunctiva.

After eversion of the upper lid, the superior palpebral conjunctiva should be likewise examined. The palpebral conjunctiva here should be smooth and satin-like. The presence of diffuse papillary hypertrophy suggests the presence of acute or chronic conjunctivitis. The presence of extremely large papillae can be suggestive of vernal conjunctivitis or of giant papillary conjunctivitis (GPC).

Bulbar Conjunctiva

The normal bulbar conjunctiva is free of hyperemia, discharge, or swelling. A common conjunctival lesion in the adult population is the pinguecula, a yellow-white nodule, sometimes highly vascularized, and located near the nasal or temporal limbus. Local elevated lesions can represent nevi, neoplastic processes, or can be benign vascularized lesions such as pterygia. Keratinization of the bulbar conjunctiva can occur in association with extreme dry-eye states and may present with or without rose bengal staining (see Chap. 38).

The normal bulbar conjunctiva may have occasional scattered petechial hemorrhages, but larger, layered subconjunctival hemorrhages can be seen spontaneously or following blunt ocular trauma.

The normal bulbar conjunctiva is generally free of pigmentation, but conjunctival pigmentation and pigmented nevi are commonly seen in darkly pigmented patients. Some drug toxicities or abnormal metabolic states can lead to abnormal coloration or pigmentation of the conjunctiva.

Active inflammation of the bulbar conjunctiva can lead to edema (chemosis). This is manifest clinically as an elevated, "glassy" appearance of the conjunctiva and can be seen in certain allergic conditions and in thyroid-related ocular disease.

Sclera

Inflammation of the anterior episclera often involves tortuous, hyperemic vessels with saccular dilatations observable under the slit lamp. Manipulation of the overlying bulbar conjunctiva with the eyelids can further assist differentiation between conjunctival and episcleral inflammation.

Scleritis involves generalized or localized areas of engorgement of deep scleral vessels, often associated with exquisite pain or tenderness on digital palpation.

Limbus

The superior limbus is usually slightly more opaque than the remainder of the limbus, and the limbal vascular arcades invade further into the cornea in the superior limbal area. Inflammation of the superior limbal area can occur in both contact lens wearers and patients with no history of lens wear. Localized elevations at the limbus can represent a hypersensitivity reaction (phlyctenular keratitis) or a congenital abnormality (e.g., limbal dermoid).

Cornea

Examination of the corneal epithelium should reveal a smooth surface free of depressions or elevations. Abrasions can be pleomorphic and represent traumatic deepithelialization of the cornea. Abrasions have bases that are transparent, unlike corneal ulcers that have milky white bases. Alterations of the corneal epithelial surface should be evaluated using topically instilled rose bengal and sodium fluorescein dyes, as discussed in Chapter 38. Denuded areas of epithelium can also represent recurrent corneal erosions, most commonly occurring in the inferior portion of the cornea. Special care should be taken to localize the area of corneal staining because its specific location serves to identify the underlying cause. For example, staining that is principally inferior is often indicative of staphylococcal keratitis or exposure keratopathy, whereas staining near the superior limbus may indicate superior limbic keratitis or vernal keratoconjunctivitis. Staining in the interpalpebral area is highly suggestive of keratoconjunctivitis sicca. Arborescent-staining patterns are usually indicative of herpes simplex infection. Contact lens-associated staining, especially with rigid gas permeable lenses, is often manifest as coalesced punctate staining in the three and nine o'clock areas at the limbus. Indeed, slit lamp examination is one of the most crucial procedures used to identify the existence of contact lens complications and to formulate an appropriate management strategy.[11]

Infiltrates, consisting principally of polymorphonuclear leukocytes, and edema are abnormal findings and may be observed in the superficial stroma. Stromal scarring may be associated with interstitial keratitis or corneal trauma and often appears as a bluish-white opacity. Stromal opacities may also be evidence of a corneal dystrophy or degeneration, and localization of the opacities to specific regions of the cornea will assist in the differential diagnosis.

The normal corneal endothelium is usually free of pigment deposits but will often be found to have scattered pigment adhering to it. Guttata are often observed in the central aspect of the cornea, but may be considered pathologic if extensive, indicating the possible development of Fuchs' dystrophy. Some drug toxicities can also be manifest as corneal endothelial pigmentation. Krukenberg's spindle represents a vertical deposition of pigment on the endothelium associated with pigmentary dispersion syndrome, a condition sometimes associated with glaucoma.

Anterior Chamber

Interpretation of the depth of the anterior chamber angle requires a simple comparison of the depth of the anterior chamber with the thickness of the cornea through which the beam travels. If the depth of the anterior chamber is equal to, or greater than, the thickness of the cornea, the anterior chamber angle is classified as grade 4, or wide open. If the depth of the anterior chamber is equal to approximately half the thickness of the cornea, the angle is classified as grade 3. An anterior chamber depth equal to one-fourth the corneal thickness is classified as grade 2, and an anterior chamber depth less than one-fourth the corneal thickness is classified as grade 1. In practical terms angles classified as grade 3 or 4 are incapable of closure upon dilatation of the pupil, angles assessed as grade 2 are narrow and may pose some risk upon pupillary dilatation, and grade 1 angles can be considered to have considerable risk for closure. Angles that are assessed as grade 1 or 2 indicate a risk of angle closure and, therefore, merit gonioscopic confirmation before the pupil is dilated.[7]

The anterior chamber should be carefully evaluated for the presence of cells and flare. The normal anterior chamber will be observed to have little or no flare and only an occasional cell. The presence of increased cells and substantial flare suggests the diagnosis of anterior uveitis. If the quantity of cells is large enough, they may be seen as depositions on the corneal endothelium, a condition known as keratic precipitates. These can be seen in both active and old anterior uveitis.

Iris

The normal iris is easily evaluated using a medium-width (1.5 mm) slit with direct illumination.[10] Any atrophy of the pigmented stroma may permit retroillumination of the iris to reveal iris sphincter atrophy or evidence of past trauma. Areas of iris atrophy will glow red when the light is reflected from the retina. Iris color, vessels, and architecture should be carefully evaluated. Iris nevi are common but must be differentiated from neoplastic processes. The pupillary border of the iris should move freely as light is shown into the pupil, and areas of adhesion between the iris and anterior lens capsule should be carefully noted and documented. A common finding representing a developmental remnant is persistent pupillary membrane (PPM). These iridopupillary membrane strands extend across the pupil from the iris collarette.

The normal iris vascular pattern should be differentiated from neovascularization presenting as fine meshwork vessels on the anterior iris surface. This condition, termed rubeosis iridis, is often found in association with conditions leading to anterior ocular ischemia, including long-standing glaucoma, diabetes, or retinal vein occlusion.

Crystalline Lens

The anterior lens surface is normally free of any pigment deposits, but is commonly observed to have pigment in the form of small spicules, a benign and stationary condition known as epicapsular stars. Some drug toxicities can be associated with pigment on the anterior lens capsule. Opacifications of the anterior subcapsular region, cortex, nucleus, or posterior subcapsular area are an indication of cataract. The precise location and character of the opacities should be carefully documented.

Anterior Vitreous

The normal fibrous framework of the vitreous is visible during routine slit lamp examination. These fibrous bands can become fragmented in the elderly. Active inflammation of the uvea may destroy the regular framework of the vitreous, and fine dustlike blood cells can be observed on the vitreous strands.[10] This can be suggestive of anterior, intermediate, or posterior uveitis. Vitreous liquifaction is common in the aging eye and increases the interval between the fibrous vitreal strands. As the eye is moved during the slit lamp examination, the strands are observed to float freely with eye movement, a condition termed *ascension phenomenon*. Another common finding, representing an acquired vitreal condition, is asteroid bodies. These are observed as small spherical white or yellow-white bodies that are firmly attached to the vitreal strands and move only with eye movement. This benign condition is usually unilateral and does not disturb vision.

There are literally hundreds of subtle variations of normal and abnormal ocular findings seen during slit lamp examination, and a great deal of patience and experience is required to master the necessary techniques to properly evaluate the anterior ocular structures.

REFERENCES

1. Keeney A. Ocular examination. St Louis: CV Mosby Co, 1970:73.
2. Vogt A. Die Sichtbarkeit des lebenden Hornhautendothels im Lichtbuschel der Gullstrandschen Spaltlampe. Klin Monatsbl Augenheilkd 1919;63:233–234.

3. Kercheval DB, Terry JE. Essentials of slit lamp biomicroscopy. J Am Optom Assoc 1977;48:1383–1389.
4. Eskridge JB, Schoessler J, Lowther G. A specific biomicroscopy procedure. J Am Optom Assoc 1973;45:400.
5. Nursall JF. An adapter to aid in slit-lamp biomicroscopy of the supine patient. Ophthalmology 1979;86:2048–2050.
6. Robboy MW, Hammack GG. Videotape recording system for use with the slit lamp biomicroscope. J Am Optom Assoc 1987;58:290–292.
7. van Herick W, Shaffer RN, Schwartz A. Estimation of width of angle of anterior chamber. Incidence and significance of the narrow angle. Am J Ophthalmol 1969;68:626–629.
8. Doggart JH. Ocular signs in slit-lamp microscopy. London: Henry Kimpton, 1967:27.
9. Dziadul J, Teague B, Oshinskie L, et al. A comparison of lens disorders using undilated and dilated biomicroscopy. N Engl J Optom 1988;40:15–17.
10. Terry JE, Kercheval DB. Interpretive biomicroscopy. J Am Optom Assoc 1979;50:793–803.
11. Josephson JE, Zantos S, Caffery B, et al. Differentiation of corneal complications observed in contact lens wearers. J Am Optom Assoc 1988;59:679–685.

Tonometry

David M. Cockburn

INTRODUCTION

Definition

Tonometry is a clinical technique that provides a measurement of the tension of the eye, which includes the combined resistance to deformity of its coats and the intraocular pressure (IOP). Only manometry is capable of providing a true measurement of IOP, but this method is not practical, since it would involve the introduction of a canula into the eye. However, it is a clinical convention to describe the results of tonometric measurements as intraocular pressure in millimeters of mercury (mmHg).

History

The first tonometers were simple applanation types credited to Weber in 1867 and the Maklakow in 1885.[1] Various designs of impression-type tonometers were produced in the latter part of the last century.[2,3] In 1905, an indentation tonometer was designed by Hjalmar August Schiøtz,[4] and this instrument, with various modifications, was to become the most widely used clinical method of estimating the IOP until the introduction of the applanation tonometer of Goldmann.[5]

Considerable ingenuity has been used to produce modifications of both applanation and indentation tonometers. These modifications have utilized the increasing sophistication of modern electronics to record precise measurements of the corneal deformity produced by the applanation or indentation forces. The McKay–Marg tonometer and applamatic tonometers made use of the electronically amplified movement of a stylus to record the extent of corneal deformity on moving paper. Microchip technology has made possible the miniaturization of the recording process as a digital display and the development of the Tono-pen.

The force necessary to deform the cornea during tonometry can be applied indirectly by gas pressure to the contact probe as used in the Tonomat. Alternatively, a carefully measured jet of air may be directed at the cornea to cause the distortion, and the extent of this distortion is measured by photoelectric cells as used in the American Optical Non Contact Tonometer. This latter method made possible the development of tonometers that did not require use of corneal anesthetics. The principle has been refined more recently by use of miniaturization and microchip technology to produce the Pulsair tonometer.

Clinical Use

Tonometry is recognized as an essential clinical procedure in the optometric examination. It is used in the diagnosis and management of glaucoma. Abnormally high intraocular pressures, abnormal asymmetric intraocular pressures, abnormal diurnal intraocular pressure variations, and an abnormal increase in the intraocular pressure over a long period, suggest the presence of glaucoma. This same information can be used in determining the effectiveness of the management of glaucoma. Tonometry can be used with all types of glaucoma and for glaucoma patients of all ages.

INSTRUMENTATION

Theory

There are two basic principles utilized in tonometry, corneal applanation and corneal indentation. In applanation tonometry, the force necessary to flatten a given area of cornea is measured or, alternatively, the area of applanation caused by a given force is

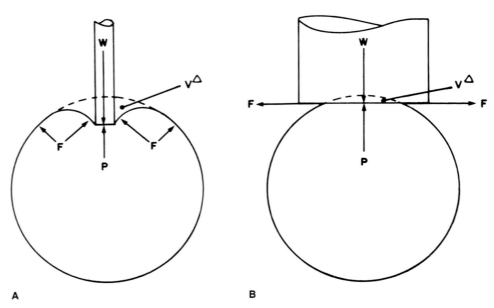

FIGURE 23–1. Comparison of impression (*A*) and applanation-type (*B*) tonometers. The weight of a tonometer *W* indents the cornea during impression tonometry and flattens it during applanation tonometry. The volume change V^Δ is greater in impression than in applanation tonometry. The volume change sets up opposing forces *F* that act tangentially to the surface of the globe during impression tonometry; those acting on the deformed portion of the cornea oppose the tonometer weight giving a falsely high estimate of IOP. During applanation tonometry the opposing force caused by V^Δ acts in the plane of flattening of the cornea and has no effect on the measured IOP.

estimated. The former method is utilized by the Goldmann, Perkins, and Draeger tonometers. Measurement of the area of applanation is the principle used in the original Maklakow tonometer and in modifications of this tonometer produced by Heine, Posner and Inglima, and others (Fig. 23–1). Indentation tonometry uses the principle of measuring the depth of impression caused by a plunger of known weight when it is resting on the cornea. Tonometers using this principle include the Schiøtz tonometer, and variations of this instrument. There are also several versions of the Schiøtz-type tonometer in which the degree of indentation of the cornea is measured electronically (see Fig. 23–1).

Applanation Tonometers

The principle of the operation of the applanation instruments may be likened to checking the pressure in a bicycle tire. One simply presses on the tire with a thumb and notes the force that is necessary to flatten an area of tire equal to the area of the ball of the thumb. The probe of the applanation tonometer acts on the eye in much the same manner as the thumb on the tire by allowing an estimate of the force necessary to flatten a standard area of cornea.

The Imbert–Fick law states that the pressure in a sphere filled with fluid and surrounded by an infinitely thin, flexible membrane, may be measured by the force that just flattens the membrane to a plane surface.[1] The applanation pressure slightly increases the pressure within the sphere and is transmitted equally in all directions. This pressure P^Δ is equal to the applanation force *W* divided by the area *A* or $P^\Delta = W/A$.

In measurements of the human eye, these requirements are not truly met because the internal volume of the eye is decreased during applanation, resulting in an increase in the pressure. The decrease in volume is partly due to reduction in blood volume in the choroid and central retinal artery system, and to a small increase in the outflow of aqueous. Some deformity of the eyeball must occur through compression of the optic disc and choroid,

together with other parts of the ocular coat that have some degree of flexibility. It is obvious that the smaller the deformity of the eye during an estimate of IOP, the less these deficiencies will contribute to error, but that the measured pressure *P* will be higher than the resting pressure of the eye.

Applanation tonometry suffers a further error that results from the physical properties of the cornea, the tear film that wets it and the anesthetic drops. This error, caused by surface tension attraction of the probe, tends to reduce the measured pressure. This has an effect opposite that caused by the decreased in volume caused by the applaning force. Goldmann and Schmidt[6] found that P_0 approx = $0.98\ P_t$, where P_0 is the undisturbed IOP and P_t is the measured pressure, and that a good approximation of $P_0 = P_t$ exists when the circle of corneal applanation has a diameter of 3.06 mm. With this diameter of applanation, the opposing errors very nearly cancel each other, and the measured pressure closely approximates the true pressure. Errors caused by variation in the rigidity of the ocular coats are kept to a minimum because of the very small distortion of the cornea when this degree of applanation is used.

Regular corneal astigmatism causes applanation mires to appear elliptical, rather than circular. If estimates of IOP are made in the normal manner, with the mires horizontal, the error is approximately 1 mmHg for every 4 diopters (D) of astigmatism, either with- or against-the-rule, and reduces almost to zero at the oblique axis positions.[7] To minimize the error induced by this distortion of the mires, the measurement should be made at approximately 43° from the flattest corneal meridian.[8] The applanation probes of the Goldmann type (Fig. 23–2) have a scale to facilitate this adjustment. Alternatively, a horizontal and vertical estimate may be made and the two readings averaged. The estimate made with the mires horizontally disposed, tends to underestimate IOP in patients who have with-the-rule astigmatism and overestimate it in patients with against-the-rule astigmatism. When the tonometer is used in both the horizontal and vertical mire locations, the averaged values

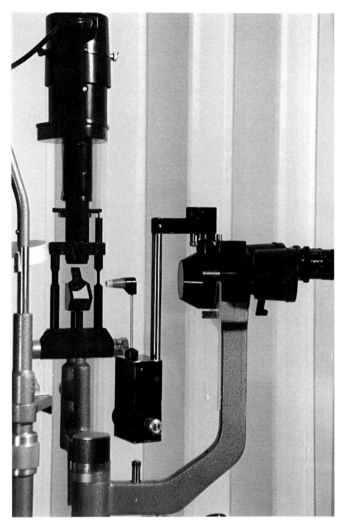

FIGURE 23–2. The Goldmann applanation tonometer shown mounted on a slit lamp and in position for use on the patient's left eye.

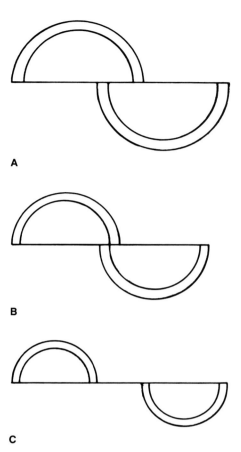

FIGURE 23–3. Appearance of the fluorescein mires in instruments using Goldmann prisms. (*A*) The rings are large and overlapped. The corneal applaned surface is greater than 3.06 mm in diameter and the pressure on the probe needs to be reduced to provide an end-point reading. (*B*) The correct appearance when the mires are aligned with their inner edges in apposition. The applanated surface is then 3.06 mm in diameter and the scale reading shows the estimate IOP. (*C*) The mires are separated and smaller than when in the correct position. The applaned surface is too small and the pressure on the probe should be increased.

provide a similar result to the method described by Holliday et al.[7] This method has the advantage of not requiring knowledge of the refraction or keratometer findings and is a more simple procedure. In practice, astigmatism of less than approximately 5 D will not cause clinically significant errors of IOP estimation, and even larger degrees of astigmatism at oblique axes can be ignored. However, horizontal and vertical estimates should be made and averaged for eyes on which the mires appear to be markedly elliptical, if the estimate is considered to be critical in the management of a patient. If excess fluid is present in the tear lake, or the lids make contact with the probe, the fluorescein mires may become much wider than shown in Figure 23–3 and the reading will be inaccurate. To correct, remove the instrument from the eye, dry the probe with a tissue, and repeat the measurement.

The applanation probe has a flattened end for corneal contact and an internal doubling prism to enable the observer to determine when a standard area of cornea of 3.06-mm diameter has been flattened. The force needed to applanate the cornea is measured against a spring (Fick tonometer) or a weight that is displaced about a horizontal axis (Goldmann tonometer manufactured by Zeiss). Hand-held applanation tonometers (Draeger, Perkins, and others) are position-independent as a result of using a balanced lever arm and spring to measure the applanation force.

The Perkins hand-held tonometer uses a Goldmann probe and provides results that are comparable with the slit lamp mounted instrument.[9]

Indentation Tonometers

The principle used in indentation tonometry is that of measuring the depth of deformity caused by a plunger of known weight when it is resting on the cornea. The amount of deformity is measured mechanically or electronically. The resistance to deformity of the eye measured by this method is the sum of the rigidity of the ocular coats and the IOP. To obtain a measure of IOP, it is necessary to assume a value for the rigidity of the eye. This has been achieved through comparison of manometrically determined pressures and those obtained from indentation tonometer readings.

Although the Schiøtz tonometer was developed in 1905, it remains popular, with only minor changes in design from the original model, because it is an inexpensive, portable, rugged, and compact instrument that, when used with care, provides satisfactory estimates of IOP. These are several versions of the Schiøtz tonometer in which the degree of indentation of the cornea is measured by electronic means.

Combined Systems

The McKay–Marg tonometer is partly an applanation-type tonometer and partly an indentation system in which the movement of an applanation plunger is measured electronically. The applanation tip on the plunger is 1.5 mm in diameter and is in contact with a spring within the hand piece. The plunger end, distal to the applaning surface, acts as part of a transducer, and its movement in a magnetic field is recorded as electronic impulses and converted into an estimate of IOP. The pressure is recorded by a stylus on paper tape in the form of a trace.

Noncontact Tonometers

The principle of operation of noncontact tonometers is that a standardized air blast is directed at the cornea and the extent of corneal deformity is measured by a photoelectric cell. In this respect, the instruments belong to the indentation class of tonometers. Noncontact tonometers have the advantage that they can be used without anesthetic, a feature that makes them suitable for operation by trained technicians as a screening procedure. They are also useful in patients who are allergic to topical anesthetics or for whom there is substantial risk of causing corneal damage through instrument contact.

COMMERCIALLY AVAILABLE INSTRUMENTS

The commercially available tonometers, listed in the order described in this chapter include the following:

Goldmann tonometer (see Fig. 23–2)
Perkins hand-held tonometer (see Fig. 23–4)
Draeger hand-held tonometer (see Fig. 23–10)
McKay–Marg tonometer
Oculab Tonopen (see Fig. 23–12)
Maklakow–Glaucotest (see Fig. 23–13)
Bausch & Lomb Applamatic tonometer (see Fig. 23–15)
Schiøtz tonometer (see Fig. 23–16)
American Optical noncontact tonometer (see Fig. 23–20)
Pulsair noncontact tonometer (see Fig. 23–22)

CLINICAL PROCEDURE

Goldmann Tonometer

The Goldmann tonometer is mounted on an arm attached to the slit lamp and is moved into the primary position when used. The illuminating system of the slit lamp, combined with the cobalt blue filter allows visibility of the fluorescein pattern that outlines the area of applanation of the cornea. Figure 23–2 shows a Goldmann tonometer on a slit lamp.

Method

1. The dry, clean tonometer probe should be inserted into the holder with its zero axis marking aligned with the reference mark on the holder.
2. The slit lamp should be adjusted and the patient comfortably positioned with the eyes approximately level with the line engraved on the headrest vertical bar. The patient may then sit back from the slit lamp and should be informed of the nature of the test. It is useful to explain that there is no discomfort other than a mild stinging as the drops are instilled.

3. Insert a suitable topical anesthetic into the lower fornices and allow approximately 30 seconds for it to take effect.
4. Place a fluorescein paper strip in the lower fornices, allowing a few seconds for some dye to enter the tear lake. If there are not sufficient tears to wet the strip, it may be moistened with sterile saline before being applied to the conjunctiva. Care should be taken to avoid contact between the strip and the cornea, since corneal staining will occur, following even light contact by the strip. The patient should be instructed to blink several times to evenly spread the fluorescein. Alternatively, a prepared solution of fluorescein or a combination of anesthetic and fluorescein may be applied, provided that sterility of the solutions can be assured. The patient should now be repositioned at the slit lamp.
5. The room lights should be dimmed or extinguished, the slit lamp illumination system opened to the wide position, and the cobalt blue filter interposed in the beam.
6. Swing the tonometer into the click stop position centered on the left microscope ocular.
7. The illumination system should be at approximately 60° to the lateral side of the eye to be measured, directed toward the engraved black line on the applanation probe, and the microscope set straight ahead. The microscope should be set at approximately 10×. The tonometer drum scale should be set to 10 mm to avoid "chattering" as it contacts the cornea.
8. Ask the patient to keep both eyes wide open and look in the direction of, but beyond, the adjustable target; this will avoid the slight change in IOP that occurs when the eye accommodates for near vision. The applanation probe is then directed onto the cornea by adjusting the slit lamp joystick and height control while observing the patient's eye directly. The applanation probe should not be allowed to touch the lids or lashes during measurement, since this may cause fluorescein-laden tears to bank up on the sides of the probe and the image of applanation to become wide, with resulting loss of precision of measurement. Should this occur, the probe should be wiped dry with a lint-free tissue kept handy for this purpose. The lids may be held apart gently if the patient is unable to keep them sufficiently wide open during the measurement. However, it is most important that no finger pressure be applied to the globe during this process, or falsely high readings will be obtained. This is probably the most common source of error when using tonometers of any kind.
9. With the prism centered on and in contact with the cornea the knurled wheel is adjusted until the fluorescein rings are apposition as shown in Figure 23–3B. Some pulsation of the rings occurs synchronous with the cardiac pulse wave. The scale reading on the drum is recorded as mmHg.
10. Repeat the measurement of the other eye.
11. After use, the tonometer should be positioned to the right of the microscope where it will not impede the normal use of the slit lamp. The applanation probe should be removed carefully from its holder, washed in clean water, and wiped with a disposable tissue. The probe should then be treated by wiping with an alcohol "prep pad," or by soaking for 15 minutes in 70% ethanol, or 3% hydrogen peroxide, or 1:10 household bleach (sodium hypochlorite). These treatments will inactivate adenovirus and probably the AIDS (HIV) virus.[10] The probe should not be stored permanently in liquid ethanol or any other solution that might cause damage to the Perspex or the bonding material used in its construction.

12. After completing the IOP measurements, the cornea should be inspected for damage. This may show as very superficial light fluorescein staining without interruption of the epithelial surface and will recover rapidly, without treatment. Significant damage occurs only rarely and may be treated with a topical antibiotic for prophylaxis and an ocular lubricant to make the eye comfortable. Patching of the eye is not necessary unless very marked trauma has occurred.

Perkins Hand-Held Tonometer

The Perkins tonometer (Fig. 23–4) is a hand-held instrument that uses the same type of applanation probe as developed for the Goldmann instrument. It applies a force on the probe through a counterbalanced arm, which in turn applies a force derived from a spiral spring. The force applied by the spring may be varied by rotation of a knurled and calibrated wheel at the rear of the hand grip. The applanated corneal surface is viewed through a magnifying lens situated behind the probe.

Because its illumination is built into the instrument, the Perkins tonometer does not require the use of a slit lamp, thereby allowing portability of the tonometer. It has the added advantage that it may be used with the patient in any position, including the prone position.

Hand-held tonometers are often easier to use than the slit lamp-mounted Goldmann instrument, since only one hand is used

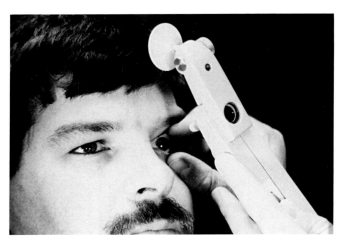

FIGURE 23–5. Perkins tonometer in use. The optometrist is gently separating the patient's lids, being careful not to press on the globe. Note that the optometrist's thumb is placed in position on the scale wheel.

to position the instrument on the cornea and adjust the applying force. This leaves the other hand free to hold the patient's lids apart. Figure 23–5 shows the optometrist holding the lids of the patient apart and preparing to place the tonometer on the cornea. Figure 23–6 shows the tonometer in contact with the cornea and being steadied by the optometrist's finger on the patient's cheek. Figure 23–7 illustrates the position of the patient and optometrist. However, after gaining experience with the instrument, many practitioners find that it can be used more comfortably and with greater speed without these rests.

If the tonometer is to be used in any position other than vertical, it is important that the prism be inserted in its holder to the correct depth. This may be checked by placing the tonometer on its test block and standing the inscribed mirror on the side of the instrument as shown in Figure 23–8. The engraved line of the mirror and that on the probe should be level. To adjust the tonometer, simply reposition the prism in its holder.

The accuracy of the instrument may be checked by placing the

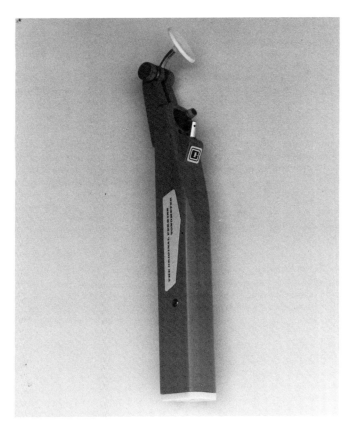

FIGURE 23–4. The Perkins hand-held tonometer with Goldmann applanation prism. The patient's forehead rest is in place, but the clinician's rest has been removed.

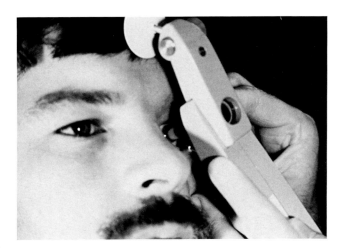

FIGURE 23–6. The Perkins tonometer in position on the cornea. The instrument is being steadied by having one finger of the hand that holds the tonometer resting on the patient's cheek.

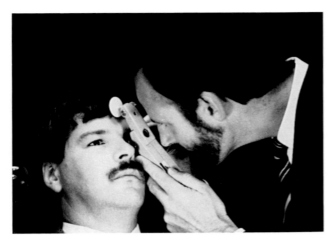

FIGURE 23–7. The Perkins hand-held tonometer in use. The patient's and optometrist's headrests are removable and, as shown here, are not needed once proficiency has been established. Note that the instrument is self-contained and portable.

tonometer on the test block provided, with its probe in position. The probe should float freely when there is no added weight and the scale is set at zero. The 20-g weight is then placed on the end of the probe, and the scale wheel is turned until the probe again floats freely. The scale should now read 20 units. The 50-g weight may be used in a similar manner to check accuracy at the high end of the scale. Figure 23–9 illustrates the Perkins tonometer on its test block with the 20-g weight in place; the 50-g weight is shown below the instrument.

Do not attempt to dismantle or to adjust the tonometer, other than described in the foregoing, if it is found to be out of adjustment. The instrument should be returned to the manufacturer for any other service.

When not in use, the scale wheel should be left in the "off scale position" below the zero setting. If the milled scale wheel is left on a scale setting, the internal spiral spring remains under tension and readings may become inaccurate over a long period.

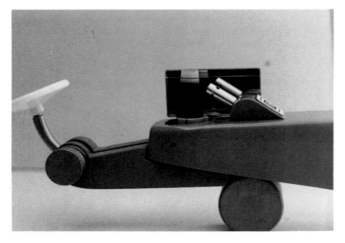

FIGURE 23–8. Setting the prism in the Perkins tonometer for use with the instrument in a position other than vertical: The prism's reference mark is set opposite the engraved line on the mirror.

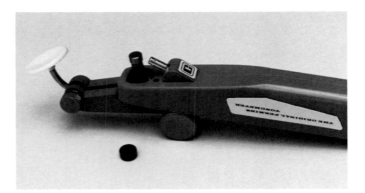

FIGURE 23–9. The Perkins tonometer being checked for calibration. The instrument is on its test block and the 20-g weight is resting on the prism. When the calibrated wheel is turned to the position at which the prism just "floats," the scale should read 20. The 50-g test weight is shown beside the tonometer.

Method

1. After preparation of the patient with corneal anesthesia and fluorescein, the Perkins tonometer is gripped in one hand (right hand for the patient's right eye and the left for the patient's left eye) with the thumb resting on the knurled wheel. The wheel is turned to approximately 10 units on the scale; this causes the lamp to illuminate when the scale reading is set at any position greater than zero. The lamp holder should be adjusted to illuminate an area immediately behind the engraved line on the prism.
2. The applanation probe may now be brought into contact with the patient's cornea, taking care to avoid contact with the lids and maintaining the area of contact as central as possible.
3. The correct reading of the end-point measurement is made in the same manner as described in step 9 for the Goldmann tonometer and illustrated in Figure 23–3. The reading of the scale is recorded.
4. After use, the applanation probe should be removed and cleaned in the same manner as described in step 11 for the Goldmann tonometer. The instrument should be returned to its case or similar safe storage, with the scale set below zero to relieve any tension on the spring mechanism and to extinguish the lamp.

Draeger Hand-Held Applanation Tonometer

This instrument is a self-contained applanation type tonometer similar to the Perkins tonometer in principle, although it uses a simpler applanation system. A change of pressure on the probe is effected by an electric motor activated by a toggle switch on the optometrist's side of the instrument. Both the cobalt blue light and the motor are powered by a transformer operated from the main electrical supply. Apart from the need to connect to the mains, the instrument is fully portable. The tonometer is illustrated in Figure 23–10. The Draeger tonometer is based in the same manner as the Perkins hand-held tonometer, and the results obtained are comparable with the Goldmann-type instrument.[11]

McKay–Marg Electronic Tonometer

Prior to its use, the instrument must be calibrated. It is also important to recalibrate the tonometer from time to time to ensure accurate performance. Detailed instructions for calibration are

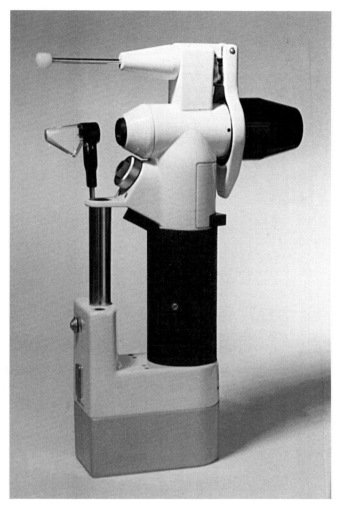

FIGURE 23–10. The Draeger hand-held tonometer. This applanation type tonometer uses a simple one-piece prism. The instrument requires an electrical connection and the applaning force is motor driven.

Method

1. Make sure that the tonometer is calibrated. Turn the instrument on and allow at least 10 minutes for the circuitry to reach operating temperature.
2. Cover the tonometer probe with a rubber cap so that the rubber is flat across the tip of the probe.
3. Place a light smear of KY Jelly, or similar water-soluble sterile gel, over the flattened end of the rubber that will contact the cornea.
4. Explain the testing procedure to the patient.
5. Anesthetize the cornea and arrange the patient in any convenient position (usually seated and with the head against a headrest) and instruct the patient to fixate a target located directly ahead.
6. Hold the body of the probe as you would a pen and place it approximately 1 to 2 mm from the corneal center with your hand supported on the patient's cheek. The lids may be gently separated, as necessary, being careful not to apply pressure to the globe.
7. Activate the foot switch to commence paper feed to the recorder.
8. Gently apply the tip briefly to the cornea, plane to its surface. Although the tip may be applied to any part of the cornea, it is preferable to make the measurement approximately at the center. Contact time should be less than 0.5 second.
9. Continue pressure on the foot switch and make four or five smoothly executed repeat probe contacts with the cornea as rapidly as is practical.
10. Check the chart to ensure that acceptable recordings have been obtained (see Fig. 23–11) and repeat if necessary.
11. Repeat steps 5 through 9 for the other eye.

A typical McKay–Marg tonometer trace is shown in Figure 23–11. The initial rise of the trace should be interrupted by a slight trough, before continuing to a peak and steep return to the baseline. The IOP estimate is recorded as the number of grid units between the lowest point of the trough in the initial slope and the baseline of the trace.

If traces similar to that shown in Figure 23–11 are not obtained, consult the fault-finding illustrations in the instruction manual and modify technique accordingly.

The Tono-Pen

The Tono-pen tonometer (Fig. 23–12), including its power source, weighs only 57 g, is 185 mm long, and 25 mm wide. It is fully portable and may be used while held in any position and with the patient in supine, seated, or prone position. In use, the tonometer is held in the same manner as a pen or pencil, and the activating

contained in the manufacturer's handbook. The McKay–Marg tonometer is in contact with the cornea for only a very brief period and measures the applanation produced by approximately 1 g of force.[12] Consequently, it is possible to use the tonometer without anesthesia. However, several repeat readings are required, and, whenever possible, anesthesia of the cornea should be used to avoid patient apprehension and resultant lid squeezing.

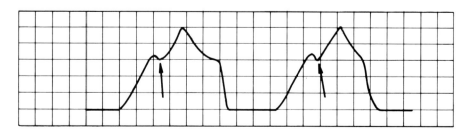

FIGURE 23–11. Typical, correctly performed trace, from the Mackay–Marg tonometer. The IOP estimate is obtained by counting the scale units from the baseline to the bottom of the notch (*arrows*) on the left side of the traces.

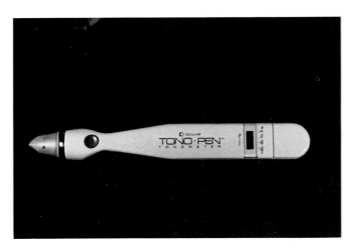

FIGURE 23–12. The Tono-pen hand-held tonometer by Intermedics. Note the latex cover on the instrument head at the left of the photograph. The operating switch is seen near the head, and the digital readout, with the reliability scale, is visible at the right hand end.

switch, located on the probe end of the body, is operated by the index finger.

The Tono-pen must be used with a latex cover over the contact probe; this cover fits into a groove machined into the probe head, approximately 20-mm behind the tip. Before its first use, and at the beginning of each day, the Tono-pen must be calibrated. This procedure is carried out after the instrument has stabilized to the room temperature and with a latex cover in place.

This instrument uses an electronic recording of a microstrain gauge, which is displayed as a digital readout located on the handle of the instrument. The optometrist applies the tonometer with several very light, brief contacts to the anesthetized cornea until the instrument receives sufficient approximately equal readings to provide an averaged measure of IOP. The resulting averaged value is displayed, together with an indication of reliability of the estimates, on a scale between 20% and 5% reliability. Readings made by the Tono-pen are not affected by corneal astigmatism.

Method

CALIBRATION PROCEDURE. Calibration need only be performed at the beginning of each day.

1. Hold down the switch until a beep sounds. The instrument will show "====." Release the switch and the display will be "– – –" followed by another beep.
2. Hold the instrument vertically with the probe down and press the switch twice in rapid succession. There will be two beeps and the display will be "CAL."
3. After a short interval, the beep will again sound and the display will read "UP."
4. Now turn the tonometer so that the probe is up and the instrument vertical. A beep will sound and the readout should be "Good." If "Bad" is displayed, repeat steps 2 through 4 until two consecutive attempts display "Good."

If several attempts at calibration are unsuccessful, check that the latex cover is not overtight and repeat the calibration check. If this also fails, consult the manufacturer's troubleshooting guide provided with the instrument.

MEASUREMENT PROCEDURE

1. Place a new latex cover over the tonometer head, ensuring that the thickened end locates in the groove machined into the head.

2. Explain the procedure to the patient and apply a corneal anesthetic.
3. Position the patient with a fixation target located so that the eyes are in the primary position and instruct the patient to look at the target.
4. Hold the Tono-pen as you would a pen and place the index finger over the switch.
5. Rest the little finger, or heel of the hand on the patient's cheek and position yourself so that you can see the patient's cornea and the probe tip. Then approach the probe to a position about 10 mm from the cornea.
6. Press and hold down the switch continuously during the remainder of these steps.
7. A beep will sound and the readout will be "====," indicating that the Tono-pen is ready to commence readings.
8. Lightly and briefly touch the cornea several times; each successful reading is signaled by a click sound and, when sufficient valid readings have been made, there will be a beep, and the averaged IOP estimate will be displayed.
9. Record the IOP estimate. Note the position of the bar located below the digital readout and its relation to the reliability scale. If the reliability is 20% or greater, a repeat estimate should be made.
10. Release the switch and wait at least 20 seconds. Press the switch and repeat steps 4 through 9 for the other eye. The instrument automatically switches off after use.

The Heine–Maklakow Glaucotest Tonometer

The Glaucotest (Fig. 23–13) is a hand-held, battery-operated instrument having the illuminating light and microscope located above a detachable head and activated by a rheostat at the top of the handle.

An adaptation of the Maklakow instrument by Heine, it allows direct viewing of a fluorescein pattern, as in Goldmann tonometry, but uses one of four fixed weights to applanate the corneal surface. These weights are 1.8, 2.2, 2.6, and 3 g. As with Goldmann tonometry, the IOP (expressed as mmHg) is given by the Imbert–Fick law.

When the applanated area has a diameter of 3.06 mm the relationship becomes: $IOP = 10 W$ so that the standard weights allow precise measurements of 18, 22, 26, and 30 mmHg. This occurs for any of the weights in use, when the diameter of the inner edge of the fluorescein circle is equal to the length of a line engraved on the applanating surface of each probe tip. Extrapolation between the 4-mmHg intervals between weights becomes reasonably accurate with experience. If the fluorescein circle appears smaller in diameter than the line, then the IOP is greater than the indicated IOP at that weight. On the other hand, if the circle is larger, the IOP is less than indicated by that weight. Figure 23–14 illustrates the appearance of the fluorescein patterns and the reference line when the IOP is less than, equal to, or greater than the weight in use.

The Glaucotest is portable, rugged, relatively simple to use, and does not require a slit lamp. It tends to read slightly higher than the Goldmann applanation tonometer; however, it has good sensitivity and is simple and quick to use.[13]

Method

1. The corneas are anesthetized and fluorescein is instilled.
2. The patient is then placed in a supine position and instructed to look at a point immediately overhead.
3. The 1.8-g weight should be attached to the collar of the Glaucotest and a sterile, plastic tip placed on the end of the applanation weight.
4. Switch on the illumination.

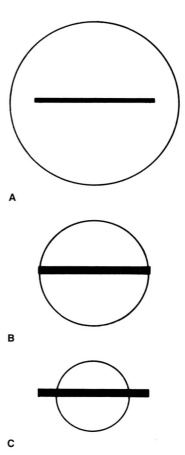

FIGURE 23–14. Fluorescein test patterns obtained with the Glaucotest tonometer. If the diameter of the fluorescein ring is equal to the length of the reference line (*B*), the IOP is equal to 10 × the weight engraved on the applaning head. If the circle is smaller than the line (*A*), the IOP is greater than the indicated pressure, and if larger (*C*), the IOP is less.

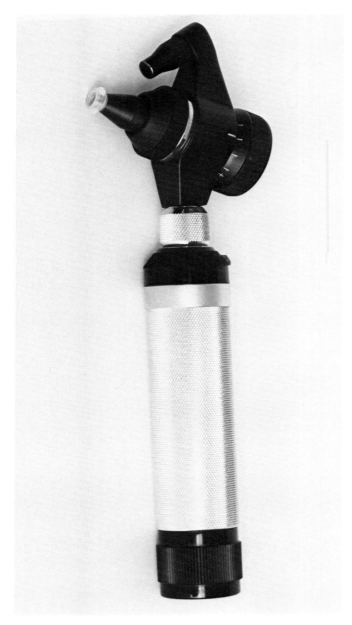

FIGURE 23–13. The Maklakow-type Glaucotest tonometer by Heine. This battery-operated tonometer is portable and rugged. It has four detachable heads of fixed weight.

5. Hold the patient's lids apart, taking care to avoid pressure on the globe. The hand that holds the instrument may be steadied by placing the fingers on the patient's forehead.
6. Lower the instrument vertically onto the center of the cornea.
7. The sliding applanation weight should be allowed to "float" so that the entire weight is resting squarely on the cornea, but the body of the instrument prevented from making contact with the weight. Take care to avoid pressure on the globe from the fingers that are holding the lids.
8. The relative sizes of the circle and the engraved line may now be assessed through the magnifier. If the illuminated fluorescein circle has a diameter equal to, or greater than, the engraved line, then the IOP is 18 nmHg or less, and no further estimate is required. If the circle is smaller than the line, increasingly heavy weights are used progressively until the IOP limits are established.
9. Record the pressure estimate limits.
10. Repeat for the other eye.

A fresh contact tip should be used for each patient. After use, the plastic tips may be washed in clean water, dried on a tissue, and disinfected with 70% ethanol or by boiling. It is important that the instrument heads be kept clean, so that the weights slide freely on the body of the instrument.

The Bausch & Lomb Applamatic Tonometer

Figure 23–15 illustrates the appearance of the Bausch & Lomb recording tonometer with the recording paper on the left and the probe and foot switch lying on the top of the instrument. This tonometer operates on the principle of using a Silastic membrane tip under gas pressure to applanate a small area of cornea. The pressure of gas necessary to applanate the cornea by a 5-mm diameter tip is maintained by a feedback system that automatically maintains this force. The applanation force is measured electronically and a readout is printed onto recording paper.

The gas used in the B&L Applamatic tonometer is a fluorohydrocarbon. Use of this gas for other than essential purposes is now illegal in some countries, owing to its reputed action in depletion

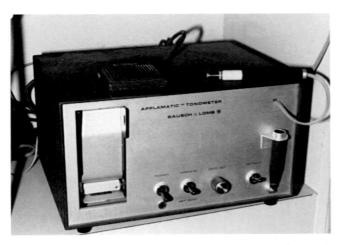

FIGURE 23–15. The Bausch & Lomb Applamatic tonometer showing the foot switch and the probe, placed on the top of the instrument. The paper trace is on the left.

of the Earth's ozone layer. It is supplied in small canisters with nonstandard fittings so that only gas packaged by the makers can be used. The Applamatic paper recording tape is also nonstandard and is obtainable only from the manufacturers. The Applamatic tonometer is accompanied by a booklet that should be consulted for correction of defects of technique or when it is necessary to use the instrument on the sclera.

The Applamatic tonometer was designed to be used on either the sclera or the anesthetized cornea. However, scleral measurement of IOP is not recommended in view of the errors that occur in this method. When used on the cornea, the instrument should be factory set for this purpose. The instrument may be used with the patient seated, supine, or standing.

Method

1. Turn the instrument on and allow 30 minutes for warmup with the "operate set" switch in the midposition. (The tonometer may conveniently be left with power switched on all day.)
2. Sterilize the tonometer membrane tip by wiping with 70% isopropyl alcohol and allow to air-dry.
3. Explain the procedure to the patient.
4. Anesthetize the patient's corneas.
5. Calibrate the tonometer by placing the sensor in its holder in a vertical position and depress the "set zero" switch. Turn the "zero set" knob until the recorder stylus is on the zero line of the chart. Release the switch.
6. Have the patient fixate on a convenient point directly ahead.
7. Separate the patient's lids, being careful not to press on the globe.
8. Observe from the patient's side, from a position level with the eye, and place the tonometer tip on the cornea.
9. Advance the tonometer tip 1 to 2 mm, being careful not to override the travel of the plunger.
10. Adjust the angle of the sensor on the cornea until an audible signal is heard. Maintain this position for 3 to 5 seconds.
11. Check the trace to ensure that a record has been made of fluctuations of 1 to 2 mmHg along an otherwise horizontal trace. (See instruction manual for evaluation of the trace.)
12. Repeat steps 6 through 11 for the other eye.
13. Turn the instrument to "standby."

The Schiøtz Tonometer

The Schiøtz tonometer has a free-floating barrel with a footplate of 10.1-mm diameter and a concavity of 15-mm radius of curvature. Because this radius is usually greater than that of the cornea on which it rests, the instrument slightly flattens the cornea when resting on it. At the center of the footplate there is a hole through which a plunger protrudes and this plunger assembly can be loaded with additional weights, so that its total weight varies from 5.5 g, in its unloaded state, to 7.5 or 15 g. The movement of the plunger as it indents the cornea is amplified mechanically to a pointer that reads over a scale at the top of the instrument, from zero through 20 units. Figure 23–16 illustrates the Schiøtz tonometer with weights and test block in its case. The scale reading is converted into an approximate value of millimeters of mercury by use of a graph or conversion table.

The scale of the Schiøtz tonometer measures with maximum accuracy when between 5 and 15 scale units. On an eye having a high IOP, the scale reading will be low, indicating that the eye is only slightly deformed by the weighted plunger. In this event, the 10-g weight is substituted, and the measurement is repeated. On the other hand, a high scale reading indicates a large deformity of the cornea and a low IOP. In this event, the auxiliary weight is removed and the plunger weight of 5 g is used in a repeat measurement. It is good practice to make estimates of IOP with two different weights and to make allowance for any gross variation from normal ocular rigidity (see following). Because there is a massage effect produced by impression-type tonometers, which reduces the true IOP, it is important that repeat measurements be kept to a minimum. Alternatively, after making more than two or three repeat readings, the eye should be allowed to recover normal pressure for approximately 5 minutes.

Estimates of IOP with an indentation-type tonometer will be inaccurate when the ocular rigidity of the eye differs from the

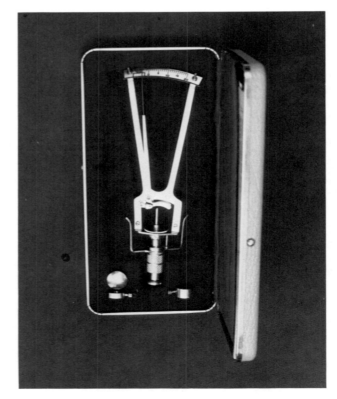

FIGURE 23–16. Schiøtz indentation-type tonometer in its case with the test block and two auxiliary weights.

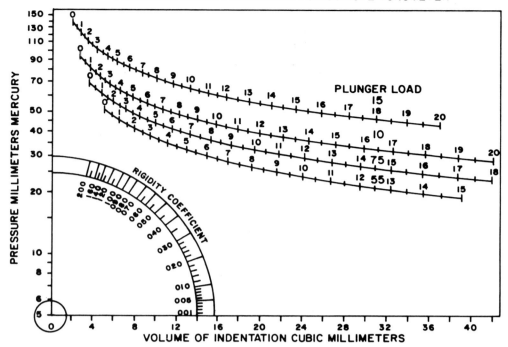

FIGURE 23–17. Friedenwald pressure–rigidity nomogram. Two scale readings are recorded using different plunger weights. A line is drawn between these points on the appropriate plunger load scales and the projection of this line gives an estimate of the IOP, allowing for ocular rigidity. The intercept of the line with the rigidity coefficient scale provides an estimate of this value. (From The Committee on Tonometer Standardization of the American Academy of Ophthalmology and Otolaryngology. Tonometry–tonography. By permission.)

value assumed in the preparation of the conversion table. If estimates of the IOP of an eye are made from two or more weights, it is possible to deduce a difference between the rigidity of that eye and the value assumed in the table. If an eye has a greater than average rigidity of ocular costs, the initial pressure will be increased by the effect of indentation of the plunger when compared with an eye having normal or a lower than average rigidity. Thus, an IOP conversion figure that becomes higher when measurements are made with increased plunger weights has a greater than average ocular rigidity. This feature was used by Friedenwald[14] to devise a pressure–rigidity nomogram (Fig. 23–17) for use with the Schiøtz tonometer.

Friedenwald reasoned that the volume of the eye was increased slightly during indentation by the tonometer and that the relationship between the initial pressure P_0 and the recorded pressure, P_t, resulting from this reduction in volume could be expressed by: $K = \log P_t - \log P_0/V_c$, where V_c is the volume of the corneal indentation by the plunger and K is the coefficient of rigidity. The average value of K is given as 0.0215.

The Friedenwald nomogram is read by taking IOP readings of an eye, using two weights. The scale reading for each weight is marked on the nomogram curve appropriate for each weight; a line joining these positions is drawn to the left, such that it intersects the vertical axis. This intersection indicates the best estimate of IOP, taking into account the variation in ocular rigidity of that eye. A value of the coefficient of rigidity of the eye is given by drawing a second line, a parallel to the first, from the origin of the nomogram to intersect the quadrant coefficient of rigidity scale.

The coefficient of ocular rigidity estimated by this method is a useful approximation, but it is not strictly accurate because it assumes (incorrectly) a constant coefficient of rigidity at both pressures. This error is greatest in the lower IOP range.

The size of the globe and the radius of curvature of the cornea affect the value of K[15] and, consequently, the IOP as measured with the indentation tonometer. Friedenwald[16] produced a chart for converting scale readings to IOP in eyes that have abnormal corneal curvature. Since correction for the corneal radius of curvature requires a keratometric reading, the method is rarely applied in clinical estimates of IOP.

Probably the most common source of error in Schiøtz tonometry arises because of a sticking plunger. If the plunger is not removed from the barrel and washed immediately after use, mucus and salt from tears dry in the barrel to leave deposits that increase friction between the plunger and its wall. This problem is exacerbated by flaming the tonometer as a sterilization procedure, without first washing to remove these residues.

Before each use, the footplate and plunger tip should be swabbed with 70% ethanol and allowed to air-dry. After use, the knurled plunger head should be unscrewed and the plunger removed. The tonometer's lower assembly and plunger should then be washed in clean running water and excess water removed by shaking. This will remove any tears or secretions.

The instrument should be checked regularly for correct scale adjustment by placing it on the test block provided. This instrument scale should read zero when placed squarely on the test block. Adjustment is achieved by loosening the screw at the base of the pointer and shifting the pointer position relative to the lever arm until it reads zero when the instrument is resting on the block.

Method

1. The Schiøtz tonometer should be sterilized by boiling or wiping with alcohol. Care should be taken to allow the instrument to cool, or the alcohol to evaporate, before contact with the cornea.

2. Explain the purpose of the tonometric procedure and reassure the patient of its harmless nature.
3. Anesthetize the patient's corneas using a short-acting topical anesthetic.
4. The patient should be arranged in an adjustable chair in a relaxed, semisupine position, with the face turned upward, without undue constriction or extension of the neck.
5. Instruct the patient to keep both eyes open and to fixate on a target placed immediately above the chair for this purpose.
6. Prepare the tonometer by placing the 7.5-g weight on the plunger extension and holding it with the thumb and first finger so that the scale is facing you.
7. Hold the patient's lids apart gently, taking care to avoid applying pressure to the globe.
8. Place the tonometer directly onto the cornea without sliding, so that the footplate rests centrally, and the instrument is truly vertical (Fig. 23–18).
9. Note the scale reading. The pointer should show slight fluctuations, and the mean position is recorded. See the foregoing discussion for selection of the weight that will provide the most accurate reading.
10. Convert the scale reading to an estimate of IOP in mmHg by reference to the conversion graph (Fig. 23–19).
11. Repeat steps 7 through 10 for the second eye.
12. Inspect the corneas by biomicroscopy to detect any corneal abrasion. Prophylactic treatment should be provided in the event of significant epithelial damage being present.

During measurement of IOP the slight pulsation of the needle over the scale results from the diastolic pulse wave affecting the pressure within the eye. The pulse wave affects chiefly the choroidal circulation, increasing its volume to a degree dependent on the ocular rigidity of that eye. The magnitude of the fluctuations, typically 1 scale unit, is greatest at low IOP, and least at higher pressures. Its presence is a reassurance that the plunger is resting on the cornea and is free from significant friction in the barrel.

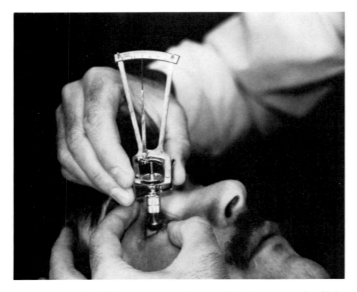

FIGURE 23–18. Schiøtz tonometer in use. The instrument should be held in a vertical position and lowered onto the patient's cornea until the instrument floats in its barrel. The scale reading shown is 5 and there are no auxiliary weights in place.

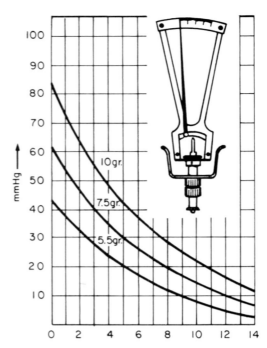

FIGURE 23–19. Table for the conversion of Schiøtz tonometer scale readings to estimates of IOP.

Noncontact Tonometer (American Optical)

The instrument is mounted on a height-adjustable table. Figure 23–20 shows the instrument from the operator's side. The base of the instrument contains most of the controls, including a joystick for horizontal movement and a centrally placed height adjustment with the firing button at its center. The function switch is on the right, as seen from the optometrist's position. Figure 23–21 illustrates the instrument from the patient's side. The instrument contains a monocular-viewing telescope, an air puff aperture, and the recording cells. There is a protective cap provided for the aperture, and this should be removed only when the instrument is in use. On the left side of the instrument there is a knurled adjustment for correction of the patient's refractive error if this is sufficient to prevent viewing of the target. When correctly positioned at the tonometer, the patient should see a red spot target in the puff aperture. The forehead rest has a pressure bar that allows pressures to be measured only when the patient is in contact with it; this function may be bypassed by use of a switch, located on the rear right-hand side of the brow bar.

The control switch on the right-hand side of the base has four positions, each having a distinctive symbol. The left-hand setting is a black disk that indicates that the instrument is switched off. The red disk is the correct setting for most IOP estimates, whereas the 'D' setting is for demonstrating to the patient the air puff and sound at firing. A disk having a crossring and target on the far right of the power switch permits use of the instrument without operation of the monitoring system. Because the air aperture is brought within a few millimeters of the eye, a safety lock is placed on the left-front part of the base. It acts to prevent the instrument from being racked too far forward where it could damage the eye.

A readout display of IOP is located at the rear and below the head, below that is a signal level indicator. After switching to the red disk position, removing the cap, and waiting 30 seconds, activation of the trigger should provide a reading of 68, as a check of calibration. The switch should then be turned to the D-position and the air blast again triggered; the reading should be 57 ± 1 and

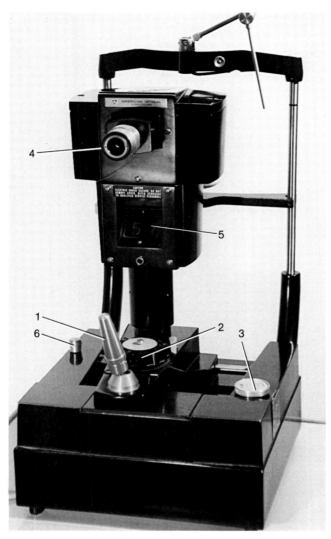

FIGURE 23–20. The American Optical noncontact tonometer. The instrument is seen from the operator's side and shows the central joystick for lateral adjustment (1) and height adjustment wheel (2). The switch is on the right of the instrument (3) as seen in this view. At the top of the instrument there is a viewing microscope (4) and below it is the readout screen (5) for the IOP estimate. The safety distance lock is the small metallic knob on the left side of the base (6).

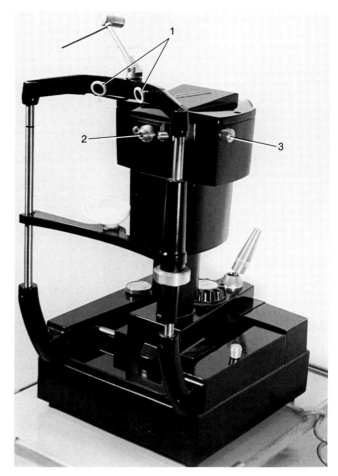

FIGURE 23–21. The American Optical noncontact tonometer. The instrument is seen from the patient's side. The two forehead pressure-monitoring buttons can be seen on the forehead rest (1). The air puff aperture, light sources, and sensors are in the center of the head (2). The refractive correction adjustment is on the right side of the head (3), as shown in this photograph.

be repeatable over several firings. The signal level indicator should not illuminate during these calibration checks.

Difficulties in the measurement of the IOP may arise when there are marked irregularities of the cornea. In these circumstances, the power switch should be turned to the crossring and target setting on the right of the power-setting knob. The instrument may now be activated, even though the alignment is not correct, and any reading other than 99 will give an indication of the IOP. The 99 reading indicates that the instrument did not obtain a signal. The manufacturer's instruction book should be consulted for other fault-solving procedures.

Although the manufacturers claim that anesthesia is not required, Draeger and Jessen found that the coefficient of correlation between this and other applanation tonometers was 0.67 when used without, and 0.78 when used with corneal anesthesia.[17]

The noncontact tonometer provides consistently lower readings than the Goldmann applanation tonometer.[18,19]

Method

1. Explain the procedure to the patient, with assurance that there is no discomfort involved, but that a puff of air will make a noise that will startle them.
2. Remove the protective cap and switch on the power. Perform the calibration checks outlined in the foregoing.
3. Rotate the switch to the D-position and have the patient place a finger approximately 10 mm from the air puff orifice. Activate the firing button to provide a demonstration of the air puff and the noise that can be expected.
4. Adjust the eyepiece of the telescope to bring the ring target into clear focus.
5. With the instrument table adjusted to a comfortable height, have the patient place the chin and brow in the appropriate positions and adjust the chin rest so that the eyes are at the level of the engraved line on the left-hand vertical chin rest–brow bar support.
6. Explain the need to keep pressure on the brow bar.

7. Switch to the red dot position (on).
8. Observe the patient's eye directly and move the aperture to approximately 10 mm from the cornea and then raise the safety lock knob.
9. Move the instrument into a position at which the red light is centrally located over the pupil; this should allow the patient to see and fixate the internal red target.
10. Switch to the red dot position (on).
11. Look through the telescope and make fine adjustments until the red spot lies in the center of the red reticule. If necessary, ask the patient to open both eyes widely and then press the firing button.
12. The readout should indicate IOP, and the signal level indicator should also be illuminated.
13. After a few blinks and approximately 10-second interval, the IOP should be measured again to confirm the first reading.
14. The procedure is repeated for the second eye.

Pulsair Noncontact Tonometer by Keeler

The Pulsair tonometer is a hand-held instrument that uses the air-puff principle to cause distortion of the cornea, the extent of which is sensed by the instrument and displaced in units corresponding to millimeters of mercury. A console, measuring 355 × 305 × 205 mm and weighing 9 kg, provides the air through an umbilical cord 3 m in length (Fig. 23–22). The console may be wall or desk-top mounted and provides a convenient stowage for the hand piece when the instrument is not in use. The hand piece weighs 1 kg and is 265 × 115 × 40 mm (Fig. 23–23). Although the tonometer is hand-held, it should not be considered portable, except to the extent of the 2-m cord.

The Tonair has a measurement range of zero to 55 mmHg equivalent, with a display accuracy of ±1 unit. When measurements exceed 30 mmHg, a switch on the hand piece allows use of an increased intensity of air jet, to improve the accuracy of readings in the higher range of IOP. In the lower-range setting, the air jet is relatively quiet, and the eye sensation quite comfortable. Measurements may be taken with the patient standing, seated, or supine, provided the instrument can be held in the same plane as the patient's face. A subflex switch allows operation of the tonometer on eyes that have reduced or distorted corneal reflexes.

Figure 23–24 illustrates the use of the Pulsair tonometer, and Figure 23–25 shows the appearance of the mires in various positions relative to the cornea.

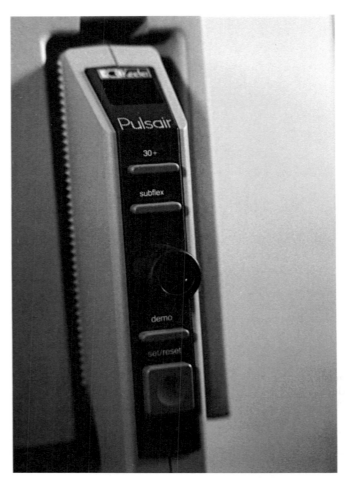

FIGURE 23–23. Closeup of the Pulsair head showing (in order from the top of the instrument) the read out screen, the 30+ and subflex switches, the sighting aperture, demonstration button, and the reset switch.

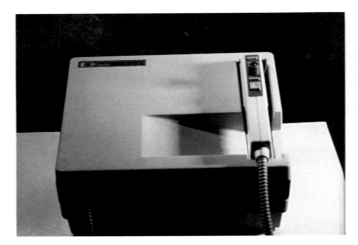

FIGURE 23–22. The Pulsair noncontact tonometer positioned on the console that contains the air pump. Note the flexible air hose.

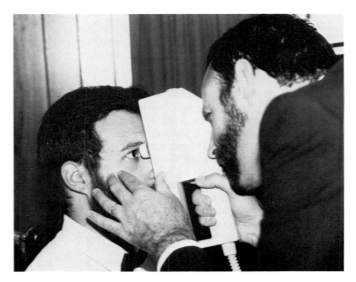

FIGURE 23–24. The Pulsair noncontact tonometer in use. Note how the optometrist's left hand is being used to steady the instrument against the patient's cheek.

Tonometer head too close to cornea (10-12 mm)

Tonometer head at correct distance from cornea (13-16 mm)

Tonometer head too far from cornea (17-20 mm)

FIGURE 23–25. Appearance of the mires seen when using the Pulsair tonometer. The appearance of these mires can be used to obtain the correct operating distance from the cornea.

Should a measurement not be made within approximately 30 seconds of activating the tonometer, the target light is extinguished; simply press the set–reset switch and restart the procedure. If the Tonair fails to fire, check that the target light is present, check the alignment of the instrument with the patient's face and eye. Do not hold down the set–reset switch or the instrument will not operate.

If the cornea of an eye to be examine is significantly scarred or irregular, the Pulsair may not fire. In this event, the subflex button is depressed and the measurement procedure repeated.

Because the Pulsair measures the IOP during a very brief time span the measurement may reflect IOP variations caused by the pulse, respirations, and patient's lid squeezing. For this reason it is recommended that four readings be made and averaged to arrive at the recorded estimate.

Method

1. Switch on the console and remove the hand piece from its cradle.
2. Check that the 30+ switch and subflex switch are off and allow approximately 5 seconds for the console pump to reach operating pressure. Press the set–reset switch. The display should now read 00.
3. Place the air jet nozzle approximately 15 mm from the patient's cheek and demonstrate to the patient the sound and air jet intensity by pressing "demo."
4. Again press the set–reset switch.
5. Locate the jet nozzle approximately 20 mm from the patient's cornea, holding the tonometer plane to the patient's face and directly along the visual axis. Instruct the patient to look at the red target light in the nozzle and to keep the eye wide open.
6. Steady the tonometer by placing one hand on both the instrument and the patient's forehead and align the red corneal reflex with the center of the eyepiece by direct observation.
7. Maintain the instrument alignment and look through the eyepiece. Note the image appearance and make suitable adjustments as shown in Figure 23–25.
8. The tonometer will activate automatically when the correct alignment is achieved; this may even occur while you

are directly observing and aligning the instrument. Such measurements are valid and should be recorded.

9. Press the set–reset switch and repeat the measurement until four estimates of IOP have been made. Calculate and record the average of these readings.
10. Repeat steps 5 through 9 on the second eye.
11. If the IOP reading exceeds 30 mm, switch to the 30+ position and repeat the estimates.
12. On completion of the measurements, return the tonometer to its cradle on the console; this will stop the air pump. The cooling fan will continue to operate until the console switch is turned off.

CLINICAL IMPLICATIONS

Clinical Significance

The significance of intraocular pressure in clinical practice is difficult to define, because many patients with open-angle glaucoma have IOP within the range that most persons tolerate without apparent visual deterioration. Determination of its significance is complicated further by the finding that up to 40% of optic nerve axons may be lost before a visual field defect is apparent.[20] This finding might be ascribed to a physiologic redundancy in the number of nerve axons, but more likely, reflects the lack of precision in the testing of visual deterioration. Whatever the explanation, it creates a dilemma, in that we cannot be certain whether an eye with raised IOP has, or has not lost vision, yet such a loss would constitute a pathologic process and, hence, merit the diagnosis of glaucoma.

Although the arguments just presented indicate a disappointingly poor efficiency of tonometry in the diagnosis of glaucoma, it is a safe, rapid, and easily applied test that yields valid and precise results. It follows that tonometry should be used extensively and considered in conjunction with the family ocular history, visual fields, optic disc assessment, and gonioscopy.

Primary open-angle glaucoma is most common in older patients, but the measurement of IOP should be part of the examination routine for all patients. Those patients who have risk factors for glaucoma have a greater need for tonometric assessment of IOP. These risk factors are detailed in Table 23–1.

Risk factors for angle-closure glaucoma differ from those of open-angle glaucoma and are shown in Table 23–2.

The current treatment of established glaucoma is aimed at reducing IOP, and tonometry is essential for monitoring the IOP. The effect of lowering IOP in modifying the progress of open-angle glaucoma is uncertain and even controversial.[21-25] Some authorities even suggest that raised IOP might be a sign, rather than a cause, of open-angle glaucoma.[26] Although it would be fallacious to treat a sign, rather than the cause of a disease, there is no alternative treatment available at present, and in patients having pressures in excess of 30 mmHg, there would appear to be sound philosophic reasons for reducing pressure. The treatment rationale is less sound in glaucoma for which pressures are in the 20s and is difficult to defend in low-tension glaucoma. However, because raised IOP is largely accepted as a cause of glaucomatous visual loss, and its reduction is the treatment objective, it follows that tonometry has an important part to play in both the diagnosis and the management of patients with glaucoma.

Clinical Interpretation

The IOP is not static, but undergoes a diurnal variation that has different amplitudes in different individuals and has been shown to reach very high levels in normal young subjects during sleep.[27] It is difficult to be certain that an individual under review for

Table 23–1
*Clinical Features Associated with Open-Angle Glaucoma**

Age 40 or over
Cup/disc ratios (vertical) greater than 0.5
Optic disc cupping asymmetric
Pallor or greyness of the discs
Hemorrhage on the disc
Family history of glaucoma
Fuchs' corneal dystrophy
Krukenberg's spindle
Pseudoexfoliation of the lens capsule
Retinal vascular occlusions, recent or long-standing
Visual field loss
Diabetes
Head- or eyeache not otherwise explained
Axenfeld's anomaly
Reiger's anomaly
Peters' anomaly
Uveitis
Iridodyalisis, eccentric pupil, or history of severe blunt trauma

* The presence of one or more of these conditions should initiate measurement of intraocular pressure. Note that a finding in the normal range of pressures does not rule out the possibility of glaucoma.

suspicion of glaucoma does not have damaging high IOP spikes at times when we are unable to detect them. It can be said with certainty that there is no single pressure level that represents a threshold for visual field loss in human subjects, either as individuals or taken as a whole. Clinical experience indicates that there is grave danger of loss of visual field when pressures remain in the mid-30s, and some visual loss seems inevitable if pressures of 40 mmHg or more are sustained. However, the outcome of long-term prospects for visual loss in subjects having IOP between 20 and 30 mmHg is less easily determined, yet the great majority of cases of open-angle glaucoma have pressures within this range. The results of several prospective studies of the outcome of IOP in this range

Table 23–2
*Clinical Features Associated with Angle-Closure Glaucoma**

Shallow anterior chamber
Gonioscopic evidence of narrow anterior chamber angle, or synechiae, or part of the trabeculae obscured
Narrow anterior chamber angle by slit lamp method (0.3 or less corneal units) or corneal–iris apposition
Moderate or high hyperopia
History of previous attack or diagnosis of angle closure
Family history of glaucoma
Halos around lights
Essential iris atrophy
Glaukomflecken
Cup/disc ratios (vertical) greater than 0.5
Asymmetric optic disc cupping
Pallor or greyness of the discs
Hemorrhage on the disc
Head- or eye-ache not otherwise explained
Intermittent visual disturbance
Vascular occlusions recent or long-standing
Visual field defect

* The presence of one or more of these conditions should initiate measurement of intraocular pressure. Note that a finding in the normal range of pressures does not rule out the possibility of angle closure glaucoma.

indicate that approximately 12% will develop visual field loss during the follow-up.[28]

It appears that the likelihood of a visual field loss occurring in association with raised IOP is directly related to the age of the patient and the level of the IOP.[29] The risk was also found to be greater when the optic discs were cupped and visual field loss became almost inevitable when IOP was above 28 mmHg, in association with optic discs having 0.6 or greater "physiologic" cupping at entry to the study.[30] Here one must ask whether the physiologic cupping was really physiologic, or alternatively, represented the first detectable damage from glaucoma. In other words, there could have been a loss of axons sufficient to cause cupping at entry to the trial, yet the visual field loss remained at a subclinical level until later in the follow-up. Regardless of the interpretation of the sequence of events, it appears that an IOP estimate considered in conjunction with optic disc assessment is a powerful combination for the detection of open-angle glaucoma.

Bengtsson[26] found IOP greater than 21.5 mmHg to have a sensitivity of approximately 0.5 in the diagnosis of open-angle glaucoma during a population survey using visual field studies, IOP, and disc assessments. He also found the efficiency of IOP as a sign appeared to be less than assessment of optic disc cupping or a disc hemorrhage. The lack of efficiency of IOP as a sign in open-angle glaucoma resulted from the many glaucoma cases of his study population having low, or normal, IOP. Much argument abounds concerning the mechanism of low-tension glaucoma and even whether or not it represents a different disease process from that of open-angle glaucoma accompanied by raised IOP. Although there may prove to be differences, the presence of progressive optic disc cupping and visual field loss of a characteristic type is a feature of both conditions. It follows that IOP has, at best, poor sensitivity in the detection of low-tension glaucoma (whatever it is called and regardless of its etiology) and in open-angle glaucoma for which the IOP is between 20 and 30 mmHg.

In angle-closure glaucoma the IOP may be extremely high; it then constitutes a diagnostic feature of the acute presentation, and neither the diagnostic nor the pathologic significance of the very high pressure is in question.[31] However the majority of cases of angle-closure glaucoma present in either subacute form, in which the IOP may be normal between attacks, or in the "creeping angle closure" or chronic form described by Lowe,[32] in which the IOP may be only slightly raised above that individual's "normal" pressure, with a gradual increase over time as further insidious angle closure takes place. In both subacute and chronic angle-closure forms there may never be an acute attack, and the patient may lose visual field in a manner identical with that which occurs in open-angle glaucoma.

Clinical judgment based on IOP assessments must be tempered with great caution in subacute and chronic angle closure, except when the pressures can be shown to rise significantly above an established baseline pressure. It must be stressed that IOP estimates in the normal range do not rule out the presence of chronic or subacute angle-closure glaucoma, nor do they indicate freedom of risk of an acute attack of the disease in the future. Gonioscopy is the only definitive diagnostic procedure in angle-closure glaucoma.

REFERENCES

1. Duke–Elder WS. System of ophthalmology, vol 7, The foundations of ophthalmology. London: Henry Kimpton, 1962:349.
2. von Graefe. Graefes Arch Ophthalmol 1863;9:215. Cited by Duke–Elder WS. System of ophthalmology, vol 7. London: Henry Kimpton, 1962:337.
3. Donders H. Klin Monatsbl Augenheilkd 1863;1:502. Cited by Duke–Elder WS. System of ophthalmology, vol 7. London: Henry Kimpton, 1962:339.
4. Schiøtz HA. Tonometry, with a description of a new tonometer. Arch Augenheilkd 1905;52:401.

5. Goldmann H. A new applanation tonometer. Bull Soc Fr Ophthalmol 1954;67:474.
6. Goldmann H, Schmidt T. Applanation tonometry. Ophthalmologica 1957;143:221.
7. Holiday JT, Allison ME, Prager TC. Goldmann applanation tonometry in patients with regular corneal astigmatism. Am J Ophthalmol 1983;96:90.
8. Schmidt T. Applanation tonometry at the slit lamp. Ophthalmologica 1957;133:337.
9. Wallace J, Lovell HG. Perkins hand-held tonometer. A clinical evaluation. Br J Ophthalmol 1968;52:568.
10. Craven ER, Butler SL, McCulley JP, Luby JP. Applanation tonometer tip sterilization for adenovirus type 8. Ophthalmology 1987;94:1538.
11. Bechrakis E, Weigelen A. Comparison of measurements made with the applanation tonometer of Goldmann and the hand tonometer of Draeger. Klin Monatsbl Augenheilkd 1987;173:835.
12. Duke–Elder WS. System of ophthalmology, vol 11, The foundation of ophthalmology. London: Henry Kimpton, 1962:339.
13. Kaiden JS, Zimmerman TJ, Worthen DM. An evaluation of the Glaucotest screening tonometer. Arch Ophthalmol 1974;92:195.
14. Friedenwald JS. Tonometer calibration. An attempt to remove discrepancies found in the 1954 calibration scale for Schiøtz tonometry. Trans Am Acad Ophthalmol 1957;61:108.
15. Duke–Elder WS. System of ophthalmology, vol 4, The physiology of the eye and of vision. London: Henry Kimpton, 1968:272.
16. Friedenwald JS. Standardization of tonometers: decennial report American Academy of Ophthalmology, 1954.
17. Draeger J, Jessen K. Tonometry and tonography. In: Bellows JG, ed. Glaucoma. Contemporary international concepts. New York: Masson Publishing, 1979:106.
18. Augsburger A, Polasky M, Walby M. Clinical tonometric measurements with the non-contact tonometer. Am J Optom Physiol Opt 1974;51:282.
19. Wittenberg S. A clinical evaluation of the non-contact tonometer. J Am Optom Assoc 1977;49:196.
20. Quigley HA, Addicks EM, Green WR. Optic nerve damage in human glaucoma: III. Quantitative corrective correlation of nerve fiber loss and visual field defect in glaucoma, ischemic optic neuropathy, papilledema and toxic neuropathy. Arch Ophthalmol 1982;100:136.
21. Holmin C, Krakau CET. Visual field decay in normal subjects and in cases of chronic glaucoma. Albrecht von Graefes Arch Klin Exp Ophthalmol 1980;213:291.
22. Kronfeld PC, McGarry HI. Five year follow up of glaucoma. JAMA 1984;136:957.
23. Cockburn DM. Does reduction of intraocular pressure prevent visual field loss in glaucoma? Am J Optom Physiol Opt 1983;60:705.
24. Phelps CD. Visual field defects in open angle glaucoma, progression and regression. Doc Ophthalmol Proc 1979;19:187.
25. Schulzer M, Mikelberg FS, Drance SM. Some observations on the relation between intraocular pressure reduction and the progression of glaucomatous field loss. Br J Ophthalmol 1987;71:486.
26. Bengtsson B. Aspects of the epidemiology of chronic glaucoma. Acta Ophthalmol Suppl 1981;146:1–48.
27. Frampton P, Rin DD, Brown B. Diurnal variation of intraocular pressure and the overriding effects of sleep. Am J Optom Physiol Opt 1987;64:54.
28. Cockburn DM. The glaucoma enigma. Am J Optom Physiol Opt 1985;63:913.
29. Armaly MF. The visual field defect and ocular pressure level in open angle glaucoma. Invest Ophthalmol 1969;8:105.
30. Yablonski ME, Zimmerman TJ, Kass MA, Becker B. Prognostic significance of optic disc cupping in ocular hypertensive patients. Am J Ophthalmol 1980;89:585.
31. David R, Tessler Z, Yassur Y. Long-term outcome of primary acute angle closure glaucoma. Br J Ophthalmol 1985;69:261.
32. Lowe RF. Primary creeping angle closure glaucoma. Br J Ophthalmol 1964;48:544.

Direct Ophthalmoscopy

Leo P. Semes

INTRODUCTION

Definition

The *direct ophthalmoscope* is an instrument for viewing the interior of the eye. It consists of a concave mirror with a hole in the center through which the observer examines the eye, a source of light that is reflected into the eye by the mirror, and lenses that can be rotated into the opening in the mirror to neutralize the refracting power of the eye being examined and thus make the image of the fundus clear.[1]

History

The fundus reflex (red reflex) was observed as early as the first century AD. Rucker[2] chronicles Pliny the Elder's description of a red reflex from animals' eyes in *Natural History*. The prevailing view was that the tapetum of nocturnal animals was self-luminous. This misconception persisted until the early 18th century.

Although Helmholtz is almost universally known for "inventing" the ophthalmoscope, credit belongs more properly to Jan Evangelista Purkinje, a Czechoslovak.[3,4] He described a technique of ophthalmoscopy as part of his habilitation theses for appointment as chair of physiology at the University of Breslau in 1823. Purkinje, better known for his description of corneal and lenticular reflections that bear his name, received his doctor of medicine degree from the University of Prague in 1819. His original description of viewing the fundus arose from his observation of the red reflex produced by the reflection of a candle from his myopic spectacle lenses directed into the eyes of dogs.[4] Purkinje had just described the technique of retroillumination. Later, he extended the observation to humans and ophthalmoscopy was born.

Because the light sources during the 19th century were gas-light or flame, bright illumination of the fundus was difficult. The infant technique of ophthalmoscopy nearly became an orphan. Charles Babbage, a London mathematician and scientific mechanician, is known to have made a model ophthalmoscope for Mr. Wharton Jones in 1847. This London ophthalmic surgeon discounted the utility of Babbage's instrument for ocular fundus examination.

Several years later, in 1850, Hermann Helmholtz, a Prussian physiologist, devised an experiment to prove to his students that light emanating from the eye follows the same course as the incident beams. He aligned the apparent light source with the observer's visual axis and rediscovered the ophthalmoscope.[2]

Helmholtz used a partially silvered mirror to achieve the coaxial condition between observer and light source. He called his instrument *Augenspiel*[5] or eye mirror. Because of his popularizing of the technique, Helmholtz is regarded as the father of ophthalmoscopy.

Dr. W. S. Dennett[6] is credited with the initial demonstration (1885) of an electric direct ophthalmoscope. Other modifications to the mirror and illumination systems led DeZeng of Camden, New Jersey, to produce a simplified direct ophthalmoscope.[2] Among the features consistent with contemporary instruments were the rotating lens bank and a sliding collar to shape the beam.

Another approach to the illuminating system was introduced, in 1914, by Charles H. May of New York City. The May prism, made of solid glass, consisted of a convex lower end, acting as a condenser, and an angled upper portion serving as the reflector.[7] The greatest advantage of May's system was the even illumination that it provided.

Contemporary instruments include the Welch–Allyn ophthalmoscope, which incorporates apertures of varying diameter, a fixation-target grid, red-free filter, and, most recently, a 4000° K filter, as well as a polarized dust cover.

Clinical Use

The direct ophthalmoscope has a number of applications in clinical practice, aside from fundus examination. For example, the demonstration of a subtle Marcus-Gunn pupil can be enhanced by using the instrument as the light stimulus.[8] The fixation target allows a test for eccentric fixation.

INSTRUMENTATION

Theory

All direct ophthalmoscopes today are self-luminous, or reflexless. Optically, the light source is reflected through the patient's pupil to illuminate an area of the fundus. This illuminated area becomes the object for the observation system of the ophthalmoscope (Fig. 24–1). The illumination and observation beams must be separated to eliminate image-obscuring reflexes.[9] Light originating from the patient's ocular fundus reaches the lens of the instrument. The examiner, whose eye is as close to the sight hole of the instrument as possible, then dials the appropriate lens into place to view the desired portion of the eye.

The direct ophthalmoscope can also be used to inspect the anterior structures of the eyes. In these cases, the lids, lashes, cornea, or iris are viewed directly. In general, the illuminated structure becomes the object for the observation system (see Fig. 24–1).

Use

The usefulness of the direct ophthalmoscope is manifold. A survey of the ocular media against the red reflex of the fundus is an initial step. Opacities interfering with this red glow in the pupillary space can be localized grossly. By applying the principle of parallax, objects anterior to the plane of the iris will show "against motion," whereas opacities of the lens or vitreous will show "with motion." A finer distinction of location can be made by observing the relative speed of movement of any opacities. For example, a Mittendorf dot on the posterior lens capsule will move more slowly than the prepapillary annular opacity from a posterior vitreous separation. In addition, iris transillumination is observable with this procedure.

If one recognizes that a high-plus lens will act as a modest magnifier and will image objects located at its focal length, the direct ophthalmoscope can be used to examine the anterior segment of the eye. By using a +20-D setting of the ophthalmoscope's lens bank and moving the instrument to 5 cm from the anterior segment structure to be examined, a clear illuminated magnified direct view of that structure can be obtained. The use of the instrument's slit beam will aid in viewing contours within the anterior segment.

To view the lens and vitreous, the ophthalmoscope can be set to decreasing values of plus power. The lens will be focused at a setting between +20 D and +12 D. The anterior and midvitreous will focus between +12 D and +8 D. By further reducing plus power in the ophthalmoscope lens bank, the examiner will focus on the posterior pole of the eye. The value of the lens bank will correspond roughly to the patient's refractive correction when a nonaccommodating examiner initially focuses on a blood vessel at the plane of the optic nerve head of a nonaccommodating patient. For all of these observations, the examiner will enjoy the greatest possible field of view when the instrument rests against his or her brow and is as close as practical to the patient's eye.

The fixation target of the instrument will allow measurement of eccentric fixation (EF). Since EF is a monocular phenomenon, the examiner must occlude the eye that is not being tested.

The red-free filter should be employed any time that a pigmented fundus lesion is encountered. Unfortunately, the limited field of view (approximately 5°), often will not allow distinction of larger lesions. When such a lesion is discovered in white light, comparison of its visibility in red-free light should be made. The monochromatic green source is absorbed by the retinal pigment

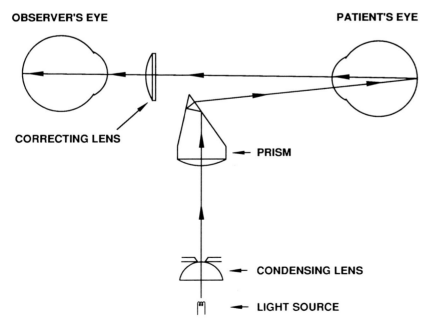

OBSERVER'S EYE   **PATIENT'S EYE**

CORRECTING LENS

← **PRISM**

← **CONDENSING LENS**

← **LIGHT SOURCE**

FIGURE 24–1. Schematic drawing of the direct ophthalmoscope. Light is directed by the prism through the patient's pupil and illuminates the ocular fundus. The illuminated area of the retina becomes the object for the correcting lens to image. The observer selects a lens power to focus the area of interest. The image is upright and virtual.

epithelium (RPE), rendering structures deep to the RPE invisible or severely attenuated from view.[10] Red-free light is also absorbed significantly by the hemoglobin pigment of the blood column, giving a striking black color to the retinal vascular tree. Red-free examination of the nerve fiber layer (NFL) of the retina can be rewarding. Early dropout of the NFL can be discovered more easily by using the red-free approach. Finally, the red-free filter can be used to enhance the estimation of cup/disc (C/D) ratio. This strategy is most useful when comparing the C/D ratio of one eye with that of its fellow.

The slit beam, as mentioned earlier, is useful for examining contours such as the cup–disc margin. In addition, the slit beam can be used to produce proximal illumination. For example, if a subretinal neovascular member (SRNVM) is suspected, directing the edge of the beam near one edge of the area of interest will cause the surrounding area to glow, whereas the SRNVM will block light reflected from the choroid and appear black.

As a general rule, the direct ophthalmoscope will be restricted to use on eyes the pupils of which have not been dilated. Patients with particularly small pupils will more easily be examined using the smaller aperture size. Similarly, patients who have larger pupils may be examined with the larger aperture. The use of a small aperture size for small pupils will help to limit or eliminate corneal reflections that interfere with the fundus image.

COMMERCIALLY AVAILABLE INSTRUMENTS

Basic Design

Observation of a patient's ocular fundus is dependent upon the clinician obtaining a conjugate focus through the ophthalmoscope. Illumination of the ocular fundus must occur along a separate axis from the observation system (see Fig. 24–1).

Welch–Allyn (11630)

The Welch–Allyn model no. 11630 direct ophthalmoscope (Fig. 24–2) is powered by a rechargable battery handle. It is available with up to five apertures. These may include various spot sizes, grid target, fixation target, red-free filter, or 4000° K slit filter. In addition, it offers a polarizing filter that doubles as a dust cover. The range of focusing lenses extends from −30 D to +38 D in 1-D steps. A combination rheostat and on-off switch controls the intensity of the light source: a 3.5-v halogen bulb. The coaxial illumination system aids in eliminating shadows of the fundus image when viewing through a small pupil.

Keeler

Keeler's Practitioner direct ophthalmoscope offers 3.5-v halogen illumination and three apertures. The lens powers range from −30 D to +29 D in 1-D steps. The Specialist version (see Fig. 24–2) offers a greater variety of apertures, which include red-free and fixation. A unique feature of this instrument is the sliding focal illuminator for focused-beam corneal examination. In addition, an increased range of lens powers from −45 D to +44 D in 1-D steps is standard.

The Medic Lux model by Keeler offers the capability of a grating acuity target. This bar resolution chart allows the clinician to perform a visual prognosis test before corneal or cataract surgery. Single-diopter steps from −30 D to +29 D and coaxial halogen illumination are standard.

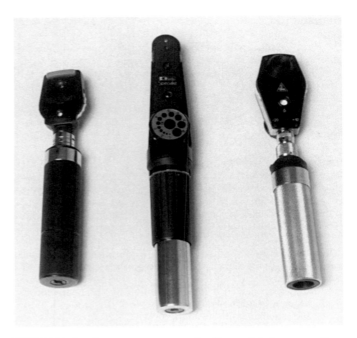

FIGURE 24–2. Contemporary monocular direct ophthalmoscopes. From left: Welch–Allyn, Keeler (specialist), and Propper.

CLINICAL PROCEDURE

1. Classic examination of the patient includes observation of the red fundus reflex from 20 to 40 cm away (Fig. 24–3). This technique shows gross media opacities or discrepancies of the red reflex.
2. The examiner then moves as close to the eye as possible to examine the anterior segment with high-plus power in the instrument's lens bank (Fig. 24–4).
3. By reducing plus power, the clinician sequentially examines the crystalline lens, vitreous, and finally, the optic nerve head.
4. At the retinal plane, the optic disc is visualized first, and then, in an ordered manner, the blood vessels can be followed to the equator and back.

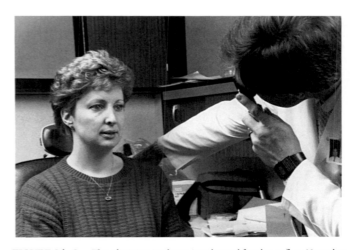

FIGURE 24–3. The clinician is observing the red fundus reflex. Note that the clinician is positioned about 15° lateral to the patient, allowing observation of the ocular media in alignment with the optic disc.

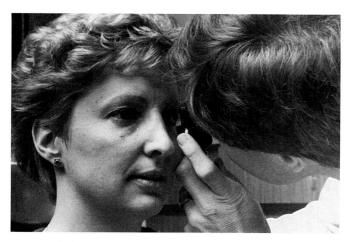

FIGURE 24–4. The clinician is positioned to observe intraocular details Note the juxtaposition of the examiner and patient.

5. Once a quadrant-by-quadrant scan of the fundus is done, the macula can be examined.
6. The slit beam is used to highlight contours in the fundus (elevations or excavations). Red-free light can be used to view pigmented lesions.

An experienced examiner will be able to examine the optic nerve head and follow the retinal vascular tree to the equatorial region of the eye through the undilated pupil of a cooperative patient. Examining the macula last is often more rewarding, since this strategy allows the patient to light adapt and the pupil to maintain its least-minimum diameter longer.

CLINICAL IMPLICATIONS

Clinical Significance

Direct ophthalmoscopy is indicated for examination of the posterior pole of the ocular fundus when the patient's pupil cannot be dilated. With the sanction of diagnostic drug use by optometrists in all 50 states and the District of Columbia, only the occasional patient will come under this heading. The increasing use of stereoscopic methods of ocular fundus examination will relegate the direct ophthalmoscope to a secondary role.

Clinical Interpretation

Although many practitioners have become quite adroit with the technique of direct ophthalmoscopy, the limited view of the fundus can be deceiving. The optics of the instrument allow a magnified view of the fundus (approximately 16×). This will vary somewhat depending on patients' refractive errors. The resulting limitation of field of view (approximately 5°) may cause the examiner to overlook even significant fundus changes.

Highly myopic refractive errors result in the greatest amount of magnification. Significant amounts of astigmia will produce a distorted clinical picture for the direct ophthalmoscopist. These two sources of error can be minimized by employing an indirect method of ophthalmoscopy. Performing direct ophthalmoscopy through the patient's refractive correction may also minimize these potential distortions.

Perhaps the most striking drawback to direct ophthalmoscopy is that it is a monocular mode of examination. The lack of stereoscopic capability forces the examiner to rely on monocular cues for depth. Because of its limited field of view, potential interference by refractive error and lack of stereopsis, the technique of monocular direct ophthalmoscopy is fraught with inherent shortcomings; these sources of error are magnified in comparison with the binocular methods of fundus examination.

REFERENCES

1. Webster's medical desk dictionary. Springfield, Mass: Merriam-Webster, Inc, 1986.
2. Rucker C. A history of the ophthalmoscope. Rochester: Whiting, 1971.
3. Albert DM, Miller WH. Jan Purkinje and the ophthalmoscope. Am J Ophthalmol 1973;76:494–499.
4. Reese PD. The neglect of Purkinje's technique of ophthalmoscopy prior to Helmholtz's invention of the ophthalmoscope. Ophthalmology 1986;93:1457–1460.
5. Helmholtz J. Cited by Friedenwald H. The history of the invention and development of the ophthalmoscope. JAMA 1902;38:549–552.
6. Dennett WS. The electric light ophthalmoscope. Trans Am Ophthalmol Soc 1885; p 156.
7. May CH. A new electric ophthalmoscope. Ophthal Rec 1914;23:386–389.
8. Cox TA. Pupillary testing using the direct ophthalmoscope. Am J Ophthalmol 1988;105:427–428.
9. Friedenwald JS. Ophthalmoscopy in yellow light. Trans Am Ophthalmol Soc 1928;26:381–426.
10. Parver LM. The clinical characteristics of presumed choroidal nevi observed in green light. Trans Am Acad Ophthalmol Otolaryngol 1979;86:1924–1930.

Monocular Indirect Ophthalmoscopy

Leo P. Semes

INTRODUCTION

Definition

Indirect ophthalmoscopy is a technique which, in its original form, combined a hand-held condensing lens with a direct ophthalmoscope.[1,2] This system provides a real, inverted ("indirect") image of the ocular fundus. The monocular indirect ophthalmoscope has evolved to an instrument that contains lenses for providing an upright wide-field image of the ocular fundus.

History

There is some confusion concerning the inventor of the method of direct ophthalmoscopy. Credit for the development of the *science* of ophthalmoscopy belongs to Helmholtz.[1] Earlier descriptions of the red reflex, the fundus, and even instrumentation and technique preceded Helmholtz (1851; see Chap. 24). It is generally agreed, however, that Ruete, in the following year, introduced the indirect method of ophthalmoscopy.[1,2] He added an additional convex lens to the system, mounted it on a table, and was able to examine patients from about a 40-cm distance.[2] The use of Helmholtz's direct ophthalmoscope in this configuration produced an inverted, reversed, real, or indirect, image of the ocular fundus. This is the origin of the adjectival prefix, *indirect,* for an ophthalmoscopic system producing such an image. The light source at the time was a flame; therefore this procedure is referred to as *reflecting* ophthalmoscopy.

In the succeeding decades of the 19th century, indirect ophthalmoscopy was generally practiced using a convex condensing lens and a direct ophthalmoscope both held by the practitioner. Gullstrand[3] was the first to recognize that the illumination and observation beams must be separated to view a fundus image that was free of reflexes. With use of his design principles, Bausch &

Lomb manufactured a *binocular* table model indirect ophthalmoscope between 1931 and 1970.

A more familiar view of the ocular fundus for practitioners accustomed to the direct magnified view would come from an instrument that gave a wide-field, real, but erect image. In 1967, the American Optical (AO) Company introduced such an instrument. The AO monocular indirect ophthalmoscope utilizes only a small portion of the patient's pupil. This strategy is intended for use when examining the ocular fundus through an undilated pupil. The instrument employs a telescopic system providing approximately 5× magnification and allowing a five times greater area to be viewed than that of the direct ophthalmoscope.[4] This offers a field of view that is more than doubled in diameter (2.23 times) over the direct ophthalmoscope. Woodruff[5] describes the usefulness of this instrument to include the wide field of view and use through small pupils. He cautions that the reduced magnification may present an initial hurdle, but that continued use is rewarding.

Clinical Use

Circumstances in the development of the monocular indirect ophthalmoscope (MIO) and the evolution of the profession of optometry have combined to relegate the MIO to a role of minimal clinical importance. In their classic paper comparing direct and indirect ophthalmoscopy, Augsburger and Reardon[6] include six indications for monocular indirect ophthalmoscopy:

1. Suspicion of peripheral retinal changes
2. Distorted field of view secondary to high myopia or astigmia
3. Absence of steady fixation by the patient
4. Dense or cloudy media
5. Unstable accommodation
6. When the depth of focus is to be maximized

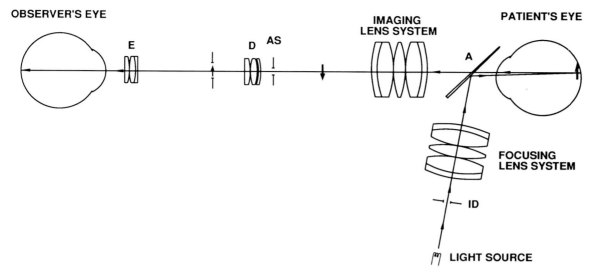

FIGURE 25–1. Schematic diagram illustrating the erect image formation system of the monocular indirect ophthalmoscope:[4] ID, iris diaphragm; A, partially silvered mirror; AS, aperture stop; D, relay lens system; E, focusing lens system.

In all cases, however, practitioners dilating the pupil would find that use of the *binocular* indirect ophthalmoscope (BIO) is superior.

One must put into perspective the time frame of this article.[6] In 1974 only two states allowed the use of mydriatics by optometrists. Indeed, all of the indications just listed could be applied equally to *binocular* indirect ophthalmoscopy.

The MIO is most useful in those clinical situations when the patient's pupil will not or cannot be dilated. For the practitioner who desires a wide field of view through small pupils, a rewarding, although not stereoscopic, view of the ocular fundus can be obtained. It is the experience of many clinicians, however, that after gaining confidence and developing expertise with the BIO, the ocular fundus can be surveyed with the binocular instrument even through undilated pupils.

With the sanction of drugs for pupillary dilation available in every jurisdiction in the United States, the MIO has been relegated to a minor role. Just as the advent of fundus biomicroscopy for examination of the posterior pole will supplant direct ophthalmoscopy, so, too, will BIO replace MIO.

INSTRUMENTATION

Theory

The optical principles of the monocular indirect ophthalmoscope include a condensing lens system to image the light source for a beam-splitter (mirror) that, in turn, illuminates the patient's ocular fundus. The observation system of the instrument consists of a telescopic arrangement to focus and present an erect image to the observer's eyepiece. In addition, an iris diaphragm acts to control the amount of light directed to the patient's eye, and the focusable eyepiece allows the examiner to overcome ametropias.

The unique feature of such an integrated monocular indirect ophthalmoscopic system is the relay lens system that presents an erect image to the eyepiece. The key feature that distinguishes the MIO from direct ophthalmoscopes is its ability to optically conjugate the pupils of observer and patient.[4] This eliminates vignetting (Fig. 25–1).

COMMERCIALLY AVAILABLE INSTRUMENTS

The only commercially available MIO is the American Optical (Reichert) Monocular Indirect Ophthalmoscope. This instrument (Fig. 25–2) is available as a cord-operated or rechargeable model. The optical systems and features are identical, except that the rechargeable model offers a 50% neutral density (ND) filter for reducing illumination.

The optical principles of this instrument have been described in the foregoing. The examiner first matches the diameter of the light source to that of the patient's pupillary diameter. This is done once the examiner has positioned the instrument close to the patient's forehead in preparation for fundus viewing. At this point, a retinal blood vessel can be selected for focusing. With the focusable eyepiece, the examiner clears the image and begins examining the retinal grounds.

The examiner can choose one of the filters available in the instrument for selected viewing of the ocular fundus. These include red-free, yellow, and, in the rechargeable model, 50% ND filters.

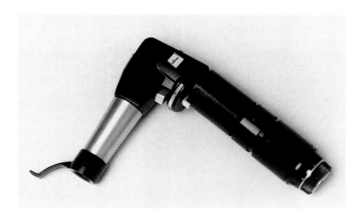

FIGURE 25–2. American Optical (Reichert) monocular indirect ophthalmoscope.

CLINICAL PROCEDURE

The clinical procedure for using the MIO for ocular fundus examination is as follows:

1. The examiner steadies the instrument against his or her forehead using the forehead rest (Fig. 25–3).
2. The patient is instructed to look across the room. Some clinicians prefer to use specific fixation targets (lights or landmarks) for patient fixation. The preferred position for examination is for the examiner to stand facing the seated patient.
3. The face of the instrument is held approximately 18 mm (3/4") from the patient's eye. This allows the light source to be focused in the pupillary plane to diffusely illuminate the ocular fundus. Orienting the fundus reflex from a few inches away as the patient is approached for examination helps to ensure centering of the fundus image once the instrument is brought close enough for retinal evaluation.
4. The continuously variable-focusing lever (upper) can then be manipulated to produce and maintain a clear view of the patient's ocular fundus (see Fig. 25–3).
5. Any examination strategy should be developed with the goals of completeness and repeatability. An effective approach would be to begin by examining the optic disc. The configuration of the margins, blood vessel contour, and size and shape of the cup–disc border should be noted. Following the retinal vascular tree around the points of an imaginary compass to their most peripheral extent and back to the disc is a useful scanning strategy for the general retinal area. Observation of blood vessel crossing changes is best made above and below the macula. This area contains arterioles and venules (small blood vessels) whose crossings are more numerous here than elsewhere in the retina. The macula, because it represents the most sensitive area of the retina, should be examined last.
6. Any pigmented lesion discovered with white light should be examined with the red-free filter. Pigmented lesions deep to the retinal pigment epithelium will disappear from view or become greatly attenuated.[7] The red-free filter enhances the appearance of the retinal blood vessels and small hemorrhages. Finally, the red-free light will provide useful contrast studies of the nerve fiber layer and cup–disc relationship.

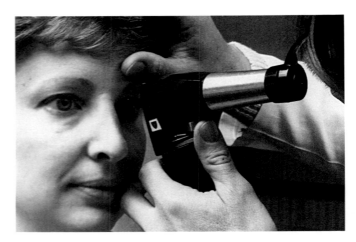

FIGURE 25–3. Proper position for the clinician to examine a patient using the MIO. Note that the examiner's thumb is placed to manipulate the focusing (upper) lever to maintain a clear view of the desired portion of the patient's ocular fundus.

The yellow filter serves to reduce chromatic aberration and scattering, providing greater contrast and perhaps enhancing details of the macula.

7. There exist as many variations on schemes for recording fundus findings as there are examiners. It is important to indicate landmarks and structural abnormalities of the fundus features observed. The cup/disc (C/D) horizontal and vertical ratio, artery/vein (A/V) ratio, and foveal reflex presence or absence represent the most salient features. In addition, a notation of unusual disc or blood vessel findings may be enhanced by a drawing. It is appropriate to note that the discs, vessels, and macula are "unremarkable for disease" in addition to the quantitative recording of the C/D and A/V ratios. As a philosophic and medicolegal imperative, the designation for within normal limits (WNL) should never be used.

A sample recording of ocular findings may, therefore,

Table 25–1
Optical and Observation Characteristics of Ophthalmoscopes

Instrument	Image	Stereopsis	Field of View	Magnification	Extent of Visible Fundus
MDO	Upright	No	≈5°*	15×†	To equator (through dilated pupils)
MIO	Upright	No	≈12°	5×	Beyond equator (through dilated pupils)
BIO	Reversed and inverted	Yes	≈30°‡	2.5×‡	Entire retinal surface and anterior with scleral indentation (through dilated pupils)

*Varies with refractive error (smaller with increasing amounts of uncorrected myopic refractive error).

†Varies with refractive error (increases with increasing amounts of uncorrected myopic refractive error).

‡Varies with condensing lens power.

appear as: "C/D 0.3 × 0.3, discs, vessels, and macula unremarkable for disease OD/OS."

CLINICAL IMPLICATIONS

Clinical Significance

The monocular indirect ophthalmoscope will be used in situations when the patient's pupil cannot or will not be dilated. Unfortunately, this limits the clinician to a monocular view of only about 70% of the retinal surface. The advantage of MIO over MDO lies in the wider field of view obtainable with the former technique. Disadvantages of all monocular instruments include lack of stereopsis and inability to conform to current standards of care. Table 25–1 compares the optical and observation characteristcs of direct and indirect ophthalmoscopes.

REFERENCES

1. Duke–Elder WS, ed. System of ophthalmology, vol 7. The foundation of ophthalmology: heredity, pathology, diagnosis, and therapeutics. London: Henry Kimpton, 1962.
2. Rucker C. A history of the ophthalmoscope. Rochester: Whiting, 1971.
3. Friedenwald JS. A critical study of the modern ophthalmoscope: contributions to its construction and use. Ophthalmoscopy in yellow light. Trans Am Ophthalmol Soc 1928;26:381–426.
4. American Optical. AO 305 monocular indirect ophthalmoscope: Model 11305 Cord Operated and 11305R Astro Cordless (rechargeable). Scientific Instrument Division. Buffalo, NY, 1974.
5. Woodruff ME. Extension of the resources for fundus examination: the monocular indirect ophthalmoscope. Optom Weekly 1968;59:24–25.
6. Augsburger A, Reardon PL. Maximizing funduscopic examination, part II: direct versus indirect ophthalmoscopy. J Am Optom Assoc 1974; 45:185–188.
7. Parver LM. The clinical characteristics of presumed choroidal nevi observed in green light. Trans Am Acad Ophthalmol Otolaryngol 1979;86:1924–1930.

Binocular Indirect Ophthalmoscopy

Leo P. Semes

INTRODUCTION

Definition

The ophthalmoscope is an instrument for viewing the interior of the eye.[1] Monocular instruments, as described in Chapters 24 and 25, offer high magnification and are self-contained units. Modern stereoscopic ophthalmoscopes consist of a headset containing the light source and viewing oculars. An additional component of the stereoscopic ophthalmoscope system is the condensing lens. It is typically a high–dioptric-power plus lens that is held by the examiner close to the patient's eye. The condensing lens concentrates light from the light source and forms a real, inverted, reversed (indirect) image to be viewed through the oculars.

History

A device for stereoscopic examination of the ocular fundus was described in 1861 by a Parisian, Girard–Teulon.[2] His instrument included a concave mirror for reflecting the light of a lamp into the patient's eye. This mirror was attached to a hand-held binocular with adjustable mirrors, to reduce the examiner's interpupillary distance, which were, in turn, imaged within the patient's dilated pupil.[2,3] A condensing lens occupied the examiner's other hand. Examiner and patient sat facing each other during the ocular fundus examination.

In 1883, Adams[4] produced a head-mounted monocular instrument for shared use by artist and examiner. The significance of Adams' development (a monocular instrument for the examiner) was its lens bank for bringing the patient's fundus into focus.

Over 50 years passed until Schepens[5] combined the early attempts at stereoscopic fundus examination and drawing of fundus findings with an electric light source. Schepens' instrument consisted of headborne oculars attached to an articulated table-mounted light source. In fact, the premier American reference[5] depicts him demonstrating the new ophthalmoscope facing a seated patient who is holding the fundus-drawing chart.

Schepens believed that examination of the entire ocular fundus was so critical in the diagnosis and management of retinal detachment that he emphasized that particular attention be paid to the ora serrata region. In addition, he described the technique of scleral indentation to examine this most peripheral portion of the sensory retina.[6]

The instrument that Schepens originally fashioned from scraps of metal and other parts from post–World War II London hospitals was refined at the Massachusetts Eye and Ear Infirmary.[7] It was first manufactured by the American Optical Company. Later, an independent company was formed to manufacture an improved version of the original design, the small-pupil binocular indirect ophthalmoscope.[8]

A decade passed from its American introduction before Elmstrom,[9] in 1958, reported the virtues of the binocular indirect ophthalmoscope (BIO). This is the earliest reference in the optometric literature. Two of his personal observations are worth noting: that the instrument is complementary to direct ophthalmoscopy, and that a portable battery pack would be useful.

In the early 1980s, Keeler introduced its second-generation spectacle-mounted BIO. It was powered by a rechargeable battery unit. Currently, this company offers a video system (single-chip camera) for use with its Fison BIO.

Clinical Use

The BIO is the single most useful instrument for examining the entire ocular fundus. Aside from meticulous stereoscopic observation of the retina, optic nerve head, and retinal vasculature, the

BIO can be used to compare quickly the red reflex in each eye, to test sluggishly responding pupils, and even to break an acute angle-closure attack.

The BIO may be particularly valuable when retinal evaluation of patients with cloudy media is necessary. Specifically, every patient deserves a stereoscopic survey of the ocular fundus. Patients who manifest symptoms suggestive of, or conditions predisposing to, retinal detachment (retinal breaks, vitreoretinal abnormalities, significant degree of myopia, or other condition) must be monitored with the BIO examination and, when indicated, scleral indentation.

INSTRUMENTATION

Theory

Binocular indirect ophthalmoscopy is designed to allow stereoscopic viewing of the ocular fundus. In addition, it provides a wide (25° or more) field of view. As with other methods of ophthalmoscopy discussed in Chapters 24 and 25, the illuminated fundus becomes the object for the observation system. For the stereoscopic system, a hand-held condensing lens of high-plus dioptric power serves three functions:[10]

1. Directs the light source of the instrument through the patient's pupil
2. Generates an indirect aerial (real) image of the illuminated retina at the lens' focal length
3. Images both of the observer's pupils within the patient's pupil, thus allowing maximum field of view and satisfying the condition for stereopsis.

Image Formation

The illuminated fundus of an emmetropic unaccommodated eye is conjugate with infinity and, therefore, will have parallel rays of light emerging from it. If these bundles of rays are intercepted by a condensing lens, a real inverted aerial image will be formed at the focal plane of the lens. This image will exist between the lens and the observer (Fig. 26–1). When using a binocular headset, the observer can view this image stereoscopically. The headset is equipped with oculars of approximately +2.00 D. This supplies some of the focusing power for observation of the aerial image.

Image Size and Depth

For the clinician to appreciate stereopsis, the interpupillary distance (IPD) must be reduced such that both of the examiner's pupils can be imaged within the patient's pupil. This condition is satisfied by mirrors or prisms, within the headset of the instrument, that optically reduce the examiner's IPD. The instrument is able to reduce the IPD to approximately 15 mm. If the patient–observer distance is 40 cm, then a +20.00-D condensing lens held at its focal length (5 cm) would image the patient's pupil 6 cm closer to the examiner. The image plane would be approximately 30 cm from the observer. This optical separation allows for a further reduction of the examiner's IPD (from 15 mm to approximately 3 mm). From geometric optics:

$$\frac{\text{Image distance}}{\text{Object distance}} = \text{magnification} = \frac{6\,\text{cm}}{30\,\text{cm}} = 1/5$$

In addition, the examiner's pupil diameter will be reduced by a similar factor. A 5-mm pupil is now reduced to 1 mm in diameter, for example. The condition established by the binocular headset and condensing lens is termed *conjugacy of pupils.*[10]

The use of a +30.00-D condensing lens would further reduce both the examiner's IPD and pupil size. A higher dioptric power condensing lens, therefore, would be advantageous when viewing through poorly dilated or small pupils.

Rubin[10] has shown that condensing lenses of approximately +15.00 D provide "normal" depth relationship images. Condensing lenses of lower dioptric power will offer an enhanced stereoscopic effect. Similarly, condensing lenses of dioptric power greater than +15.00 D would show increasingly flatter images. The dioptric power of the eye under examination has relatively little influence on the observed size of its image. Note that this is in contrast with direct ophthalmoscopy, in which more myopic eyes give larger images.

Field of View

Optical considerations show that the larger the diameter of the lens, the larger the field of view.[10] As the examiner attempts to view portions of the peripheral ocular fundus, certain limitations infringe upon the field of view. The apparent narrowing of the pupillary aperture as the patient looks in oblique directions is chief among these. This effect can be overcome if the examiner aligns the instrument with the long axis of the patient's apparently elliptical pupil. This allows a greater chance for the examiner's pupils and light source to be imaged within the patient's pupil. Recall that this condition must be satisfied for stereopsis.

All condensing lenses used for BIO have two differently curved convex aspheric surfaces. Asphericity permits a clear image over the entire lens surface.[11] The lens should be held so that the more steeply curved surface faces the examiner.[10] This position maximally reduces the effect of spherical aberration as well as the magnitude of reflection from the lens surface.

One final consideration of angular field of view is the influence of axial refractive error. This will vary only slightly as angular field is limited by the viewing lens aperture. In myopia, the field will be slightly smaller, compared with the emmetropic condition; the field will be slightly larger in hyperopia (Fig. 26–2).[10]

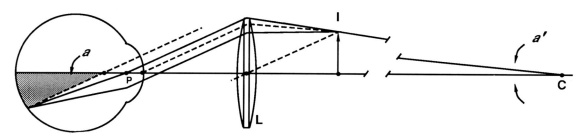

FIGURE 26–1. The lens aperture is the limiting factor for field of view: *a* represents one-half the extent of the fundus visible to the clinician (*C*). *a'* is one-half the extent of the aerial fundus image (*I*) formed at the focal length (*F*) of the lens (*L*). The clinician's pupil is imaged at *P*. (Adapted from Rubin ML. The optics of indirect ophthalmoscopy. Surv Ophthalmol 1964;9:449–464)

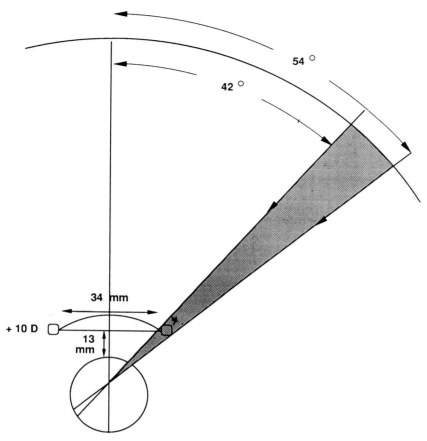

FIGURE 28–3. Trial lens scotoma.

such as those associated with pituitary tumor, are perhaps better sought using the perimeter, as this instrument may reveal them while they are still relatively peripheral, thereby leading to earlier neurologic consultation.

Clinical Interpretation

There is a portion of the visual field in which test objects are normally not seen: the blindspot. With remarkably little variation from individual to individual, the center of the blindspot will be found to lie at a point slightly more than 15° temporal to the fixation point.[4] The usual stimulus for blindspot testing is a 5-mm diameter white pin on the tangent screen. The target to be used for blindspot testing should be visible at a point 25° straight temporal from fixation. Thus, of the tests listed in Table 27–1, only those for which the radius of testing exceeds 15° will be useful. Chen and Frenkel[5] have pointed out how the Amsler grid may also be used to assess the blindspot.

In a clinical setting, a 2-m tangent screen offers considerable ease in measurement of the blindspot because the linear size of the blindspot on the screen's surface is about 341 × 261 mm. The blindspot may also be conveniently measured at the 1-m tangent screen, where its dimensions will be about 170 × 130 mm. There is some difference in the variability of bindspot measurements when perimetric and tangent screen data are compared, with the perimeter showing slightly more variability. This is likely due to the mechanical problems of working with the smaller physical size

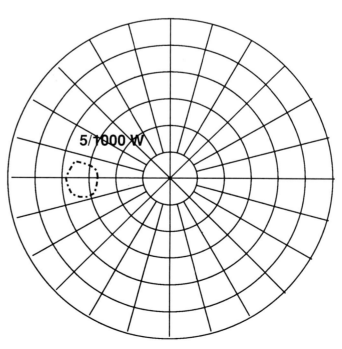

FIGURE 28–4. Normal blindspot.

of the blindspot. The clinician is occasionally faced with a patient who claims to have a visual field defect when one is not actually present. In this situation, it is useful to test the patient at different test distances (at 2 m and at 1 m, or at a tangent screen and at a perimeter). It will be difficult for the malingering patient to accurately reproduce the angular size of the defect under these different test conditions.

Figure 28–4 shows a normal blindspot assessed at the tangent screen. This patient was slightly hyperopic. The blindspot tends to be smaller and more centrally located in hyperopes, and larger and more peripherally located in myopes.

REFERENCES

1. Long WF, Woo GCS. Measuring light levels with photographic meters. Am J Optom Physiol Opt 1980;57:51–55.
2. Graham CH, ed. Vision and visual perceptions. New York: John Wiley & Sons, 1965:329.
3. Williams TD. Malformations of the optic nerve head. Am J Optom Physiol Opt 1978;55:706–718.
4. Williams TD. Correlation of nerve head and blind spot elliptical features. Am J Optom Physiol Opt 1988;65:29–36.
5. Chen KFS, Frenkel M. Dynamic visual field testing using the Amsler grid patterns. Trans Am Acad Ophthalmol Otol 1975;79:761–771.

Sphygmomanometry

Linda Casser Locke

INTRODUCTION

Definition

Sphygmomanometry (*sphygmos,* pulse, + *manos,* rare, thin, + *metron,* measure) is the determination of blood pressure through the use of a sphygmomanometer.[1]

History

The discovery of blood pressure has been attributed to the Englishman Stephen Hales who made the first measurements of this vital sign during experiments on a horse in 1733.[2] The accurate study of blood pressure did not resume until 1828, when the French physician–physicist Poiseuille completed his doctoral dissertation on the use of a mercury manometer for blood pressure measurement through direct arterial cannulation of laboratory animals. In 1856, Faivre made the first accurate direct assessment of a human patient's blood pressure by connecting an artery to a mercury manometer during surgery.

Beginning in the mid-19th century, several elaborate, but clinically unwieldy, techniques were devised to measure blood pressure by indirect, noninvasive means through the application of unilateral pressure to the arm to obliterate the radial pulse.[2] These methods included the use of weights (Vierordt, 1854), a water chamber (Etienne Jules Marey, 1860), a rubber bag filled with water (von Basch, late 1870s), and a bulb inflated with air (Potain, 1889).

The forefather of modern sphygmomanometry was Riva-Rocci.[2] In 1896, this Italian physician reported his technique of measuring blood pressure by using a 5-cm wide cuff containing an inflatable rubber bag that was wrapped around the circumference of the arm. The resultant inaccuracies inherent in using this nar-row cuff were corrected by von Recklinghausen, in 1901, through the use of a 12-cm wide armband.

In 1905, the Russian physician N. C. Korotkoff first reported the auscultatory method of indirectly measuring blood pressure.[2] Since that time, blood pressure measurement has been an important component of physical diagnosis to aid in indirectly assessing the cardiovascular system.

Clinical Use

Essential hypertension, that is, hypertension of unknown cause, accounts for over 90% of the cases of high blood pressure in the United States. Patients with essential hypertension are usually asymptomatic, but have an increased risk of stroke, heart attack, and premature death.[3] The target organs within the body that sustain damage caused by hypertension are the eyes, the heart, the brain, and the kidneys. Risk factors that have been linked to the development of essential hypertension include heredity, cigarette smoking, high cholesterol levels, obesity, excessive caffeine consumption, stress, and alcohol ingestion.[4]

It is estimated that nearly 58 million people in the United States have high blood pressure or are taking antihypertensive medication.[5] Just under half of these individuals (46.1%) are unaware that they have the disease, and, of the patients who know they are hypertensive, 43% have inadequate control of their blood pressure.[6] The prevalence rate of hypertension increases with age, and the prevalence of hypertension in the black population is considerably higher than in the white population. Blacks develop hypertension at an earlier age, and it is likely to be more severe than in other racial groups.[7] Studies have shown that mild elevations in blood pressure are more common in children than was previously recognized, especially among adolescents. Thus, the blood pressure status of the pediatric population, from which the

Table 29–1
Some Clinical Applications of Blood Pressure Measurement in the Optometric Setting

To screen for hypertension during routine examination
In conjunction with diagnostic and therapeutic drug use
   Topical ophthalmic phenylephrine
   Topical ophthalmic hydroxyamphetamine
   Topical ophthalmic epinephrine and related compounds
   Topical ophthalmic β-adrenergic blocking agents
To aid in or augment clinical diagnosis
   Chronic open-angle glaucoma
   Low-tension glaucoma
   Repeated spontaneous subconjunctival hemorrhages
   Hypertensive retinopathy
   Retinal embolic phenomena
   Transient ischemic attacks
   Amaurosis fugax
   Headache
   Papilledema

Table 29–2
Effects of Cardiac Output and Peripheral Vascular Resistance on Blood Pressure ($BP = CO \times R$)

Cause	Clinical Example	Effect
Increased CO	Heavy exertion, such as exercise	Increased BP
Decreased CO	Myocardial infarction	Decreased BP
Increased R	Peripheral vasoconstriction from sympathomimetics such as phenylephrine or epinephrine	Increased BP
Decreased R	Peripheral vasodilation from sublingual nitroglycerin use	Decreased BP

Table 29–3
Other Factors Contributing to Arterial Blood Pressure Levels

Cause	Clinical Example	Effect
Blood volume	If reduced by major blood loss from trauma or surgery	Decreased BP
Blood viscosity	If elevated as measured by hematocrit in polycythemia	Increased BP
Arterial wall elasticity	If reduced because of atherosclerosis	Increased BP

hypertensive patients of the future will derive, is recently receiving more intensive study.[8]

Optometry provides most of primary eye care and, in many instances, may be the only health care professional that an individual may consult.[9] Thus, the doctor of optometry is in an excellent position to serve the overall health care needs of his or her patients by screening for hypertension in the course of delivering eye and vision care.[10–12] Optometry has been identified as an underutilized professional resource for hypertension screening.[13] Screening for hypertension can and should be routinely included in the optometrist's patient diagnostic procedures, with appropriate referrals made for further medical evaluation.[14–18] Besides the goals of detecting undiagnosed or uncontrolled hypertensives, blood pressure screening in the optometric setting, along with thorough medical history-taking, will help to reinforce patient compliance with treatment regimens, physician visits, and home monitoring, and will help to foster interprofessional communication and referrals.[19–21]

In addition to the use of sphygmomanometry to screen for hypertension during routine examination, the optometrist's knowledge of the blood pressure level may be important in the use of several diagnostic and therapeutic agents, and may aid in or augment the diagnostic process of several ophthalmic conditions.[22–29] Table 29–1 summarizes the clinical applications of blood pressure measurement in the optometric setting.

INSTRUMENTATION

Theory

The circulatory mechanism is a closed system comprised of the cardiac pump that forces a finite supply of blood through a complex arterial tree.[30] The systemic arterial blood pressure represents the force applied against blood vessel walls resulting from the direct effects of cardiac output (CO) and peripheral vascular resistance (R).[31] Specific alterations in cardiac output or peripheral vascular resistance may cause the blood pressure to increase or decrease (Table 29–2). Other factors that contribute to the level of arterial blood pressure include blood volume, blood viscosity, and arterial wall elasticity (Table 29–3). The body employs a variety of complex, and not yet fully delineated, internal regulatory mechanisms to maintain blood pressure at a relatively constant level. These regulatory devices provide for the efficient supply of blood to tissues that constantly vary in their circulatory needs.[32]

The *systolic pressure* is the pressure in the arteries, at the height of pulsation, caused by cardiac contraction as the left ventricle pumps blood into the aorta. The *diastolic pressure* is the pressure in the arteries during ventricular relaxation between cardiac contractions.[33] These pressures are expressed in millimeters of mercury (mmHg), indicating the height to which the blood pressure will raise a column of mercury against the force of gravity.[34] The blood pressure is recorded in ratio form with the systolic reading preceding the diastolic. A blood pressure reading of 140/90 is verbally referred to as "140 over 90."

Indirect Versus Direct Blood Pressure Measurement

The blood pressure of a patient who has sustained severe and extensive trauma, who is in the operating room undergoing major surgery, or who is critically ill in the intensive care unit can be measured directly. This is accomplished through the use of a catheter inserted into a major artery that is usually connected to an electronic-recording system.[35] The very familiar auscultatory technique to measure blood pressure that uses a stethoscope and sphygmomanometer is known as an *indirect method.*[36] Although not as accurate as the direct method, the indirect auscultatory method for determining systolic and diastolic pressures usually results in values that are within 10% of those obtained by direct measurement.[37]

The Korotkoff Sounds

With use of the narrow inflatable cuff described by Riva-Rocci in 1896, Korotkoff described the sounds produced from the time the artery was completely compressed until initial refilling occurred.[2] The first and last phases of these sounds, corresponding to their first audible detection to their disappearance, determine the systolic and diastolic readings, respectively (Table 29–4). The interim sounds between systole and diastole are probably produced by the spurting of arterial blood beneath the cuff to cause turbulence and vessel wall vibration (Fig. 29–1).[38]

Table 29–4
The Korotkoff Sounds

Phase I	Sudden appearance of clear, regular tapping sounds (systolic pressure; SP)
Phase II	A swishing softening of sounds
Phase III	Crisper sounds, increasing in intensity
Phase IV	Abrupt damping or muffling of sounds (diastolic pressure I; DP I)
Phase V	Complete disappearance of sound (diastolic pressure II; DP II)

COMMERCIALLY AVAILABLE INSTRUMENTS

There is a variety of sources for sphygmomanometers and stethoscopes. Sphygmomanometers are manufactured by such companies as Sargent-Welch, Bauman, Trimline, and Tycos. Stethoscopes are manufactured by Tycos and Littman, among others. To purchase either of these diagnostic instruments, contact a local medical equipment distributor for details about model features, cost, and availability.

Stethoscope

By preventing the dissipation of sound waves as they reach the body's surface and amplifying them for the clinician, the stethoscope is used to determine the systolic and diastolic readings through auscultation of the Korotkoff sounds. Although they may vary in construction and configuration, most stethoscopes are comprised of earpieces, binaurals, plastic or rubber tubing, and a chestpiece. The rubber- or plastic-coated earpieces should fit comfortably, but snugly, to block out external noises. To best receive the sound, the binaurals are angled to follow the contour of the auditory canal so that for most individuals the earpieces should point toward the face when the stethoscope is in place. A spring clamp connecting the binaurals is often present to help maintain tight contact with the auditory openings (Fig. 29–2).[34]

The chestpiece usually has two components, a bell and a diaphragm. It may, however, have a single surface or up to four surfaces (Fig. 29–3). The diaphragm is the circular, flat-surfaced

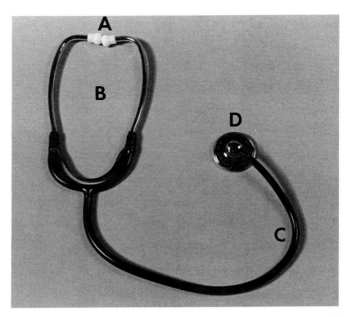

FIGURE 29–2. This single-head stethoscope comprises earpieces (*A*), binaurals (*B*), plastic or rubber tubing (*C*), and a chestpiece (*D*).

portion ending in a thin plastic disk that best transmits high-frequency sounds. A modification of the diaphragm, known as the corrugated diaphragm, increases the sound frequency range that can be efficiently received by the diaphragm and has been a favorably recommended chestpiece for blood pressure measurement.[39]

The bell side of the chestpiece transmits low-frequency sounds, such as heart or vascular sounds. Firmer pressure of the bell against the patient's skin will more efficiently detect high-frequency sounds. Depending on the need of the examiner, either the bell or diaphragm portion of the chestpiece is rotated or "clicked" into position so that sounds are transmitted.

Sphygmomanometer

The blood pressure cuff, or sphygmomanometer, is comprised of a nonstretchable fabric bag that joins at the ends by Velcro cloth strips and contains an inflatable rubber bladder. Connected to the

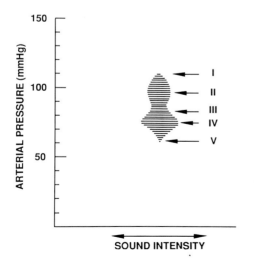

FIGURE 29–1. Intensity of the Korotkoff sounds corresponding to a theoretical blood pressure measurement of 116/62. (Modified with permission from Sykes MK, Vickers MD, Hull CJ. Principles of clinical measurement. Oxford, Engl: Blackwell Scientific Publications, 1981:173)

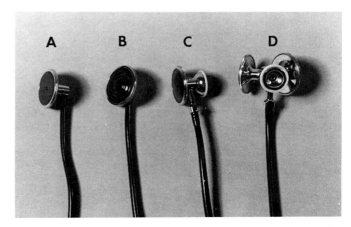

FIGURE 29–3. Sample available chestpieces: a single-head diaphragm (*A*), a corrugated diaphragm (*B*), a double-head with a bell and diaphragm (*C*), and a triple-head (*D*).

cuff by one or more rubber tubes are an inflating bulb, with a pressure-release valve, and a manometer gauge for measuring the pressure in the bladder.

Currently, in the clinical setting, the cuff pressure is usually registered by either a mercury or an aneroid manometer. The mercury manometer contains a narrow vertical column of mercury within a glass or unbreakable plastic tube that is set upright on a table top, is wall-mounted, or is on a floor stand[40] (Fig. 29–4). When the examiner notes the appropriate Korotkoff sounds, the meniscus level of the mercury is read at eye level from the adjacent millimeter scale. Although less conveniently portable than many aneroid types, the mercury manometer is generally viewed to be the standard against which all other blood pressure measurement devices are compared.[41] Accuracy is generally ensured when the meniscus level reads "zero" when no pressure is applied and when the column is observed to fall freely as the cuff pressure is released.[42]

The aneroid manometer contains a small metal bellows or spring that moves a needle across a calibrated dial to register changes in pressure. Although most aneroid manometers have a small oval, rectangular, or similarly shaped area at the 6 o'clock position on the dial to mark the normal "zero" position of the uninflated cuff, the nature of their construction makes them subject to drift and somewhat less reliable than the mercury manometers. Although the needle may rest at the appropriate zero position, this does not guarantee that the reading will be accurate throughout cuff deflation. It is suggested that the aneroid manometer be recalibrated against a perfectly working mercury manometer at least annually.[41,43] Various styles of aneroid sphygmomanometers are available, including hand (combined manometer gauge and inflation bulb), pocket (separate manometer gauge and inflation bulb), wall-mounted, and stand-mounted (Fig. 29–5).

The length of the arterial segment that is compressed by the inflated cuff during blood pressure measurement is one of the most important factors influencing the accuracy of the reading.[44] Thus, over the years, numerous studies have been conducted to determine the optimum cuff width and length. It has been determined that sphygmomanometry in the average-sized adult is most accurate when performed with a cuff 12 to 14 cm wide.[28] This will generally correspond to a cuff size that is approximately 40% of the arm's circumference.[44] In clinical practice it is unusual for the practitioner to measure arm circumference to determine the correct cuff size, although the relationship of cuff width to arm circumference can be grossly assessed by wrapping the cuff sideways around the patient's arm.[45]

Usually, clinical judgment and common sense will dictate cuff size needs along with ensuring that the rubber bladder encircles at least two-thirds of the arm circumference.[5] If the patient is obese or extremely muscular, the regular adult size cuff will not fit around the arm adequately, especially as the bladder is inflated. The six standardly available cuff sizes are newborn, infant, child, adult, large adult, and thigh for taking blood pressure of the leg. The cuff sizes most commonly used in optometric practice are child, adult, and large adult (Fig. 29–6). Alternatively, the practitioner will have on hand several-sized cuff and inflatable bladder combinations that can be interchanged with the aneroid or mercurial manometers and inflation bulbs as needed.

In the mid- to late-1960s techniques were described that used Doppler ultrasonic methods to measure the pulsatile movement of the brachial artery during deflation of the pneumatic cuff.[44] A number of electronic sphygmomanometers are now commercially available that are based on the Doppler ultrasonic principle, oscillometry, or they incorporate small microphones to detect the Korotkoff sounds.[46] The sensor is usually built into the cuff, eliminating the need for the stethoscope, and the readings are frequently registered by flashing lights, beeping sounds, or digital readouts (Fig. 29–7).[47]

Although electronic devices have some applicability, particu-

Table 29–5
Categories of Available Sphygmomanometers

Mercury manometer
Aneroid manometer
Electronic
Stationary automated
Automatic ambulatory

larly as in-home monitoring devices, and are easy to use, they are currently not widely utilized in-office. They are often more expensive than aneroid or mercury sphygmomanometers, require precise alignment of the sensor or microphone over the artery, will be affected by excess arm movement, are frequently less accurate, and require greater maintenance.[28,48] The value of in-home automatic or semiautomatic blood pressure measurement devices is maximized if the manufacturer has documented the validity and reliability of the unit and if it is periodically calibrated and maintained.[41] Further technological advancement, however, may enhance the reliability of this instrumentation, leading to more widespread use among health care professionals.

Stationary automated machines have been installed in many public places such as work sites, airports, and shopping malls. They are usually fully automated so that a push of the button will trigger inflation and deflation of the cuff. Concerns have been expressed about the reliability of the readings obtained and the frequency of calibration of these instruments.[41]

Since the mid-1970s, noninvasive, automatic ambulatory blood pressure monitors have been studied as a method to assess blood pressure around-the-clock as the patient pursues his normal activities. These prescription-only devices are utilized under physician supervision and can be programmed to measure between 12 to 200 readings in a 24-hour period.[49] Guidelines suggested by the National High Blood Pressure Education Program indicate that the ambulatory monitors are not yet intended as a routine, practical, or cost-effective means for monitoring most patients.[41] However, substantial research data support the use of these units to aid in the diagnosis and management of hypertension, specifically as it relates to the response of blood pressure to medication, as a prognostic indicator relating to target organ damage and clinical outcome, and in verifying discrepancies in blood pressure readings obtained in and out of the health care setting.[50,51] Table 29–5 lists the various categories of available sphygmomanometers.

CLINICAL PROCEDURE

Patient Preparation

Before measurement of the blood pressure is begun, the patient should be as comfortable and relaxed as possible. It is recommended that the measurement be taken after 5 minutes of quiet rest and that caffeine consumption, smoking, and exercise be avoided in the 30 minutes before the measurement is taken.[5] The arm to be measured should be slightly bent with the palm turned upward and supported on the arm of a chair or table, slightly above waist level, so that the stethoscope head will be positioned at the level of the heart.[43] The forearm is usually freed of clothing, and care should be taken that a rolled up sleeve does not excessively constrict the upper arm (Fig. 29–8).[52] Blood pressure readings have been successfully obtained through a single layer of thin fabric, such as the sleeve of a nylon jacket or blouse.[53]

1. *Localizing the brachial artery and applying the cuff.* The brachial artery is palpated just below the antecubital
(*Text continues on page 273*)

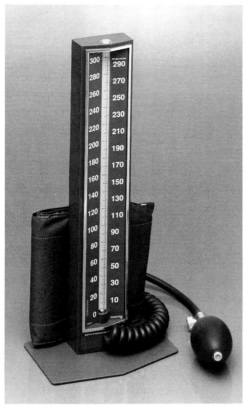

A

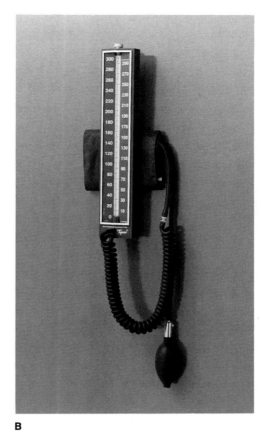

B

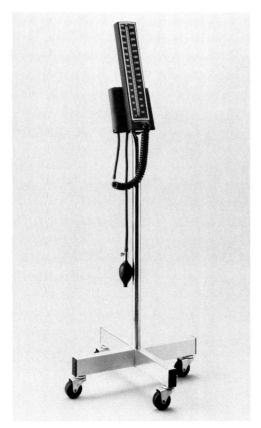

C

FIGURE 29–4. The mercurial sphygmomanometer may be set on a table top (*A*), wall-mounted (*B*), or on a floor stand (*C*). (Courtesy Tycos Instruments, Inc., a Welch–Allyn Company)

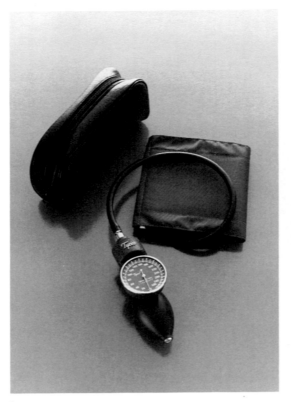

A

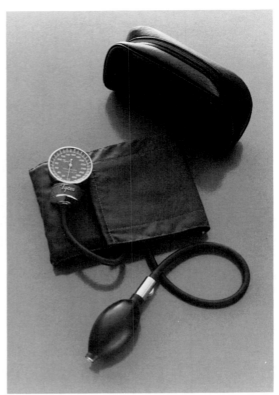

B

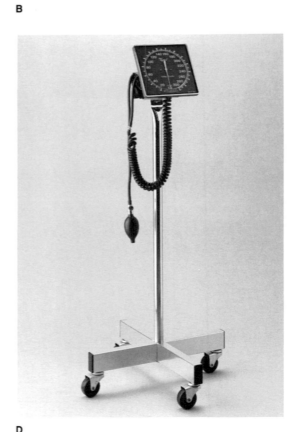

C

D

FIGURE 29–5. Various available aneroid sphygmomanometers: hand (*A*), pocket (*B*), wall-mounted (*C*), and stand-mounted (*D*). (Courtesy Tycos Instruments, Inc., a Welch–Allyn Company)

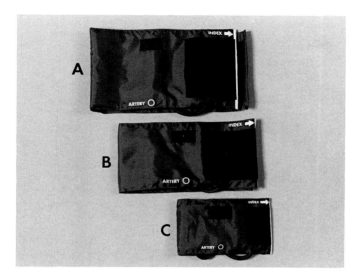

FIGURE 29–6. Blood pressure cuffs: large adult size (*A*), regular adult size (*B*), and child size (*C*).

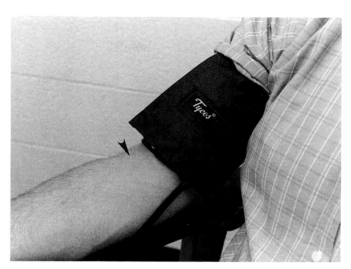

FIGURE 29–9. The lower border of the blood pressure cuff should lie approximately 2.5 cm (1 in.) above the antecubital crease (*arrowhead*).

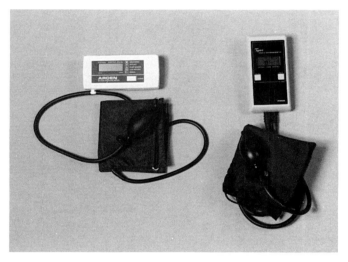

FIGURE 29–7. An electronic home blood pressure unit (*left*), and an in-office electronic unit (*right*).

crease, the bend of the elbow (see Fig. 29–8). The bladder of the cuff is centered on the upper arm overlying the brachial artery, lining up the appropriate arrow on the cuff for the right or left arm. The lower border of the cuff should lie approximately 2.5 cm (1 in.) above the antecubital crease. The cuff should be wrapped smoothly and secured snugly (Fig. 29–9).[39,54]

2. *Palpation for systolic pressure.* In most procedure descriptions of blood pressure measurement, it is recommended that the clinician palpate the systsolic pressure to avoid an artificially low reading produced by auscultatory gap. With the forefinger and middle-finger of one hand gently palpating the radial artery at the wrist, the cuff is inflated to approximately 30 mmHg above the level at which the pulse disappears (Fig. 29–10). The cuff is deflated smoothly at a rate of approximately 2–3 mmHg/sec until the pulse is first palpated, and the clinician makes a mental note of the manometer reading. The cuff is then rapidly and steadily deflated completely (see Fig. 29–7).[43,55]

3. *Placing the stethoscope.* The clinician sets the binaurals of the stethoscope in place as previously described. The dia-

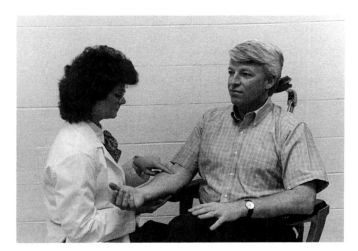

FIGURE 29–8. With the patient's arm in proper position, the brachial artery is palpated just below the antecubital crease, the bend of the elbow.

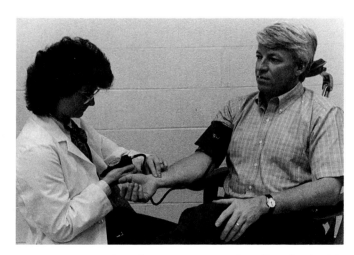

FIGURE 29–10. Before taking a measurement, the cuff is inflated and the systolic pressure is palpated.

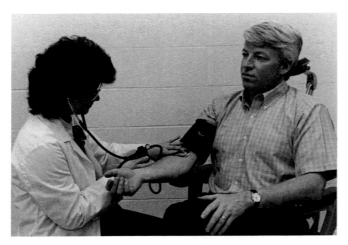

FIGURE 29–11. To measure the blood pressure, the chestpiece diaphragm is placed over the brachial artery between the antecubital crease and the lower edge of the cuff. The cuff is inflated and the Korotkoff sounds are auscultated.

phragm of the chestpiece is placed gently but firmly over the brachial artery between the antecubital crease and the lower edge of the cuff. Contact between the chestpiece and the cuff should be avoided to prevent the production of confusing frictional noises.[56] Although the bell side of the chestpiece may more effectively detect the low-frequency Korotkoff sounds, better skin–chestpiece contact can usually be achieved when the diaphragm is used (Fig. 29–11).[43,45]

4. *Taking the measurement.* To measure the blood pressure by auscultation, the cuff is inflated to approximately 20 to 30 mmHg above the systolic pressure determined by palpation. By using the manometer release valve, the air in the bladder is smoothly released at the rate of approximately 2–3 mmHg/sec. The first audible (Phase I) Korotkoff sound corresponds to the systolic reading, and the clinician mentally notes the manometer reading when the Phase I sound is heard.

The various other Korotkoff sounds will be audible with continued deflation of the cuff and, then, will disappear. The disappearance of sounds (Phase V) is the generally accepted diastolic reading for most patients. The examiner mentally notes the manometer reading when Phase V is noted, listens for an additional 10 to 20 mmHg below Phase V, to confirm sound disappearance, then rapidly deflates the cuff completely. If a repeat reading is necessary, it is recommended that this be done after 1 to 2 minutes to permit the release of blood trapped in the brachial venous system.[43]

By convention in the medical community, both the systolic and diastolic readings are recorded to the nearest 2 mmHg.[57] The blood pressure reading is entered in the patient record, indicating the position of the patient and which arm was used for measurement. For example, an entry of 150/90 R.A. Sit. would indicate that the measurement was done "right arm, sitting."[58] If a cuff size other than the regular adult was used, this information is noted as well.[43] Kaplan has suggested that the time of day the measurement was taken also be recorded.[59] Table 29–6 is a step-by-step procedural listing for measuring blood pressure.

Table 29–6
Procedural Steps for Measuring Blood Pressure by Indirect Auscultation

1. Put the patient at ease as best possible
2. Prepare the patient's arm to be used for measurement
   Arm is slightly bent, palm upward
   Arm is fully supported at heart level
   Forearm is freed of excess clothing
3. Palpate the brachial artery below the antecubital crease
4. Center the cuff bladder over the brachial artery, wrap snugly
5. Determine the systolic pressure by palpation; deflate
6. Place the stethoscope diaphragm over the brachial artery
7. Reinflate the cuff 30-mm above the systolic pressure
8. Auscultate for Phase I and Phase V sounds, deflating 2–3 mmHg/sec, noting manometer readings
9. Rapidly deflate the cuff fully
10. Wait 1–2 min before repeating the reading if necessary
11. Record SP/DP, arm used, patient position, pertinent cuff size

CLINICAL IMPLICATIONS

Clinical Significance

The diagnosis of hypertension is not made on the basis of one elevated in-office reading. Usually two to three readings taken at several different visits are considered necessary to diagnose essential or primary hypertension.[59,60] Two readings taken during a visit are averaged, and if these first two measurements differ by more than 5 mmHg, additional readings are taken and averaged in.[5] However, if the blood pressure is severely elevated (see Table 29–7) the patient is referred immediately for medical care.

Over the years the accepted upper limits of normal blood pressure measurements have lowered as the relationship of even minimally elevated blood pressure (mild hypertension) and the risk of cerebrovascular accident (stroke), myocardial infarction (heart attack), congestive heart failure, chronic occlusive peripheral vascular disease, aortic aneurysms, and renal failure in all age groups has been more clearly elucidated.[61–64] Research has indicated that even isolated systolic hypertension in the elderly with normal diastolic readings should be evaluated for possible treatment.[65]

Guidelines for normal blood pressure readings, the classification of hypertension, and the recommended guidelines for medical follow-up are shown in Table 29–7.

Clinical Interpretation

Diurnal Variation

Similar to the observed phenomenon of diurnal variation of intraocular pressure readings, blood pressure measurements will naturally vary over a 24-hour period. With use of an intra-arterial (direct) device continuously over a 24-hour period in 20 untreated ambulatory hypertensives, Millar-Craig et al. reported the highest blood pressure values in the midmorning, a progressive fall throughout the day, and lowest readings during sleep.[66] The variation from the lowest to the highest systolic or diastolic reading was observed to be as much as 40 mm. Higher blood pressure levels will exhibit greater diurnal variability.[67] As anticipated, isolated spikes of pressure rise will occur throughout the day in response to particular stimuli and environmental effects, such as pain, excitement, exercise, and such.[68,69]

Table 29-7
Classification of BP with the Recommended Guidelines for Medical Follow-up Based on Initial Readings

BP Range (mmHg)	Category	Recommended Follow-up
Adults (Over Age 18 Years)		
≤95/60	Hypotension	Routine unless symptomatic
Diastolic		
<85	Normal BP	Recheck within 2 years
85–89	High-normal BP	Recheck within 1 year
90–104	Mild hypertension	Confirm within 2 months
105–115	Moderate hypertension	Medical care should be obtained within 2 weeks
≥115	Severe hypertension	Medical care should be obtained immediately
Systolic, when diastolic <90		
<140	Normal BP	Recheck within 2 years
140–159	Borderline isolated systolic hypertension	Confirm within 2 months
≥160	Isolated systolic hypertension	Confirm within 2 months
≥200	None given	Medical care should be obtained within 2 weeks
Children		
<135/90	Ages 14–18 years	Routine
<125/85	Ages 10–14 years	Routine
<120/80	Ages 6–10 years	Routine
<110/75	Less than 6 years	Routine

(Adapted from the 1988 Report of the Joint National Committee on Detection, Evaluation, and Treatment of High Blood Pressure. Arch Intern Med 1988;148, and Kaplan NM. Hypertension in the population at large. Clinical hypertension. Baltimore: Williams & Wilkins, 1986:13.)

Interobserver Variability

Certain skill levels are required of the observer to allow for accurate blood pressure measurement. These include adequate hearing to recognize the Korotkoff sounds; adequate vision to read the manometer calibration marks; adequate coordination of eye, hand, and ear skills; and an ability to recall the readings and record them accurately.[70]

For a variety of reasons, including errors in technique, inadequate training, carelessness, digit preferencing, and preconceived expectations, blood pressure readings have been found to vary widely between different observers.[71] Mitchell and Van Meter, in comparing sphygmomanometry readings obtained by nursing personnel and the investigators, found differences of more than 15 mmHg in 21% to 27% of the readings.[72] Scherwitz et al. noted that 14% of the diastolic blood pressure readings taken by physicians varied by more than 15 mmHg.[73]

Diastolic End Point

Some controversy persists over the correct and more accurate diastolic reading, either Phase IV Korotkoff (Diastolic I), when the muffling of sound first occurs, or the complete disappearance of sounds of Phase V Korotkoff (Diastolic II).[74,75] The average difference between Phase IV and Phase V diastolic values for most patients is approximately 5 mmHg.[76] It is probably somewhat easier to subjectively interpret the disappearance of sound as the end point, rather than the muffling of sound. Although most clinicians

record the disappearance of sound (Phase V) as the diastolic reading, some practitioners elect to record both end points (e.g., 150/90/70). The American Heart Association recommends that Phase V be used for the diastolic blood pressure reading for adults, except for those with hyperkinetic conditions, such as hyperthyroidism, or following exercise. For the hyperkinetic adult and for children Phase IV is recommended as the diastolic end point.[58]

Difference in Right and Left Arm Readings

Many authors suggest that, during at least the initial visit to the physician's office, the blood pressure of both arms should be measured. If a difference in the readings between the two arms is noted, the arm with the higher reading is used for future measurements.[59] A 5- to 10-mmHg discrepancy between the two arm readings is viewed to be within normal limits.[57] Differences in the readings between the right and left arms greater than 10 to 15 mmHg could be indicative of atherosclerotic narrowing of the subclavian or brachiocephalic arteries, as an age-related change consistent with more diffuse atherosclerotic involvement or, specifically, as part of the subclavian steal syndrome. In the latter condition, marked stenosis of the subclavian or brachiocephalic artery occurs proximal to the origin of the vertebral artery so that blood flows in a retrograde direction from the contralateral vertebral artery through the basilar artery. Because of subclavian steal, the difference in blood pressure between the right and left arms will be marked. In evaluating the blood pressure of 155 patients with subclavian steal, Fields and Lemak found the average systolic blood pressure differential between the right and left arms to be 45 mmHg.[77] For most patients, however, there is probably no significant average difference between the right and left arm blood pressure readings.[46]

Weak or Inaudible Korotkoff Sounds

Attempting to assess weak or inaudible Korotkoff sounds may result in variable blood pressure readings. Accentuation of the Korotkoff sounds may be accomplished by several techniques, used singly or in combination.[45] Blood flow within the brachial artery may be enhanced by asking the patient to open and clench his fist approximately ten times, either just before or during cuff inflation. Elevating the patient's arm before inflating the cuff will empty the blood from the forearm and will increase the gradient in flow between the portions of the artery proximal and distal to the cuff. The clinician should lift the patient's arm, as isometric exercise by the patient to hold the arm up may elevate the diastolic blood pressure by slightly over 10%.[78] Finally, inflating the cuff quickly will minimize the amount of blood trapped in the forearm due to venous congestion that decreases the flow gradient of the arterial blood passing under the cuff during deflation and may reduce the audibility of the Korotkoff sounds.

Orthostatic (Postural) Hypotension

An adult whose blood pressure is 95/60 or less, without a postural change, is considered to be hypotensive. In the healthy adult patient with no symptoms, a systolic blood pressure that persists in the range of 90 to 100 mmHg is not clinically significant.[55]

As a patient changes from a lying or sitting position to a standing position, the systolic pressure drops slightly or remains unchanged, whereas the diastolic pressure rises slightly.[57] A patient under treatment with antihypertensive medication or who has a history of fainting or postural dizziness may have orthostatic (postural) hypotension caused by a substantial drop in blood pressure upon rising. The fall in blood pressure is usually at least 25 mmHg systolic and 10 mmHg diastolic.[79] Orthostatic hypertension

Table 29–8
Possible Sources of Variability in Blood Pressure Measurement

Diurnal variation
Interobserver variability
Diastolic end point
Difference in right and left arm readings
Weak or inaudible Korotkoff sounds
Orthostatic hypotension

will be apparent by the changes in blood pressure measured in the supine, sitting, and standing positions.

Table 29–8 lists possible sources of variability in blood pressure measurement.

Besides the multiple factors that contribute to blood pressure variability, several factors may result in blood pressure readings that are artificially low or high (Table 29–9).

Falsely Low Readings

The use of a cuff that is too wide for the patient's arm will produce an artificially low reading because less pressure will be needed to collapse the artery. Deflating the cuff too fast will result in an underestimation of the systolic pressure.[57] If the patient's arm is positioned above the level of the heart, the blood pressure reading will be artificially low.[80]

Auscultatory gap refers to the silence caused by the disappearance of the Korotkoff sounds between Phase I and Phase II that may occur in some hypertensive patients. This sound gap may cover a range of 10 to 40 mmHg. If the examiner does not inflate the cuff sufficiently, this auscultatory gap may be misinterpreted as the absence of sound preceding Korotkoff Phase I and the systolic pressure will be underestimated.[34] If the cuff is inflated until the brachial artery pulse is palpably obliterated, this misinterpretation of the gap will be avoided.[36]

Constant[45] describes a somewhat more practical approach to avoiding auscultatory gap. He contends that the gap can be prevented by rapidly inflating the cuff after having the patient open and clench his fist ten times. Constant then inflates the cuff to 140 mmHg. If Korotkoff sounds are heard at this level, the cuff is inflated another 20 mmHg. Listening and inflating are repeated until no Korotkoff sounds are heard and the systolic and diastolic readings are taken as usual.

Table 29–9
Possible Sources of Error in Blood Pressure Measurement

Falsely Low Readings
Cuff too wide
Deflating the cuff too rapidly (systolic)
Patient's arm above heart level
Auscultatory gap

Falsely High Readings
Patient anxiety, fear, emotional distress
Cuff too narrow
Cuff too loose
Deflating the cuff too slowly (diastolic)
Deflating the cuff too rapidly (diastolic)
Patient's arm below heart level
Pseudohypertension

Falsely High Readings

Patient anxiety, fear, and emotional distress produce an elevation of blood pressure. Patient anxiety is common during medical examinations of all types, particularly when the doctor is present. This iatrogenic, in-office anxiety has led some observers to describe the phenomenon known as "office" or "white coat" hypertension. In-home measurements have been found to be consistently lower than in-office measurements by as much as 5 to 10 mmHg and will generally continue to reduce over time.[81,82] The iatrogenic anxiety factor has been shown to elevate blood pressure by as much as 30 to 50 mmHg.[83] To minimize this effect on elevating the blood pressure, the examiner, as with all procedures, should put the patient at ease as much as possible. It may be advisable to postpone the blood pressure measurement to later in the course of the examination, for the anxiety effect has been shown to dampen after approximately 10 minutes of contact with even an unfamiliar doctor.[84] Blood pressure measurement by trained personnel other than the doctor may also help to reduce the anxiety factor.[83] It has also been suggested that two or three blood pressure readings be taken at each medical office visit and that the average of the three should be taken.[59,85]

Use of a cuff that is either too narrow for the size of the patient's arm or a cuff that is too loose will result in readings that are artificially high because additional pressure will be needed to compress the artery.[86] Deflating the cuff too slowly produces venous congestion, which falsely elevates the diastolic pressure and may also produce patient discomfort.[42] Deflating the cuff too rapidly will also elevate the diastolic reading.[57] If the arm is positioned below the level of the heart, the reading will be slightly high.[80] If an elderly patient has very rigid, calcified arteries excessive pressure within the cuff bladder may be required to collapse the brachial artery and a high reading will result. This phenomenon is known as pseudohypertension.[87]

ACKNOWLEDGMENTS

Appreciation is extended to Tycos Instruments, Inc., a Welch–Allyn Company, for the loan of instruments used in Figures 29–2, 29–3, and 29–6 through 29–11 and to Jacque Kubley for photographic assistance.

REFERENCES

1. Stedman's medical dictionary, 24th ed. Baltimore: Williams & Wilkins Co, 1982:1173.
2. Booth J. A short history of BP measurement. Proc R Soc Med 1977;70:793–799.
3. Kleinstein RN. New screening criterion for systemic hypertension. Optom Monthly 1980;71:89–91.
4. Kaplan NM. Treatment of hypertension: nondrug therapy and the rationale for therapy. In: Clinical hypertension, 4th ed. Baltimore: Williams & Wilkins Co, 1986:147–179.
5. Joint National Committee on Detection, Evaluation, and Treatment of High Blood Pressure. 1988 report. Arch Intern Med 1988;148:1023–1038.
6. Joint National Committee on Detection, Evaluation, and Treatment of High Blood Pressure. Hypertension prevalence and the status of awareness, treatment and control in the United States: final report of the Subcommittee on Definition and Prevalence, 1984.
7. Prineas RJ, Gillum R. Epidemiology of hypertension in blacks. In: Hall WD, Saunders E, Shulman NB, eds. Hypertension in blacks: epidemiology, pathophysiology and treatment. Chicago: Yearbook Medical Publishers, Inc, 1985:17–36.
8. Horan MJ, Sinaiko AR. Synopsis of the report of the Second Task Force on Blood Pressure Control in Children. Hypertension 1987;10:115–121.
9. Kleinstein RN, Maxwell L, Wayne JB, et al. Screening for hypertension. J Am Optom Assoc 1982;53:379–381.

10. Augsburger AR, Good GW. Hypertension: an optometric problem for the 80's. J Am Optom Assoc 1986;57:355–359.

11. Guerrein RL. Who's screening for what . . . and who should be. Rev Optom 1977;114:68–73.

12. Lenfant C, Roccella EJ. National high blood pressure education program. J Am Optom Assoc 1986;57:347–348.

13. Pierce JR, Kleinstein RN. Screening for hypertension by optometrists. Am J Public Health 1977;67:977–979.

14. Daubs JG. A protocol for hypertension screening and referral. Am J Optom Physiol Opt 1975;52:351–357.

15. Terry JE. Screening for hypertension during the eye examination. Rev Optom 1977;114:45–47.

16. Walls LL, Pheiffer CH, VanVeen H. A simple guide to high blood pressure screening. Rev Optom 1981;118:57–61.

17. Werner DL, Podell S. Effectiveness of hypertension screening in an urban optometric setting. J Am Optom Assoc 1978;49:1393–1397.

18. Werthamer ER. Blood pressure measurement and patient satisfaction with the optometric examination. J Am Optom Assoc 1984;55:333–336.

19. Good GW, Augsburger AR. Role of optometrists in combating high blood pressure. J Am Optom Assoc 1989;5:352–355.

20. Levy RI, Ward GW. The optometrist and hypertension control: a cooperative effort is the key. J Am Optom Assoc 1979;50:529–530.

21. McQuarrie CW. Optometry, a preventive profession. J Am Optom Assoc 1979;50:526–528.

22. Drance SM, et al. Studies of factors involved in the production of low tension glaucoma. Arch Ophthalmol 1963;89:457–465.

23. Jaanus SD, Pagano VT, Bartlett JD. Drugs affecting the automatic nervous system. In: Bartlett JD, Jaanus SD, eds. Clinical ocular pharmacology, 2nd ed. Boston: Butterworths, 1989:69–148.

24. Kaplan NM. Hypertensive crises. In: Clinical hypertension, 4th ed. Baltimore: Williams & Wilkins Co, 1986:273–291.

25. Lieberman E. Hypertension in childhood and adolescence. In: Kaplan NM. Clinical hypertension, 4th ed. Baltimore: Williams & Wilkins Co, 1986:447–472.

26. Locke LC. Induced refractive and visual changes. In: Amos JF, ed. Diagnosis and management in vision care. Boston: Butterworths, 1987:313–368.

27. Stelmack TR. Headache. In: Amos JF, ed. Diagnosis and management in vision care. Boston: Butterworths, 1987:9–42.

28. Terry JE. Sphygmomanometry. In: Terry JE, ed. Ocular disease (detection, diagnosis and treatment). Springfield, Ill: Charles C Thomas, 1984:242–287.

29. Wallace W. Diseases of the conjunctiva. In: Bartlett JD, Jaanus SD, eds. Clinical ocular pharmacology, 2nd ed. Boston: Butterworths, 1989:515–566.

30. Weller H, Wiley RL. Cardiovascular and lymphatic systems. In: Basic human physiology, 2nd ed. Boston: Prindle, Weber & Schmidt, 1985:381–427.

31. Guyton AC. Physics of blood, blood flow, and pressure: hemodynamics. In: Textbook of medical physiology, 6th ed. Philadelphia: WB Saunders Co, 1981:206–218.

32. Page, IH. Measurement of blood pressure. In: Hypertension mechanisms. Orlando, Fla: Grune & Stratton, 1987:14–15.

33. Tortora GJ, Evans RL. Cardiovascular physiology. In: Principles of human physiology, 2nd ed. New York: Harper & Row, 1986:511–546.

34. Potter PA, Perry AG. Vital signs. In: Basic nursing theory and practice. St Louis: CV Mosby Co, 1987:202–211.

35. Sykes MK, Vickers MD, Hull CJ. Direct measurement of intravascular pressure. In: Principles of clinical measurement, 2nd ed. Oxford, Engl: Blackwell Scientific Publications, 1981:159–172.

36. Narrow BW, Buschle KB. The assessment phase of nursing process. In: Fundamentals of nursing practice. New York: John Wiley & Sons, 1987:296–299.

37. Guyton AC. Short-term regulation of mean arterial pressure: nervous reflex and hormonal mechanisms for rapid pressure control. In: Textbook of medical physiology, 6th ed. Philadelphia: WB Saunders Co, 1981:246–258.

38. Berne RM, Levy MN. The arterial system. In: Cardiovascular physiology, 5th ed. St Louis, CV Mosby Co, 1986:134–135.

39. Ballard PD. Office procedures for the indirect determination of blood pressure. Rev Optom 1977;114:46–55.

40. Fedder DO, Frohlich ED, Zweifler AJ. Sphygmomanometers: which to choose? Patient Care 1987;21:67–76.

41. Hunt JC, Frohlich ED, Moser M, et al. Devices used for self-measurement of blood pressure. Arch Intern Med 1985;145:2231–2234.

42. Jarvis CM. Assessing pulse, respiration and blood pressure. In: Sorensen KC, Luckmann J, eds. Basic nursing. Philadelphia: WB Saunders Co, 1986:538–550.

43. American Heart Association. Recommendations for human blood pressure determination by sphygmomanometers, report of a special task force appointed by the steering committee, 1987.

44. Geddes LA. The indirect measurement of blood pressure in man. In: The direct and indirect measurement of blood pressure. Chicago: Yearbook Medical Publishers Inc, 1970:98–134.

45. Constant J. Accurate blood pressure measurement. Postgrad Med 1987;81:73–86.

46. O'Brien E, Fitzgerald D, O'Malley K. Blood pressure measurement: current practice and future trends. Br Med J 1985;290:729–734.

47. Buyer's guide to sphygmomanometers and stethoscopes. Rev Optom 1977;114:59–66.

48. Guirlani BP, Obie LG, Petersen CG, et al. A comparison of a semiautomated sphygmomanometer with a conventional sphygmomanometer for estimation of blood pressure. Optom Weekly 1977;68:1431–1434.

49. White WB. Ambulatory blood pressure monitoring. Physicians Comput 1987;5:32–35.

50. Perloff D, Sokolow M, Cowan R. The prognostic value of ambulatory blood pressures. JAMA 1983;249:2792–2798.

51. White WB. Assessment of patients with office hypertension by 24-hour noninvasive ambulatory blood pressure monitoring. Arch Intern Med 1986;146:2196–2199.

52. Delp MH, Manning RT. The cardiovascular system. In: Major's physical diagnosis, 9th ed. Philadelphia: WB Saunders Co, 1981:235–237.

53. Goldwater S. Blood pressure measurement [Letter]. Br Med J 1979;2:1443.

54. O'Brien ET, O'Malley K. ABC of blood pressure measurement: the sphygmomanometer. Br Med J 1979;2:851–853.

55. Judge RD, Zuidema GD, Fitzgerald FT. Vital signs. In: Clinical diagnosis, 4th ed. Boston: Little, Brown & Co, 1982:55–58.

56. O'Brien ET, O'Malley K. ABC of blood pressure measurement: technique. Br Med J 1979;2:982–983.

57. Bates B. The cardiovascular system. In: Examination and history taking, 4th ed. Philadelphia: JB Lippencott Co, 1987:271–276.

58. Kirkendall WM, Feinleib M, Freis ED, et al. AHA recommendations for human blood pressure determination by sphygmomanometers. Circulation 1980;62:1146A–1155A.

59. Kaplan NM. Hypertension in the individual patient. In: Clinical hypertension, 4th ed. Baltimore: Williams & Wilkins Co, 1986:29–55.

60. Hartley RM, Velez R, Morris RW, et al. Confirming the diagnosis of mild hypertension. Br Med J 1983;286:287–289.

61. Amery A, Brixko P, Clement D, et al. Mortality and morbidity results from the European Working Party on High Blood Pressure in the Elderly Trial. Lancet 1985;1:1349–1354.

62. Kannel WB, Doyle JT, Ostfeld AM, et al: Optimal resources for primary prevention of atherosclerotic diseases: atherosclerosis study group. Circulation 1984;70:153A–205A.

63. Breckenridge A. Treating mild hypertension. Br Med J 1985;291:89–90.

64. Medical Research Council Working Party. MRC trial of treatment of mild hypertension: principal results. Br Med J 1985;291:97–104.

65. The Working Group on Hypertension in the Elderly. 1985 statement. JAMA 1986;256:70–74.

66. Millar–Craig MW, Bishop CN, Raftery EB. Circadian variation of blood-pressure. Lancet 1978;1:795–797.

67. Watson RDS, Stallard TH, Flinn RM, et al. Hypertension 1980;2:333–341.

68. Bevan AT, Honour AJ, Stott FH. Direct arterial pressure recording in unrestricted man. Clin Sci 1969;36:329–344.

69. Littler WA, Honour Aj, Pugsley DJ, et al. Continuous recording of the direct arterial pressure in unrestricted patients. Circulation 1975;51:1101–1106.

70. Curb JD, Labarthe DR, Cooper SP, et al. Training and certification of blood pressure observers. Hypertension 1984;5:610–614.

71. O'Brien ET, O'Malley K. ABC of blood pressure measurement: the observer. Br Med J 1979;2:775–776.

72. Mitchell PW, VanMeter M. Reproducibility of blood pressures recorded on patients' records by nursing personnel. Nurs Res 1971;20:348–352.

73. Scherwitz LW, Evans LA, Hennrikus DJ, et al. Med Care 1982;20:727–738.

74. Manek S, Rutherford J, Jackson SHD, et al. Persistence of divergent views of hospital staff in detecting and managing hypertension. Br Med J 1984;289:1433–1434.

75. Rose G. Standardization of observers in blood pressure measurement. Lancet 1965;1:673–674.

76. Sykes MK, Vickers MD, Hull CJ. Indirect methods for measuring arterial pressure. In: Principles of clinical measurement, 2nd ed. Oxford, Engl: Blackwell Scientific Publications, 1981:173–181.

77. Fields WS, Lemak NA. Joint study of extracranial arterial occlusion VII subclavian steal—a review of 168 cases. JAMA 1972;222:1139–1143.

78. Silverberg DS, Shemesh E, Iaina A. The unsupported arm: a cause of falsely raised blood pressure readings. Br Med J 1977;2:1331.

79. Schulz IJ. Clinical diagnosis. In: Orthostatic hypotension. Philadelphia: FA Davis Co, 1986:67–89.

80. Mitchell PL, Parlin RW, Blackburn H. Effect of vertical displacement of the arm in indirect blood-pressure measurement. N Engl J Med 1964;271:72–74.

81. Laughlin KD, Fisher L, Sherrard DJ. Blood pressure reductions during self-recording of home blood pressure. Am Heart J 1979;98:629–634.

82. Pickering TG, Harshfield GA, Devereux RB, et al. What is the role of ambulatory blood pressure monitoring in the management of hypertensive patients? Hypertension 1985;7:171–177.

83. Mancia G, Parati G, Pomidossi G, et al. Alerting reaction and rise in blood pressure during measurement by physician and nurse. Hypertension 1987;9:209–215.

84. Mancia G, Grassi G, Pomidossi G, et al. Effects of blood pressure measurement by the doctor on the patient's blood pressure and heart rate. Lancet 1983;2:695–698.

85. Souchek J, Stamler J, Dyer AR, et al. The value of 2 or 3 versus a single reading of blood pressure at a first visit. J Chronic Dis 1979;32:197–210.

86. Maxwell MH, Waks AU, Schroth PC, et al. Error in blood-pressure measurement due to incorrect cuff size in obese patients. Lancet 1982;2:33–36.

87. Kaplan NM. Hypertension in the population at large. In: Clinical hypertension, 4th ed. Baltimore: Williams & Wilkins Co, 1986:1–28.

Lensometry

Clifford W. Brooks

INTRODUCTION

Definition

Lensometry is the clinical procedure to measure the sphere, cylinder, and axis of an optical prescription, to locate the optical center or the major reference point of a lens, and to determine the base, the direction, and the amount of prism present.

History

According to Hirschberg,[1] the oldest device used to measure the refractive power of a spectacle lens was the *phakometer of Snellen* in 1876. The instrument was made of wood and looked like an optical bench. A cross consisting of holes and located at one end of the rail was illuminated by an oil lamp. The image of this cross was focused through the lens of unknown power and onto a frosted glass located at the other end of the rail. Both the cross and the frosted glass were moveable. Two auxiliary lenses on either side of the unknown lens were used to shorten the focal distance required in measuring. To measure a negative lens, a positive lens of known power had to be employed. The plus lens was of greater dioptric value than the unknown negative lens. This permitted a real image to be created and its location measured.

Because the phakometer of Snellen was time-consuming and awkward to use, about the end of the 1800s and the beginning of the 1900s, lens power was also being measured by using a *lens measure* or *lens clock*. The lens clock is designed to find the curvature of a surface. From surface curvature, surface powers and lens power can be calculated (see Chap. 31 for more on the use of the lens clock).

The first instrument that used the principles of the optometer, and the forerunner of today's lensmeter, was built in 1912 by Troppmann.[1] Patents were taken out by Zeiss and American Optical in 1914 and 1918 and by J. Trotter in 1918.[2] Changes have followed, including the introduction of a target using a circle of dots for ease of determining the cylinder axis, and a cross as a test target. Both of these target types are still in use.

The lensmeter is referred to by a variety of names, depending upon manufacturer. Such names include vertex focimeter, refractionometer, lensometer, focimeter, vertometer, lensmeter, and vertexometer.

Clinical Use

When a patient presents for an eye examination, one of the necessary pieces of information is the ophthalmic lens prescription they are presently wearing. Knowledge of the current prescription will enable the clinician to have a comparison between what the patient has been wearing and the new refractive findings. If this is known, a determination can be made of whether the chief complaint stems from an uncorrected refractive problem or whether alternative causes are more likely. To do this, the power of the patient's ophthalmic lenses needs to be determined.

INSTRUMENTATION

Theory and Use

Manual lens-measuring devices work by neutralizing the refracting power of the lens so that a viewing target comes into clear view. Consequently, the process of evaluating a pair of glasses is sometimes referred to as *neutralization*.

The optics of a standard, manual lensmeter are shown in Figure 30–1. When the instrument is set at zero, an illuminated

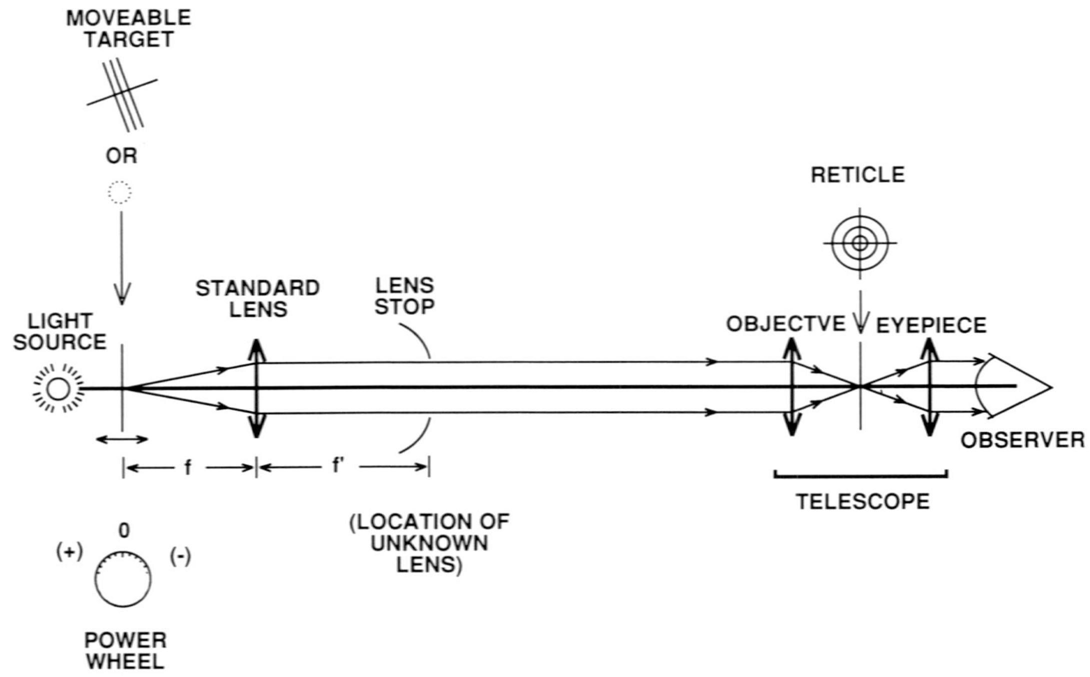

MOVEABLE
TARGET

OR

RETICLE

LIGHT
SOURCE

STANDARD
LENS

LENS
STOP

OBJECTVE ↓ EYEPIECE

|← f →|← f' →|

OBSERVER

(+)   0   (-)

(LOCATION OF
UNKNOWN
LENS)

TELESCOPE

POWER
WHEEL

FIGURE 30–1. Optics of a standard lensmeter. (Modified from Fannin T, Grosvenor T. Clinical optics. Stoneham, Mass: Butterworth Publishers, 1987:76)

target is positioned at the focal length of a plus lens. The lens is referred to as the *standard lens*. Diverging rays of light from the target are bent by the lens so that they emerge from the lens in parallel. The target may now be viewed through a telescope consisting of two plus lenses. The telescope allows the introduction of a reticle used in determining prismatic effect. The two plus lenses of the telescope, an objective and an eyepiece, are positioned so that their two focal points are coincident with one another. The reticle is located at the intersection of these points.

The lens stop, at which the lens of unknown power is positioned, is at the secondary focal plane of the standard lens. The stop is located between the standard lens and the telescope. When the lens of unknown power is introduced, the image of the target is thrown out of focus. The target itself is moveable. By moving it closer to or farther from the standard lens, the refractive effect of the unknown lens can be "neutralized." The physical distance forward or backward that the target moves directly indicates the power of the unknown lens for the meridian being measured.

COMMERCIALLY AVAILABLE INSTRUMENTS

Cambridge Instruments

(AO) Reichert Lensometer (Fig. 30–2)
B & L Vertometer (Fig. 30–3)

Marco

Lensmeter 101 (Fig. 30–4)
Lensmeter 201

Topcon

Lensmeter Model LM-6 (Fig. 30–5)

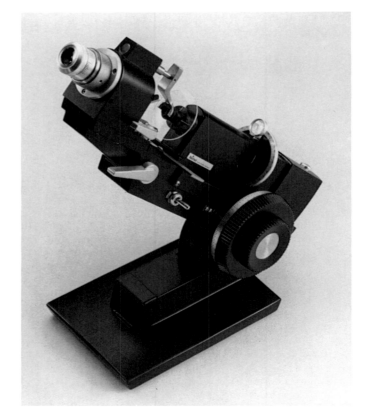

FIGURE 30–2. Cambridge AO Reichert Lensometer. (Courtesy of Reichert Ophthalmic Inst.)

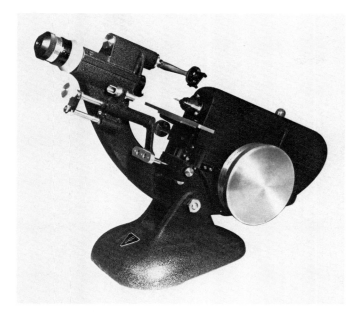

FIGURE 30–3. Cambridge B & L Vertometer. (Courtesy of Reichert Ophthalmic Inst.)

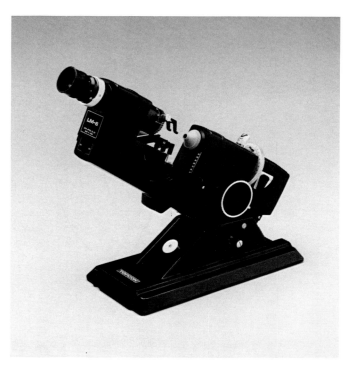

FIGURE 30–5. Topcon Lensmeter Model LM-6. (Courtesy of Topcon Inst. Corp.)

RH Burton

2020 Lensmeter (Fig. 30–6)

Basic Design

Although these instruments appear different externally and have noticeable and distinctive differences in design, the mode of operation is similar in that all use conventional *crossed-line targets.* The nature of these targets and how they are used is explained in the "Clinical Procedure" section.

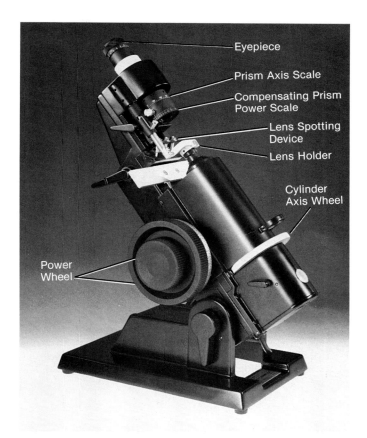

FIGURE 30–4. Marco Lensmeter Model 101. There are a great variety of lensmeter brands available, but many features such as those labeled in the picture are common. (Courtesy of Marco Equipment Inc.)

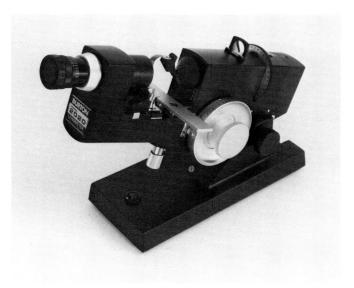

FIGURE 30–6. Burton 2020 Lensmeter. (Courtesy of R. H. Burton Co.)

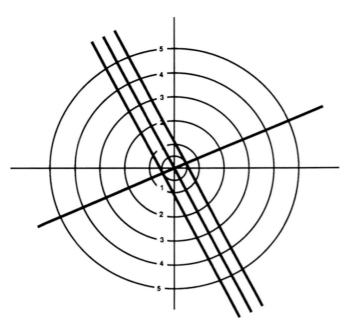

FIGURE 30–7. When a lensmeter is focused with no lens in place, it appears the same as when a spherical lens is focused. With spheres, the illuminated lines can be at any angle, as there is no axis to a spherical lens.

As seen in Figure 30–4, the instrument consists of an *eyepiece,* through which the internal target may be viewed; a *power wheel,* by which the sphere and cylinder powers are found; and an *axis wheel,* which rotates the target to find the cylinder axis. An example of a typical illuminated target is shown in Figure 30–7. It is shown as it would look if the instrument were empty and focused, or if a spherically powered lens were in place and correctly focused. In this same figure, narrowly spaced lines relate to the sphere power of the lens and are called the *sphere lines.* (Most lensmeters have a set of closely spaced triple lines, but some may have a single line for the sphere meridian.) The set of three widely spaced lines are known as the *cylinder lines.*

Some instruments have a set of rotary prisms mounted on the instrument so that large amounts of prism may be found without using an externally mounted auxiliary prism.

Zeiss Vertex Refractionometer (Fig. 30–8)

Topcon Lensmeter Model LM-T3 (Fig. 30–9)

Basic Design

These two instruments are distinctively different in appearance, but both use a *corona*-type viewing target. The corona target is a circle of dots. Such a target is shown in Figure 30–10. Because such a target does not need to be physically rotated, these instruments are often smaller than other types.

Topcon Digital Projection Lensmeter Model LM-P5 (Fig. 30–11)

Basic Design

The Topcon Digital Projection Lensmeter uses a conventional crossed-line target combined with a corona target. Both are projected onto the screen of the lensmeter which is externally placed on the instrument. Although the instrument works much like manual, nonprojection models, it displays results digitally and, if the

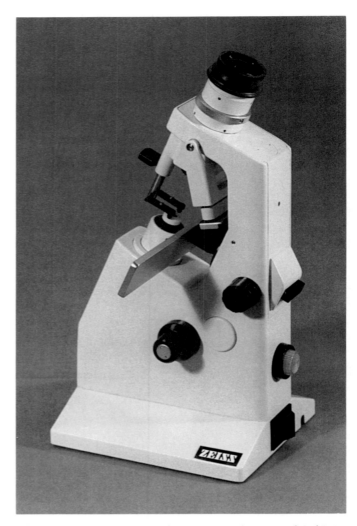

FIGURE 30–8. Zeiss Vertex Refractionometer. (Courtesy of Carl Zeiss, Inc.)

results have been found in minus cylinder form, they are easily transposed to plus cylinder form with the touch of a button.

In addition, the lensmeter may be equipped with an optional printer for a permanent record of results.

Marco Digital Projection Lensmeter Model LM 770 (Fig. 30–12)

Basic Design

The Marco Model LM 770 is a computer-assisted, manual projection lensmeter. It is computer assisted in that it automatically selects which target lines should be focused first. It is manual in that the lines denoting the two meridians must be focused by the operator. The instrument contains a printer, and it automatically calculates the multifocal add power.

Allergan Humphrey Lens Analyzer, Models 306, 330, 340

Basic Design

The external appearance of the three Allergan Humphrey Lens Analyzers appears in Figure 30–13. All three look the same from

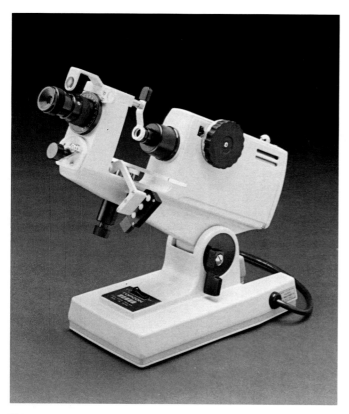

FIGURE 30–9. Topcon Lensmeter Model LM-T3. (Courtesy of Topcon Inst. Corp.)

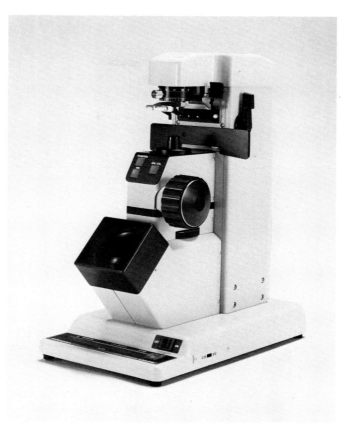

FIGURE 30–11. Topcon Digital Projection Lensmeter Model LM-P5. (Courtesy of Topcon Inst. Corp.)

the outside. The difference is in what the three models can do. Feature comparison is summarized in Table 30–1.

The lens analyzer does not require visual judgments of crossed-line or corona targets, as do the manual models. With models 330 and 340, the instrument will display the pupillary distance (PD) without having to move the lens to find the optical center (OC). When used in this PD-at-OC mode, the speed of operation increases, and operator error decreases. However, if the PD is known, the operator can neutralize the lenses at the position of the PD and find the net prismatic effect for the spectacle lens pair.

The Allergan Humphrey Lens Analyzer has only one internal moving part. The light used is from a white, full-spectrum source. All models will measure in either plus or minus cylinder form,

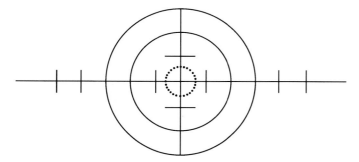

FIGURE 30–10. When a lensmeter using a circle of dots system is set for zero without a lens in place, the target appears as shown. This is also how the target will appear with a spherical lens in place and properly neutralized.

Table 30–1
Allergan Humphrey Models 306, 340 Feature Comparison

Feature	306	330	340
Automatic lens identification (left or right)	*	*	*
Contact lens measurement	*	*	*
Digital display	*	*	*
Preselectable modes of operation for cylinder, round-off, and prism	*	*	—
Footswitch	—	*	*
Instantaneous readout	*	*	*
Automatic lens detection	—	*	*
Thermal printer	*	*	*
Automatic PD measurement	—	*	*
Calculation of PD at optical center	—	*	*
Automatic layout function	—	—	*
Lens marker	*	*	*
Automatic wave detection	—	—	—
Automatic detection of add power	—	*	*
Prism recall	—	*	*
Measurement in 0.1-D, 0.12-D, 0.25-D increments	—	—	*
Results in prescription notation	*	*	*
Portable	*	*	*

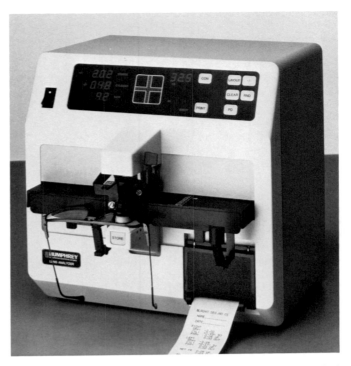

FIGURE 30–13. Allergan Humphrey Lens Analyzer. (Courtesy of Allergan Humphrey)

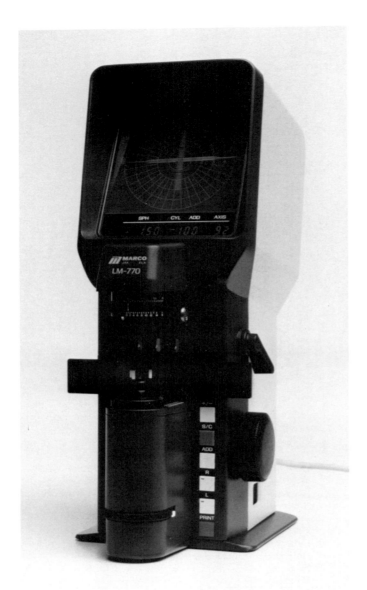

FIGURE 30–12. Marco Digital Projection Lensmeter Model 770. (Courtesy of Marco Equipment, Inc.)

depending upon the frame selected. Prism base direction will be displayed as either rectangular (base-up, down, in, out) or polar (in degrees). Power will display rounded to either 0.25, 0.125, or 0.001 diopters. Readings are printed out upon completion of the measurement.

Topcon Computerized Lensmeter, Model CL-1500

Basic Design

The Topcon Computerized Lensmeter shown in Figure 30–14 has an appearance similar to that of a projection lensmeter. The difference is that the optical screen that would be in a projection lensmeter is a monitor (CRT) for the Topcon Computerized Lensmeter. The lensmeter target appears on the left side of the screen. The right and left lens readings appear on the right side of the screen. It should be noted that after the second lens has been measured, the sphere, cylinder, axis, horizontal and vertical prism,

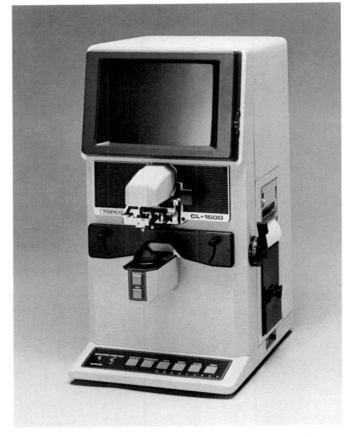

FIGURE 30–14. Topcon Computerized Lensmeter. (Courtesy of Topcon Inst. Corp.)

and near addition all appear on the screen simultaneously for both left and right lenses. As would be expected for a computerized lensmeter, the instrument has a printer.

The target is similar to that of the standard, manual, crossed-line target. It has one long line intersected at right angles by one short line. However, since the instrument is computerized, the lines are not used for focusing. Instead they are used in lens centering and alignment.

Marco Automatic Lensmeter, Models LM-850 and LM-870 (Fig. 30–15)

Basic Design

The Marco Automatic Lensmeter has a CRT screen that shows the alignment targets on the left half of the screen. It shows sphere, cylinder, axis, and prism for the right and left lens on the right half of the screen. There is also a digital readout display to the right of the CRT screen. This is a continuous-reading display and can also be used for speed when a printout is not needed.

The pressure-sensitive lens table automatically senses which lens in the pair of glasses is being measured.

Model LM-870 will allow an interface to the Marco objective/subjective Auto-Refractor so that the refraction may begin with the old prescription as read by the lensmeter. The Model LM-870 also extends the prism power range to ± 10 D.

CLINICAL PROCEDURE

Cambridge Instruments

(AO) Reichert Lensometer
B & L Vertometer

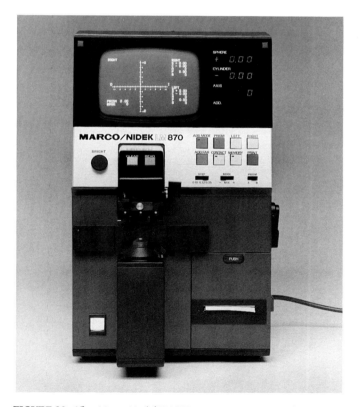

FIGURE 30–15. Marco Model LM 870 Automatic Lensmeter. (Courtesy of Marco Equipment, Inc.)

Marco

Lensmeter 101
Lensmeter 201

Topcon

Lensmeter Model LM-6

RH Burton

2020 Lensmeter

Procedure for Measuring the Refraction Power of Single Vision Lenses

The following procedure is used for measuring sphere and cylinder power and cylinder axis for single-vision lenses when using manual instruments having standard *crossed-line targets*.[3–6]

1. *Focus the eyepiece.* Before measurements can be accurately done, the lensmeter eyepiece must first be focused. This is done as follows:
   a. Turn the eyepiece outward.
   b. Set the lensmeter power wheel at zero.
   c. Look into the instrument and relax accommodation by imagining that the point being looked at is off in the distance.
   d. Slowly turn the eyepiece inward until the cross hairs and concentric circles *first* come into clear focus.
2. *Position the spectacles in the lensmeter.* Choose the lens of highest power and begin with that lens. When in doubt begin with the right lens.
3. *Find the sphere line.* Turn the lensmeter power wheel in the high plus direction. Slowly turn the power wheel in the minus direction until the sphere line of the illuminated target first begins to clear (Fig. 30–16). If the entire target clears at one time, the lens is a sphere. If this is the case, go on to step 4, then skip to step 8.
4. *Center the lens.* Move the lens up and down, left and right until the illuminated target centers.
5. *Find the cylinder axis.* Rock the axis wheel back and forth in an attempt to bring more clarity to the sphere line and focus the sphere line with the power wheel (Fig. 30–17).
6. *Record the sphere power and cylinder axis.* Read the sphere power from the power wheel and the axis direction from the axis wheel.
7. *Find the cylinder power.* Turn the sphere wheel farther in the minus direction until the cylinder lines clear (Fig. 30–18). The difference between the new power reading shown on the power wheel and the original sphere power is the power of the minus cylinder.
8. *Spot the optical center of the lens.* Make certain that the lens is centered and the spectacles are sitting on the lens table. Use the spotting mechanism on the lensmeter and spot the lens (Fig. 30–19). Three dots will be marked. The center dot is the optical center. The other two indicate the 180° line.
9. *Position and read the second lens.* Without moving the lens table, slide the spectacles over to the other lens. Repeat steps 3 through 7, but do not move the lenses up or down as was stated in step 4—only left and right.
10. *Spot the second lens.* Move the spectacles left or right until the illuminated target is in the same vertical plane as the center of the cross hairs. Use the spotting mechanism on the lensmeter and spot the lens.

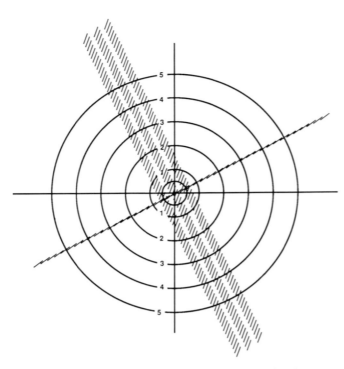

FIGURE 30–16. When the sphere line appears almost clear, but cannot quite be made to focus because of a diagonal brokenness, the axis is off slightly, and the axis wheel needs to be turned.

    If the illuminated target is above or below the center of the cross hairs, record the amount and base direction of this vertical prism. If there is vertical prism present which is greater than or equal to 1/3 Δ, use the lens table

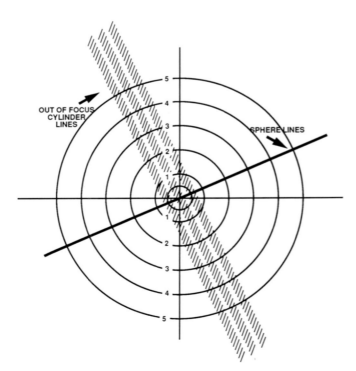

FIGURE 30–17. When the sphere line is in sharp focus, the sphere power may be read from the lensmeter.

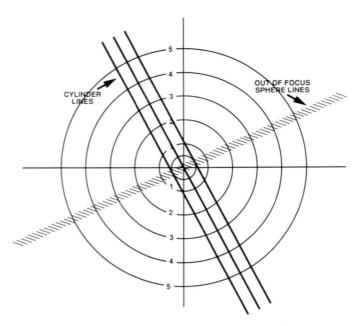

FIGURE 30–18. When cylinder lines are clear, the difference between the power wheel readings obtained for sphere and cylinder lines is the cylinder power.

and move the glasses up or down until the target is centered. Spot the lens a second time. If these two dots are farther than 1-mm apart, the unwanted vertical prism exceeds accepted quality standards. (Procedures for measuring vertical prism are explained in more detail in the section following.)

11. *Measure the distance between OCs.* Remove the lenses from the lensmeter and using a millimeter ruler, measure the horizontal distance between the center dots on the two lenses. This should be equal to the wearer's PD when no prescribed prism is present. If the distance between spotted centers is within 2.5 mm of the ordered PD, the prescription passes American National Standards quality specifications, and step 12 is not necessary.

12. *Test for PD and horizontal prism tolerance limits.* If the distance between centers is not within 2.5 mm of what

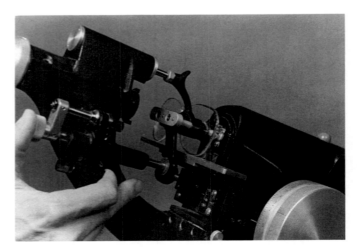

FIGURE 30–19. The optical center or major reference point is spotted using the lensmeter spotting mechanism.

was specified, put the lenses back in the lensmeter and do the following:

    a. For the first lens, move the spectacles *away* from the original center dot in the direction of the wearer's PD until 1/3rd prism diopter results. Redot the lens.

    b. Do the same thing for the second lens, redotting it in the same manner.

    c. If the distance between the two newly dotted center points is equal to or overshoots the wearer's PD by any amount, the lens pair passes American National Standards horizontal prism tolerances.

Here is an example of how these types of instruments are used to find the sphere, cylinder, and axis for a single-vision prescription.

Suppose the right lens of a pair of lenses is positioned in the lensmeter. The power wheel is turned into the high plus. As the power wheel is being turned back in the minus direction, find the sphere lines first. The axis is rocked until the axis wheel is 30. As the power wheel is turned more in the minus direction, it becomes evident that the sphere line appears somewhat diagonally broken (as was shown in Fig. 30–16). This is an indication that the axis reading is not exact. To correct this the axis wheel is adjusted to remove the diagonal brokenness seen in the sphere line. This is done by rocking the axis wheel while slowly moving the power wheel in the minus direction. The first focus is obtained and the power wheel reads +1.75. The axis wheel is now found to be on 35. At this point, part of the prescription can be written as:

$$+1.75 - \underline{\hspace{1.5cm}} \times 35$$

To find the cylinder power, the lensmeter power wheel is slowly turned farther into the minus direction until the three cylinder lines come into focus. Now the power wheel reads +1.00. The cylinder power is the difference between the two readings and is expressed as a minus value.

$$- \text{cyl power} = -(\text{first reading} - \text{second reading})$$

or

$$- \text{cyl power} = -(+1.75 - +1.00) = -0.75$$

Now the full refractive power may be written as

$$+1.75 - 0.75 \times 35$$

To Verify Prescribed Prism

When the prescription contains a desired prismatic effect, the verification of that prescription is done in a manner nearly identical with what has been previously prescribed. The only difference is in how the target is positioned in the lensmeter.

The following procedure is used when verifying prescribed prism:[7]

1. *Focus the eyepiece.* Use same method as in step 1 a–d of the foregoing basic procedure.
2. *Position the lenses in the lensmeter.* Choose the lens of highest power and begin with that lens.
3. *Preset the sphere and cylinder axis.* When the prescription is known, the sphere and axis wheels are preset at their expected values.
4. *Position the lens for the correct prismatic effect.* The lens is positioned in the lensmeter so that the center of the illuminated target is at the place on the circular mires corresponding to the prism called for.

    For example, if the right lens calls for 1 prism diopter base-up, then the illuminated target would be positioned at the "1" ring directly above the center of the mires (Fig. 30–20).

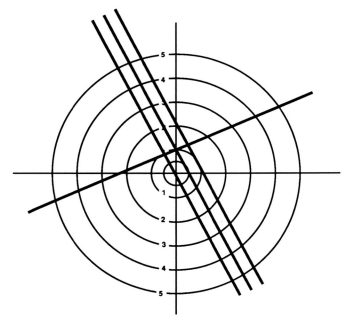

FIGURE 30–20. When a lens has 1^Δ of base-up prism, the lens must be centered in the lensmeter so the target appears as shown. This assures that the lens' major reference point (MRP) is correctly centered.

If, however, the right lens called for 2 prism diopters base-in, then the illuminated target would be positioned on the "2" ring where it crosses the horizontal line to the right of the center of the mires (Fig. 30–21).

Suppose that the prescription for the right lens calls for both 1 prism diopter base-up and 2 prism diopters base-in. Then the illuminated target would be centered at the height of the "1" ring and to the right by a distance equal to the radius of the "2" ring. In other words, 1 unit up and 2 units to the right (Fig. 30–22).

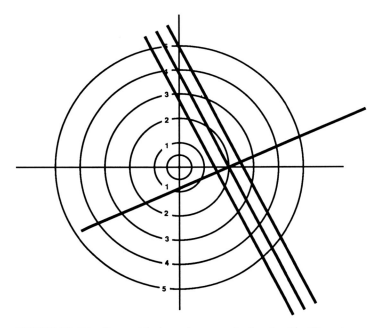

FIGURE 30–21. For a right lens, the target is showing 2^Δ of base-in prism. If the lens were a left lens, the prism would be base-out.

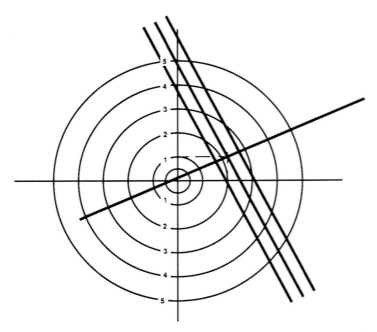

FIGURE 30–22. The center of the illuminated target is positioned for 1^Δ base-up and 2^Δ base-in, assuming the lens is a right lens.

5. *Spot the lens.* Once the lens has been centered in this manner, the lens is spotted.
6. *Read the second lens.* The spectacles are slid across the lensmeter table so that the second lens can be checked.
    Note: The point on the lens at which the amount of prescribed prism is correct is called the *major reference point* (MRP). When there is no prescribed prism, the major reference point and the optical center are one and the same point.

When there is an unusually high amount of prism present in a lens, the target may fail to center. Here, either auxiliary prisms or a prism-compensating device may be used. This moves the target back onto the screen where it may be read. The use of the prism-compensating device is explained later in the section on the Marco Digital Projection Lensmeter.

To Measure Multifocal Lenses

To use these instruments to measure bi- and trifocal lenses, *front* vertex powers must be found. Therefore, the following procedure is used:

1. *Measure the distance portion.* Measure the distance portion in the same manner as was used with single-vision lenses. (This was previously shown in Fig. 30–19.)
2. *Reposition the lenses in the lensmeter.* Turn the spectacles around backward so that the temples face the operator.
3. *Find distance front vertex power.* The distance power is read as front vertex power at a point as far above the major reference point of the lens as the segment is below the major reference point of the lens (Fig. 30–23). (This is so that front vertex powers are being compared, instead of one front vertex power and one back vertex power. It also assures that any power difference caused by lens thickness and peripheral lens aberrations will be identical, canceling each other out.) It should be noted that when there is a cylinder in the prescription, the cylinder axis will be the

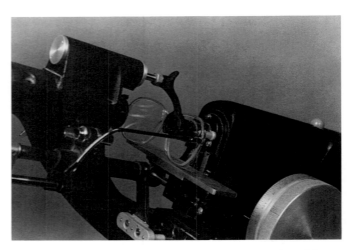

FIGURE 30–23. If the distance or near power of a multifocal lens is moderate to high, to find the measure add accurately, the lenses must be turned around so that the front vertex power is read. The first step is to obtain a distance front vertex power, since the add power is the difference between distance and near powers.

mirror image of what it was before. If the prescription is axis 30, it will now read axis 150.
4. *Find near front vertex power.* Move the lenses upward until the lens stop is on the segment portion. Now the sphere power reading through the near portion is found (Fig. 30–24).
5. *Record the add power.* The difference between the distance front vertex power and the near front vertex power is the add power.

Although the foregoing procedure for turning the glasses around in the lensmeter is correct, it is not always used. When the distance power and near add power are both small, most people do not bother to turn the glasses around. The results for small powers will be almost identical when comparing the two methods. However, when powers increase, significant differences can and do occur. For other than lower-powered lenses, the more cumbersome front vertex power method is important.

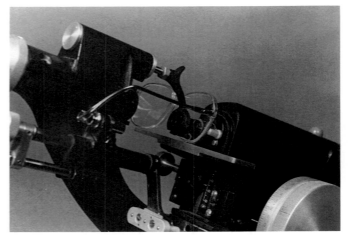

FIGURE 30–24. After the distance power is found with the lenses in backwards, the near power is found; the lenses are still in backwards. The difference between these two readings will give an accurate add power.

Verifying Progressive Addition Lenses

1. *Verify distance power.* Progressive addition lenses are verified for sphere, cylinder, and axis at a point slightly above the MRP (major reference point). [Remember that when there is no prescribed prism, the OC (optical center) and MRP coincide.] This is necessary because the power of the lens begins to change at the MRP. The MRP marks the beginning of the progressive corridor of the lens. This corridor moves downward and slightly nasalward, increasing in power the farther down the eye travels, until full add power is reached (Fig. 30–25).

2. *Verify PD.* The progressive add lens must be checked right at the MRP for PD and the presence of unwanted prism. Therefore, once the refractive power of the distance portion has been found, the lens is centered at the MRP as if it were a single-vision lens, then spotted. It is normal for the target to be somewhat out of focus, since the lower half of the lensmeter aperture will be reading slightly more plus than the upper half.

3. *Find the near power.* A progressive addition lens is checked for near power at a point well into the near portion. This point is usually indicated by yellow markings on the lens which were applied by the optical laboratory. If no markings are present, they may be redrawn. Each manufacturer has its own recommended system for recreating these marks so that verification can be done more easily.

4. *Figure the near add.* As with other multifocals, find the difference between the distance and near powers by subtracting the difference between the sphere value found in the near portion from the sphere value found in the distance portion of the lens.

To Verify Contact Lenses

For *hard contact lenses,* the lens is held against the lens stop between the thumb and index finger and measured in the same manner as single-vision lenses. Some instruments have a second, interchangeable lens stop for contact lenses. This lens stop has a smaller aperture for the smaller optic zone of the contact lens. To help prevent lens loss, place the instrument in a vertical position, if possible. With the instrument straight up and down, the contact lens is less likely to slip off the lens stop.

For *soft contact lenses,* the instrument should be angled upward until it is in a fully vertical position. (This is not possible with all models.) With use of lens tweezers, the soft contact lens is rinsed and excess solution removed by gently shaking the lens. The lens is placed on the lens stop using the tweezers and gently balanced there while the power is read.

Zeiss Vertex Refractionometer

Topcon Lensmeter Model LM-T3

Both of these instruments use the corona-style target.

Procedure for Measuring the Refractive Power of Single-Vision Lenses [8,9]

1. *Focus the eye piece.* This is done as was described for the previous group of instruments.

2. *Turn the sphere wheel in the plus direction.* Turn the sphere wheel in the plus direction until the circle of dots blurs out.

3. *Find the sphere power.* Slowly return the power wheel in the minus direction. If all dots clear into a well-defined circle the lens is a sphere. Read the power. Steps 4 and 5 are not needed, since the lens is a sphere and the power has been found.

   If the dots elongate and focus into lines, the lens has cylinder power as shown in Figure 30–26. Record the sphere power and proceed on to step 4.

4. *Find the cylinder power.* Turn the power wheel farther in the minus direction, until the lines reform at right angles to their original direction. Record the difference between the first reading and the second reading as the power of the minus cylinder.

5. *Find the cylinder axis.* Measure the dot-line angle using the moveable hair line in the eyepiece. Turn the hair line until it parallels the direction of the focal dot-lines. Note where

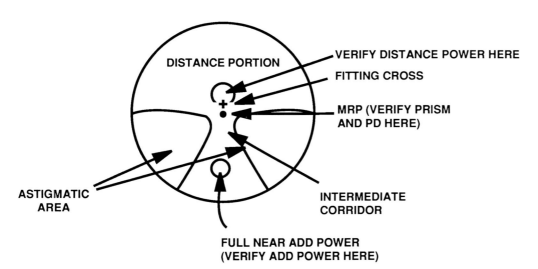

FIGURE 30–25. Not all progressive addition lenses look exactly like the one shown here. Some have a wider or narrower near portion. Some have a shorter or longer intermediate corridor. With some lenses, the astigmatic area extends higher into the distance portion.

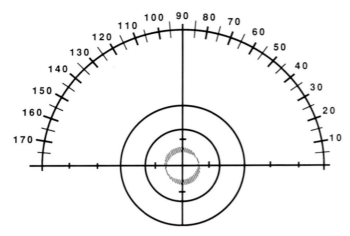

FIGURE 30–26. The first time the elongated dots come into focus indicates the sphere power of the lens.

the hair line crosses the degree scale (Fig. 30–27). Record this as the cylinder axis.

Using the Corona-Type Instrument to Verify a Prescription When Prescribed Prism Is Present

When measuring prescribed prism, the following procedure is used:

1. *Focus the eyepiece.* This is done as previously described.
2. *Position the lenses* in the lensmeter, so that the highest powered lens well be measured first.
3. *Preset the sphere value.*
4. *Position the lens for the prescribed prismatic effect.* The center of the corona target is positioned on the reticle at the horizontal and vertical prismatic position called for in the prescription. When using the *cartesian or rectangular*

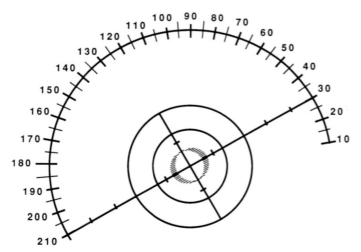

FIGURE 30–27. When the power wheel is turned farther into the minus direction, the elongated dots will refocus 90° away from their original focus direction. The difference between the first power and second power reading is the minus cylinder power of the lens. The cylinder axis is found by turning the rotating cross hair until it parallels the elongated lines. The axis of the cylinder corresponds to where the cross hair crosses the degree scale.

coordinate system, this procedure is carried out in the same manner as was described for *crossed-line* instruments. When using the *polar coordinate system* for specifying prism, the hair line in the reticle is rotated to the specified base direction and the corona target positioned on the hair line at the prism diopter reading called for. (The polar coordinate system combines horizontal and vertical prismatic components into one single prism. Its base direction is specified in degrees instead of just up, down, in, or out.)

5. *Spot the lens.*
6. *Read and spot the second lens* in like manner.

Multifocals, progressive add, and contact lenses are verified in the same manner as was described for crossed-line instruments.

Topcon Digital Projection Lensmeter Model LM-P5

Procedure for Measuring the Refractive Power of Single-Vision Lenses[10]

1. *Position the lenses in the lensmeter.* Choose the lens of highest power and begin with that lens. When in doubt begin with the right lens.
2. *Find the sphere lines.* Turn the lensmeter power wheel in the high-plus direction. Slowly turn the power wheel in the minus direction until the thin, triple sphere lines of the illuminated target first begin to clear.
3. *Center the lens.* Move the lens forward and backward, left and right until the illuminated target centers.
4. *Find the cylinder axis.* Use the stretched-out corona target to help in locating the direction of the cylinder axis as described in the section on corona-type instruments. Rock the axis wheel back and forth in an attempt to bring more clarity to the sphere lines while focusing the sphere lines with the power wheel.
5. *Press the SPH/CYL button.* There is a red light that had been illuminated above the "sphere" reading to indicate that the sphere power was being measured. When the SPH/CYL button is pressed, this light goes off and the red light above the "cylinder" reading lights up.
6. *Find the cylinder power.* Turn the sphere wheel farther in the minus direction until the cylinder lines clear. The sphere, cylinder, and axis can now be read from the digital display.
7. If desired, *spot the lens optical center.*
8. *Press the SPH/CYL button a second time.* This clears the sphere/cylinder/axis display so that the second lens can be read.
9. *Move to the second lens* and repeat the procedure.

To Find the Add Power

Carry out steps 1 through 6 as previously described for single-vision lenses. Next proceed as follows:

1. *Press the ADD button.* The red light will light up next to the "add" on the display panel.
2. *Reposition the lenses.* Move the lens table and lenses so that the bifocal section is over the lens stop.
3. *Refocus the sphere lines.* Once the sphere lines have been refocused, the "add" reading is correct.

It should be noted that for accuracy with high-powered distance or near powers, the lenses must be turned and front vertex power measured using the procedure as described in the section on standard crossed-line target instruments.

To Measure Prism Values

Prism can be measured in one of two ways. The first is just as was described in the section on standard crossed-line instruments. This uses the rectangular coordinate system of base-in, base-out, base-up, and base-down.

The second method of measuring prism uses the polar coordinate system. In the polar coordinate system a single prism is specified in conjunction with a prism axis. The base direction is given in degrees. (The polar coordinate system was described previously in the section on corona target instruments.) The Topcon Digital Projection Lensmeter is different from the manual corona target instrument. Instead of finding a prism base direction by using a rotating cross hair, the axis wheel of the Topcon Projection Lensmeter is rotated until the sphere line crosses the center of the screen. Thus, the axis reading on the digital display shows the prism axis, whereas the position of the center of the illuminated target shows the amount of prism.

For contact lenses an accessory contact lens support is used. Readings are performed in the same manner as described for ordinary single-vision lenses.

Marco Digital Projection Lensmeter Model LM 770

Procedure for Measuring the Refractive Power of Single-Vision Lenses[11,12]

1. *Position the lenses in the lensmeter.* Choose the lens of highest power and begin with that lens. When in doubt about power, begin with the right lens. The spectacles are placed against the lensmeter table, temples down, with the top of the lens against the surface of the table. (This is different from many other lensmeters that position the bottom of the lenses against the lensmeter table.)
2. *Precenter the lens over the lens stop.* The lens should be approximately centered over the lens stop in preparation for reading the lens power. The top of the spectacles should remain against the lensmeter table. In other words, to center the lens, the table may have to be moved. (This step is preliminary and is not an optical centering of the lens.)
3. *Set the desired instrument modes.* The instrument allows the operator to preselect plus or minus cylinder mode. Rounding is for quarters, eighths, or hundredths of a diopter. Simply press the corresponding selection button.
4. *Prepare the instrument to read the sphere power.* The display area should show 0.00 in the sphere display. There should be no reading showing in the cylinder display area. If there is a reading in the cylinder display (even a 0.00 reading), the S-C button should be pushed showing that only the sphere display is registering.
5. *Find the sphere lines.* Assuming that the reading is to be done in minus cylinder form, the lensmeter power wheel is first turned in the high-plus direction. Then it is slowly turned in the minus direction until the three thin sphere lines of the target first begin to clear. (The instrument has sphere and cylinder indicator lights just below the screen. These lights help in reminding the operator which set of lines is being focused.)
6. *Center the lens.* Move the lens forward and backward, left and right until the illuminated target centers.
7. *Find the cylinder axis.* Because the target is a combination of the line and corona types, the stretched-out corona target may be used to help in locating the direction of the cylinder axis. (This procedure was described in the section on corona-type instruments.) To bring more clarity

to the sphere lines the axis wheel may be rocked back and forth somewhat while simultaneously focusing the sphere lines with the power wheel.
8. *Press the S-C button.* Once the sphere power and cylinder axis have been located, the S-C button is pressed. This holds the sphere power in memory and sets the cylinder display at 0.00.
9. *Find the cylinder power.* Turn the power wheel until the cylinder lines clear.
10. *Spot the optical center.* If desired, the lens optical center may be spotted.
11. *Print.* If a printout is desired, press the print button.
12. *Repeat for the second lens.* Move to the second lens and repeat the procedure.

To Find the Add Power

Follow steps 1 through 10, then proceed as follows:

1. *Press the "add" button.* Once the sphere, cylinder, and axis have been found and the optical center or major reference point spotted, press the "add" button.
2. *Reposition the lenses.* Move the lens table and lenses so that the bifocal section is over the lens stop.
3. *Refocus the sphere lines.* Once the sphere lines have been refocused, the "add" reading is correct. Results will show in the cylinder/add display.

As with other instruments, for accuracy in reading high-powered distance or near powers the glasses must be turned around. Front vertex power is measured using the procedure that was described in the section on standard crossed-line target instruments.

To Measure Prism Values

MEASURING PRISM VALUES USING THE RECTANGULAR COORDINATE SYSTEM. When the prismatic effect being measured is low, prism values are found in the same manner as was described for standard crossed-line instruments. The common rectangular coordinate system of specifying prism as base-up, down, in, or out is used.

MEASURING PRISM VALUES USING THE POLAR COORDINATE SYSTEM. With a polar coordinate system prism base direction is given in degrees. It may be read directly from the screen. However, when read from the screen, accuracy will only be ±5°. For higher accuracy, press the S-C button and turn the axis wheel until the axis line goes through the center of the screen. Prism base direction will appear in the axis display area. If the target is above the midline of the screen, the reading in the axis display is the base direction of the prism. If the target is below the midline of the screen, the base direction is the reading in the axis display, plus 180°.

When prism values are higher than 5 prism diopters, regardless of whether a rectangular or polar coordinate system is being used, the target will disappear from the screen. When this happens the prism-compensating device on the instrument must be used.

MEASURING PRISMATIC EFFECT USING THE PRISM-COMPENSATING DEVICE. To use the prism compensating device, follow these steps:

1. *Set the power wheel* at the sphere power of the prescription.
2. *Place the point of reference over the lens stop.* The point of reference is usually the expected location of the major reference point of the lens. The MRP will correspond to the location of the monocular PD or to one-half the binocular PD for a given pair of glasses.

3. *Center the target by using the prism compensator.* The prism-compensating device is a Risley prism positioned in the optical axis of the lensmeter. Compensating prism power is increased or decreased by turning the knob on the compensating device. In this instance the knob is turned around its own axis. However, the base direction of the compensating prism is changed by physically moving the knob so that the knob rotates around the axis of the lensmeter. The compensating operation is complete when the target is centered in the middle of the screen where the cross hairs intersect.

4. *Read the amount of prism present.* Once the target has been centered, prism power is read from the power scale on the prism-compensating device and prism axis from the degree scale. The Risley prism in the compensating device is like a number line, increasing in power in either direction from the zero mark. On the other hand, when the compensating prism axis is on zero, one direction on the prism power scale is base-in and the other base-out. When the compensating prism axis is on 90, one direction on the prism power scale is base-up and the other base-down.

When the prism-compensating axis ends up at an oblique angle and power reading is on the "positive" side of the prism power scale (usually white), then the prism axis is correct as shown. But if the power reading is on the "negative" side of the scale (usually red), then either 180° must be added to the prism axis shown, or the base direction reading must be marked as DN. For example, if the prism power shows 7Δ on the red part of the scale and the prism axis shows 45, the prism is 7Δ base 225 or 7Δ base 45 DN.

Note: It is possible to leave the base direction of the prism-compensating device at either 90 or 180 if most of the prismatic effect in the spectacle lens is either just horizontal or just vertical. If the base direction of the prism-compensating device is left at 90 or 180, the rectangular coordinate system (base-up, down, in, or out) can be used without having to convert from the polar coordinate system. If the prism compensator is left at 90 or 180, then the target is moved so that it intersects either the horizontal or the vertical cross hair. This means that either the vertical component is read from the screen and the horizontal component from the prism compensating device, or vice versa.

To Measure Contact Lenses

Contact lenses are measured with the Marco Digital Projection Lensmeter in the way a spectacle lens is measured. The only difference is that the 9-mm aperture is replaced with a 5-mm aperture, and the lens holder is not used on the contact lens.

Table 30–2
Clinical Procedure for the Allergan Humphrey Lens Analyzer

1. Power on
2. Position spectacles
3. Read first lens
4. Read add
5. Read second lens
6. Print Rx

Allergan Humphrey Lens Analyzer, Models 306, 330, 340

Procedure for Measuring the Refractive Power of Single-Vision Lenses[13]

1. *Power on.* Turn the power on with the switch on the front of the instrument. Verify that the following modes are as desired:

   Plus/minus cylinder convention
   Round-off precision (0.12 or 0.25)
   PD measurement mode

   Pull the lens table forward so that it is ready for the lenses.

2. *Position lenses.* The spectacles are positioned in the instrument with the bridge against the nose piece of the instrument and the temples downward. The instrument immediately begins reading the sphere, cylinder axis, and PD. (Model 306 does not read the PD.)

   The lenses must press against the lens table to assure an accurate axis reading. For lenses over 8.00 D, the lens clamp should be used to hold the lens in a stable position. Final positioning is done with either the *PD mode* or the *PD-at-OC mode.*

   In the *PD mode* the lens analyzer shows the monocular PD as being the point on the lens at which the instrument is reading (at the read head). It also shows the prismatic effect at that point on the lens. The PD mode is used when the patient PD is known and the operator wants to measure refractive power and prismatic effect at the patient's PD. To use the PD mode:
   a. Choose the PD mode by pressing the PD button until the *PD* light comes on.
   b. Move the lenses until the desired monocular PD is shown in the PD display window.

   In the *PD-at-OC mode,* the instrument calculates the PD. It does this by using the power and prismatic effect of the lens found at the read head, and the distance from the center of the bridge of the frame to the read head. After the second lens has been read it also calculates vertical prism present. To use PD-at-OC:
   a. Select this mode using the PD button.
   b. Since the initial positioning of the lenses in the lens analyzer has already been done, for the PD-at-OC mode no further positioning is required.

   To mark the patient's PD on the spectacles use the *PD mode* and watch the cross in the center of the instrument panel. As soon as the instrument begins continuous reading, a read cross appears on the display. Move the spectacles until the read cross reaches the fixed, hollow-center cross. When it does, the fixed cross will light up (Fig. 30–28). Mark the OC of the lens by pushing the marking pen arm back, then down onto the lens. (This procedure is later repeated for the second lens.)

3. *Read the first lens.* Once the lens has been positioned as described in step 2, press the *store* button or a foot switch. If the *right* or *left* indicator light does not come on, the lenses have not been pressed against the table firmly enough and the results will not print. While pressing the spectacles against the table again, press *store.*

4. *Read the add.* Move the lens so that the add is over the read head, as close to the top of the segment (seg) as possible. The *add 1* light will come on. Press the *store* button or foot switch. If a second add is present in the same lens, the procedure is repeated, the *add 2* light comes on and the *store* button is pressed again.

5. *Read the second lens.* The lens is positioned as was done for the first lens. The lens table must still be in the original

A simple layout design facilitates speed and ensures accuracy.

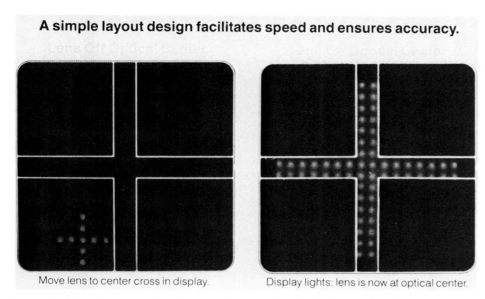

Move lens to center cross in display.　Display lights; lens is now at optical center.

FIGURE 30–28. The left half of the figure shows how the display looks in the Allergan Humphrey Lens Analyzer when the lens is not centered. The right half shows how the display appears when the lens is centered.

position as set for the first lens so that prism and PD readings will be correct. The lens and add are read as was described for the first lens.

6. *Print the Rx.* A printout appears as soon as the print button is pressed. The printout appears as shown in Figure 30–29. An "XXX" on the printout indicates that when the measurement was taken, the lens showed considerable distortion. This could be caused by taking a reading on the bifocal line. When "XXX" appears, the reading should be repeated.

To Measure Adds for High-Plus Lenses

For high-plus lenses, the multifocal add must be measured using front vertex power. (Actually, for *all* adds situated on the front surface of the lens, front vertex powers should be used. But because, for thin lenses, there is not much difference between front and back vertex powers when the add is measured, this method is not necessary every time.) To measure front vertex power for the add, the following steps are used:

1. Measure the distance Rx as if the lenses were single vision. Print the results.
2. Turn the glasses over so that the concave side is facing upward instead of downward.
3. Measure the distance Rx a second time, but this time from the front. Move the multifocal segment as close to the read head as possible, without allowing the segment line to cross over onto the read head. After making certain that the lens is flat on the lens stop, press the *store* button.
4. Now move the lens so that the read head is just into the multifocal segment. Make certain the lens is flat on the lens stop and press the *store* button. (Model 306 requires that an *add* button be pressed first.)

To Measure Progressive Addition Lenses

Because the power of the lens varies in the various regions of the progressive addition lens, it is necessary to be certain that the

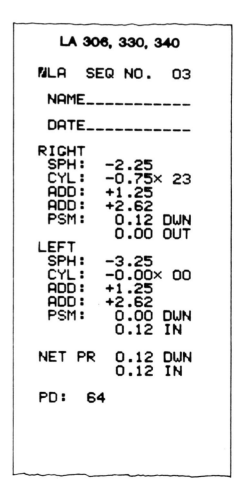

```
    LA 306, 330, 340

  ▮LA   SEQ NO.   03

  NAME_____

  DATE_____

  RIGHT
    SPH:   -2.25
    CYL:   -0.75× 23
    ADD:   +1.25
    ADD:   +2.62
    PSM:    0.12 DWN
            0.00 OUT
  LEFT
    SPH:   -3.25
    CYL:   -0.00× 00
    ADD:   +1.25
    ADD:   +2.62
    PSM:    0.00 DWN
            0.12 IN

  NET PR   0.12 DWN
           0.12 IN

  PD:   64
```

FIGURE 30–29. A typical printout for the Allergan Humphrey Lens Analyzer.

correct locations on the lens are used in finding the distance power and near add. The procedure is as follows:

1. *Measure the distance Rx.* Measure the distance Rx, but *not* at the optical center. Instead measure the lens *above* the distance optical center, in the upper third of the lens. Press *store.*
2. *Measure the add power.* Move the lens so that the read head begins to enter into the progressive channel of the lens. The progressive channel leads to the lower, nasal portion of the lens, where the full near power of the lens is found. As the read head enters the progressive channel, the changing lens power will activate the *ADD 1* indicator. The instrument will start a continuous reading, but the *NON-TOR* (non-toric) indicator light will come on, showing that there is a rapid change in lens power, or distortion present. This light will stay on until the full add power is reached and the power stabilizes. When full add power is reached, press store.

To Measure Contact Lenses

To use tne Allergan Humphrey Lens Analyzer to measure contact lenses the following steps are used:

1. *Move the table.* Move the lens table back out of the way.
2. *Choose the correct mode.* Press the *CON* (contact lens) button. Choose either *hard* or *soft* mode, depending on which type of contact lens is to be measured. The hard lens mode restricts the measure to the central area of the lens only. The soft lens mode measures the lens, but reports only the spherical equivalent of the power found.
3. *Find the optical center.* Place the lens on the read head and find its optical center by using the centering cross found in the middle of the control panel. When the optical center is located, the hollow cross will light up.
4. *Press* store. To have the instrument print *left* or *right,* the spectacle frame table must be pressed. Pressing on the right side of the table while pressing store will cause "left" to print. Pressing on the left side of the table while pressing store will cause "right" to print.
5. Press *print* to record results.

Topcon Computerized Lensmeter, Model CL-1500

Procedure for Measuring the Refractive Power of Single-Vision Lenses[14]

1. *Power on.* Do not place any lens in the lensmeter before turning on the power! Doing so will result in inaccurate readings. Turn on the power and check to be certain that both the sphere (S) and the cylinder (C) values are zero. Set the Measuring/Marking switch to *Measuring.*
2. *Position the lenses.* Turn the lens table lever to move the lens table into the forward position. Place the spectacles with the temples down and the top of the spectacles toward the operator so that the bottoms of the spectacle lens rims rest against the lens table. If the right lens is the stronger lens, measure it first. The left lens is hooked over the lever on the left which is built into the lens table. Hooking the left side of the glasses over the lever depresses it so that the instrument knows which lens is being measured. (If the frame will not depress or reach the lever, press the button on the lower panel marked "Right" instead.) The lens clamp (lens holder) is then lowered into place to hold the lens securely.
3. *Read the first lens.* Move the lens and frame until the center of the target on the CRT screen falls within the 0.5-prism diopter ring. (The 0.5 ring is the smallest circle.) When the target center falls within this circle, "ALIGNMENT OK" will appear in the lower left hand portion of the screen. The best method is to first slide the glasses left or right until horizontal alignment is achieved, then move the glasses vertically using the lens table. When satisfied with the alignment, press the *memory* button. (The lens may be spotted for PD by pressing the axis-marking lever against the lens.)
4. *Read the second lens.* Lift the lens clamp, move the left lens into place and hook the right lens over the lever on the right. Slide the glasses left and right until "ALIGNMENT OK" appears. Press the *memory* button.
5. *Print.* Once both lenses have been measured, press the *print* button. Before measuring a new Rx, the instrument's memory must be cleared by pressing the *clear* button.

To Measure Multifocal Add Power

1. *Measure the distance power of the first lens.* When multifocals are measured, the same process is followed as was used for measuring single-vision lenses. After the distance portion of the first lens is measured, press the *memory* button.
2. *Measure the add power.* Press the *add* button. Move the lens so that the segment is in the measuring position. The add power should be displayed. Press *memory.* (If there is more than one segment that must be measured in the same lens, press the add button again and repeat the process.)
3. *Move to the second lens.* Repeat steps 1 and 2.

To Measure Progressive Addition Lenses

1. Set the instrument so that it is in the *marking* mode. This will allow the operator to find the optical center. (This method will not work if there is Rx prism present or if equal bilateral base-down prism has been ground in an effort to thin the lens.)
2. Move the lens until the centering mark is lined up in the middle of the target. The OC is now centered.
3. With the lens table handle, move the lens table against the bottom of the frame (this may have already been done in the course of centering the lens).
4. Turn the scale ring at the base of the lens table handle until the "OC" mark is lined up.
5. Move the lens by turning the lens table handle until the scale ring reads "FAR." This shifts the lens so that a point above the OC is measured.
6. Press *memory.*
7. Press *add.*
8. Move the lens by turning the lens table handle until the scale ring reads "ADD."
9. Move the frame 2 to 3 mm laterally so that a point in the lower add portion of the lens and slightly nasalward is being measured.
10. Press *memory.*
11. Repeat for the second lens.

To Measure Contact Lenses

For measuring *hard* contact lenses using the Topcon Computerized Lensmeter Model CL-1500, use the following procedure:

1. Press the *contact* button.
2. Remove the regular measuring head that supports the lens in the instrument and replace it with the hard contact lens support.
3. Press *clear.*

4. When *HARD C* appears on the screen, proceed in the same manner as was described for measuring a normal single-vision lens.
5. Press *contact*.
6. Replace the contact lens support with the regular lens support.
7. Press *clear*.

For measuring *soft* contact lenses, use the following procedure:

1. Press *contact*.
2. Change the regular lens support for the soft contact lens support.
3. Press the *contact* button.
4. Use tweezers and shake any excess contact lens solution from the lens. Place the lens on the soft contact lens support.
5. Proceed as with single-vision spectacle lenses.
6. Replace the soft contact lens support with the regular lens support.
7. Press *clear*.

Note: In the soft contact lens mode, the spherical equivalent will be read. This may be overridden only by changing a preset switch under a slide panel.

Marco Automatic Lensmeter, Models LM-850 and LM-870

Procedure for Measuring Single-Vision Lenses[15]

1. Position the lenses with the approximate center of the first lens in front of the lens stop. The spectacles are placed with temples down and the lower edge of the lenses away from the operator.
2. Press the side of the spectacles *not* being measured against the lens table firmly enough to cause the instrument to beep. "Right" or "left" should appear in the upper left-hand corner of the screen.
3. Using the cross hair target on the CRT screen, move the lens until it is centered. The prism display should read zero. (For information on how to measure lenses having Rx prism, see the section on prism that appears later.)
4. Press *read*. The measurement is displayed in the right half of the CRT screen.
5. Move the lenses over horizontally so that the second lens may be read. Repeat steps 2 through 4 for the second lens.
6. Press the *read* button.
7. Press the *print* button, if a printed copy is desired.

To Measure Prism in Lenses

1. Place a dot on the lens at the location at which prism is to be measured. This usually corresponds to the distance PD.
2. Put the lenses in the instrument, with the newly marked dot centered over the lens stop.
3. Press the *prism* button.
4. Make certain that the instrument knows whether the right or left lens is being read. This is done by either pressing the *right* or *left* button, or by pressing the opposite lens against the lens table until a beep is elicited.
5. Press the *read* button.
6. Repeat for the second lens.
7. Press *print*.

The prism can be read using the base-up, down, in, or out system, or as a single prism oriented to a specific axis. The prism switch should be set for delta (δ) for the former and theta (θ) for the latter.

To Measure Low-Powered Multifocal Lenses

1. Measure the first lens as was described for a single-vision lens and press *read*.
2. Press the *add mode* button.
3. Move the lens so that the lens stop is over the add.
4. Press *read* again.
5. Repeat for the second lens.

To Measure High-Plus Multifocal Lenses

1. Read the distance portion in the normal manner and press *read*.
2. Press the *add mode* button.
3. Turn the lenses so that the temples are up, the bottom of the lenses are toward the operator and the same lens is over the lens stop.
4. Move the lenses so that the lens stop will be read through a position as far above the lens optical center as the add is below the lens center. (The lens stop should be positioned at a point above the lens OC which is equal in thickness to the point on the segment at which the add will be read.)
5. Press the *Add Far* button.
6. Move the lens until it is over the multifocal segment. (For multisegmented lenses, start with the segment portion that is lowest in power.)
7. Press the *read* button. (Repeat steps 6 and 7 for each segment in the lens.)
8. Repeat steps 1 through 7 for the second lens.

This method is, by far, the more accurate method for reading a multifocal lens of any power. The reason it is used only for high-plus lenses is because of the extra steps involved.

To Measure Progressive Addition Lenses

The procedure used to measure progressive addition lenses with the Marco Automatic Lensmeter is basically the same as was described for measuring low-powered multifocal lenses. However, the following points should be noted:

1. Read the distance portion 5-mm above the lens optical center.
2. Watch the digital display to be certain that the progressive zone is being followed as the near addition zone is being located.
3. Once the maximum add has been encountered and the power reading stabilized, the add power may be read.

To Read Contact Lenses

1. Replace the standard 9-mm lens stop with a 7-mm lens stop.
2. Choose the correct measuring mode. For powers up to +5.00 diopters, leave the instrument in the normal mode. For powers from +5.00 to +20.00 diopters, press the *contact* button.
3. Press the *LEFT* or *RIGHT* buttons if a printed copy is desired. This identifies the correct power with the correct lens.
4. Proceed as for single-vision spectacle lenses.

CLINICAL IMPLICATIONS

Clinical Significance and Interpretation

Clinical significance for lens refractive and prism powers, as well as placement of lenses in the wearer's frame, should be approached from the aspect of possible consequences of errors. Some guidelines are presented, but ultimately the practitioner must simply ask what the particular error would mean for the patient. An individual clinical interpretation is made. Here are some guidelines.

Sphere Power

The higher the minus sphere power, the higher the ability of the wearer to tolerate a small variation in sphere power without serious consequences. (With young people this is true, particularly if the deviation is in the minus direction.)

Variations in sphere power for individuals with low refractive errors are more bothersome, since their uncorrected vision is especially sharp at certain distances anyway.

Cylinder Power

If the cylinder power is off, an error on the low side is less serious than an error on the high side. However, this would *not* be true if the clinician has purposely cut the power of the cylinder from the refractive value found during the examination.

Errors in low cylinder powers when combined with low spherical powers can be troublesome. These should remain as prescribed.

Cylinder Axis

The higher the cylinder power, the more serious the result will be if the axis is off. (This is evident in the American National Standards Institute (ANSI) guidelines.)

Prescribed Prism

Errors in prescribed prism may be checked against the full phoria or tropia value found during the examination. The clinician might have chosen to correct a condition with a 5 diopter prism, for example, when the tests were indicating a possible range of from 4.5 to 7.0 prism diopters. If the prism came back as 4.5 instead of 5.0, the practitioner may wish to consider whether this would fulfill the intent of the prescription.

Wrong Distance PDs

Errors in lens optical center placement (PD) resulting in horizontal prism greater than ANSI guidelines are usually not acceptable. In certain instances the clinician may wish to check the phoria or tropia findings of the individual to see if an error would compound or possibly alleviate a problem. The only time when such an error would be acceptable, for example, would be if the induced prism were in a certain base direction and the clinician had been contemplating giving the individual some prism in this base direction anyway.

Errors in PD will cause the wearer to have to converge or diverge the eyes continually to keep from seeing double. In some instances, when the individual was at the limit of their vergence abilities, this could produce headaches, diplopia, a pulling sensation, or eyes that seem to "tire" easily.

Wrong Near PD

An error in the horizontal placement of bi- or trifocal segments will result in an incorrect near PD. Consequences will vary. They are:

1. When the add power is low: An error in the near PD for those who have a low-powered near addition may not be of great consequence *if* the bifocal width is large enough to avoid decreasing the field of view.
2. When the power of the distance lens is plus:
   a. A near PD that is slightly small simply counteracts some of the base-out effect induced by the distance lens at near.
   b. A near PD that is too large, however, worsens the base-out effect and is to be avoided.
3. When the power of the distance lens is minus:
   a. A near PD that is small worsens the base-in effect of the distance lenses at near and is to be avoided.
   b. A near PD that is slightly large counteracts some of the base-in effects induced by the distance lens at near and may not be too serious.

In all of the foregoing instances, caution should be used. Prism amounts induced at near can be calculated using Prentice's rule to help make a better judgment.

Unwanted Vertical Prism

Vertical prism is usually one of the most troublesome of problems. Even small amounts of vertical prism may not be well tolerated, unless there is a vertical difference in the anatomic placement of the two eyes which, if measured, would also result in one eye having a higher vertical MRP height in the glasses. Even then, the vertical prism would have to be in a complementary direction. If no vertical phoria or fixation disparity appeared during the examination, problems may still develop if an erroneous prescription were accepted.

REFERENCES

1. Hirschberg J. The history of ophthalmology, vol 11, part 2. Haugwitz T. Optical instruments. 1981:A49. (First English Edition, 1986, Wayenborgh Verlag, Bonn, West Germany).
2. Emsley HH, Swain W. Ophthalmic lenses. London: Hatton Press Ltd, 1951:183.
3. Reichert. 12603 lensometer lens measuring instrument, instructions. Buffalo: Cambridge Instruments Company, 1986.
4. Reichert. Bausch & Lomb vertometer instruction manual, Cat. No. 21-65-70. Buffalo: Cambridge Instruments Company.
5. Marco. Marco lensmeter instruction handbook. Jacksonville, Fla: Marco Equipment Inc.
6. Topcon. Topcon Lensmeter Model LM-6 (Instrument Manual). Tokyo, Japan.
7. Brooks CW. Essentials for ophthalmic lens work. New York: Professional Press, 1984.
8. Zeiss. Vertex refractionometer with B-eyepiece for spectacle wearers, operating instructions. Oberkochen, West Germany.
9. Topcon. Topcon Lensmeter Model LM-T3 (instrument manual). Tokyo, Japan.
10. Topcon. Topcon Digital Projection Lensmeter Model LM-P5 (instrument manual). Tokyo, Japan.
11. Marco. Marco Digital Projection Lensmeter 750-C Instruction Manual. Jacksonville, Fla: Marco Equipment Inc.
12. Marco. Interum instructional supplement for operating the Marco LM-770C Lensmeter. Jacksonville, Fla: Marco Equipment Inc.
13. Allergan Humphrey. Humphrey Lens Analyzer, Models 306, 330, 340, owner's manual. San Leandro, Calif: June 1986.
14. Topcon. Topcon Computerized Lensmeter Model CL-1500 (instrument manual). Tokyo, Japan.
15. Marco. LM850 Automatic Lensmeter instruction manual. Jacksonville, Fla: Marco Equipment Inc.

Ophthalmic Materials Evaluation

Clifford W. Brooks

INTRODUCTION

Definition

An ophthalmic lens prescription has several parameters which are nonrefractive but are vital elements of the ophthalmic lens correction. The nonrefractive parameters that need to be considered are the lens material; frame and lens size; lens base curve; lens thickness; and multifocal style, size, and position. The *base curve* of a lens is "the surface curve of a lens that becomes the basis from which the other remaining curves are calculated."[1]

The base curve of a lens is almost always on the front. The main notable exception would be when the lens is a bifocal with the segment on the back of the lens. Generally, the front side of an ophthalmic lens is spherical. If the lens has a toric front surface, the base curve is the front curve of least power. (It should be noted that there are some slight differences between the United States and Britain as to what is defined as the base curve.)

Clinical Use

An ophthalmic lens prescription is not properly ordered or filled unless all of the parameters of the lenses are specified and properly evaluated. This information is needed to determine the type of lenses that the patient is presently wearing and to properly prescribe and evaluate the ophthalmic lenses that the patient needs.

INSTRUMENTATION

Theory and Use

The instruments that are used for verifying the nonrefractive parameters of an ophthalmic lens prescription are rulers, lens clocks, and lens calipers.

To measure the base curve, a *lens measure* or *lens clock* is used. The lens measure is a dial-reading instrument that measures the sagittal depth of the lens surface. The *sagittal depth* is the depth of an arc of a circle. If a straight line is drawn parallel to the equator of a circle, the distance from the highest point of the arc of the circle to the straight line is the sagittal depth (Fig. 31–1). The closer the line is to the equator, the wider the arc and the deeper the sagittal depth will be. Thus, it can be seen that the sagittal depth depends upon the width of the arc. The width of this arc is called the *chord*.

The lens clock measures the sagittal depth by using two stationary pins and one movable pin (Fig. 31–2). The instrument converts the sagittal depth directly into surface power and is calibrated in diopters (D). The relationship between sagittal depth (sag) in millimeters and surface power in diopters is found by first using the sag formula.[1]

$$r = (y^2/2s) + s/2$$

where r is the radius of curvature of the surface in millimeters, y is the semidiameter of the chord (half the chord size), and s is the sagittal depth. Once the radius of curvature is known, then the power of the surface can be found using the Lensmaker's formula which is

$$F = (n' - n)/r$$

where F is the power of the lens surface in diopters, n' is the index of refraction of the lens material, and n is the index of the surround. The index of the surround is air and is taken to be 1.

The diopters indicated by the lens clock are based on a theoretical index of refraction of 1.53. Since crown glass has an index of 1.523, there will be little difference between what the instrument reads and the refractive power of the surface. For tool consistency in the optical laboratory, lens base curves are given in terms

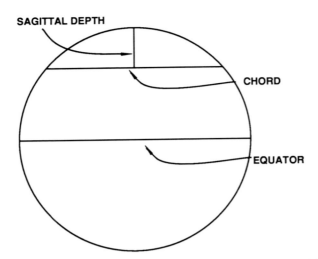

FIGURE 31–1. The horizontal line that crosses the circle is called the *chord*. The depth of the arc for this chord is called the *sagittal depth*.

of a theoretical 1.53 index curve, regardless of whether they are crown glass, high-index glass, or plastic. Base curve values are used for reference only. They are not normally used for their refractive values. For ordering a specific lens form, differences between lens clock readings and lens surface refractive values are of no consequence.

There are two types of measuring points available. The pointed-type tips are the oldest and were used exclusively when all lenses were glass (Fig. 31–3A). When plastic lenses came to be commonly used, ball tips were introduced to keep from scratching the lens surfaces (see Fig. 31–3B). Much confusion has ensued

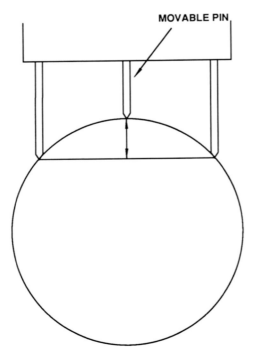

FIGURE 31–2. The sagittal depth for a given chord size is physically measured by the distance the central movable pin travels in relationship to the fixed positions of the two outer pins. This distance is then converted into a dioptric value.

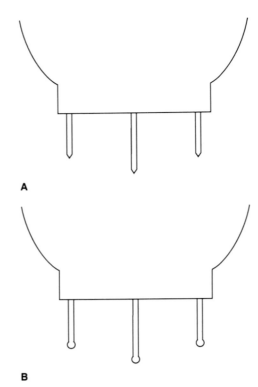

FIGURE 31–3. (A) Lens measures are available with pointed tips. These are best used on glass lenses, which are not as prone to scratching. (B) Lens measures with ball tips are used on plastic lenses. They are less likely to scratch the surface. Even when ball-tipped lens measures are used, they should not be dragged across the lens surface when searching for the meridian of highest or lowest power.

because ball-tipped lens measures are often thought to be exclusively for plastic lenses. Many believe that all lens clocks with pointed tips are calibrated for 1.53 glass, and all lens clocks with ball tips are calibrated for 1.498 plastic. This is not true. As a general rule in the United States, all lens clocks are calibrated for 1.53, regardless of the shape of the measuring tip.

The *lens caliper* is an instrument that physically measures the thickness of a lens. By using a leverlike extension, as the caliper tips physically touch the surface of the lens, the extension sweeps a scale that is six to ten times larger than the actual thickness measurement.

Lens calipers close automatically with the help of a spring. When closed the instrument must read zero. By squeezing the leverlike extension, the jaws of the calipers open. Caliper points are positioned at the location on the lens where the thickness is to be read. As the jaws close, the pointer on the extension sweeps the enlarged, graduated scale until the lens is firmly clamped by the calipers. Because the graduated scale is proportionally enlarged, lens thickness can be read with more accuracy.

COMMERCIALLY AVAILABLE INSTRUMENTS

Rulers

Optical rulers are available from a variety of sources. One should be aware, however, that inexpensive rulers may not be reproduced exactly. All rulers must be checked against an exact, known standard. The more accurate rulers have traditionally been made from either metal or a wood–plastic combination. These are available from suppliers such as Franel, Hilco, Sadler, Vigor, and Western (see the Appendix).

Lens Measures

Lens measures are available from a variety of sources such as those provided in the Appendix. Individual instruments vary in their measuring ranges. Ranges include plus or minus 10 D, plus or minus 14 D, plus or minus 17 D, and plus or minus 20 D.

Lens Calipers

There are a large variety of lens thickness-measuring calipers available. When looking for a caliper, the following characteristics should be sought:

1. The tips should be padded with nylon or plastic to avoid scratching the lenses.
2. The "throat" of the caliper should be deep enough to allow the tips of the caliper to get all the way to the center of the lens. Because calipers are not always made just for the optical industry, but may be used in a variety of industries, it is possible to get an instrument that will not allow the very center of a large lens to be measured.

CLINICAL PROCEDURE

Identification of Lens Material

Following is a list of the most commonly available lens materials:

Glass

- Crown (index 1.523).
- Photochromic (index 1.523).
- High-index glass (Indices are most commonly 1.60, 1.70, or 1.80, but may vary, depending upon manufacturer).

Plastic

- CR-39 (Index of about 1.498 or 1.499, depending upon additives used by individual lens manufacturers.)
- Polycarbonate (index 1.586).
- High-index plastic (such as index 1.56, 1.58, and 1.60. Again, indices may vary by manufacturer).

Lens materials are most easily identified as either glass or plastic. If the material is light in weight and has a dull sound and feel when lightly tapped with a hard object such as a ring, the lens material is plastic. It is easy to tell the difference between glass and plastic. Only one or two practice tries are necessary for the practitioner to develop an ability to distinguish these two categories of materials from one another.

Photochromic materials are made from glass and are easily identified by their color and ability to darken when exposed to sunlight.

High-index glass materials are comparatively thinner than their conventional crown glass counterparts of equal power. High-index glass lenses are no lighter in weight than an equal-powered crown glass lens, unless they are above about 7 D in power. This is due to their high density. However, even an experienced individual would be hard pressed to identify a high-index lens on the basis of weight reduction alone.

A plastic minus lens may be suspected of being made from polycarbonate material if the center thickness is below 1.9 mm. Some with a practiced eye may pick up a slight variation in the cast of the clear polycarbonate lens material. However, differences in cast are more easily seen in the laboratory before the lens blank has ever been worked and is still large and thick.

It is helpful to ask the patient about the lens material they are currently wearing. They may know if they are wearing polycarbonate or a special high-index material.

Identification of Frame or Lens Size

Frame or lens eyesize can be measured with a millimeter ruler. The *boxing system* of frame and lens measurement is generally used. The boxing system measures the lens or the frame's lens opening by constructing the smallest rectangle that encloses the lens shape (Fig. 31–4). The horizontal measurement of this rectangle or box is the *eyesize* or *A* dimension. In the United States, the eyesize of a frame is *not* the width of the lens in the middle of the shape. (This would be the eyesize if the Datum system were being used, as in Britain.) Rather the eyesize is the width of the enclosing box. However, because many lens shapes are widest in the middle of the lens, the eyesize may sometimes be the same in both the boxing and the Datum systems.

The bridge size of a frame is the shortest distance between the two lenses. This is the distance between the imaginary boxes that enclose the right and left lenses (see Fig. 31–4).

The frame eyesize and bridge size markings are usually

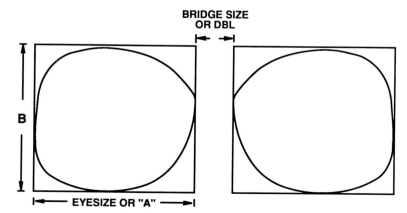

FIGURE 31–4. The boxing system for measuring frames and lenses defines the eyesize as the horizontal dimension of the smallest rectangle that just encloses the frame or lens shape. The vertical dimension of this box is called the B dimension.

stamped on the frame front behind the bridge, behind the nose-pads, or on the backs of the endpieces. Temple length is stamped on the inside of the temple. In some instances, there may be a color identification number found on the inside of the temple as well.

It should be noted that, although the frame should be marked with the accurate boxing eyesize and bridge size, the marked sizes do not always correspond exactly. This results from either failure to adhere to the accepted boxing standards or to manufacturing that falls out of tolerance.

Temple length is most often measured beginning at the butt end of the temple, progressing on back and around the temple bend, and on to the end of the temple. The length is measured in a manner similar to that of driving on a road with a curve. Thus, the temple length is measured *around* the curve and not in a straight line from the butt to the tip.

Verifying Base Curve

To determine the base curve of a lens with a lens clock, position the clock on the front surface of the lens. Be certain it is held perpendicular to the surface, and that the two stationary pins are pressed firmly against the lens (Fig. 31–5). If there is a protruding bi- or trifocal segment, the segment area must be avoided. If the lens has an aspheric portion, as in the lower area of a progressive addition lens, this area too must be avoided.

Base curve values found on the front surface of the lens are recorded exactly as read on the instrument, using the convex (black) scale on the lens measure.

Verifying Lens Center Thickness

Lens center thickness is verified using thickness calipers. It is best to use a pair that have plastic tips, rather than leave the bare metal tips exposed. It is easy to scratch a lens, especially a plastic lens, when the tips are not padded.

The center thickness for a minus lens will be the thinnest part of the lens, and the center thickness of a plus lens will be the thickest part of the lens. This corresponds to the optical center of the lens. The optical center of the lens is determined by placing the lens in a lensmeter and positioning the lens so that the lens-meter target is centered. This point can then be marked on the lens. The lens is removed from the lensmeter and the tips of the

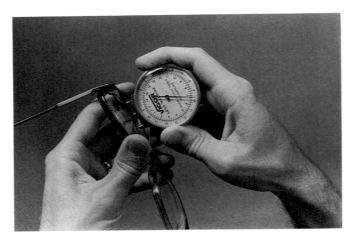

FIGURE 31–5. A lens clock measures the base curve of a lens, referencing the reading to a 1.53 index of refraction. (Base curves are given in 1.53 index terms, regardless of the actual index of the lens.) The lens clock must be held perpendicular to the lens surface.

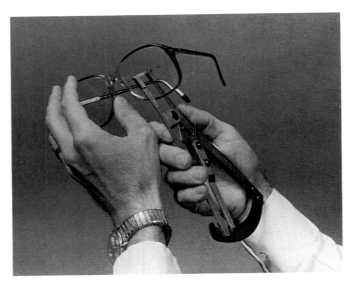

FIGURE 31–6. Lens thicknesses are read using calipers. It is best to use calipers that have plastic tips and are large enough to reach the center of the larger lens shapes.

lens caliper are placed at this point. Be certain that the tips are pressed firmly against the lens. The thickness of the lens is read in millimeters directly from the caliper scale (Fig. 31–6).

Identifying Multifocal Styles

Styles of multifocal lenses are presented in tabular form in Tables 31–1 through 31–3 and in corresponding Figures 31–7 through 31–9. These tables are not meant to be all-inclusive. Not all segment types and sizes come in all materials. Because of the number of new glass and plastic materials available, the local laboratory or a lens catalogue should be consulted.

Verifying Multifocal Segment Positioning

Segment Height

When verifying segment height for bi- or trifocals, the height is measured from the lowest portion of the inside bevel of the lower eyewire (the bottom of the box in the boxing system) up to the top of the segment. If the glasses are constructed so that the lower shape of the lens is flat on the bottom, the measurement is easy to perform (Fig. 31–10). However, if the lens shape slopes, as with the aviator shape, then measuring straight down from the segment top will give an artificially low reading (Fig. 31–11).

Near Pupillary Distance

When verifying the near PD,* the distance between the near segments are measured using a millimeter ruler. This is *not* done by means of a lensmeter. The correct method is to measure the distance from the left side of one segment to the left side of the other segment (Fig. 31–12). Sometimes the segments are decentered so far nasally that they are cut off. If this happens the physical centers of the segments can be dotted and the distance between these dots measured.

---

* The interpupillary distance (IPD), commonly referred to as the PD, is the distance between the center of the pupils measured in millimeters with the patient fixating at distance or near.

Table 31–1
A Summary of Available Bifocal Lens Styles

Type of Segment	Segment Width	Location of Seg OC	Physical Description of the Segment
Flat top or D style segment	22 25 28 35 40	5 below 5 below 5 below 4.5 below or on line On line	This segment looks like a circle with the top cut off either 5-mm above the center of the circle or, in the flat top 40, cut off right in the middle of the circle.
Curve top	22 25 28	4.5 below	This segment resembles a flat top, but the top line of the segment is arched upward in a slight curve.
Panoptik or "P" style lens	24 28	4.5 below	Panoptik segments resemble curve top segments, except that the top edge corners are rounded.
Franklin or Executive	Full lens width	On line	The top of the segment is a straight line that transverses the whole lens. The segment occupies the whole bottom half of the lens.
Ribbon B R	 22 wide 9 deep 22 and 26 wide 14 deep	 4.5 below 7 below	A ribbon segment looks like a round segment with both the top and bottom cut off.
Blended bifocals	22 25 28	11 below 12.5 below 14 below	Blended or "invisible" bifocals are basically a type of one-piece round segment bifocal that does not have a sharp definition at the edge of the segment; rather, it is smoothed or blurred out.
Round			One-piece round segments (made by changing the curve of the lens in the segment area rather than by fusing another material into the lens) are often referred to as "ultex" segments.
22 round	22	11 below	The segment is circular in appearance. The 22 round is often referred to as a "kryptok" seg, although kryptok technically refers only to a certain type of fused glass lens. One-piece 22 round seg glass lenses are sometimes referred to as "ultex B" segs.
24 round 25 round	24 25	12 below 12.5 below	
A style	38	19 below	This segment is listed as being semicircular in appearance, since the full circle is not available in the lens blank. (The bottom half of the circle is cut off.) The "A" designation is often listed for any 38- or 40-mm semicircular segment, regardless of segment location (i.e., front or back, top or bottom half of the lens), as long as the segment depth is half width. In other words, the total seg height available for a 38-mm round is 19 mm.
AA or AL or R-40 style	38 40	19 below 20 below	This lens has the full circle of the 38- or 40-mm round segment available. They would only be used if a very high segment height were desired.
Rede-Rite or minus add upcurve	38	19 above	A semicircular upcurve design with the near power located in the main lens and the distance power in the "add," which is located at the top of the lens. It is a "minus add" lens.

Table 31–2
A Summary of Available Trifocal Styles

Type of Segment	Segment Dimensions	Physical Description of the Segment
Flat-top trifocal	6 × 22 6 × 28 7 × 23 7 × 25 7 × 28 7 × 35 8 × 25 8 × 35 9 × 35 10 × 25 10 × 35	These lenses look like a flat-top bifocal, except with an intermediate portion in the upper half of the lens segment. The first number refers to the vertical intermediate depth, the second, the horizontal segment width at the widest part of the seg. Not all segments are available in both glass and plastic. The underlined sizes are the most commonly used.
	14 × 35 CRT	A flat-top style lens designed for computer or other uses requiring an especially wide intermediate portion.
Franklin style	Full width of the lens, 7-mm intermediate seg depth	Franklin, or Executive trifocals are one piece in design, have the segment optical centers on the lines and are very visible. The higher the add, the thicker the lens, the greater the lens weight and the more obvious the seg line appears.
CRT	Full width of the lens, 14-mm intermediate seg depth	Has the appearance of a Franklin style trifocal lens, but with a deeper intermediate portion. For computer and other near situations for which a deep, wide intermediate viewing distance is required.
ED	Full width intermediate, D 25 style near.	The ED trifocal has a full-width, Franklin style lower half that is of intermediate power; 8-mm below the intermediate line and positioned within the lower intermediate area is a flat top, "D" style segment with a 25-mm width.
Round	7 × 22 × 36	This trifocal has a 22-mm round near segment portion surrounded by a 36-mm diameter intermediate, leaving the intermediate with a 7-mm "rim" around the 22-mm near seg.
X or A style	8 × 32 × 48	Same style as the above round trifocal, except with different dimensions. Blank size allows the seg height to be only 24-mm maximum.
AL style	8 × 32 × 48	Blank allows the seg height to be as high as 35-mm maximum.
Ribbon	6 × 22	This segment style is the same as the bifocal ribbon segment with both top and bottom of the segment being flat, except that there is a 6-mm deep intermediate area.
Curve top	7 × 24	Same as the bifocal version of the curve-top segment, except with a 7-mm deep intermediate portion.
Progressive addition lenses	Seg begins at MRP. Near progressive zone width varies.	Progressive addition lenses have a progressive corridor that begins at the major reference point of the lens. The farther down into the progressive corridor the eye drops, the higher the add power becomes, until the full prescribed add power is reached.
Smart seg	Flat-top 30	The lens has the appearance of a conventional flat-top bifocal that is 30 mm wide. However, the optics within the segment area are progressive.

CLINICAL IMPLICATIONS

Clinical Significance and Interpretation

Lens Material

Inadvertently switching a patient out of a high-index material can be a costly mistake. The lenses will come back thicker and more unsightly than the patient will tolerate.

Mistakenly switching the patient out of highly impact-resistant polycarbonate material can be serious. Should the replacement lenses break while being worn, a possible lawsuit could result.

Frame or Lens Size

Inaccurately identifying frame size when ordering "lenses only" will result in lenses that will not fit the frames. A reorder will be

Table 31–3
A Summary of Available Occupational and Other Styles

Type of Segment	Segment Dimensions	Physical Description of the Segment
Occupational flat top or "double D"	22/22 25/25 28/28 28/25 35/35	These lenses appear to be a flat-top bifocal on the bottom with an inverted flat top on the top. Top and bottom segments are separated by from 12 to 15 mm; 13- and 14-mm separations are the most commonly used. Segment dimensions listed are for the width of the lower segment, followed by the width of the upper segment. The upper segment add power may be a. The full value of the add, like the lower seg. b. One-half diopter less than the lower seg add power. c. A percentage of the full add power such as 60% or 50%.
Double round	22/22 25/25	Standard upper and lower segment separations are 13 or 14 mm, although for glass, factory orders can be made for separations from 11 to 20 mm.
Franklin double-segment bifocals	Full width	Most common segment separations are 10 and 14 mm.
Quadrafocal	7/25 (25 upper) 7/28 (28 upper)	A quadrafocal is a lens with a flat-top trifocal in the lower portion and an inverted flat-top bifocal in the upper portion; 10- and 13-mm segment separations are normal. Special order segment separations may be available, varying from 9 to 20 mm.
ED occupational	Full width intermediate, D 25 style near.	The ED occupational trifocal has a full-width, Franklin style lower half that has a 50% intermediate power; 13-mm below the intermediate line and positioned within the lower intermediate area is a flat-top, "D" style segment with a 25-mm width.
FD Trifocal	Full width intermediate, D 28 style near.	The FD occupational trifocal has a full-width, Franklin style lower half, which has a 60% intermediate power; 11-mm below the intermediate line and positioned within the lower intermediate area is a flat-top, "D" style segment with a 28-mm width.
Varilux overview	Progressive add lower, 40-mm round upper.	This lens has a progressive addition lower portion with a 40-mm upcurve round segment at the top of the lens at a point 9-mm above the fitting cross. The upper segment add power is always 0.50-D less than the prescribed add power in the lower portion.
Prism segment	Extended R style	This bifocal lens looks like a ribbon segment having a 10-mm depth that extends to the nasal edge of the lens blank. Horizontal prism available is from 1.00 to 3.5 prism diopters in adds ranging from 1.00 D to 3.00 D in 0.25-D steps.

necessary. It is safest to send a patient's frame to the laboratory for an exact fit.

Failure to identify a wrong frame size on an incoming order will result in patient dissatisfaction and a decreased level of esteem for the practice in general. Even though, from an optical point of view, the results may not be serious if the lens centers and seg heights are still properly situated, the prescription should be rejected and the proper frame size reordered.

Base Curve

Some patients will wear their ophthalmic lenses for a period of time and then decide they need a second pair. If this second pair is ordered and difficulty in adaptation experienced, the problem may be due to a difference in base curve.

Different base curves will cause viewing differences in the periphery of the lens. Switching back and forth between two pair of glasses with two different ways of "distorting" the peripheral

view may prove problematic for some. When reordering a second pair of glasses it is advisable to use the same optical laboratory as before and to specify the same base curve.

If there are unequal base curves on the right and left lenses without a correspondingly large difference in lens powers, difficulty in adaptation can occur. This difficulty is not just due to peripheral aberration differences, but is also a result of magnification differences caused by a change in front surface curvatures. The more steeply the front surface of the lens is curved, the more that lens will magnify the image size. Different base curves on the right and left lenses which are not accompanied by corresponding differences in refractive power between the right and left eyes will result in aniseikonia.

Lens Center Thickness

Unless center thickness was specified on the original order, there are only limited circumstances in which the prescription should

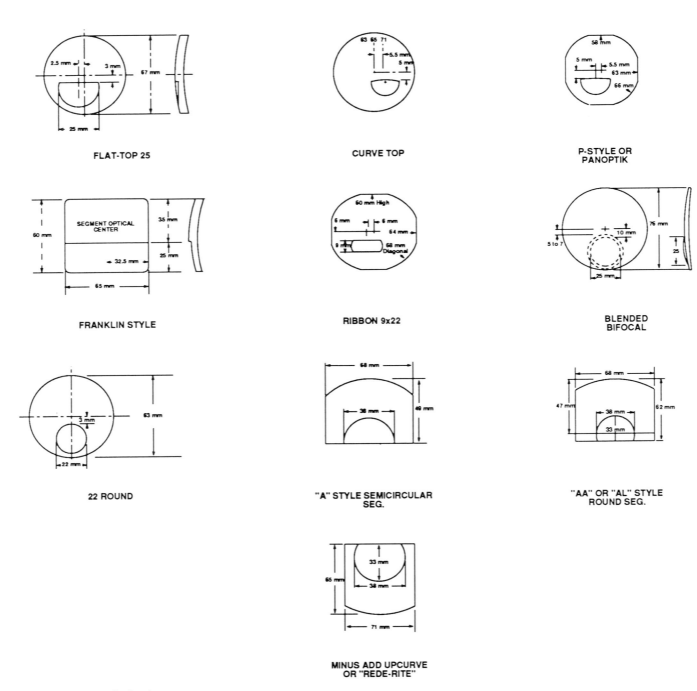

FIGURE 31–7. Bifocal styles.

be rejected. These circumstances might be

1. When the lens is plus in, but still has an excessively thick *edge,* even at its thinnest point.
2. When the lens is a crown glass or CR-39 lens and is less than 1.9-mm thick. (There is no minimum thickness required by the FDA as long as the lens can pass the drop ball test for impact resistance. Nonetheless, most laboratories will not deliver a crown glass or conventional plastic lens that is much less than the commonly accepted United States' standard of 2.2 mm.)
3. When the lens is an "industrial thickness" lens. Here, the

minimum center thickness for plus or minus is 3.0 mm. (Most laboratories use a 3.2-mm minimum thickness, just to be safe.)

Polycarbonate lenses may be thinner than others, because of their superior impact resistance. The exception is when these lenses are being used for "safety glasses" as defined by Z87 American National Standards Institute guidelines for "Occupational and Educational Eye and Face Protection." Safety lenses must be 3.0-mm thick, even if they are polycarbonate.

Failure to identify a lens that is unacceptably *thin* has definite legal ramifications if the person wearing the lens experiences an

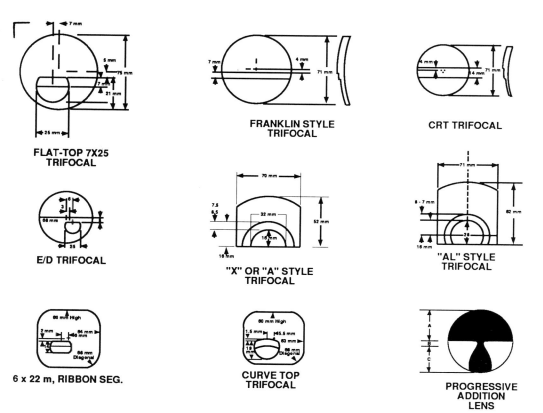

FIGURE 31-8. Trifocal styles.

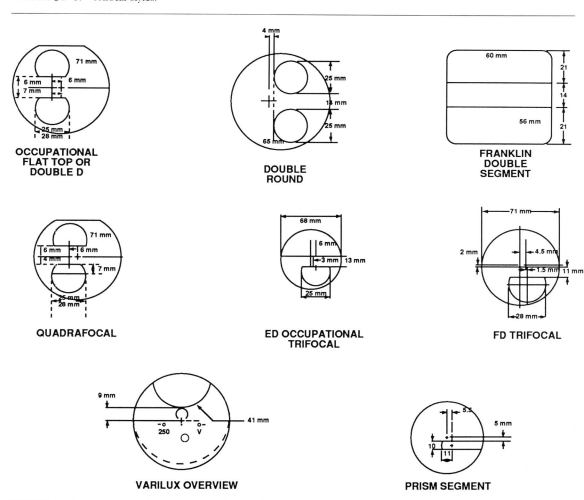

FIGURE 31-9. Occupational and other multifocal styles.

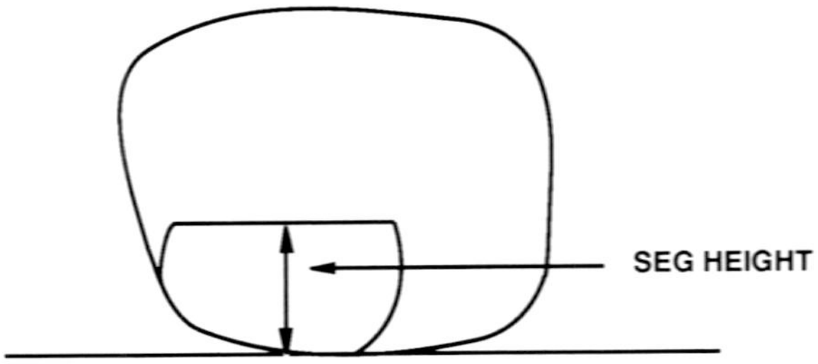

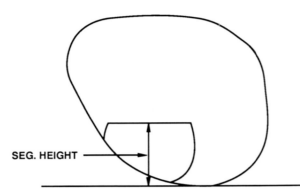

FIGURE 31–10. The segment height is measured vertically from the segment top to the lowest portion of the inside bevel of the lower eyewire. For lens shapes with flat lower rims, the measure is straightforward.

FIGURE 31–11. Measuring segment height for bi- or trifocals can easily be done in error. With the boxing system of lens measuring, the height is always referenced to the lowest level of the lens, regardless of where the lens is cut off below the middle of the segment top. The height as shown above is correct, but could easily be measured as being smaller than it really is.

eye injury. If the injury could have been prevented had the lens been properly inspected and found to be unacceptably thin, the optometric practice could be named in a lawsuit.

If a lens is *thicker* than it would need to be, the glasses will weigh more and be cosmetically inferior. In addition, plus lenses that are thicker than necessary will cause the patient's eyes to look bigger to an observer. Objects seen by the wearer will be magnified. Increased lens thickness for plus lenses cause increased magnification.

Differences in lens thickness between right and left lenses of equal powers will result in differential magnifications for the two eyes. This can cause an aniseikonia and may cause the wearer difficulty in fusing the images comfortably.

Multifocal Style

Incorrect identification of lens multifocal style can mean an incorrect order. Incorrect orders mean costly reorders.

What if the person verifying a new pair of glasses fails to note that the multifocal style is not what was ordered? When this happens, there is a high probability that there will be an inability on the part of the wearer to use the glasses as intended. For example, a multifocal segment that is narrower than needed will constrict the wearer's reading field. A segment that is wider than planned may interfere with distance vision in the inferior periphery of the field of view.

Multifocal Segment Positioning

Sometimes *unequal segment heights* are ordered because of anatomic differences in the height of the two eyes. Yet sometimes an order comes back from the laboratory with the segments unequally high when they were ordered for the same height. If the eyes are at the same level, but the bifocal lines are not, the unequal segment heights will cause the line to be much more noticeable to the wearer.

Segments that are too high or low can cause a temporary clumsiness on the part of the wearer or an inability to see or use the lenses as desired. If the patient does not complain, but tries to adapt to the problem, postural problems involving the body or head may result. These postural abnormalities result from the patient attempting to use or see over a poorly located multifocal segment.

REFERENCE

1. Brooks CW, Borish IM. System for ophthalmic dispensing. Stoneham, Mass: Butterworths, 1979:376, 462.

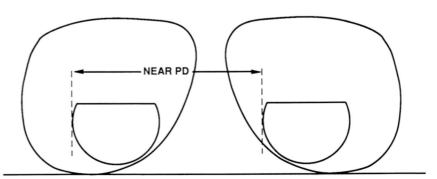

FIGURE 31–12. The near PD is measured from one side of the lens segment to the same side of the other segment.

APPENDIX

Optical rulers, lens measurers and lens calipers are available from a variety of sources. Selected manufacturers of dispensing equipment are provide below.

Franel Optical Supply Co.
111 Atlantic Dr.
P.O. Box 96
Maitland, FL 32751

Hilco
Division of the Hilsinger Corp.
33 W. Bacon St.
Plainville, MA 02762

Sadler Bros., Inc.
561 Newport Ave.
South Attleboro, MA 02703

Vigor Optical Co.
Division of B. Jadow and Sons, Inc.
53 West 23rd St.
New York, NY 10010

Western Optical Supply, Inc.
11200 Chandler Blvd.
P.O. Box 266
North Hollywood, CA 91601

PART 2

Ocular Disease Procedures

Gonioscopy

David M. Cockburn

INTRODUCTION

Definition

Gonioscopy is a procedure that enables the clinical examination of the periphery of the anterior chamber angle.

History

The periphery of the anterior chamber is not normally available for direct inspection because light reflected by the structures posterior to the limbus is totally reflected within the chamber. Trantas[1] used limbal indentation, together with an ophthalmoscope, to obtain a view of the angle, and coined the term gonioscopy to describe the technique. Troncoso[2] was responsible for the introduction of a practical technique, using a contact lens to neutralize the anterior corneal surface as a refracting medium, thereby permitting visual inspection of the angle, without distortion of associated structures.

The technique of gonioscopy was further simplified by Goldmann[3] who developed a contact lens having an enclosed mirror, a modification that allowed the use of a slit lamp. The binocular features of modern slit lamps, their excellent optics and variable magnification, permit the clinician to view the undisturbed structures of the chamber angle under stereoscopic conditions, with a variety of magnifications and types of illumination. Figure 32–1 shows a single-mirror goniolens similar to the original Goldmann lens. Today the most commonly used goniolens is the Goldmann three-mirror lens (Fig. 32–2).

Clinical Use

Table 32–1 shows the clinical indications for gonioscopic examination. The list of clinical indications includes signs and symptoms suggesting the presence of angle closure glaucoma; neovascularization or other forms of neoplasia of the angle; anterior chamber inflammation, pigment dispersion, exfoliation, synechiae, trauma, and degeneration.

In addition to these signs it is necessary to exclude angle closure as a cause of ocular hypertension or of an increase in intraocular pressure (IOP) from a previously established base pressure. Gonioscopy is required for the management of such patients and is an essential part of the diagnosis of glaucoma, because it is not otherwise possible to distinguish between open-angle glaucoma and angle closure glaucoma and, consequently, to initiate the appropriate treatment or referral.

INSTRUMENTATION

Theory

The anterior chamber angle is concealed from direct observation by the projection of opaque scleral tissue over its anterior wall as far as the limbus and Schwalbe's line. Light reflected from structures within the angle is totally reflected within the anterior chamber because of the curvature of the cornea, so that attempted observations made obliquely through the cornea are unable to include these structures.

All goniolenses use the principle of eliminating the cornea as a refracting surface by use of a concave contact surface that is placed against the cornea. Any small difference in curvature between the lens and the cornea is minimized by interposing a fluid between the two surfaces. As a result, corneal refraction is virtually eliminated, and an observer is able to view the angle recess through an obliquely inclined mirror (Goldmann, see Figs. 32–1, 32–2; and Zeiss, Fig. 32–3) or directly through a curved hemispherical dome (Koeppe, Fig. 32–4).

Goniolenses that use mirrors may have the mirror embedded within the body of the lens, as in the Goldmann and the Allen–

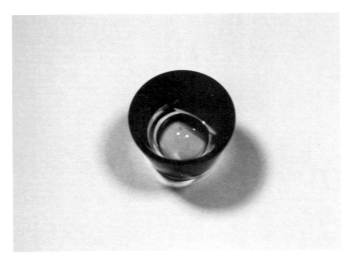

FIGURE 32–1. Single-mirror Goldmann goniolens similar to the original lens introduced by Goldmann in 1938.

Thorpe lenses, or have prismatic sides that are externally silvered, as in the Zeiss system. These goniolenses all have plano-front surfaces and are referred to as indirect types because they involve reflection of the image in a mirror. They also utilize the adjustable illumination system and variable magnification of the slit lamp. However, in a situation for which a slit lamp cannot be used, a direct ophthalmoscope will provide a useful view of the angle through these goniolenses.

The Koeppe goniolens provides a direct view of the angle with 1.5× magnification. Additional magnification is obtained through a ceiling-suspended, low-powered binocular microscope, and illumination by means of a separate illuminating system. In less critical circumstances, or when the patient cannot be suitably arranged for this system, an indirect ophthalmoscope provides a quite adequate view, with greater magnification than available with the indirect goniolenses.

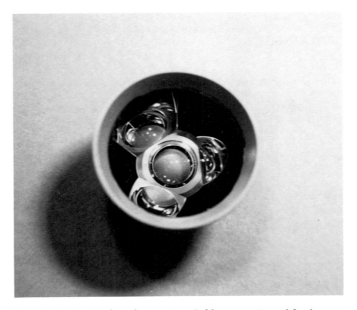

FIGURE 32–2. Modern three-mirror Goldmann gonio and fundus contact lens seen from the clinician's side. The oval mirror is for gonioscopy.

Table 32–1
Indications for Gonioscopy

Narrowness or Closure of the Anterior Chamber Angle
  Slit lamp estimate of angle width of 0.3 or less corneal units
  Shallowness of anterior chamber by shadow test or pachometry
Historical Evidence of Angle Closure
  Symptoms of intermittent blur, frontal pain or headaches (not otherwise explained), or halos around lights
  History of a previous attack of angle closure
Other Clinical Evidence
  Glaukomflecken
  Documented increased intraocular pressure from previous base or IOP greater than 21 mmHg
  Cup/disc ratio equal to or greater than 0.6 or observed increase in ratio
Evidence Suggesting Possible Anterior Chamber Neovascularization
  Diabetes, particularly severe background, early or established proliferative diabetic retinopathy
  Recent or previous central, or hemispherical retinal vein occlusion
  Naked vessels on the iris or pupil margin
Evidence of Neoplastic Activity in the Anterior Chamber
  Localized bulging of the iris surface
  Enlarged or proliferated iris blood vessels
  Iris naevi extending beyond the limbus
  Documented evidence of iris naevus enlargement
  Unusual pigmentation of the iris
Evidence of Active or Past Inflammation in the Anterior Chamber
  Keratic precipitates, flare or cells in the aqueous, synechial attachments of the iris to the lens or cornea
  Ciliary flush
  Irregular or poorly responsive pupil
History or Evidence of Trauma
  Iridodialysis, eccentric pupil, anisocoria, ruptures of the pupil margin, iris transillumination, hyphema, or unusual sectoral variation in anterior chamber depth
  History, or signs of penetrating ocular foreign body
Degenerative Conditions Affecting the Anterior Segment of the Eye
  Iris transillumination
  Iris heterochromia
  Irregularity of the pupil, or topography of the iris surface
  Corneal edema
  Krukenberg's spindle or free pigment in the aqueous
  Pseudoexfoliation of the lens capsule

(Adapted from Cockburn DM. Indications for gonioscopy and assessment of gonioscopic signs in optometric practice. Am J Optom Physiol Opt 58:706, 1981)

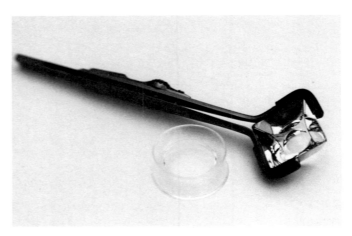

FIGURE 32–3. Zeiss goniolens in holding forceps. The lid speculum is shown below the goniolens.

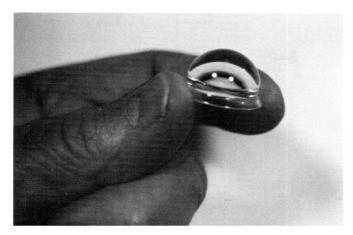

FIGURE 32–4. The Koeppe goniolens. Note the flange that retains the lens in place during gonioscopy.

Use

The first view through the gonioscope presents some difficulty of orientation. Figure 32–5 is a diagram showing both the gonioscopic features of the angle and their equivalent anatomic section. Note the anatomic features at the left of the diagram, with their corresponding gonioscopic appearances toward the right-hand side. It will assist in interpreting the gonioscopic view if the clinician imagines that he or she is looking from a position within the anterior chamber and sighting across the pupil and the anterior surface of the iris toward the opposite side of the angle.

The appearance of the anterior chamber angle varies according to congenital individual differences and with acquired changes due to age, injury, or disease. In addition, the extent to which any, or all, of its structures are visible during gonioscopy, depends upon the width of the angle and the convexity of the iris diaphragm. Recognition of the landmarks of the gonioscopic examination allows interpretation of these factors and lays the foundation for clinical diagnosis.

From anterior to posterior, the gonioscopic landmarks consist of Schwalbe's line, the trabeculae (divided somewhat arbitrarily into anterior and posterior portions), the scleral spur, and the ciliary body. The last roll of the iris (Fuch's roll) appears opposite the pupil margin. Iris processes may bridge the space between the peripheral iris and the internal wall of the chamber angle, usually inserting into the ciliary body, but occasionally bridging to the trabeculae or Schwalbe's line. These structures and the technique for their identification will be described in the foregoing listed order.

Schwalbe's Line

Schwalbe's line forms the termination of Descemet's membrane and marks the transition from transparent cornea to opaque scleral tissue. It also forms the anterior boundary of the trabeculae.

When the broad slit lamp beam is used, it is not easy to identify Schwalbe's line, unless it is particularly prominent. Prominence of Schwalbe's line is a feature of posterior embryotoxon, and when it is dusted with pigment, as occurs in pseudoexfoliation of the lens capsule and in the anterior chamber pigment dispersion syndromes. In most other cases, Schwalbe's line is best identified by using the narrow light beam of the slit lamp. The anterior and posterior corneal bright bands of the cornea, being unable to pass through the opaque scleral tissue, appear to merge at the transition zone between cornea and sclera. The gonioscopist should seek the point at which the bands become confluent, as shown in the diagram (see Fig. 32–5). This point of confluence of the corneal bright bands marks Schwalbe's line.

The Trabeculum

The trabeculum is bounded anteriorly by Schwalbe's line and posteriorly by the anterior edge of the scleral spur. They are somewhat arbitrarily divided into anterior and posterior portions. The anterior trabeculum appears amorphous, more pale in youth, and more pigmented with age, although it is usually paler than the posterior trabeculum. It occupies approximately half the width of the trabecular band.

The posterior trabeculum varies in appearance within and between individuals, being heavily pigmented in some subjects and almost colorless in others, but with a general tendency to increased pigmentation in subjects having darker complexions and with age. Labile pigment in the anterior chamber tends to accumulate in the posterior trabecular meshwork and on the surface of Schlemm's canal, particularly in the inferior angle, where it may cause these tissues to be very dark. In addition, the presence or absence of blood in Schlemm's canal influences the color of the posterior trabeculum. Reflux of blood in Schlemm's canal is a normal condition, and its presence imparts a pink hue to an otherwise pale trabeculum.

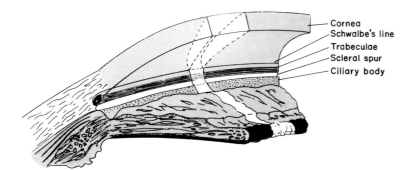

Cornea
Schwalbe's line
Trabeculae
Scleral spur
Ciliary body

FIGURE 32–5. Diagram showing the anatomic and corresponding gonioscopic view of the anterior chamber angle. Note that the scleral spur is an extension of the sclera under the trabeculae and appears starkly white by comparison with the other angle features. The corneal anterior and posterior bright bands converge at Schwalbe's line and the trabeculae lie between this point and the anterior border of the scleral spur. Schlemm's canal occupies the posterior half of the trabecule. The tissue posterior to the scleral spur is the ciliary body.

It is important to recognize that the canal of Schlemm, on gonioscopic examination, lies underneath the posterior trabeculum and thus occupies approximately half the trabecular tissue, as seen in gonioscopy. The posterior border of the trabeculae is at the scleral spur and, in practice, is most easily identified by first seeking the scleral spur and, then, looking for the trabeculum at its anterior margin.

The Scleral Spur

The scleral spur is a projection of the sclera beneath the trabeculae and the canal of Schlemm. It forms an annulus of dense tissue that may be thought of as providing physical support for the rather loose, spongy tissue of the trabeculae and for the underlying canal of Schlemm. Its scleral origin is apparent from its gonioscopic appearance, where it is seen as solid in form and clearly whiter than any other angle structure. This white band of scleral spur is the most constant gonioscopic finding, making it the most readily recognized landmark, assuming that it is not hidden by the iris in an eye having a narrow angle.

Having located the scleral spur, it follows that all structures anterior to it are trabeculae, Schwalbe's line, or cornea, whereas all structures posterior are ciliary body (with or without iris processes) and the iris.

The Ciliary Body

The ciliary body lies posterior to the scleral spur and varies from pink to dark brown. It generally tends to be pigmented according to the patients' overall complexion, but becomes darker with age and is often darkest in the inferior portion, at which pigment tends to be deposited more heavily. The iris inserts into the ciliary body slightly medial to the wall of the chamber, and the sulcus so formed is termed the *angle recess*. The insertion point of the iris varies somewhat, and extreme anterior insertion leads to the anatomic state referred to as *plateau iris*. This rather rare anatomic variation predisposes to the occurrence of angle closure during mydriasis, since iris tissue crowds into the limited sulcus and is likely to occlude the angle.

Iris Processes

The iris processes are variably present in the angle and form fine wispy (occasionally course) strands between the peripheral face of the iris and the ciliary body; occasionally, some strands may extend to the trabeculae or the line of Schwalbe. Usually, these iris processes are very fine and have the appearance of teased cotton wool strands. Course iris processes are less common and may be mistaken for anterior synechiae. However, synechiae are more broadly based in their attachment to the wall of the chamber angle and consist of solid iris tissue that tends to be distorted by the attachment. Iris processes are probably the atavistic remains of the pectinate ligament which, in lower animals, replaces the trabeculae.

COMMERCIALLY AVAILABLE INSTRUMENTS

Commercially available diagnostic goniolenses include the Goldmann single-mirror and three-mirror lenses (see Figs. 32–1 and 32–2), the Zeiss (see Fig. 32–3), and the Koeppe lens (see Fig. 32–4). Instruments similar to the Goldmann lens include the Carl Zeiss three- and four-mirror lenses, Barkan lenses, the Wilson three-mirror, and a series of lenses by Thorpe.

Several goniolenses have been specially developed for anterior chamber angle surgery; these include the Swan–Jacob lens, which has an inclined plano outer surface that permits a wide undistorted view of the angle during surgery. The Worst, Barkan, and Troncoso goniolenses are also commonly used for surgical purposes. The Koeppe lens is also an excellent lens for surgical procedures and is modified for this purpose by the addition of a dimple at its outer surface center to permit manipulation of the lens by an assistant.

CLINICAL PROCEDURE

Only Goldmann, Zeiss, and Koeppe gonioscopic lenses will be discussed because they are the most commonly used lenses, and the techniques required for the use of other instruments are essentially similar. The Goldmann lens provides a somewhat clearer view of the angle than the Zeiss system. However, the Zeiss lens is much more simple and convenient to use, and, because there is no viscous fluid used, it causes less blurring for the patient after the examination.

It is good practice to explain to the patient the nature of any procedure that is about to be undertaken, so that anxiety is reduced and the patient is able to cooperate fully. Before commencing gonioscopy, the patient should be told that the examination permits the optometrist to examine an important part of the eye that cannot be seen by other methods and that a special form of contact lens will be used.

Goldmann Gonioscopic Lens

The Goldmann gonioscopic lens is the most popular lens in use, since, in its three-mirror form, it permits gonioscopic examination, viewing of the mid and far periphery of the fundus, and examination of the macular region. It has excellent optics and is easily handled. The Goldmann three-mirror lens provides a view of the anterior chamber angle through an arc-shaped internal mirror forming a 62° angle with the frontal plane surface. The corneal surface of the three-mirror lens has a 7.4-mm concave radius of curvature, a 12-mm internal diameter, and an 18-mm overall diameter, to form a scleral lip. Two additional mirrors and the central lens are used for ocular fundus examination.

Method

1. Anesthetize the patient's corneas with 1 or 2 drops of 0.5% proparacaine.
2. Position the patient comfortably at the slit lamp, so that the eyes are at the level of the guide marks on the headrest vertical bars. The fixation target should be adjusted to enable the patient to maintain fixation in the straight-ahead position.
3. Set the microscope at a power of approximately 15× and the illuminating slit to its wide-open position.
4. Ask the patient to maintain gentle pressure on the chin rest and brow bar of the instrument.
5. Place one or two drops of bubble-free methylcellulose, or similar fluid, into the concavity of the Goldmann goniolens.
6. Sit comfortably at the slit lamp. Hold the Goldmann lens between thumb and first finger of one hand (left hand for patient's right eye and right hand for patient's left eye), with the goniomirror (D-shaped mirror) located superiorly.
7. Instruct the patient to look directly ahead toward the fixation light and then place the lip of the goniolens into the lower fornix, using the thumb to partly evert the lower lid (Fig. 32–6). Use the index finger again to gently lift the upper lid over the lip of the goniolens (Fig. 32–7). Main-

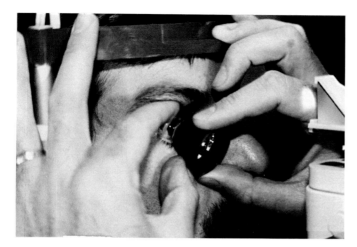

FIGURE 32–6. Inserting the Goldmann three-mirror lens with the patient in position at the slit lamp. The lens is inserted under the lower lid, while the patient's upper lid is held clear of the lens, which is tilted out at the top.

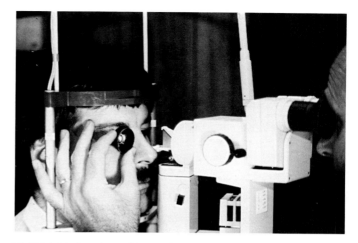

FIGURE 32–8. The Goldmann lens in position ready for gonioscopic examination. Note that the clinician's hand is steadied against the headrest upright bar.

tain steady and gentle pressure of the lens against the cornea to avoid the introduction of an air bubble. The inferior angle should now be available for inspection in the oval mirror (Fig. 32–8). Other parts of the angle may be inspected by rotating the lens through 360°.

8. When performing gonioscopy in the lateral angles with a slit lamp illumination, the lamp should be tilted from the vertical to allow separation of the light and viewing axes in a horizontal plane. The Goldmann and similarly designed slit lamps have this facility, whereas other slit lamps have adjustable mirrors in the illumination path to achieve the same result.

9. Remove the lens by parting the lids so that they are clear of the lip of the goniolens; in most instances, the lens will then drop out into the cupped hand of the optometrist. If the lens remains attached to the cornea by capillary attraction, simply press firmly with one finger tip on the lateral sclera, adjacent to the rim of the lens. This will allow air into the concavity of the lens and will break the capillary attraction that is holding the lens against the cornea. Do *not* apply force to the lens in an attempt to remove it from the eye, since corneal trauma is likely to occur.

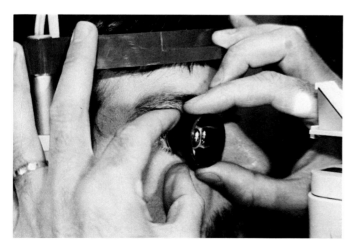

FIGURE 32–7. The lens is rotated back against the eye, while the upper lid is eased over the lip of the lens.

10. Inform the patient that any blurring of vision is temporary and is due to the retention of some of the gonioscopic fluid used in the examination. Saline flushing of the fornices can be used to remove excess fluid if desired.

11. After use, the lens should be washed in soap and water, dried with lint-free tissue or cotton towel, and replaced in the lens container.

The Zeiss Gonioscopic Lens

The Zeiss gonioprism has four externally silvered mirrors and is supplied with a holder and speculum (see Fig. 32–3). This system is probably the most simple with which to commence the practice of gonioscopy, because the speculum keeps the patient's lids separated, allowing the prism to rest on the cornea without being partly under the lids, as with the Goldmann lens. Because the corneal surface of the Zeiss lens has approximately the same curvature as the average cornea, it is not necessary to use gonioscopic fluid. However, a single drop of saline will facilitate maintaining a bubble-free contact with the cornea and help prevent corneal drying should the examination be protracted.

The Zeiss gonioscopic lens requires only very light pressure to seal against the cornea, with the result that there is little distortion of the angle structures. It follows that the view obtained of the angle is very nearly the normal appearance, unless the lens is deliberately used to distort the chamber.

Method

1. Anesthetize the patient's corneas with 1 drop of a suitable short-acting corneal anesthetic.

2. Position the patient comfortably at the slit lamp, so that the eyes are at the level of the guide marks on the headrest vertical bars. The fixation target should be adjusted to enable the patient to maintain fixation in the straight-ahead position.

3. Set the microscope at a power of approximately 15× and the illuminating slit to its wide-open position.

4. The patient should then sit back from the slit lamp to allow insertion of the speculum (Figs. 32–9, 32–10, and 32–11 illustrate the technique for insertion of the speculum).

5. The patient is repositioned at the slit lamp and the Zeiss gonioscopy prism placed lightly on the cornea, using just

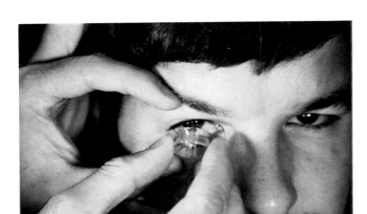

FIGURE 32–9. Inserting the Zeiss lid speculum. The patient looks upward and the speculum is inserted under the lower lid.

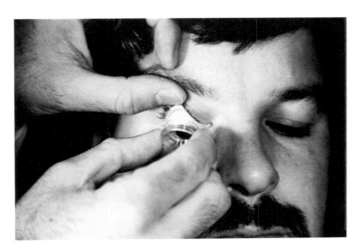

FIGURE 32–10. The patient looks down while the upper lid is held up, and the speculum is inserted against the superior bulbar conjunctiva.

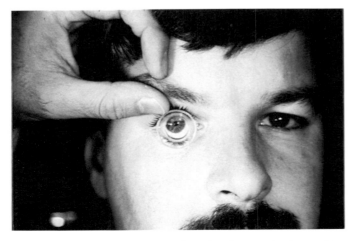

FIGURE 32–11. The upper lid is allowed to slip over the flange of the speculum, and the patient looks directly ahead.

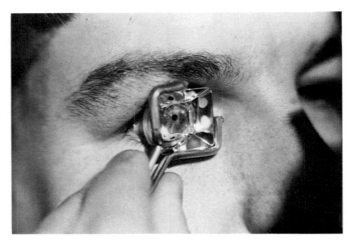

FIGURE 32–12. With the speculum in position, the Zeiss goniolens is placed lightly against the cornea in preparation for the gonioscopic examination.

sufficient pressure to eliminate air bubbles. Keep the edges of the gonioprism horizontal and vertical. A little practice will soon enable the goniolens to be maintained with its concavity in the same plane as the patient's cornea and with bubble-free contact uniformly over the lens contact surface. The prism and its holder are held as shown in Figure 32–12. The little finger of the hand that holds the goniolens may be rested on the patient's cheek.

6. Look first in the top mirror at the image of the inferior angle, then in the bottom mirror to inspect the superior portion of the angle. Rotate the goniolens so that the mirrors are oblique and inspect the lateral angles. The width of the mirror of the Zeiss lens is not sufficient to accommodate both the slit lamp illumination beam and the microscope ray path when the lens is held horizontally and vertically and the side mirrors are being used to inspect the lateral and nasal angles. It is necessary to rotate the mirrors slightly one way and then the other to enable inspection of the most lateral and nasal sectors of the angle.

7. After completing the gonioscopic examination, the Zeiss goniolens is simply backed away from the cornea; it will not adhere to the cornea, so removal is uncomplicated.

8. The speculum is removed by having the patient look up and slipping the lower lid from the lip of the speculum and then having the patient look down. The speculum will then fall into the optometrist's cupped hand.

9. After use, the goniolens and speculum should be cleaned with soap and water and dried with lint-free tissue or a cotton towel. Care should be taken in handling the Zeiss lens, since the mirroring is on the outside of the lens and is readily scratched if roughly handled or subjected to chemicals. Always store the prism in a protective container when not in use.

The appearance of the angle through the Zeiss goniolens is distorted slightly at the far edges of the mirror in a manner that makes the angle appear narrower than it does in the central portion. Rotate the mirror to check that this is an artifact, until you are familiar with the technique.

The Koeppe Gonioscopic Lens

Since there are no mirrors, the Koeppe lens (see Fig. 32–4) provides a direct method of examining the anterior chamber angle. It relies on neutralizing the corneal surface as a refracting medium and its spherical outer surface to permit an almost direct line of sight into the angle. The image magnification provided is approximately half that seen with the Zeiss or Goldmann systems. However, the field of view is correspondingly wider and the image less distorted toward its extreme edges. The Koeppe lens is usually used in the operating room in conjunction with a binocular magnifier suspended from the ceiling or an overhead beam.

Although not the preferred system for optometric clinical use, the Koeppe lens is ideal for anterior chamber angle surgery because of the wide, undistorted field of view and the ability to see into the entire angle by the clinician moving around the patient.

Method

1. Anesthetize the patient's corneas with 1 drop of a suitable short-acting corneal anesthetic.
2. Place the patient in a recumbent position.
3. Place 1 or 2 drops of methylcellulose or similar viscous fluid in the concavity of the Koeppe lens and then place the lens on the patient's anesthetized cornea, in much the same manner as described for the Goldmann lens.
4. Inspect the angle through a magnifying system with an associated light source, through an operating microscope, or through an ophthalmoscope with auxiliary plus lenses.
5. Remove the lens by separating the lids beyond the edge of the lip and allowing it to fall out into the cupped hand. If the lens does not remove easily after use, use a finger tip to depress the sclera adjacent to the lens margin to allow air to pass between the lens and cornea.

Examination Procedure

Once the gonioscope is in place, you are ready for the clinical examination of the periphery of the anterior chamber. A typical gonioscopic view is shown in Figure 32–13. Proceed as follows:

1. Locate the pupil margin and follow the iris across to its last visible roll, the angle recess lies immediately beyond this roll. Provided the angle is open and reasonably wide, the scleral spur will be seen beyond the last iris roll as a white band having darker bands on either side.

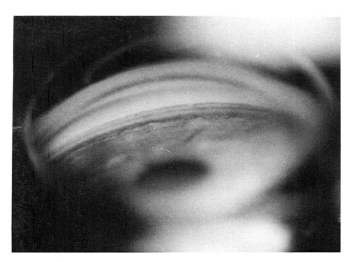

FIGURE 32–13. A normal wide anterior chamber angle with some pigment attached to Schwalbe's line and overlying Schlemm's canal. Note the contrasting white band of the scleral spur above the iris and ciliary body band.

2. Now locate the dark band immediately posterior to the scleral spur. This is the ciliary body. Fluffy strands may bridge the iris and ciliary body.
3. The band immediately anterior to the scleral spur is the posterior trabecular tissue, with Schlemm's canal lying beneath. In all but the young subject, this will appear pink to dark brown, owing to reflux of blood into the canal and increased pigmentation during life. Remember that this darker band of the posterior trabeculae occupies approximately half the total trabecular width.
4. Anterior to the posterior trabeculum and approximately equal to it in width is the anterior trabeculum. It is generally lighter in color than the posterior band.
5. The most anterior portion of the trabeculae is bounded by Schwalbe's line. It may be faintly outlined with pigment granules. If Schwalbe's line is not visible, or its position is in doubt, proceed as follows:
   a. Reduce the illumination to a narrow slit and have approximately 20° separation between lamp and microscope.
   b. Look in the clear cornea to locate the anterior and posterior corneal bright bands of the slit lamp beam. Remember that these are being seen, as it were, from the inside of the anterior chamber. They will converge at a point that marks the transition from cornea to sclera; this point of convergence also identifies Schwalbe's line.
   c. When the angle structures are partly hidden, as in a narrow angle, the optometrist should rotate the prism about a horizontal axis to obtain the highest view point that allows visibility into the angle.
   d. Now inspect the superior angle in the lower mirror of the Zeiss goniolens, or rotate the Goldmann lens into the inferior position. In most subjects, the superior angle will be narrower and less pigmented than the inferior angle.

For photography of the anterior chamber angle, use the Goldmann lens for maximum clarity of the image. Keep the slit lamp magnification to not more than 15× and enlarge the result if necessary after film processing. This magnification provides a good compromise between depth of focus and magnification. Although it is necessary to experiment with film speeds and flash settings, a good starting point is to use a color film having a rating 100 ASA, a fully open lamp aperture, and the lowest flash setting available. Expose a test film using each flash setting provided for your slit lamp camera, keeping a record of the various settings. Alternatively, commence with the exposure recommended in the instruction book for iris photographs. Narrow-beam aperture settings do not usually provide useful photographs, but if required, they can be obtained by using flash settings two or three steps higher than prove correct for photographs using the full beam.

The angle width may be assessed and described as the apparent angular separation of the iris and posterior wall of the chamber, as a description of the angle's structures visible with gonioscopy, or in terms of a numerical grading system. The best system to use is one in which the extent of the visibility of the angle structures is recorded; its width is described simply in terms of wide, intermediate, narrow, or closed; and the possibility of closure is described in words.

Several systems have been proposed for recording the appearance of the anterior chamber angle as viewed during gonioscopy. Gradle and Sugar[4] utilized the graticule in the microscope objective of a slit lamp to measure the length of an imaginary line from Schwalbe's line to the perpendicularly opposite point on the iris. Measurements made with this device are subject to modification by the combined optics of the gonioprism and the eye, as well

Table 32–2
Grading System for the Gonioscopic Appearance of the Anterior Chamber Angle

Angle Grade	Degrees	Numeric Grade	Clinical Interpretation
Wide open	30–45	3–4	Closure impossible
Moderately narrow	20	2	Closure possible
Extremely narrow	10	1	Closure probable
Extremely narrow with complete or partial closure		0	Closure present or imminent

(Adapted from Kolker AE, Hetherington J. Diagnosis and therapy of the glaucoma, 5th ed. St Louis: CV Mosby Co, 1983:42)

as being affected by artifacts produced by the various types of gonioprisms. This method is useful for measuring and documenting the changes that may occur in an individual eye as the result of treatment, but it does not lend itself to comparisons between different individuals.

Several grading systems depend upon the categorization determined by the visibility of anatomic landmarks.[5,6] Probably the most widely used is the classification of Kolker and Hetherington,[7] in which the widest angles are designated grade 4, through narrower angles, to the occluded angle, which is graded as zero. The variations between gradings are also identified by the angular separation of the iris and the trabeculae, and clinical interpretations are assigned to these grades. Table 32–2 illustrates this system.

A quantitative grading that utilizes the visibility of the gonio-structures has been developed[8] and is useful for statistical purposes; the system is both reliable and valid. However, it is more practical in the clinical setting to describe in words, the extent of visibility of the structures seen, and the presence of iris corneal or trabecular contact, if this is present. In very narrow angles, the angle structures may be partly or completely hidden beyond the last roll of the iris. In these cases, it is important to determine whether the angle is open or closed at the last visible point as described in the foregoing.

When the cornea is deformed by pressure on the gonioprism, lines of distortion appear in Descemet's membrane. These inhibit clear viewing of the angle; therefore, in normal goniscopy, excessive pressure on the cornea should be avoided. However, distortion of the cornea and, in turn, the iris diaphragm, may be used to permit a gonioscopic view of a narrow and otherwise hidden angle recess. This is achieved, using the Zeiss prism, by applying pressure to the edge of the gonioprism opposite the part of the angle being viewed. The iris will then be forced away from the posterior wall of the chamber and will allow a somewhat distorted view of the sulcus. If there are fresh synechial attachments, these may be broken by the forces caused by the corneal distortion; however, if the attachments are well established and firm, the iris and trabeculae will not separate. The method may also be used to break a recent angle closure glaucoma attack if ophthalmologic assistance is not available or will be delayed.[4]

Examination Hints

Optometrists who require presbyopic correction may find that a look-over spectacle correction designed for use at approximately 30 cm will allow use of the microscope, yet the ability to see the patient's eyes when carrying out the preliminary placement of the gonioprism (and speculum if used) on the cornea.

Under low magnification (10× to 15×) the depth of focus is improved, and the larger field of view allows easier orientation within the angle. Magnifications over approximately 25× are not

generally useful, since the increased magnification is offset by the loss of clarity of the image and the decreased depth of focus.

It is more difficult to view the lateral parts of the angle than the superior and inferior parts, because the slit and observation beams may not fit together on the lateral mirrors. When using the Zeiss system, either rotate the mirror 45° from the normal position and view the lateral aspects alternatively through all four mirrors, or keep the prism edges horizontal and vertical and use only one microscope ocular. The vertical tilt facility on the slit lamp light source allows sectional viewing of the lateral angles with a slit illumination, in a manner similar to that possible in the superior and inferior angles.

The view through the extreme edges of the Zeiss gonioprism and, to a lesser extent the Goldmann lens, is slightly distorted, giving the impression that the angle narrows toward the extreme edge of the field of view under inspection. To check that this is an artifact, simply rotate the gonioprism on the cornea to view these parts through the more central part of the mirror.

Lacrimal and lid secretions may cause wetting problems on the surface of the gonioprism, especially if contact is made with the lids. Keep a fiber-free tissue and normal saline handy for cleaning the corneal surface of the lens.

The metal holder provided with the Zeiss gonioprism set may cause chipping of the rather sharp outer edge of the glass prism. This can be avoided by threading fine polythene tubing over the holder prongs before using them to clasp the gonioprism. The tube from a saline intravenous drip bag is ideal for this purpose (see Fig. 32–3).

When using a Goldmann or Koeppe gonioprism, it is necessary to use a viscous fluid between the lens and the gonioprism. Even with quite viscous fluids, it may be difficult to keep bubbles from forming beneath the lens. Lacrilube or KY Jelly is a readily obtainable water-soluble jelly that remains on the lens during insertion and is harmless to the eye provided sterility is maintained.

It is possible to perform gonioscopy at the bedside, or during out-of-office visits, by substituting a direct ophthalmoscope for the slit lamp and using a high-plus correcting lens in the ophthalmoscope viewing system.

CLINICAL IMPLICATIONS

Clinical Significance

Gonioscopy is the best clinical procedure for evaluating the anterior chamber angle to assess the risk of angle closure associated with pupillary dilatation. Although the prevalence of narrow angles is low—6% of eyes have significantly narrowed angles, and 2% of eyes have critically narrowed angles—it is essential to know the status of the anterior chamber angle before the pupils are dilated.[9]

Gonioscopy also provides visualization of the anterior chamber angle for the assessment of anatomic anomalies, disease, or the effects of trauma. The presence and the extent of pigment, exfoliation material, iris processes, synechiae, and the depth of the angle recess can provide important information for the care of the patient. The results of glaucoma surgery can also be evaluated.

Clinical Interpretation

The normal anterior chamber angle is generally wider inferiorly and narrower superiorly.[10] When parts of the angle structures are hidden from view in a narrow angle, the assessment of the risk of angle closure becomes important. If only half or less than half of the trabeculum is visible in all of the quadrants, the eye should be considered at risk for angle closure during dilatation of the pupil.[9] Figures 32–14, 32–15, and 32–16 illustrate the gonioscopic ap-

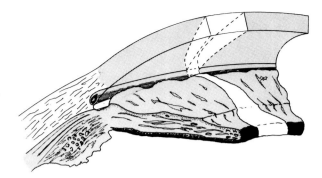

FIGURE 32–14. Anatomic and gonioscopic correlations in a narrow angle in which only the anterior trabeculum is visible during gonioscopy. Since the scleral spur is not visible, orientation is obtained by finding Schwalbe's line, which is marked by the point at which the corneal bright bands come together. Note that the light band on the iris and that on the wall of the anterior chamber are not aligned; this indicates that the angle is open at the last gonioscopically visible point.

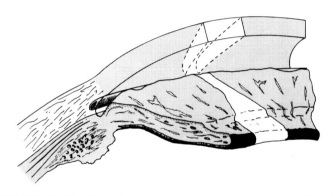

FIGURE 32–15. An angle that is narrower than that in Figure 32–14. Note that no gonioscopic angle landmarks are visible. The slit beam on the iris remains offset from the beam on the chamber wall, indicating that, although very narrow, the angle is still open at the last gonioscopically visible point.

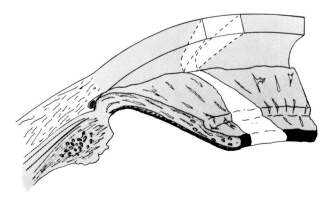

FIGURE 32–16. The anatomic and gonioscopic view of an angle that is closed. No gonioscopic angle structures are visible, the anterior and posterior corneal bright bands do not become confluent. The posterior corneal and iris bands are aligned, indicating that the angle is closed at this point.

pearance of the angle features and their anatomic correlations as the angle width decreases.

In Figure 32–14, the posterior trabeculum is hidden from gonioscopic view, as are the scleral spur and ciliary body. Schwalbe's line and the last roll of the iris are the only useful gonioscopic landmarks visible in this illustration. Notice that the bright bands on the iris and those on the posterior wall of the chamber do not coincide at the point where they dip down into the angle recess. This indicates that the angle is open at the point at which visibility is lost. Of course, from the gonioscopic view, this illustration does not tell us whether the angle is open or closed beyond this last visible point. This angle could be described in the following terms: "Angle narrow, with only Schwalbe's line and the anterior trabeculum visible. The angle is open at the last gonioscopically visible point."

Figure 32–15 illustrates an angle that is narrower than that shown in Figure 32–14; note that no angle structures are visible and that the corneal bright bands do not quite converge at Schwalbe's line, but rather dip below the last roll of the iris still separated. However, the posterior bright corneal band is not coincident with its equivalent band on the iris, but separated slightly from it. This indicates that the angle is still open at the last roll of the iris, but provides no information on whether it remains open over the entire depth of the sulcus. This angle would be described as: "Angle very narrow, no angle structures seen, but the angle remains open at the last gonioscopically visible point."

Figure 32–16 illustrates a closed angle. As in Figure 32–15 the corneal bright bands remain separated as they dip beyond the last roll of the iris. However, the posterior corneal bright band edges are now seen to be coincident with their equivalent bands on the iris surface. This indicates a closed angle and the appearance could be described as: "Very narrow angle in which no structures are visible and the angle is closed anterior to Schwalbe's line."

Although this angle is closed at the last visible point, it is possible that it becomes open again within the angle recess, at a point not accessible to normal gonioscopic view. It is possible that aqueous has access to the trabeculae through a gap between the iris and posterior wall of the chamber situated elsewhere around the circumference. However, this is a dangerous situation in which total angle closure is likely under provocation. The clinician would wish to know more about the state of an angle that appears to be closed on examination.

The degree of pigmentation of the ciliary body usually reflects the skin coloration; however, this is not invariable and a dark ciliary body is occasionally seen in a lightly pigmented subject. With increasing age, iris pigment tends to lodge on the slight inward projection of Schwalbe's line, is trapped in the trabecular spaces, and appears particularly in the region over the wall of Schlemm's canal. The inferior angle is most heavily dusted with pigment, which is more prolific in eyes having pigmentary glaucoma, pseudoexfoliation of the lens capsule, or iris atrophy. The degree of pigmentation of the anterior chamber angle structures provides a rough clinical guide to the severity of the underlying condition. It may be recorded in terms of a scale in which a dense, dark band of pigment is recorded as grade 4 through to light pigmentation as grade 1.[7]

Iris processes can be present in normal eyes, but if there are many of them and if they insert above the scleral spur around the entire circumference of the angle, they could decrease the aqueous outflow and be abnormal. Iris processes can also be confused with peripheral anterior synechiae.

After even quite mild ocular trauma, the iris may be torn from its insertion at the ciliary body to form an iridodialysis (Fig. 32–17). This may not be visible on slit lamp examination, but requires gonioscopy for its identification. More serious trauma may cause a split in the ciliary body, which is termed angle recession, because the angle appears unusually deep as a result of the

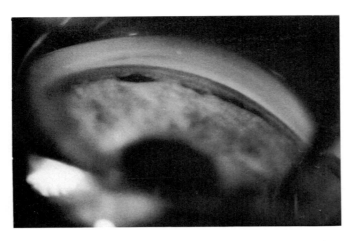

FIGURE 32–17. Iridodialysis following mild trauma. The iris has been torn from its insertion in the ciliary body. This lesion was not visible by other than gonioscopic examination.

tear in the gonioscopically visible face of the ciliary body. The importance of these gonioscopic signs is that glaucoma may occur months, or even years, after the trauma.[11] It follows that all cases presenting with a history of recent or old trauma should have a gonioscopic examination to exclude this type of injury.

The most common causes of neovascularization of the anterior chamber angle are ischemic central retinal vein occlusion and proliferative diabetic retinopathy; other less common causes are trauma, uveitis, sickle cell disease, retinal detachment, intraocular tumors, and Eales disease. The mechanism of this complication is believed to be the production of a neovascular stimulus by a hypoxic retina, which then stimulates new vessel growth on the retina, in the vitreous, on the iris and anterior chamber angle. The new vessels are accompanied by a fibrovascular membrane that covers and occludes the angle leading to raised IOP. Contraction of the neovascular membrane pulls the iris into contact with the anterior wall of the angle and results in a form of angle closure glaucoma that is difficult to treat effectively. Gonioscopy is a mandatory procedure when there is evidence, or risk, of ocular neovascularization.

REFERENCES

1. Trantas A. Ophthalmoscopie de las région ciliare et rétrociliaire. Arch D'Ophthalmol Paris 1907;27:581.
2. Troncoso MU. Gonioscopy and its clinical applications. Am J Ophthalmol 1925;8:433.
3. Goldmann H. Zur technik der spaltlampenmikroskopie. Ophthalmologica 1938;96:90–97.
4. Gradle HS, Sugar HS. Concerning the chamber angle: a clinical method of gonioscopy. Am J Ophthalmol 1940;23:1135.
5. Scheie HG. Gonioscopy. In: Clarke WD, ed. Symposium on glaucoma. St Louis: CV Mosby Co, 1959.
6. Spaeth GL. The normal development of the human anterior chamber angle: a new system of descriptive grading. Trans Ophthalmol Soc UK 1971;91:709.
7. Kolker AE, Hetherington J. Becker and Shaffer's diagnosis and therapy of the glaucomas, 5th ed. St Louis: CV Mosby Co, 1983.
8. Cockburn DM. A new method of gonioscopic grading of the anterior chamber angle. Am J Optom Physiol Opt 1980;57:258.
9. Cockburn DM. Prevalence and significance of narrow anterior chamber angles in optometric practice. Am J Optom Physiol Opt 1981;58:171–175.
10. Cockburn DM. Slit lamp estimate of anterior chamber depth as a predictor of the gonioscopic visibility of the angle structure. Am J Optom Physiol Opt 1982;59:904–908.
11. Jenson OA. Contusive angle recession: A histopathological study of Danish material. Acta Ophthalmol 1968;46:1207.

External Photography

William F. Long

INTRODUCTION

Definition

External photography is the use of a conventional hand-held camera to photograph external ocular and surrounding features.

History

Photography really started with the *camera obscura,* an instrument described by della Porta and others, in the 16th century.[1] The first chemical recording of a photographic image is credited to Nicephore Niepce in 1827.[2,p12] The asphaltlike substance he used required an 8-hour exposure.

The remainder of the 19th century saw rapid advances in the new technology. In 1835, William Henry Fox Talbot introduced the calotype process, the first to use a photographic negative.[2,p16–17] George Eastman democratized photography with the introduction of the Kodak box camera in 1889. That camera used cellulose-based roll film, much like that in current use. The 35-mm film format used in most of today's clinical cameras was incorporated in the Simplex camera in 1914.[2,p54] In 1949, the Contax 'S' became the first pentaprism reflex camera, the prototype for cameras most commonly used today.

Early photography was handicapped not only because film was black and white, but also because it was orthochromatic; that is, it was sensitive to only short-wavelength light, much like black and white printing papers and some graphic arts materials today. Sensitization to long-wavelength light was achieved by chemists gradually over the last quarter of the 19th century and, by 1905, panchromatic film, sensitive to the entire visible spectrum had been developed.[3,p8–9]

Generations of experiments with color photography culminated in the development of Kodachrome film by the musicians Leopold D. Mannes and Leopold Godowski in 1935.[2,p39–40] Their Kodachrome film produced a colored positive image on a transparent film base (i.e., a slide). It is still in wide use in clinical and general photography a half century after its introduction. A dozen years later came the last great film innovation, Polaroid instant picture film, developed by Edward H. Land in 1947.[2,p43]

Although Fox Talbot did the first photography using an electric flash as light source in 1851,[3,p22] the era of the electronic flash did not really start until nearly a century later, with Harold Edgerton's experiments in 1931. Use of electronic flash became increasingly widespread in the 1940s, and the inexpensive strobe has become commonplace today.

In 1900, Druener reported procedures for external photography of the eye.[4] Contemporary external photography has benefited from the rapid developments in photographic technology at the beginning of this century.

Clinical Use

The main purposes for photographing the eye and its adnexa are as follows:

1. *Patient management.* Anomalies, suspicious lesions, or irregularities may be recorded. Evanescent conditions such as intermittent strabismus or bruising and hemorrhage in trauma can be documented for later evaluation and comparison. Finally, the photographic record may be useful in comparing a case with literature descriptions or in discussions of a case with other practitioners.
2. *Legal purposes.* A photograph may be a valuable supplement to a carefully documented clinical record.

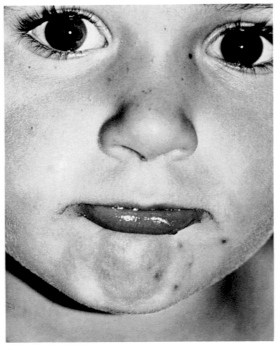

A

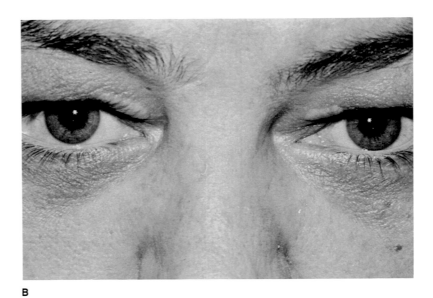

B

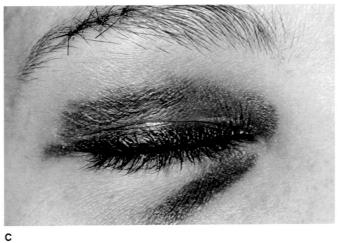

C

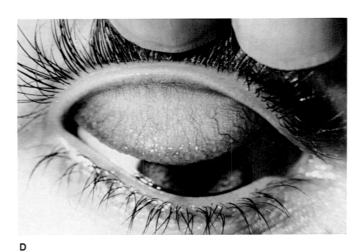

D

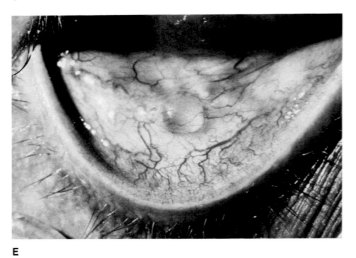

E

FIGURE 33–1. Photographs taken with a hand-held camera: (*A*) facial infection transferred from the patient's fingers after scratching an infected vaccination on the arm; (*B*) bilateral xanthelasma; (*C*) orbital trauma photographed at about half life-size (1 : 2 magnification); (*D*) conjunctival papillae shot at about two-thirds life-size (2 : 3 magnification); (*E*) conjunctival cyst photographed life-size (1 : 1 magnification).

3. *Educational purposes.* Photographs of clinical anomalies and the changes with different viewing conditions and with time are extremely valuable in helping practitioners understand disease and anomalies. The slide carousel has become a commonplace at classroom lectures or grand rounds.
4. *Research applications.* Photography has been used to advance the understanding of disease and anomalies and in the care of such conditions.

A hand-held camera may be used for portraiture, binocular photography, and close-up photography of the eye and adnexa with magnifications up to 1:1 (life-size). Portraits such as that in Figure 33–1A are useful in showing large distributions of lesions, facial asymmetry, and asymmetric lesions, or to illustrate facies characteristics of a particular disease entity. Binocular photographs like Figure 33–1B allow detailed comparison of the two eyes and are useful in strabismus or when there is differential involvement of the two eyes in a condition. The most frequent need in external ocular photography is pictures of a single eye and its adnexa at magnifications from 1:2 (half life-size) to 1:1 (life-size) such as Figures 33–1C, D, and E. Such photographs can show lumps and bumps, trauma, infections, congenital malformation, and other problems.

With appropriate film and filters, a hand-held camera can also document the fluorescein pooling or staining that can be seen with a conventional Burton lamp.

A glossary of photography terms is appended to this chapter for the convenience of the reader.

INSTRUMENTATION

Theory and Use

Except for a couple of external photography systems built around simple box cameras, the 35-mm single-lens reflex camera (SLR), the staple of the professional or serious amateur photographer, is the basis for all ophthalmic photographic instruments. As Figure 33–2 shows, its principal advantage is that the viewing and taking lens are identical, so there is no parallax error. This is especially helpful in close-up photography and makes it easy to fit the camera with a variety of lenses and attachments. Several external photographic systems are possible with a reflex camera.[5] In this chapter we will describe a simple system that uses relatively inexpensive and readily available components.[6]

Just about any reliable SLR camera will do for external photography. A basic camera, with or without autoexposure or autofocus, will work just fine. The simplest lens for clinical purposes is a normal lens of about 50-mm focal length, the basic lens for 35-mm photography. A 50-mm macrolens, a lens especially designed for close focusing, will simplify some jobs, but is not essential. Additionally, an ocular photographer needs a 2× teleconverter, an optical attachment of negative power that mounts behind the photographic objective to double the image size.

If a macrolens is *not* used, supplementary devices for close focusing will be necessary. The best choice is a set of extension tubes, opaque tubes, devoid of optics, that mount between objective and camera. A less expensive choice is a set of close-up lenses,

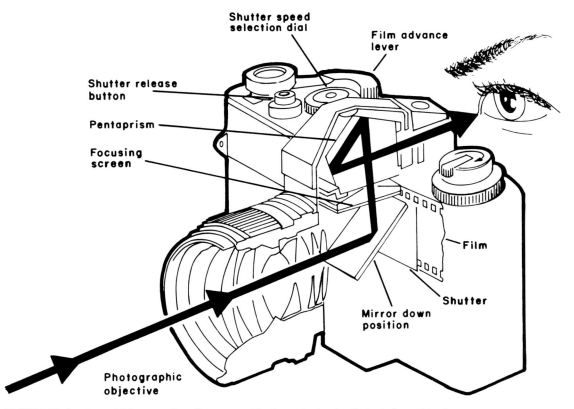

FIGURE 33–2. Essential features of a reflex camera. The image in the viewfinder is formed by the same optical system that forms the image on the film. Film and focusing screen are conjugate. When the shutter is triggered the mirror flips up to allow the image to reach the film.

thin lenses of positive dioptric power, which mount in front of the camera lens.

The light source for virtually all external photography is a small strobe (Fig. 33–3). Other lights may be on in the examination room, but they are sufficiently dim that only the brief intense pulse from the strobe will register in the picture. That pulse is so brief (less than 1/1000 second) that all motion is frozen. Crisp photos of even nystagmoid eyes are possible.

Automatic exposure and coupling features of a strobe are irrelevant. It *is* important that it be possible to use the strobe off the camera. It should be possible to connect the strobe electronically to the camera by a PC cord running from the strobe to a jack on the camera body. If there is no PC jack on the camera, one can be produced with a hot-shoe adaptor (Fig. 33–4). When using electronic flash, the shutter speed of the camera should be set for the strobe synchronization indicated in the camera manual, usually either 1/60 second or 1/125 second.

The strobe can be hand-held by the photographer or an assistant; but, generally, it is better to use brackets to hold the strobe away from the camera in close-up photography (Fig. 33–5).

An alternative to a reflex system is a framing system that focuses and aligns the subject by placing it inside a rectangle conjugate to the film plane, as shown in Figure 33–6. Framing systems are very easy to use, although they lack the versatility of reflex systems.

Most clinical photography is done with 35-mm film, a small-format film that produces a 24-mm × 36-mm slide or negative. Slide film is preferable to color print film because it is less expen-

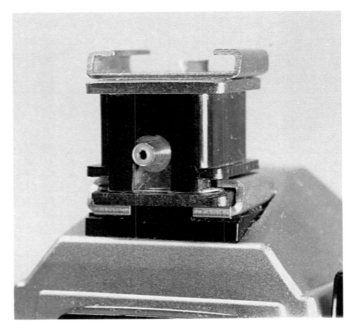

FIGURE 33–4. A hot-shoe adaptor slides into the shoe on top of the camera and provides a jack to connect with a PC cord.

sive per frame and permits the photographer greater control of the final product. Almost all slide films can be processed in-office with minimal equipment, but, since 24- to 36-hour slide processing is available nearly everywhere, few can justify going through this tedious and time-consuming procedure.

If extremely rapid turnaround *is* important, it might be worthwhile to consider Polachrome, a 35-mm slide color film marketed by Polaroid. With the aid of some modestly priced special equipment, a roll of this film may be developed in 2 minutes. At this writing, the image quality of the color film is just fair. It is suitable mainly for emergencies and for teaching purposes.

Polaroid instant picture film gives the fastest turnaround— color prints within a few minutes. It must be used with special cameras or adaptor backs that accommodate the large-format film and contain the mechanical appurtenances requisite to development. Instant picture film has a number of obvious advantages, but its expense and relatively poor picture quality (compared with 35-mm film) have limited its clinical use.

Color balance and exposure can be adjusted with filters that can be screwed into the threads at the front of the camera lens or attached to the strobe (Fig. 33–7). Most photographers like to put a UV haze filter over the camera objective to protect it and improve color rendition very slightly. Sometimes, filters are used to improve color rendition (e.g., the Wratten 81B, a yellow warming filter). Fluorescein photography requires two filters, one over the strobe, the other in front of the lens (see later discussion).

COMMERCIALLY AVAILABLE INSTRUMENTS

Excellent reflex cameras suitable for ocular photography are made by a great many manufacturers including Nikon, Pentax, Minolta, Olympus, Canon, and others. Lenses and other optical accessories are made by the manufacturers or by independent companies such as Vivitar, Tamron, and Soligor. These can be obtained from any commercial photographic outlet.

Filters that screw onto the camera objective are made by Hoya, Toshiba, and many others. These and Kodak Wratten gel filters can also be obtained from ordinary commercial sources.

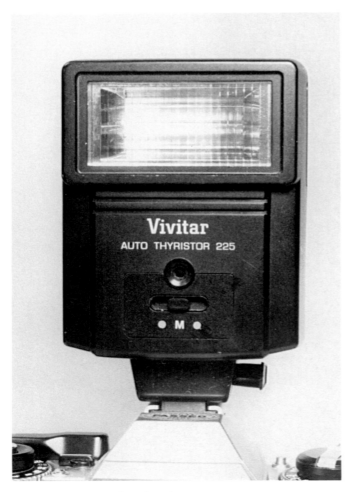

FIGURE 33–3. Typical small strobe.

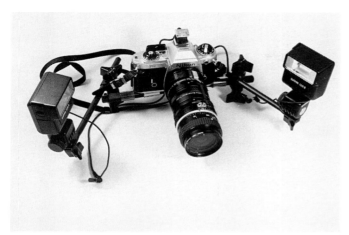

A

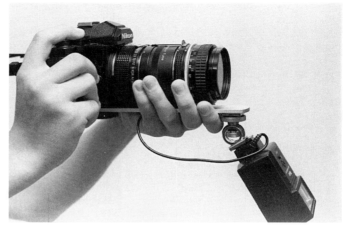

B

FIGURE 33–5. Two kinds of brackets for mounting a strobe on a camera. (*A*) The Lepp macrobracket* mounted on a Nikon camera equipped with normal lens, extension tubes, and teleconverter. Note the hot-shoe adaptor which connects the two strobes to the camera. (*B*) A strobe may be mounted beneath the camera with a straight flash bracket and a bounce shoe. It may be necessary to peel the rubber cushion off the top of the flash bracket and attach it to the other side with rubber cement to cushion the interface between camera and bracket or to remount the shoe of the bracket onto the side of the bracket with the cushion.

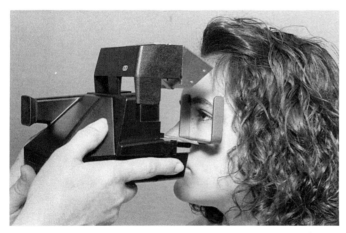

FIGURE 33–6. The Polaroid version of the Kodak Instatech used with the blue frame.

The best bracket for fundus photography is the Lepp macro-bracket that holds one or two strobes securely and allows them to be aimed in any direction (see Fig. 33–5A). A satisfactory arrangement can be constructed from a straight flash bracket and a bounce shoe, small items available at a well-equipped camera store (see Fig. 33–5B).

A typical framing system is the Kodak Instatech Camera, a specially modified Kodak Instamatic Camera, a fixed focus box camera. It uses easy-to-load 126 Film Cartridges that produce a square slide or negative, 24 mm on a side. It comes with a series of color-coded frames that attach to color-coded shields that screw onto the front of the camera. The shields include a close-up lens, which sits in front of the camera objective and baffles to attenuate the flash light to the appropriate level. Light is provided by flash-cubes, although an optional electronic flash is available. The objec-

* The Lepp bracket can be obtained from Lepp and Associates, PO Box 6224, Los Osos, CA 93402.

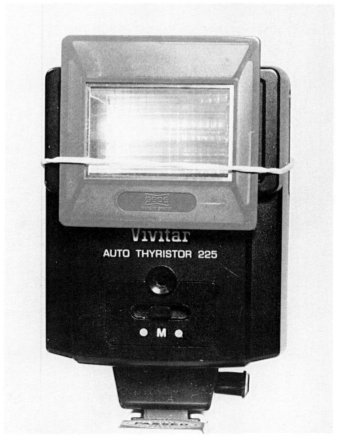

FIGURE 33–7. Filter material in a slide mount can be attached to a strobe head with a rubber band.

tive is a simple lens with a tiny, 1-mm diameter aperture stop. Another version of the camera is based on the Pocket Instamatic, which uses small format 110 film cartridges. There is also a Polaroid Instatech camera for instant pictures (see Fig. 33–6).

CLINICAL PROCEDURE

Reflex Systems

Portraiture

A portrait photographer must be about 1.5 m from his subject to avoid foreshortening.[5,pp26-28] To fill the picture frame with the patient's face at this distance requires a lens of about 100-mm focal length. Use either a short telephoto lens or a 50-mm lens with 2× teleconverter.

The strobe should be mounted straight ahead in the hot-shoe on top of the camera. Use a slow, fine-grain film, like Kodachrome 64 or Ektachrome 100. For most strobes, the best exposure using a 50-mm lens with a 2× teleconverter will be with a stop setting around f/5.6. With a short telephoto lens, try f/11.

After the camera has been loaded and prepared and the starting exposure settings dialed in, the clinical procedure is as follows:

1. Place the patient comfortably in the examination chair, facing straight ahead. If the patient is fidgety, use the headrest for stability.
2. Standing about 1.5 m from the patient, adjust camera-to-patient distance and the focusing ring of the camera until the patient's face fills the frame and the patient's irides are in sharp focus. The camera should be held with the longer dimension of the film frame vertical (see Fig. 33–1A).
3. Press the shutter release.
4. After the indicator light on the flash shows that it has recycled, take several more shots, bracketing exposures at least one stop.

Binocular Photography

Binocular photography is done with a normal lens combined with a 2× teleconverter; set the lens for 40 to 50 cm, the closest focus of standard normal lenses.

As in portraiture, the strobe should be mounted straight ahead in the hot-shoe on top of the camera. The Purkinje image of the strobe illustrates ocular alignment. Use a slow film, like Kodachrome 64 or Ektachrome 100. For most strobes, best exposure will be with a stop setting around f/11.

After the camera has been loaded and prepared and the starting exposure settings dialed in, the clinical procedure is as follows:

1. Place the patient comfortably in the examination chair, supporting his head with the headrest if necessary.
2. Set the lens distance for 40 cm or the closest focus of the camera lens. Adjust camera-to-patient distance until the patient's irides are in sharp focus. The camera should be held horizontally (see Fig. 33–1B).
3. Press the shutter release.
4. After the flash has recycled, take several more shots, bracketing exposures at least one stop.

Close-up Photography

For close-up photography of the eye, use a normal lens mounted with a 2× teleconverter. No additional attachments are necessary if a 50-mm macrolens is used. If a standard lens is used, either mount an extension tube between lens and teleconverter or mount a close-up lens in front of the camera lens. For a single eye with adnexa, use either a 15-mm extension tube or +4.00-diopter close-up lens. For an isolated single eye, use either a 25-mm extension tube or +6.00-diopter close-up lens.

The strobe should be mounted 20 to 30 cm from the patient at or beneath eye level. Take care that the Purkinje image of the flash does not obscure anything important (e.g., if the subject is a pigmented lesion on the temporal iris, do not place the flash temporal to the patient). Usually one flash will do, although two flashes provide more uniform illumination.

If necessary, a strobe can be hand-held by the photographer or an assistant. It is better to use a bracket to hold the strobe or strobes, which must then be connected to the camera with a PC cord. The Lepp Macro Bracket makes it easy to mount one or two strobes in any position. The bracket screws into the tripod mount of the camera and comes with strobes and electrical connections. Alternatively, a strobe may be mounted with a straight flash bracket and a bounce shoe. The flash bracket is a flat piece of metal that attaches to the tripod mount. At one end is a shoe for the strobe. The strobe may be mounted directly in the shoe or mounted through a bounce shoe that permits the strobe to be pivoted. Vertical mounting of the older style "flat-iron" strobes with vertical flash tubes worked well. The newer strobes with horizontal tubes generally work better mounted beneath the camera shooting upward (see Fig. 33–5B).

Use a slow, fine-grain film, like Kodachrome 64 or Ektachrome 100. A stop setting around f/11 will be satisfactory with most strobes. After the camera has been loaded and prepared with starting exposure settings dialed in, the clinical procedure is as follows:

1. Place the patient comfortably in the examination chair. It is usually best if the patient leans forward slightly, but a fidgety patient can be placed in the headrest. Illuminate the patient's face and eyes with the stand light.
2. With a macrolens, set the lens focus at 10 to 20 cm, depending on the desired magnification. With a standard lens with close-up attachments, set the lens focus at infinity. (The attachments are doing the focusing for you.)
3. Have the patient move his eye and lid to the position that best illustrates the condition in question. For most conditions, it is best if the eye is wide open to minimize lid shadows in the final picture.
4. While you are holding the camera horizontally, focus by moving back and forth until the patient's irides are clear; then move back just slightly (1 to 2 mm) to place the focus in the anterior chamber. Depth of field will allow the iris and more anterior features to simultaneously appear in sharp focus. Since the optical attachments make the image in the viewfinder dim, a useful alternative is to focus on the first Purkinje image of the stand light. Then pull back 5 to 6 mm.
5. Press the shutter release.
6. After the flash has recycled, take several more shots, bracketing exposures at least one stop.

Fluorescein Photography

In fluorescence, short-wavelength light goes in and long-wavelength light comes out. In fluorescein photography (see Chaps. 38 and 63) the blue light is strobe light filtered by a blue Wratten 47A filter, the "exciter filter."[7] Since film is so sensitive to short-wavelength light, fluorescein patterns and staining do not show up well in pictures unless a yellow K2 filter, the "barrier filter," is screwed onto the front of the camera objective. This filter combination absorbs a lot of light. The amount of light lost makes it necessary to use a fast film, such as Ektachrome 200 or, better, Ektachrome 400.

Fluorescein photography is almost always close-up photography, but occasionally it might be binocular photography. The optical setups used in white light photography work here also.

Exposure in fluorescein photography is rather unpredictable, so it is especially important to bracket exposures. Start exposures with a setting of about f/5.6.

The clinical procedure for fluorescein photography is much the same as that for the corresponding white-light photography. After the camera has been loaded and prepared and the starting exposure settings are dialed in, the procedure is as follows:

1. Place a generous amount of fluorescein dye in the eye in the usual way.
2. Preview the staining or fluorescein pattern with a Burton lamp or slit lamp.
3. Turn the room lights *on* and take the picture in the regular way. The film will see the fluorescence, not the room lights. The lower f/number decreases depth of field, so focus as precisely as possible on the cornea.
4. Press the shutter release.
5. After the strobe recycles, take several more shots, bracketing exposures at least two stops.

Kodak Instatech Camera

Procedures are almost the same for all three versions of the camera. Before a photography session, prepare the camera and load the film. While 110- and 126-format slide films exist, it is best to use print films because of the greater exposure latitude, bracketing being impossible with these cameras. Only print film may be used with the Polaroid version of the Instatech. For the 110 and 126 versions of the camera, insert a flashcube. For the Polaroid version, touch the shutter switch lightly to turn on the strobe. Select the frame appropriate for the subject (e.g., the gold frame for close-up photography). Mount the corresponding shield and frame on the camera. The clinical procedure is simple:

1. Place the frame against or around the subject of interest. If the gold frame is used, turn the camera upside down to avoid shadows. For portraiture, mount the green lens and measure camera-to-subject distance with the attached chain and frame the picture in the viewfinder. For portraiture with the Polaroid version, flip the flash bar up.
2. Press the shutter release. With the Polaroid version, it is a good idea to move the camera away from the patient's face right after the flash to keep the picture from hitting him when it is ejected.
3. Repeat steps 1 and 2 only if additional photos are desired. Since exposure cannot be changed with the 110 and 120 version of the camera, bracketing is impossible. With the Polaroid Instatech, exposure can be altered with a slide switch on the back of the camera. If exposure is not satisfactory, make the indicated adjustment and repeat steps 1 and 2.

CLINICAL IMPLICATIONS

Clinical Significance

As in all clinical photography, the chief value of external photography is in providing an objective record of the appearance of a clinical condition at a particular time.

Clinical Interpretation

Clinical interpretation of photographs is the same as that for corresponding observations with the naked eye. To get the maximum benefit from the photographic record, certain information should be written on the back of every print or the margin of every slide. It should include the date, the patient's name and file number, the patient's sex, the laterality of the eye in the picture, an arrow indicating the orientation of the picture, the patient's visual acuity, and a diagnosis.

APPENDIX

aperture stop, the stop within a lens that determines the image illuminance.

bracketing, taking multiple photos with exposure settings around the estimated exposure setting to assure some perfectly exposed shots.

camera back, camera body.

dedicated, designed to work with only one kind of equipment, as a dedicated strobe or dedicated camera back.

entrance pupil, the image of the aperture stop of a lens seen from object space.

f/number, the ratio between the diameter of the focal length of a lens to the diameter of its entrance pupil. In photography, the standard f/numbers lie in a sequence such that each higher number halves exposure one stop. That sequence is: f/0.5, f/0.7, f/1, f/1.4, f/2, f/2.8, f/4, f/5.6, f/8, f/11, f/16, f/22, f/32, . . .

film speed, film sensitivity. A "fast" film is more sensitive than a "slow" film.

foreshortening, a spatial distortion produced when a camera is too close to its subject.

grain, the microscopic silver halide crystals or dye droplets that constitute a photograph or negative.

hot-shoe, the slot, usually on top of a camera, that mounts the strobe while simultaneously connecting it to the camera body electrically.

illuminance, the light flux incident per unit area.

ISO, a measure of film speed, replacing the older ASA measure. The higher the ISO, the more sensitive the film.

latitude, the margin of error a film allows in exposure. A film with a one-stop latitude will give acceptable results in pictures over- or underexposed one stop.

lens, photographic objective.

luminance, the "brightness" of a source that determines the illuminance of its film plane image and, hence, its photographic exposure.

PC cord, a cord that may be used to connect camera and strobe electrically.

shutter speed, the length of time, in seconds, that the camera shutter is open.

stop, 1. Aperture stop. 2. f/number 3. a 2× exposure change (e.g., a one-stop increase in film exposure doubles it). Such an increase might be achieved by opening the aperture stop one f/number, leaving the shutter open twice as long, doubling the illuminance of the object, or doubling film ISO.

strobe, electronic flash unit.

REFERENCES

1. Porta JB. Natural magick. New York: Basic Books 1957:355. (facsimile edition edited by Derek J. Price of the English translation of Magica Naturalis originally published in 1658.)
2. Wills C, Wills D. History of photography techniques and equipment. New York: Exeter Books, 1980:12, 16–17, 39–40, 43, 54.
3. Neblette CB. Photography, its materials and processes, 6th ed. New York: van Nostrand Reinhold, 1962:8–9, 22.
4. Druener L. Ueber Mikrosteropsie und eine neue vergroessernde Steroskopcomera. Z Wissensch Mikros 1900;17:281.
5. Long W. Ocular photography. Chicago: Professional Press, 1984:25–50, 26–28.
6. Long W. A simple system for external ophthalmic photography. Can J Optom 1979;41:67–71.
7. Bailey N. Blacklight photography of the eye. Contacto 1961;5:91–96.

Slit Lamp Photography

William F. Long

INTRODUCTION

Definition

Slit lamp photography is a clinical procedure adapted from standard biomicroscopy, designed to record photographically what may be seen with the slit lamp.

History

Slit lamp photography was first attempted with some success by R. Thiel as early as 1930. The low luminance of the image and the shallow depth of field, however, presented significant problems. Goldmann attempted to solve the latter problem with an ingenious photographic system that moved along the optic section.[1] But practical photographic slit lamp photography had to wait for faster photographic media and the electronic flash unit. It was not until the manufacture of the Carl Zeiss photo slit lamp in 1965 that routine slit lamp photodocumentation became practical.[2]

Clinical Use

A photographic slit lamp is used to obtain high-magnification photos of the anterior segment of the eye. The instrument may be used to take external photographs at magnifications of 1:1 or greater and is especially useful for documenting anomalies of the cornea and crystalline lens. Filters make fluorescein photography possible and, with appropriate auxilliary lenses, the photographic slit lamp can be used for goniophotography and some fundus photography.

INSTRUMENTATION

Theory and Use

Modern photographic slit lamps have not evolved far in form or function from the standard clinical biomicroscope (Fig. 34–1). The photographic slit lamp differs from the conventional instrument only in having a flash tube somewhere in the illumination system and a reflex camera back mounted on a tube[3,pp57–60] beside or beneath the oculars. The photographic slit lamp can function as a conventional biomicroscope when photographs are not desired.

All photographic slit lamps more-or-less closely resemble the corresponding conventional slit lamps of the same manufacturer. Before using a particular instrument, use the camera manual and experiment a little to become familiar with the following photographic features:

1. *Power supply.* There will be an on–off switch and a knob to determine flash settings. Somewhere on the power supply or on the instrument itself will be the on–off switch and rheostat for the observation light.
2. *Illumination system light housing.* In addition to the usual red-free and cobalt blue filters in the light housing, there may be neutral-density filters to regulate exposure. In the original Nikon model, there is an aperture stop in the illumination system that accomplishes the same thing.
3. Most instruments have a "fill flash" that can produce a diffuse general illumination over the whole eye.[4] Typically, light for the fill flash is deviated from the strobe by means of a fiberoptics bundle, its intensity regulated by an aperture stop.
4. *Beam splitter.* In the newer cameras, a beam splitter sends about half the light entering one of the objective lenses to a

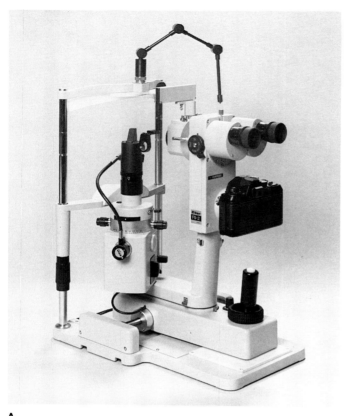

A

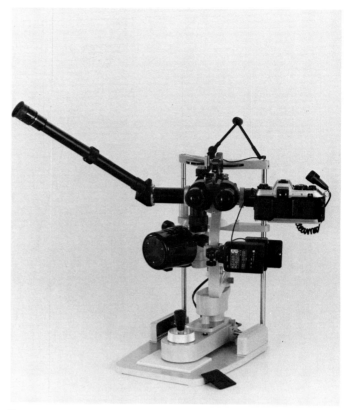

B

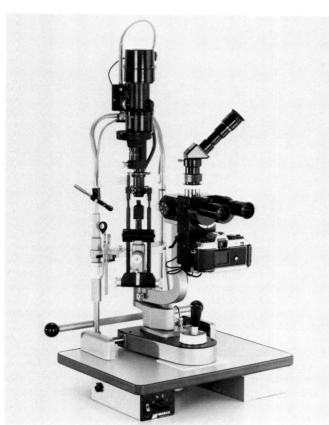

C

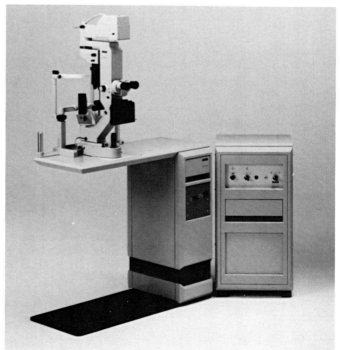

D

FIGURE 34–1. Some of the photographic slit lamps currently on the market: (*A*) Nikon FS-2 (courtesy Nikon Inc); (*B*) Marco 4 (courtesy Marco Equipment, Inc); (*C*) Marco 5G (courtesy Marco Equipment, Inc); (*D*) Zeiss 40 SL/P (courtesy Carl Zeiss, Inc); (*E*) Topcon SL-6E (courtesy Topcon Instrument Corporation of America).

E

FIGURE 34–1, *continued*

camera back. The beam splitter may be permanently in position or it may be removable. As a safety feature, removing the beam splitter disables the shutter release on most cameras. On a couple of older photographic slit lamps, there is a sliding mirror arrangement instead of a beam splitter. It is important to determine which ocular contains the beam splitter, since the picture should be focused and framed with that ocular.

5. *Camera back.* Most manufacturers use a conventional reflex camera back with their photographic slit lamps, the slit lamp becoming, in effect, the camera objective and flash. The camera back can be removed for use in external clinical photography or general photography. Some manufacturers use less versatile dedicated camera backs designed solely for use with the photographic slit lamp. In modern instruments, film is advanced automatically. In some older photographic slit lamps, film must be advanced by hand with a lever on the camera back.

6. *Shutter release.* The camera shutter release is most commonly located at the top of the joystick. It may also be triggered by a foot pedal[5] or by a button on the camera body or autowinder.

Components of a typical photo slit lamp are shown in Figure 34–2.

A film of ISO 200 is the best general-purpose film for most photographic slit lamps. A slower film would be preferable for documenting external features and a faster one for fluorescein photography, but in most clinical settings it is easier to stick to one all-purpose film.

The primary means of regulating exposure with a photo-graphic slit lamp is by a knob on the power supply, which determines the flash intensity. This knob usually has a series of click positions, each of which changes the flash output 40% or a half stop. The click positions are labeled numerically, the higher numbers corresponding to brighter flash intensities. In many cameras, these numbers stand in the sequence 1, 1.4, 2, 2.8, . . . Alternatively, they may simply be labeled 1, 2, 3, 4, . . .; or I, II, III, IV.

An aperture in the observation tube gives additional exposure control in a few cameras. There is little consistency in the labeling of these aperture settings. In some Marco photographic slit lamps the apertures are labelled 1.0, 1.4, 2.0, . . . , but those numbers are inversely proportional to the *area* of the aperture and are not, as one might guess, f/numbers. The labeling of the apertures on the side-arm version of the Zeiss photographic slit lamp *does* give real f/numbers—unless vignetting places the aperture stop in the microscope objective, in which case the aperture setting on the side arm is irrelevant to exposure.[6]

Finally, filters or apertures in the illumination housing may diminish the light reaching the patient.

There is no standardization among photographic slit lamps, and instrument manuals frequently leave out critical information. It is possible to analyze the optics of a photographic slit lamp in about 1 hour with ordinary optometric equipment.[3,pp85–87] Ultimately, however, the optimal exposure settings must be determined by trial exposures.

Two sets of trial exposures should be taken; one set of a narrow corneal slit; and one set of a blue iris. The best exposures of all other subjects lie within a stop or two of one of these two (Table 34–1). The camera manual can be used to obtain starting

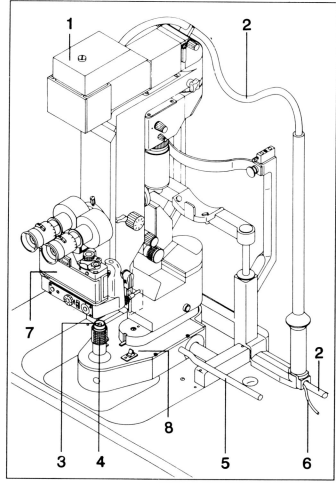

FIGURE 34–2. Key components of a typical photo slit lamp, the Zeiss 40 SL/P. The components numbered in the diagram are as follows: 1, lamp housing; 2, 5, 6, electrical connections; 3, shutter release button; 4, joystick; 7, camera back; 8, on–off switch for fill flash. (Courtesy Carl Zeiss, Inc.)

points for trial exposures. In clinical practice, it is imperative to bracket exposures.

COMMERCIALLY AVAILABLE INSTRUMENTS

Every major optical manufacturer makes a photographic slit lamp and discontinued models are still in active use in many clinics.

Table 34–1
Exposure Recommendations

Subject	Exposure
Sclera	Blue iris exposure − 2 stops
Caucasian lid	Blue iris exposure
Negroid lid	Blue iris exposure + 1 stop
Blue iris	Blue iris exposure
Brown iris	Blue iris exposure + 1 stop
Corneal parallelepiped	Corneal section exposure − 1 stop
Corneal section	Corneal section exposure
Lens section	Corneal section exposure + 1 stop

Models currently marketed include the Bausch & Lomb PSL-3000; Kowa SC-6; Marco 4 and Marco 5G; Mentor 22-4600; Nikon FS-2; Rodenstock RO 2002; Topcon SL-6E; Zeiss Standard and Zeiss 40 SL/P. All these can do basic slit lamp photography with 35-mm or Polaroid film. A few offer special features of interest to a few photographers, such as the endothelial specular microscope attachment on the Zeiss cameras, the Scheimpflug attachment on the Rodenstock camera that increases depth of field in optic section photos, or the-photo keratoscope of the Topcon instrument.

CLINICAL PROCEDURE

The clinical procedures for slit lamp photography are:

1. Load film and make the exposure settings appropriate to the subject.
2. Focus in the eyepieces of the instrument to make the focus of the illumination beam conjugate to the observer's retina. Take special care with the ocular behind the beam splitter. Confirm the focus through the observation system of the camera back, if it has one.
3. Since most photographic slit lamps do not have data backs, start any sequence of pictures with a photograph of the patient's identification (e.g., a name, file number, and such). This is best done at low magnification using the fill flash without a slit.
4. Place the patient comfortably in the chin rest of the instrument.
5. Experiment to find the illumination and magnification that best illustrates the patient's condition. Close your eye behind the ocular *without* the beam splitter to preview the photograph. Adjust exposure settings if necessary.
6. When the view seems satisfactory, press the shutter release.
7. When the strobe has recharged, repeat steps 5 and 6 bracketing exposures at least a half stop around the estimated best exposure.

Although the operation of the photographic slit lamp presents no fundamental difficulties to the experienced biomicroscopist, obtaining properly exposed, psychologically clear photos *does* often require a modification of conventional examination techniques. The reasons are twofold: first, the photographer is required to show in a single view (or small number of discrete views) the information a biomicroscopist can integrate from a variety of perspectives; second, photographic film can record only a fraction of the range of luminances the observer's eye can see.

Selection of the proper illumination is especially important. The illumination in slit lamp photography is more subtle than in most other kinds of ocular photography, and general rules are less easy to develop. Here are recommendations for some specific cases:

1. *External eye at low (1:1) magnification.* Light from the illumination beam will not fill the frame, so take the picture with light from the fill flash. Use a narrow slit to focus and align the picture. Close the slit completely just before the picture is taken.
2. *Details of the external eye at high magnification.* Use a wide-open focal beam.
3. *Corneal scars and dystrophies.* There are a variety of choices here. If the cornea is generally transparent with many lesions, retroillumination from the fundus shot through a dilated pupil shows the lateral distribution of lesions very well. A parallelepiped used to provide direct, proximal, or retroillumination from the iris may provide an alternative or supplemental view showing the longitudinal distribution of lesions. But beware the optical section that looks great through the eyepiece, but provides very poor photodocumentation.

4. *Corneal endothelium.* Severe defects can sometimes be successfully documented with retroillumination or specular reflection at high magnification. Photographs of individual cells can be accomplished with a conventional photographic slit lamp, using special optical and darkroom techniques,[7,8] but are best done with special instruments or attachments.

5. *The iris.* Use a wide-open focal beam. A beam making a large angle with the observation system will show iris topography very effectively.

6. *Pigment on the anterior lens.* Photograph as with the iris.

7. *Cataracts and vitreous opacities.* As with corneal opacities, use retroillumination from the fundus or a parallelepiped. Dilatation is essential in most cases.

8. *Fluorescein photography (see Chap. 38).* Use the cobalt blue filter of the illumination system with a K2 barrier filter held in front of, or taped onto, the microscope objective. Set the strobe for maximum output and, if possible, use fast film. Exposure varies considerably with the amount of pooling or staining; hence, it is especially important to bracket exposures. Use the highest magnification and the widest beam that will illustrate the condition well.

9. *Goniophotography.* Use the gonioprism in the usual way, with the exposure settings for the iris.

10. *Fundus photography with auxilliary lenses.* Be especially careful to eliminate distracting reflections and use the exposure appropriate for lenticular slits. Although fundus pictures with a slit lamp are occasionally helpful in demonstrating the topography of lesions, results of this kind of photography are usually disappointing. Fundus photographs with a fundus camera—especially stereo photographs—are far preferable.

Examples of some of these techniques are shown in Figure 34–3.

Photographers are generally tempted to shoot with somewhat larger fields of view than they should. A good rule of thumb is to choose a magnification one-step larger than seems really comfortable.

CLINICAL IMPLICATIONS

Clinical Significance

As in all clinical photography, the chief value of slit lamp photography is in providing an objective record of the appearance of a clinical condition at a particular time.

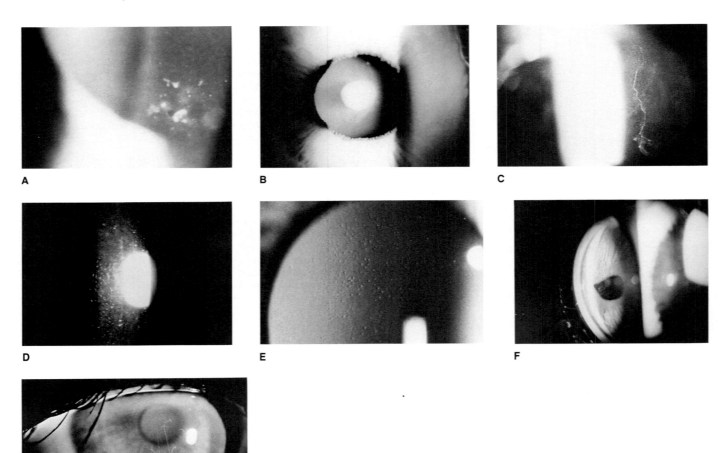

FIGURE 34–3. Examples of the use of photo slit lamp illuminations: (*A*) direct illumination of a corneal scar; (*B*) direct illumination of a pyramidal cataract; (*C*) a parallelepiped used to show a vitreous floater; (*D*) corneal guttata shown with specular reflection; (*E*) the corneal guttata of Figure 34-3*D* shown with retroillumination from the fundus; (*F*) iris degeneration photographed through a gonioprism; (*G*) fluorescein photography of a corneal abrasion.

Clinical Interpretation

Clinical interpretation of slit lamp photographs is the same as that for corresponding biomicroscopic observations. Since it is difficult to take physiologically clear slit lamp pictures, photos should be considered an adjunct to, and an extension of, conventional biomicroscopic documentation.

As in all ocular photography, slides or prints should be labeled with the date of the photography session, the patient's name and file numbers, the patient's sex, the laterality of the eye in the picture, an arrow indicating orientation, a visual acuity, and a diagnosis.

REFERENCES

1. Goldmann H. Spaltlampenphotogrphie und photometrie. Opthalmolica 1939;98, 257.
2. Justice J. Ophthalmic photography. Boston: Little, Brown & Co, 1976:12–14.
3. Long W. Ocular photography. Chicago: Professional Press 1984:57–60, 85–87.
4. Cummings RW, Clompus RJ, Ellis RJ. An accessory fill-in flash for the Nikon photo-slit lamp. Am J Optom Physiol Opt 1971;56:128–132.
5. Cockburn DM. A foot-operated camera trip for the Nikon photo slit lamp. Am J Optom Physiol Opt 1978;55:62–63.
6. Long W, Wessel J. Determination of photo slit lamp exposure settings. Am J Optom Physiol Opt 1982;59:72–82.
7. Holden BA, Zantos SG, Jacobs K. The Holden–Zantos technique for endothelial and high magnification slit lamp photography. Rochester: Bausch and Lomb Soflens International, 1978.
8. Long WF, Murphy M. Alternative technique for photographing the corneal endothelium with a conventional photo slitlamp 1987; Am J Optom Physiol Opt 64:217–220.

Fundus Photography

William F. Long

INTRODUCTION

Definition

Fundus photography is a clinical procedure designed to photograph the ocular fundus.

History

Experiments in retinal photography originated with J. D. Webster in 1886.[1] A half-century of development culminated in the excellent Carl Zeiss fundus camera, introduced in 1955. It used electronic flash and 35-mm color film.[2] It set the standard for future instruments. Photographers and clinicians showed much ingenuity in adapting this sturdy machine for a variety of special applications. By far the most important of these was the pioneering fluorescein angiography work of Harold R. Novotny and David L. Alvis.[3] Many of these modifications have found their way into the production model cameras currently available.

Clinical Use

The main use of the fundus camera is to photograph retinal conditions observed ophthalmoscopically. Most fundus cameras can also be used to document retroilluminated views of cataracts or corneal opacities and to take anterior segment photos. Even portraiture is possible with some fundus cameras. Not surprisingly, the closer a lesion is to the retina, the better a fundus camera will document it.

INSTRUMENTATION

Theory and Use

Optically, a fundus camera is an indirect ophthalmoscope in which a camera and film replace the clinician's eye and retina. The essential features of the fundus camera are illustrated in Figure 35–1.

There are two optical subsystems in a fundus camera: an illumination system that sends light to the fundus, and an observation system that forms the photographic image of the fundus. In most fundus cameras, the illumination system is in the bottom part of the camera and consists of elements 1–11 in Figure 35–1. Light for observing and focusing the retina comes from tungsten lamp 1 and is relayed by mirrors and lenses until it passes through lens 11 on the way to the patient's retina. Lens 11 serves the same function as the condenser lens of a clinical indirect ophthalmoscope. A needle pointer may be inserted into the illumination beam at 21. The patient can see the image of the pointer, and by adjusting the pointer's position, the eye can be lined up. When the photograph is taken, the light from the tungsten filament is supplemented by a light from flash tube 4, reflected into the illumination beam by half-silvered mirror 3.

Light entering the patient's eye is reflected through lens 11 to form a real and inverted image of the retina. That image is observed and photographed with a reflex camera system consisting of elements 12–20 of the camera. Since the retinal image is so dim, the ground glass screen, which would usually be at 16 in a reflex camera, is replaced by a clear screen upon which there is a focusing cross. When the observer sees both cross and retinal image clearly, the retinal image is conjugate to the film plane and the picture may be taken.

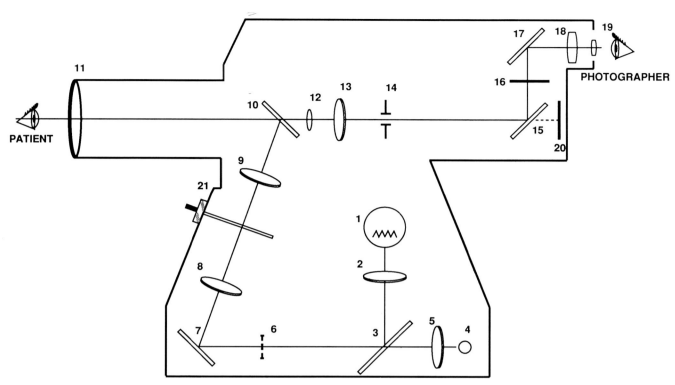

FIGURE 35–1. Optical arrangement of a typical fundus camera. The components are as follows: 1, tungsten focusing light; 2, condenser lens; 3, half-silvered mirror; 4, flash tube; 5, condenser lens; 6, donut-shaped aperture stop; 7, half-silvered mirror; 8, 9, relay lenses; 10, half-silvered mirror; 11, lens analogous to the binocular indirect ophthalmoscope condenser; 12, ametropia correction lens; 13, lens that determines field size; 14, field stop; 15, mirror that rotates upward when film is exposed; 16, focusing screen, usually a clear screen with a cross-hair target; 17, mirror; 18, 19, focusing system to render photographer's retina conjugate with focusing screen 16; 20, film; 21, fixation target.

An alternative focusing scheme sends light from an aerial image formed at 16 *toward* the retina. When the photographer sees that image focused on the retina, the retinal image is conjugate to the film plane.[4] This method is used in most nonmydriatic cameras and can be adapted to permit autofocus.

As in ordinary direct ophthalmoscopy, white light reflected from the cornea can swamp the fundus image. Designers have solved this problem by modifying the illuminating system one of two ways. Hand-held fundus cameras incorporate the simpler method in which light is simply sent through the bottom part of the patient's pupil. In most stand-mounted cameras, a donut-shaped aperture is placed in the illuminating system (at 6 in Fig. 35–1), positioned so that it will be roughly conjugate to the patient's cornea. The resulting illumination beam then has a double–cone-shaped light-free zone centered on the cornea (Fig. 35–2). The base of the double cone is the exit pupil of the illumination system. Since most of the crystalline lens is also within the light-free region, the picture is largely uncontaminated by bluish light scattered by the crystalline lens.[5]

All fundus cameras are constructed similarly (Fig. 35–3). Before using a particular instrument, use the camera manual and experiment a little to become familiar with the following photographic features:

1. *Power supply.* Typically there is an on–off switch, a rheostat for the focusing light, and a knob determining flash settings. Somewhere on the instrument or power supply is a warning light indicating when the strobe has recharged.
2. *Ametropia correction.* There is a changer that places a lens in the observation system which selects for the degree of ametropia, allowing settings for high myopes, high hyperopes, and, sometimes, for anterior segment photography. A few cameras also have an astigmatism correction.[6]
3. *Filters.* It may be possible to insert filters in the light path (e.g., a red-free filter, fluorescein exciter, and barrier filters). Determine what filter is appropriate for the film you have chosen.

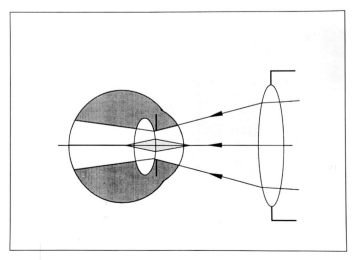

FIGURE 35–2. Illumination beam of a fundus camera.

A

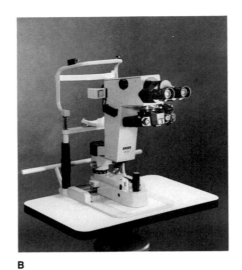

B

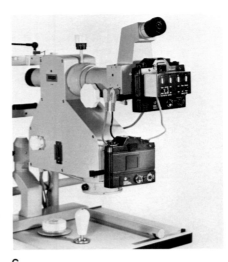

C

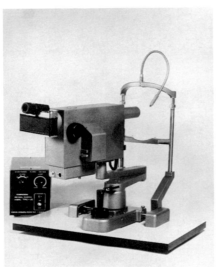

D

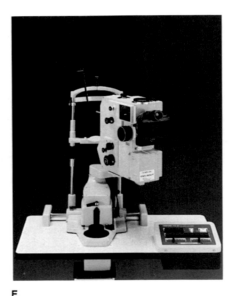

E

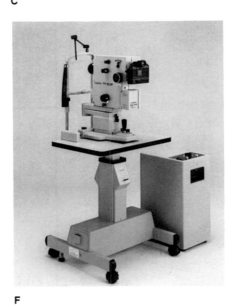

F

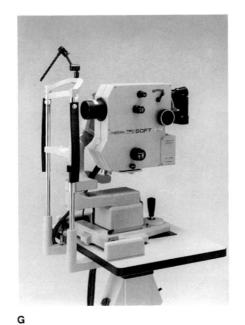

G

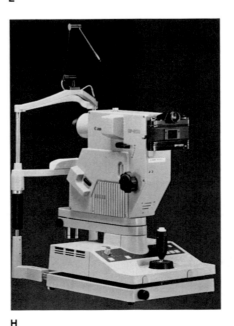

H

FIGURE 35–3. Some of the stand-mounted mydriatic fundus cameras currently on the market: (*A*) Nikon NFC-50 (courtesy Nikon, Inc); (*B*) Zeiss FK 30 (courtesy Carl Zeiss, Inc); (*C*) Zeiss FF-4 (courtesy Carl Zeiss Inc); (*D*) Topcon TRC-JE (courtesy Topcon Instrument Corporation of America); (*E*) Topcon TRC-50VT (courtesy Topcon Instrument Corporation of America); (*F*) Topcon TRC-50F (courtesy Topcon Instrument Corporation of America); (*G*) Topcon TRC-50FT (courtesy Topcon Instrument Corporation of America); (*H*) Canon CF-60U (courtesy Canon USA Inc).

4. *Field of view.* Cameras used in ordinary photodocumentation have fields of view ranging from 15° to 45°. The most common fields of view are 30° and 45°, and almost all cameras will provide one or the other, or both. Many will also have a 15° or 20° field as well (Fig. 35–4). Wide-angle fields of 50° to 60° are possible on several cameras. On most cameras, there is a lever determining the field of view. On some cameras, the field of view is changed with auxiliary optics (e.g., a teleconverter placed in front of the camera back). In a few, only one field of view is possible.

5. *Focusing knob.* This is generally on the side of the instrument.

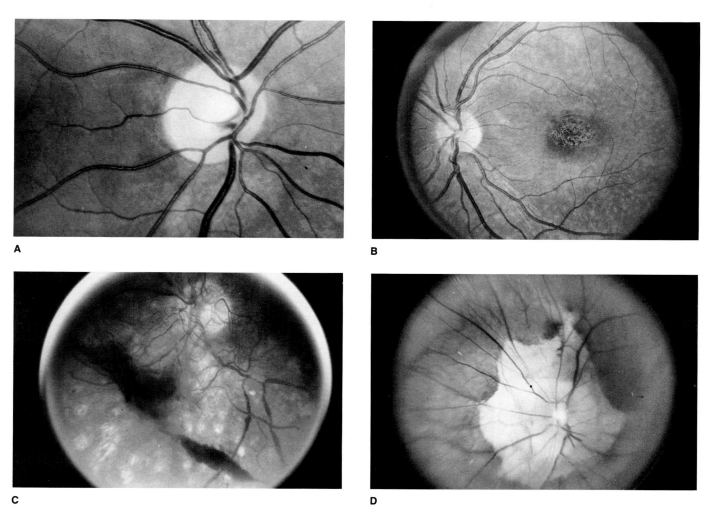

A

B

C

D

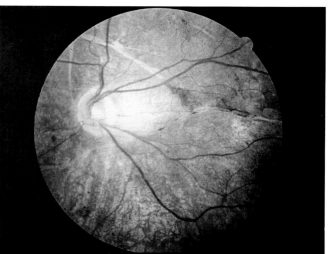

E

FIGURE 35–4. Fields of view in ordinary fundus photography: (*A*) 15° field: disk pallor in optic atrophy subsequent to trauma; (*B*) 30° field: macular degeneration and fundus flavimaculatus; (*C*) 30° field: vitreous hemorrhage in diabetic retinopathy; (*D*) 30° field: retinal degeneration in high myopia; (*E*) 45° field: dragged disc in retinopathy of prematurity. (Courtesy Linda Trick, O.D.)

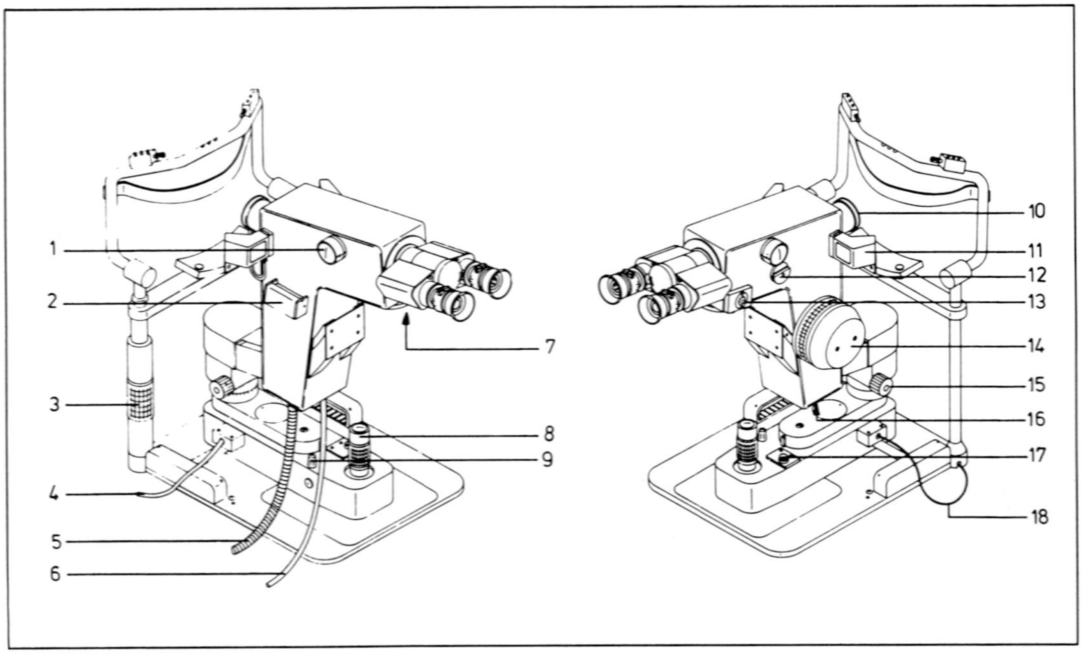

FIGURE 35–5. Features of a typical stand-mounted, mydriatic fundus camera, the Zeiss FK 30 (courtesy Carl Zeiss Inc). Numbered features are: 1, focusing knob (on both sides); 2, filter insert; 3, height adjustment for chin rest; 4, 5, 6, connections to power supply unit; 7, clamping screw for photographic system; 8, joystick; 9, locking knob for instrument base; 10, objective lens; 11, sighting device (on both sides); 12, level; 13, jack for camera systems; 14, vertical swivel adjustment drive; 15, lateral swivel locking screw; 16, control ring for pupil diaphragm; 17, electrical camera release; 18, electrical connection for fixation light.

6. *Name tag.* Often there is a slot into which a label with the patient's name or identification number may be inserted. The name then appears on the film. Some cameras have alternative methods of identifying pictures, such as an identification number that appears in the frame.
7. *Shutter release.* On the newer cameras this is on top of the joystick. On hand-held cameras the shutter release is operated by the thumb or forefinger.
8. *Camera back.* Almost all fundus cameras are equipped with dedicated camera backs. These come equipped with a keyhole-shaped field stop to give a crisp edge to fundus pictures and to help orient them. Newer cameras have autowinders that advance film automatically. Manual advance is necessary on some older models.

Figure 35–5 shows these features on a typical fundus camera.

Most fundus cameras can be used with either Polaroid film or 35-mm film. Generally, photographers prefer to take advantage of the high resolution of modern fundus cameras by using a low-speed, fine-grain 35-mm film, such as Kodachrome or Ektachrome 100. The final choice depends on taste, availability, and processing turnaround.

Exposure is controlled by the flash setting on the power supply. There is little variation from patient to patient in the exposure of retinas. The difference between the palest and darkest fundi lie within the exposure latitude of slide film. Camera manuals usually give fairly accurate exposure settings. Find what flash settings the manufacturer recommends for the film you have chosen. These should be confirmed with trial photographs.

COMMERCIALLY AVAILABLE INSTRUMENTS

Fundus cameras may be stand-mounted or hand-held. Either type of camera can be mydriatic, requiring a pharmacologic agent to

dilate the patient's pupil; or nonmydriatic, permitting retinal photography through the patient's natural pupil.

Every major optical manufacturer makes at least one fundus camera. At this writing, over a dozen models are manufactured, and many discontinued models are still in active use in eye care clinics. Some of the mydriatic cameras currently in production include the Canon CF-60U; Kowa RC-X, RC-Xf, RC-Xv; Nikon NFC-50 and NFC-60; Topcon TRC-JE, TRC-F, TRC-50FT, TRC-50V, TRC-50VT; Zeiss FF4 and FK-30. All these cameras permit color photography with 35-mm or Polaroid film. The Zeiss instruments and the Topcon TRC-JE have a fixed 30° field. The other cameras permit a variety of fields including, for the Canon, Nikon, and Topcon TRC-50V and TRC-50VT, wide-angle fields of 50° or 60°. Two nonmydriatic cameras are readily available in North America, the Canon CR4-45NM and the Topcon TRC-NW3. The Kowa RC-2 and Reichert Docustar are hand-held fundus cameras.

CLINICAL PROCEDURE

Mydriatic Stand-Mounted Fundus Cameras

Mydriatic stand-mounted fundus cameras are the standard clinical instruments. They permit quick, relatively easy, high-quality fundus photography.

The procedure for fundus photography is as follows:

1. Dilate the patient using your usual regimen. A drop or two of 0.5% or 1.0% tropicamide suffices in almost all cases.[7]
2. Load film and make preliminary camera adjustments, adjusting for the patient's ametropia, the field of view, setting the flash unit power supply according to the film chosen, and placing patient identification in the appropriate slot (if available). Focus the eyepiece mires much as you would the mires on a lensometer or keratometer.

3. Place the patient comfortably in the chin rest of the instrument.

4. From outside the camera, focus the donut-shaped exit pupil of the fundus camera illumination system in the plane of the patient's pupil and then center the exit pupil in the patient's pupil.

5. Adjust the orientation of the camera or the direction of the patient's fixation to line up the photo. The fixation can be directed with the fixation light attached to the headrest or with the internal fixation pointer. If the internal pointer is used, it should be withdrawn just before the photograph is taken, unless it is desired to document fixation.[8]

6. While looking through the camera focusing system, adjust the focusing wheel on the side of the camera until both the eyepiece mires and the patient's retina are clear.

7. Eliminate artifacts (i.e., blue or yellow casts or fringes) by moving the camera with the joystick. If the picture appears blue or desaturated, move the camera closer to the patient. If there is a yellow fringe, move away from it (e.g., move the camera to the right if there is a fringe on the left) (Fig. 35–6).

8. When a crisp, artifact-free retinal image has been obtained, trigger the shutter.

9. When the strobe has recharged, repeat steps 4 through 8 until about five photographs are taken. You may want to bracket exposures, although that is usually not necessary.

In practice, steps 5 through 8 proceed more or less simultaneously, with the photographer making constant small adjustments until he or she is satisfied.

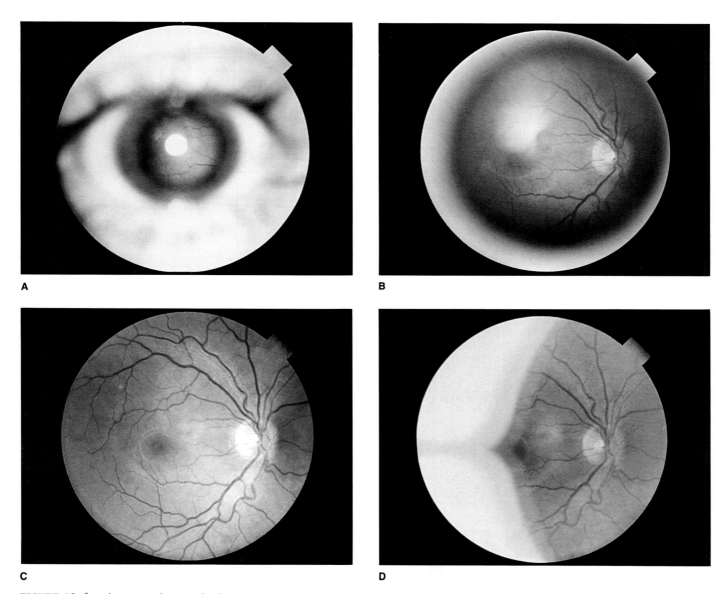

FIGURE 35–6. Alignment of an eye for fundus photography as seen through the camera viewfinder. (*A*) When first approaching the eye, the retina can be seen through the pupil. (*B*) As the camera moves nearer the eye, the retina becomes larger, but increasingly obscured by the bright corneal reflex. A blue circle surrounds the retina owing to scattering from the crystalline lens. (*C*) Continuing to approach the eye produces a clear, high-contrast image, devoid of artifacts. At this point the shutter should be triggered. (*D*) Moving too far to one side will produce a characteristic white or orange reflex, like the one at the left of this picture. Eliminate this artifact by moving away from it (e.g., to the right, in this example).

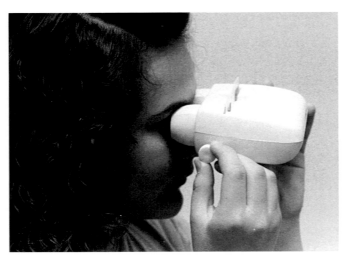

FIGURE 35–7. LIFE-LIKE stereo viewer allows the observer to fuse the images of two 35-mm slides. (Courtesy DEEP-VUE Corporation)

The procedure for anterior segment photography is identical, except the anterior segment setting of the ametropia correction should be dialed in, if the camera has one. Exposure is about the same as that for the fundus.

Stereoscopic fundus pictures can be taken by photographing the retina sequentially from two different perspectives through a widely dilated pupil.[9] The resultant stereo pairs can most easily be observed through a stereo viewer (Fig. 35–7). The stereo effect in these sequential pairs will be satisfactory. More consistent stereo is possible with the addition of special attachments.[10]

Nonmydriatic Stand-Mounted Cameras

Two stand-mounted nonmydriatic cameras (Fig. 35–8) are now in production, the Canon CR4-45NM and the Topcon TRC-NW3, and the Canon CR3-45NM is still in wide use. All have very similar designs. They require a natural pupil at least 4 mm in diameter for photographs. The dilatation is facilitated by performing photography in a dark room. Focusing is done by infrared light outside the visible spectrum so that miosis is not stimulated. Electronics convert the infrared fundus image to a visible black and white image on a television monitor for the photographer. Infrared alignment lights visible on the monitor show when the working distance is correct. Because of the low resolution of the monitor, fine focusing is done with a projection system using a vernier criterion. Photography is done by the light of a strobe, as with a mydriatic camera. Either 35-mm or Polaroid film may be used, with the appropriate camera backs. The Canon cameras have a 45° field of view, and the Topcon has a 20° field of view, as well as a 45° field. All have a slot for an identification tag, which will appear in the picture.

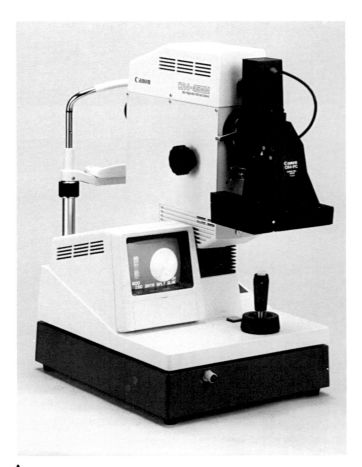

A

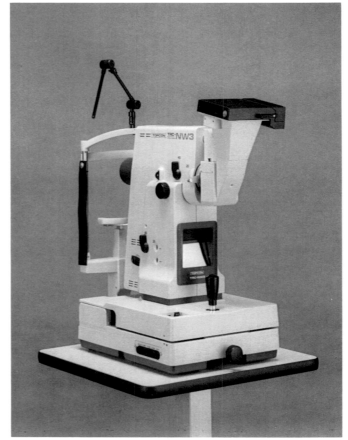

B

FIGURE 35–8. Stand-mounted nonmydriatic cameras: (*A*) Canon CR4-45NM (courtesy Canon USA Inc); (*B*) Topcon TRC-NW3 (courtesy Topcon Instrument Corporation of America).

The procedures for the two instruments are quite similar:

1. Place the patient in the darkened photography area long enough for him or her to obtain sufficient natural dilatation.
2. Load film and make preliminary camera adjustments, adjusting for the patient's ametropia with the slide on the right-hand side of the Canon instruments (or the left-hand side of the Topcon), setting the flash unit power supply, and placing patient identification in the appropriate slot. The field of view on the Topcon is selected by setting the angle-changing selector and diaphragm selector levers on the left-hand side of the camera.
3. Place the patient comfortably in the chin rest of the instrument.
4. Line up the camera with the patient's pupil. On the Canon CR3-45NM, place the green switch on the control panel in the upper position and adjust camera position until the external eye is visible on the television screen. Center the eye within the black circle on the screen using joystick movements and adjusting the camera height with the knurled knob centered under the camera housing. On the

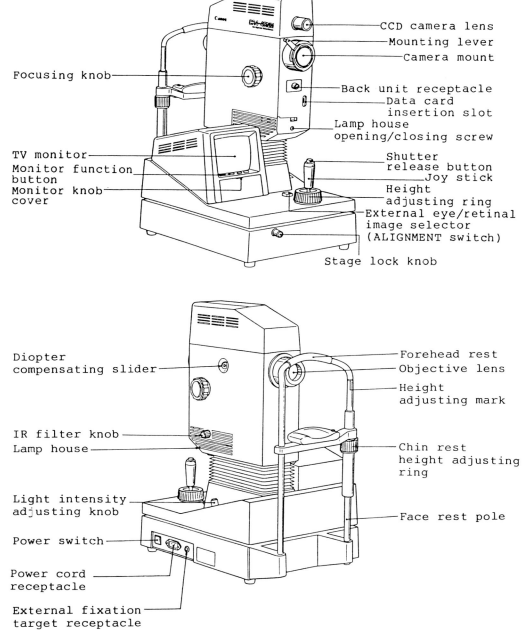

FIGURE 35–9. Components of the Canon CR4-45NM nonmydriatic fundus camera. (Courtesy Canon USA Inc)

CR4-5NM Canon camera (Fig. 35–9) move the joystick to align the pupil image which is split horizontally. On the Topcon simply pull the camera away from the patient with the joystick and turn the focusing knob on the left all the way counterclockwise. Center the eye behind the I-shaped marker.

5. Focus on the retina. For the Canon CR3-45NM, just flip the green switch to its other position. The retina should come into view on the television screen. On the Canon CR4-45NM, the ALIGNMENT switch performs the same function. The Topcon instrument should be moved forward, as with a nonmydriatic camera. Adjustment of the focus ring will clear up the picture on the video monitor.

6. Continue manipulating the position of the camera to obtain proper alignment. This occurs when two small bright lights at the left and right of the screen (two with the Canon and three with the Topcon) are visible and superimposed on the image of the retina. The image is now aligned without artifacts.

7. Manipulate the focusing knob until the two bright horizontal lines in the center of the screen (within the tongue–depresser-shaped dark area) are aligned. The fundus is now focused. In practice, this step and the previous one proceed simultaneously.

8. When the fundus is focused and aligned, trigger the shutter release on the joystick.

Hand-Held Mydriatic Cameras

The compact optics of the hand-held instruments require extremely short working distances, typically less than a centimeter. This combined with the weight of the camera makes alignment and focus rather more difficult than with stand-mounted fundus cameras.

The Kowa RC-2 is the only mydriatic hand-held camera currently marketed in North America. This instrument is held in the right hand with the thumb on the shutter release and the forefinger on the focusing wheel. Alignment is achieved very much as with a monocular indirect ophthalmoscope. Alternatively, it may be used with a stand to function as a stand-mounted camera. Two fields of view are possible: 15° and 30°. A back is available for 35-mm or Polaroid film. Consult the instrument manual for the exposure setting, which depends on the power supply that came with the instrument as well as the film. Pictures may be identified by a number from 1 to 40, which will appear on film.

The procedure for fundus photography is as follows:

1. Dilate the patient using your usual regimen. A drop or two of 0.5% or 1.0% tropicamide usually suffices.

2. Load film and make preliminary camera adjustments, adjusting for the patient's ametropia, the field of view, setting the flash unit power supply, and setting the patient identification number by repeatedly pressing the shiny button on the upper left side of the camera. Focus the eyepiece mires much as you would the mires in a lensometer or keratometer.

3. Seat the patient comfortably in a straight-backed chair or in the examination chair, leaning slightly forward.

4. Grasp the handle of the instrument with the right hand, the thumb on the silver shutter switch on the left side of the camera, the forefinger on the knurled focus knob on the right side of the camera. Place the left hand on top of the camera to steady it (Fig. 35–10).

5. With the last two fingers of the left hand extended to touch the patient's forehead, cautiously approach the patient's eye until the camera is about 1 cm from it. Through the viewfinder you should initially see the external eye with a

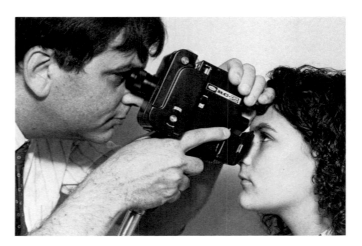

FIGURE 35–10. The Kowa RC2 fundus camera in use. The right hand grasps the handle with the right forefinger on the focusing knob and the left thumb (not shown) on the trigger. The left hand rests on the camera and the patient's forehead to facilitate alignment.

bright-red fundus reflex. As you move closer the fundus will become visible.

6. While looking through the camera focusing system, adjust the focusing wheel on the side of the camera until both the eyepiece mires and the patient's retina are clear.

7. Eliminate artifacts (i.e., blue or yellow casts or fringes) by moving the camera.

8. When a crisp, artifact-free retinal image has been obtained, trigger the shutter.

9. When the strobe has recharged, repeat steps 5 through 8 until about five photographs have been taken. You may want to bracket exposures.

The procedure for anterior segment photography is essentially the same as the foregoing, with a greater, more comfortable working distance. Exposure of the external eye is about the same as that of the fundus.

Nonmydriatic Hand-Held Camera

Only one hand-held nonmydriatic camera has been marketed in recent years, the Docustar (Fig. 35–11). It is modeled after, and handles like, the American Optical monocular indirect ophthalmoscope. The focusing light is sufficiently dim that most subjects will retain sufficient mydriasis for fundus photography. If not, the focusing light can be dimmed still further with a filter and aperture operated by a trigger next to the shutter trigger. The instrument is restricted to a 20° field of view. It uses only Polaroid film, placing two fundus photos in a picture.

The steps in using it are as follows:

1. Load the Polaroid film pack.

2. Adjust the focusing knob on the back of the camera to the zero position. While looking at a distant object, adjust the eyepiece by twisting it clockwise until the object is clear in the viewfinder. (This unfogs it.) A viewfinder screen that can be slid into the viewing system may be helpful.

3. Seat the patient comfortably in a straight-backed chair or in the examination chair, leaning slightly forward.

4. With the right hand holding the back handle of the camera and the fingers of the right hand on the triggers, with the thumb on the knurled focusing knob, and the left hand

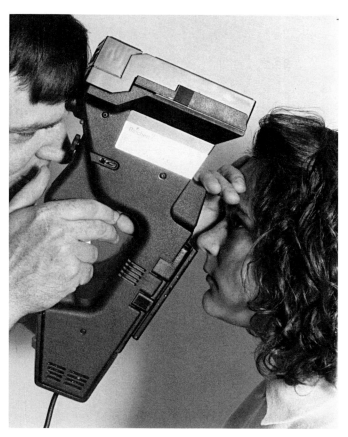

FIGURE 35–11. The Docustar camera in use. The thumb of the left hand hooks around the camera while the fingers of the left hand rest between the camera and the patient's forehead. The weight of the camera is borne mainly by the right hand. The fingers of the right hand rest on the trigger, which engages an aperture and filter to facilitate nonmydriatic photography, and also triggers the shutter.

with its thumb hooked behind the camera body and fingers projecting in front of the camera, move toward the patient while observing the eye. You should initially see the external eye with a bright-red fundus reflex. As you move closer you will see the retina.

5. Adjust the orientation of the camera to get rid of any corneal reflexes. If inadequate dilatation is present, pull the lower trigger to throw an aperture and red filter into the system, cutting down on the light reaching the retina.
6. When a crisp, reflex-free retinal image has been obtained, take the picture by pulling the upper trigger.

CLINICAL IMPLICATIONS

Clinical Significance

As in all clinical photography, the chief value of fundus photography is in providing an objective record of the appearance of a clinical condition at a particular time.

Clinical Interpretation

Clinical interpretation of fundus photographs is the same as that for corresponding ophthalmoscopic observations. It is tempting to think of photographs as definitive documentation of the retina, but pictures do suffer from some limitations. Reflections from the retina may sometimes produce misleading artifacts (e.g., spurious arterial plaques). These can be identified by comparison with other photographs or the ophthalmoscopic record. While it is fairly easy to get consistently good documentation of the central 45° of the retina, it is difficult to photograph lesions in the far periphery.

Most fundus pictures are of a particular localized lesion. These are typically taken with 30° or 45° fields of view, with enough additional shots, usually about five, to be sure of getting a good picture despite artifacts, blinking, focus misjudgment, and so

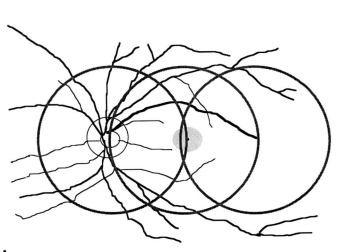

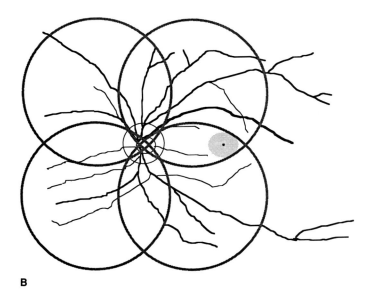

A   B

FIGURE 35–12. Parr's seven standardized fields of view for baseline documentation. Each circle represents a photograph taken with 30° field of view: (*A*) three photos taken along the horizontal meridian; (*B*) four photos clustered around the optic disc. Note that each photograph includes a portion of the optic disc or macula to facilitate orientation.

on. If the lesion is not too peripheral, it is a good idea to include at least a corner of the optic disc or macular region for orientation purposes in these pictures.

Sometimes, however, a lesion extends beyond the field of view of a conventional camera, or baseline photography of an extended area of the retina is desired. In the absence of a large-field fundus camera, such as the Canon CF-60U, large areas of the retina can be documented by means of fundus composites. Such composites either follow the lesion or follow some standard layout such as that suggested by Parr in documenting diabetic retinopathy[11] (Fig. 35–12).

As in all ocular photography, slides or prints should be labeled with the date of the photography session, the patient's name and file numbers, the patient's sex, the laterality of the eye in the picture, and a diagnosis. The keyhole-shaped exit pupil of the camera frames the photograph and indicates its orientation, but it is still a good idea to include an arrow showing which way is up. When a portion of the optic disk or macular area is included in the picture, it is easy to determine the location of the retinal area photographed. In more peripheral shots, be sure to indicate the location on the picture.

As in all clinical photography, retinal photographs should be regarded as a supplement to—not a substitute for—conventional means of recording funduscopic observations.

REFERENCES

1. Jackman WT, Webster JD. On photographing the retina of the living human eye. Phil Photogr 1886;23:275.
2. Litmann H. Die Zeiss-Funduskamera. Bericht Ophthalm Ges 1955;59:318–321.
3. Novotny HR, Alvis D. A method of photographing fluorescence in circulating blood in the human retina. Circulation 1961;24:82–86.
4. Long W. Ocular photography. Chicago: Professional Press, 1984:110–111.
5. Bengtsson B, Krakau C. Some essential optical features of the Zeiss fundus camera. Acta Ophthalmol 1977;55:123–131.
6. Busse B, Mittelman D. Use of the astigmatism correction device on the Zeiss fundus camera for peripheral retinal photography. In: Justice J, ed. Ophthalmic photography. Boston: Little Brown & Co, 1976:63–74.
7. Mordi J, Lyle W, Mousa G. Does prior instillation of a topical anesthetic enhance the effect of tropicamide? Am J Optom Physiol Opt 1986;63:290–293.
8. Steiger R, Wuerth A. Die Fixationsphotographie und die Elektroenzephalographie in der Beurtailung der Schielamblyopie. Ophthalmology 1958;129:240–244.
9. Allen L. Ocular fundus photography. Ophthalmol 1964;57:13–28.
10. Stenstrom WJ. A modification of the new Zeiss fundus camera. Arch Ophthalmology 1960;64:935–938.
11. Parr J, Spears G. Grading of diabetic retinopathy by point-counting on a standardized photographic sample of the retina. J Ophthalmol 1972;74:459–465.

Lacrimal System Evaluation

Leo P. Semes

INTRODUCTION

Definition

The lacrimal system can be divided conceptually into three components. Physiologically the production, distribution, and drainage systems interact in a continuous dynamic fashion to maintain the integrity and comfort of the exposed ocular surface. The artificial separation, however, is a convenient device for categorizing lacrimal system procedures.

The production system is responsible for secretory activity and includes the main and accessory lacrimal glands that produce reflex (aqueous) tears. The basic secretory glands of the conjunctiva and lids continuously produce the tear film under normal physiologic conditions. Specific measures of reflex and basic tear activity are available.

The lids represent the distribution system for the tear film. They are assessed by observation with the slit lamp biomicroscope.

Finally, the lacrimal drainage system is responsible for equilibrating the quantity of tears presented at its origin, the punctum. Although the punctum is observable directly, the remainder of the excretory portion of the lacrimal system must be assessed indirectly.

The reader is cautioned to accept this division as an artificial device for understanding lacrimal system assessment. Integration of subjective assessment with a logical approach to the patient with a history of tearing can result in a rewardingly confident diagnosis and basis for treatment plans[1] (Fig. 36–1).

History

Our understanding of the anatomy and physiology of the lacrimal system forms the basis for evaluation procedures. Three groups have made major contributions to this foundation. Schirmer[2] described a series of tests for measuring basic and reflex lacrimal secretions, as well as a rudimentary approach to assessing the integrity of the efferent reflex pathway. These well-known tests have borne his name for nearly a century. The evolution of the science of tear film physiology led to a categorization of such disorders in the mid-1970s by Holly and Lemp.[3] Their familiar LAMBS mnemonic for localization of production and distribution system disorders serves as a guide to diagnosis and management. The mnemonic translates to disorders of lipid layer (L), aqueous dysfunction (A), mucin deficiency (M), blepharitic disorders (B), and surface abnormalities (S).[3] Assessment of the lacrimal drainage system is based on the work of Lester Jones.[4] His careful anatomic descriptions of the lacrimal drainage pathways and their interactions with the lids remain classics. The tests of lacrimal drainage patency have borne his name since their introduction in the early 1960s.

Clinical Use

The Schirmer tests for lacrimal secretory function should follow the original description, for sake of consistency.[2] In a practical sense, the *basic secretion test* is probably most useful. This segment of the hierarchy is performed after the instillation of a topical anesthetic. It is intended to measure the basal tear film quantitatively, but practically, it assesses the continuous aqueous portion of the tear film.[1] An overview of the procedure for Schirmer tear testing is shown in Figure 36–2.

Stability of the trilayered tear film can be measured by the tear breakup time (TBUT) using fluorescein dye.[5] Surface epithelial integrity is assessed with the aid of another dye, rose bengal.[6] Staining by rose bengal is specific for dead or diseased epithelial cells.

Fluorescein dye is the marker used to stain the tears in the

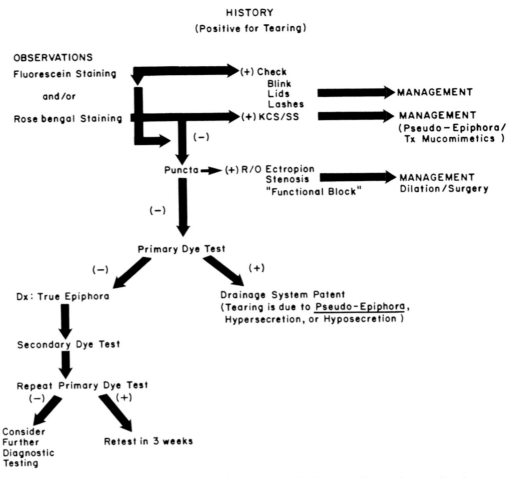

FIGURE 36–1. Flow chart outlining recommended procedures for diagnosis of lacrimal system disorders when the patient presents with a history of tearing. (From Semes L, Clompus RJ. Diseases of the lacrimal system. In: Bartlett JD, Jaanus SD, eds. Clinical ocular pharmacology, 2nd ed. Boston: Butterworth, 1989:491–511, with permission)

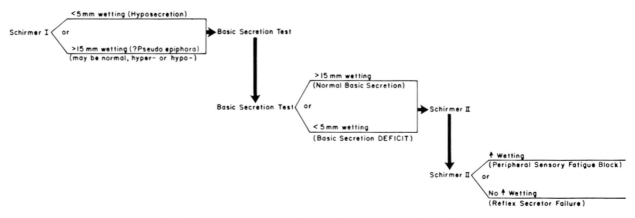

FIGURE 36–2. Flow diagram of the Schirmer test sequence. See text for interpretation. (From Semes L, Clompus RJ. Diseases of the lacrimal system. In: Bartlett JD, Jaanus SD, eds. Clinical ocular pharmacology, 2nd ed. Boston: Butterworth, 1989:491–511, with permission)

diagnosis of drainage system disorders. When instilled into the conjunctival cul-de-sac, its presence can be sought at appropriate points along the drainage pathway. The presence of the dye marker among the drained tears indicates a physiologically patent system.[1,4] Diagnostic localization of drainage system disorders can be carried out using specifically designed probes and lacrimal cannulae. In addition, sophisticated assessments of tear film content and lacrimal drainage function are available.

Objective assessment of the distribution system, the lids, is performed with the slit lamp biomicroscope. Irregularities or blepharitic conditions can be directly observed.[1,3]

Both subjective and objective data are considered together when making decisions about the status of the lacrimal system.[1]

INSTRUMENTATION

Theory

Secretory Function

The dyes used in lacrimal procedures are fluorescein and rose bengal. Fluorescein will stain areas of the cornea and conjunctiva that have been disrupted. The basis may be pH difference or cellular alteration.[6,7] The TBUT test uses fluorescein as a marker for the evaluation of tear film stability. The TBUT test is a nonspecific qualitative assessment of tear film integrity. A reduced TBUT can result from deficiencies of any layer of the tear film (see Fig. 36–1).

Rose bengal dye will stain dead or devitalized cells. Rose bengal staining is thought to be consistent with a diagnosis of aqueous deficiency.[6] It is, therefore, more specific than the staining or premature breakup observed with fluorescein.

The Schirmer[2] tests are carried out with 5-mm × 50-mm strips of Whatman No. 41 filter paper placed in the inferior cul-de-sac. Capillary action is responsible for wetting the strip within a given time.[1,2,8] The amount of wetting for each of the tests is useful for comparison purposes (see Figs. 36–2 and 36–3).

Another aqueous tear assessment is the lysozyme assay.[9] Lysozyme constitutes one-fourth of total tear protein and will be reduced in hypersecretion (by dilution) as well as in aqueous-deficiency disorders. The test is based on inhibition of microbial growth of the bacterium *Micrococcus luteus* (*lysodeikticus*).[9]

The protein lactoferrin may also be measured as a yardstick for aqueous function. A tear sample is placed in a small incubator, and the amount of diffusion (corresponding to lactoferrin content of the tears) is measured 2 to 3 days later.[10] This procedure may

represent a reliable marker for the diagnosis of aqueous deficiency in moderate to severe keratoconjunctivitis sicca (KCS).[11]

Cellulose acetate strips have been used for the direct assessment of goblet cell counts.[12] The MF Millipore Filter Paper VS is pressed gently to the conjunctiva, removed, and stained with Schiff's reagent and hematoxylin. The specimen is examined under a microscope.

Distribution Function

The lids are assessed by direct observation. The slit lamp biomicroscope is used to examine the lashes, lid margins, and to evaluate the blink. In addition, the tear prism can be evaluated qualitatively.

Drainage Function

A patent lacrimal drainage system accommodates normal tear production and distribution. Upset of the delicate balance among any of the components, however, can result in tearing. Access to the drainage system, the puncta, may be directly evaluated at the slit lamp biomicroscope. A normal punctum is apposed to the globe and the lower lid must be everted to view it. Since the remainder of the drainage system is not observable directly, fluorescein dye is instilled to serve as a marker for draining tears. The secondary dye test (Jones no. 2 test) consists of a saline lavage of the lacrimal drainage pathway.[13]

Use

The general indication for lacrimal system testing is the symptom of tearing. Following the flow diagrams presented in Figures 36–1 and 36–2 will assist the clinician in the application of these procedures. Fluorescein dye will be the most widely applied test. It is used for the assessment of tear film stability as well as for lacrimal drainage testing. Rose bengal dye is applied to confirm the diagnosis of aqueous deficiency. Schirmer tests can be used to demonstrate an insufficient tear secretion rate.

When a patient's medical history includes rheumatoid arthritis, the clinician should suspect aqueous deficiency. Additional probing concerning dry mouth, for example, may crystallize the tentative diagnosis of keratoconjunctivitis sicca. Confirmatory tests, as mentioned earlier, as well as tear protein or goblet cell investigations may be invoked for equivocal cases.

All patients with a complaint of tearing should be examined with the slit lamp biomicroscope. When the history includes lid trauma, neurologic dysfunction (e.g., Bell's palsy), other lid disease (e.g., blepharitis), incomplete lid closure, ectropion, or systemic health problems (e.g., Graves' disease), special attention should be given to assessment of the tear prism, punctum position, and lid apposition.

COMMERCIALLY AVAILABLE INSTRUMENTS

Dyes

Fluorescein dye is available in sterile impregnated-strip and solution form. The fluorescein-impregnated strips are moistened with sterile saline before being touched to the cul-de-sac (see Fig. 36–3).

Rose bengal dye is also available in these two formulations. A note of caution is in order concerning liquid rose bengal dye. The 1% solution represents a saturated concentration. Evaporation may result in crystallization at the opening of

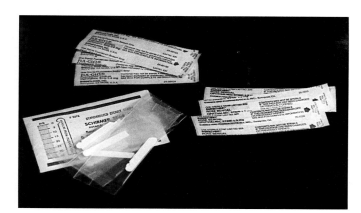

FIGURE 36–3. Diagnostic materials for lacrimal system procedures. Clockwise from top: fluorescein-impregnated strips, rose bengal-impregnated strips, and Schirmer tear test strips.

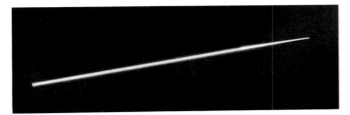

FIGURE 36–4. Ruedemann lacrimal dilator. The fine tip and gentle taper allow this instrument to be admitted to almost any punctum for dilatation.

the dispensing tip. Care is urged for the clinician in forcing the dispensing at this point. A portion of the crystallized material or a rush of the liquid under pressure may reach the patient's eye (and adnexa).

Schirmer strips: Schirmer strips are 5-mm × 50-mm pieces of Whatman No. 41 filter paper. The standardized design has a notch at 5 mm from one end for folding over the lid margin. Each pair of strips is packaged in a sterile, sealed plastic bag. Five pairs are contained in an envelope, which has a millimeter scale for measurement of wetting (see Fig. 36–3).

Tear Protein Measurements

The measurement of lactoferrin is the most clinically useful of the tear protein assays, and the Lactoplate is the diagnostic instrument used. It consists of a plastic incubation chamber with two reagent–gel cells. A small piece of filter paper is used to collect a tear sample, which is then transferred to the reagent cell. After a period of 2 to 3 days, diffusion is complete and the results are read.

Dilators and Cannulae

Instrumentation for investigation of the integrity of the lacrimal drainage apparatus is highly personalized. Congenital epiphora may be assessed by using a variety of Bowman probes. Typically, these are used in attempts at finding bony malformations or as a curative strategy in cases of incomplete cannulization of the drainage pathway.

Diagnostic dilation and irrigation[13–17] in the primary care setting can be accomplished with a few instruments. The dilator may be any of a variety of designs with fine to blunt tips. They also are available in a range of tapers. The most useful is the Ruedemann (Storz No. E3466), with a very fine tip and narrow taper, or others of this design (Fig. 36–4).

Lacrimal cannulae are available from several sources in a variety of styles and a range of gauges. Nasolacrimal cannulae may have blunt tips with the needle hole on one side. The West cannula has a straight shaft; the most useful size is 23 gauge (Fig. 36–5). Sources include Storz Instruments,* Katena Eye Instruments,† and i-Tech Industries, Inc.‡

Another approach to diagnostic lacrimal lavage is to use an open-ended cannula, some of which are reinforced. In addition, curved cannulae are preferred by some clinicians.

Whichever cannula is chosen, it must be attached to a syringe. Plastic disposable syringes of 5-mL capacity are adequate for this purpose. This size allows a good balance between volume and ease of use.

* 3365 Tree Court Industrial Blvd., St. Louis, MO 63122

† 4 Stewart Ct., Denville, NJ 07834

‡ 849 Westwood Avenue, Addison, IL 60101

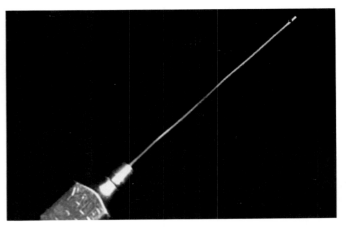

FIGURE 36–5. The 23-g West straight lachrymal cannula. The blunt tip allows this instrument to be advanced through the delicate lacrimal drainage tissues without tearing them. The hole in the side is aligned with the nasolacrimal duct. This cannula is fitted to a 2- or 3-mL syringe for lacrimal lavage.

CLINICAL PROCEDURE

Secretory Function

There are three Schirmer's[2] tests. The Schirmer 1 test is performed before the instillation of a topical anesthetic. Total tear flow—reflex or stimulated tears in addition to basal secretions—wets the filter paper. The basic secretion test (BST) was designed to measure only the continuous tear flow. Following instillation of a topical anesthetic, the cul-de-sac is dried and a fresh filter paper strip is inserted over the lower lid margin. The amount of wetting is measured. The Schirmer 2 test was designed to assess the efferent reflex pathway from the lacrimal nucleus. With the (dry) strip in place from the BST, the nasal mucosa is stimulated with a cotton-tipped wire. Increased wetting is taken as evidence of an intact reflex arc.[2] The sequence of Schirmer testing is shown in Figure 36–2.

The TBUT test is performed by measuring the time (in seconds) to the appearance of the first randomly distributed dry spot after fluorescein dye is placed in the inferior cul-de-sac to stain the tears. The clinician seats the patient at the slit lamp biomicroscope, asks the patient to blink several times and to stare straight ahead without blinking. The clinician then commences counting while observing for tear film breakup.

Perhaps the best estimate of tear film integrity is qualitative. The clinician observes whether a dry spot appears (representing tear film breakup) before a reflex blink renews the tear film.[1] Quantitative guidelines, however, are useful, since applying quantitative measures represents a consistent intraexaminer estimate of tear film integrity.

Observation for rose bengal staining at the slit lamp biomicroscope is performed with white light. Generally the staining pattern will be found in the intrapalpebral area on the cornea or conjunctiva.

Other measurements of the aqueous fraction attempt to correlate tear protein concentration with aqueous function. The measurements of lysozyme and lactoferrin are not part of universal clinical practice.

Mucus function may be specifically assessed by a pseudohistologic technique. The Millipore filter paper system is used to make a goblet cell impression from the inferior cul-de-sac. This is transferred to a glass slide for staining, and the specimen is examined under a microscope.

Distribution Function

The lids are assessed by direct observation. The slit lamp biomicroscope is used to examine the lashes and lid margins. In addition, the tear prism can be evaluated qualitatively. Incomplete lid closure, ectropion, or entropion may be observed during the patient interview and examined in more detail with the slit lamp biomicroscope.

Drainage Function

The primary dye test (Jones no. 1 test)[4] is used to test lacrimal drainage patency. Fluorescein dye is placed into the inferior cul-de-sac to serve as a marker to stain the tears. A physiologically patent lacrimal drainage system will show the presence of the marker. The presence of dye is most conveniently observed, after an interval of 5 minutes, by asking the patient to clear his or her nose into a white tissue. Whether bilateral or unilateral involvement is suspected, each side should be evaluated independently. Other methods of dye recovery are more tedious and need not be covered here.

A negative result (no dye present) would indicate that the dye either entered the drainage system and became obstructed in its passage or never arrived at the entry point (the punctum). A negative primary dye test is the indication for diagnostic dilation and irrigation of the lacrimal drainage system.[4,13]

Initially, dilation of the punctum is carried out under topical anesthesia, and the primary test is repeated to confirm a negative result. A specifically designed lacrimal cannula is then used to rinse 2 to 3 mL of sterile saline through the nasolacrimal duct. When the patient is inclined forward about 30° from the vertical, the effluent can be collected in an emesis basin. The presence of dye at this stage indicates reestablishment of drainage patency. The presence of clear fluid confirms a proximal location for the obstruction, suggesting that fluorescein dye never entered the drainage pathway[4,13] (see Fig. 36–1).

CLINICAL IMPLICATIONS

Clinical Significance

Lacrimal function testing follows the logical anatomy of the secretory glands, lids, and drainage pathway.[1,3,4,16] Evaluation of the aqueous secretors by the Schirmer's[2] tests, tear film stability investigation by the TBUT, lid and lash inspection with the slit lamp biomicroscope, and indirect evaluation of the drainage system, all contribute a confident diagnosis and basis for treatment plans[1] (see Fig. 36–1).

The diagnosis of a dry-eye problem typically indicates treatment initially with mucomimetics. "Dry eye," unfortunately, may be used to describe aqueous deficiencies (keratoconjunctivitis sicca) as well as abnormalities of the tear film. For the clinician to make the best choice of a management plan, judicious use of a logical approach to diagnosis must be made. Often mild dry-eye conditions and tear film deficiencies can be managed with mucomimetics. The clinician, however, should be aware of the numerous causes of tearing. A thorough workup of patients whose subjective complaint is tearing cannot be emphasized strongly enough.

Clinical Interpretation

Values of less than 5 mm on the Schirmer[2] tests generally indicate aqueous deficiency.[1] Initial therapy should be with mucomimetics

or bland ointments at night if compliance is a problem. The trend is toward quaternary ammonium salt preservatives and nonpreserved unit-dose formulations.

Breakup times less than the blink interval indicate an unstable tear film and may be treated with mucomimetics as well. Unless the clinician can determine the presence of blepharitis or mucus deficiency at slit-lamp examination, this is appropriate. The observation of lid disease, however, demands attention to that underlying cause of tear film instability.

The observation of rose bengal staining can be interpreted as evidence of dead or devitalized cells.[6] Positive rose bengal staining is typically taken as evidence of an aqueous deficiency. Other conditions that produce rose bengal staining include viral (herpes simplex) ulceration and the mucus fishing syndrome.[17]

The presence of tearing may indicate epiphora, tearing due to obstruction. The entry to the drainage system, the punctum, may be the causal factor. Stenosis, or closure by collapse, is usually a problem encountered among the elderly. This can be observed and confirmed by the primary dye test. The absence of dye indicates a negative result and a proximal drainage system deficiency.[1,14–17] A positive dye test indicates physiologic patency of the drainage pathway and should prompt the clinician to review the observable portions of the lacrimal system.

A negative primary dye test (no dye detection) following punctal dilation, indicates a blockage in the distal portion of the drainage pathway.[1,15–18] The secondary dye test is then performed in an attempt to localize the site of the obstruction, as well as to force the obstruction through the drainage system.

REFERENCES

1. Semes L, Clompus RJ. Diseases of the lacrimal system. In: Bartlett JD, Jaanus SD, eds. Clinical ocular pharmacology, 2nd ed. Stoneham, Mass: Butterworths, 1989:491–511.
2. Schirmer O. Studien zur physiologie und pathologie der tränenabsonderung und tranenabfuhr. Arch Klin Ophthalmol 1903;56:197–291.
3. Holly FJ, Lemp MA. Tear physiology and dry eyes. Surv Ophthalmol 1977;22:69–87.
4. Jones LT. An anatomical approach to problems of the eyelids and lacrimal apparatus. Arch Ophthalmol 1961;66:111–124.
5. Lemp MA, Hamill JR. Factors affecting tear film breakup in normal eyes. Arch Ophthalmol 1973;89:103–105.
6. Norn MS. Vital staining of the cornea and conjunctiva. Acta Ophthalmol Suppl 1972;13:9–65.
7. Romanchuk KG. Fluorescein: physicochemical factors affecting its fluorescence. Surv Ophthalmol 1982;26:269–283.
8. van Bijsterveld OP. Diagnostic tests in the sicca syndrome. Arch Ophthalmol 1969;82:10–14.
9. de Luise VP, Tabbara KF. Quantitation of tear lysozyme levels in dry-eye disorders. Arch Ophthalmol 1983;101:634–635.
10. Boersma HGM, van Bijsterveld OP. The lactoferrin test for the diagnosis of keratoconjunctivitis sicca in clinical practice. Ann Ophthalmol 1987;19:152–154.
11. Goren MB, Goren SB. Diagnostic tests in patients with symptoms of keratoconjunctivitis sicca. Am J Ophthalmol 1988;106:570–574.
12. Nelson JD, Havener VR, Cameron JD. Cellulose acetate impressions of the ocular surface. Arch Ophthalmol 1983;101:1869–1872.
13. Jones LT, Linn ML. The diagnosis and causes of epiphora. Am J Ophthalmol 1969;67:751–754.
14. Campbell HS, Smith JL, Richman DW, et al. A simple test for lacrimal obstruction. Am J Ophthalmol 1962;53:611–613.
15. Zappia RJ, Milder B. Lacrimal drainage function. I: The Jones fluorescein test. Am J Ophthalmol 1972;74:154–159.
16. Hecht SD. Evaluation of the lacrimal drainage system. Am Acad Ophthalmol Otolaryngol 1978;85:1250–1258.
17. McCully JP, Moore MB, Matoba AY. Mucus fishing syndrome. Ophthalmology 1985;92:1262–1265.
18. Semes L, Melore GG. Dilation and diagnostic irrigation of the lacrimal drainage system. J Am Optom Assoc 1986;57:518–525.

Exophthalmometry

George W. Comer

INTRODUCTION

Definition

Exophthalmometry is the clinical procedure used to measure the anteroposterior position of the globe in the orbit relative to some orbital landmark, most commonly the lateral angle of the orbital rim.

The term exophthalmometry was coined in 1867 by Cohn,[1] who originated the concept of measuring the distance from the orbital rim to the anterior surface of the cornea. Other terms have been used to describe this measurement over the years including the terms "proptometry" and "ophthalmostatometry."[2,3] However, exophthalmometry is almost exclusively used today.

The name, exophthalmometry, is derived from the orbital condition that an exophthalmometer is most commonly utilized to detect, exophthalmos. *Exophthalmos,* or proptosis, is an abnormal forward displacement or protrusion of the globe within the orbit (Fig. 37–1). Exophthalmos occurs when there is an imbalance between the volume of the orbit and volume of orbital contents. Since the orbit is essentially a cavity surrounded on three sides by bone, the volume of the orbit is relatively fixed, and any increase in the volume of orbit results in a forward displacement of the globe.

Enophthalmos is an abnormal posterior displacement of the globe or a relative sinking of the globe posteriorly into the orbit. Enophthalmos is typically caused by a degeneration and shrinking of orbital fat. A herniation of orbital contents, particularly orbital fat, through a break in the orbital wall, such as in blow-out fracture may also result in a posterior displacement of the globe.

History

Cohn originated the term exophthalmometry and the concept of specifying the anteroposterior position of the globe in the orbit by measuring the distance from the lateral orbital rim to the anterior surface of the cornea or to the corneal apex. In 1837 he designed an elaborate instrument to measure the distance from the superior orbital rim to the corneal apex and collected data on the normal position of the globe.[1]

Numerous instruments based on the concepts of Cohn's original instrument have been developed over the years.[4] The instrument that has gained widest acceptance is the Hertel exophthalmometer, developed by Hertel in 1905.[5] The Hertel exophthalmometer incorporates mirrors inclined at about 45° from the patient's line of vision. This allows an image of the corneal apex to be projected onto a millimeter rule so that the examiner could measure and compare the anteroposterior positions of both eyes almost simultaneously from a position anterior to the subject (Fig. 37–2). The Hertel exophthalmometer has evolved with only minor modifications over the years.

Although the use of a millimeter rule to roughly determine the amount of forward displacement of the globe was widespread, in 1938, Luedde described a transparent ruler that could be placed against the angle of the lateral orbital rim.[6] There have been numerous modifications of the Luedde exophthalmometer over the years.[4,7,8] This simple device, the Luedde exophthalmometer (Fig. 37–3), is the second most commonly used exophthalmometer today.

In 1967, Watson described an instrument that measures not only the anteroposterior positioning of the globe, but also the

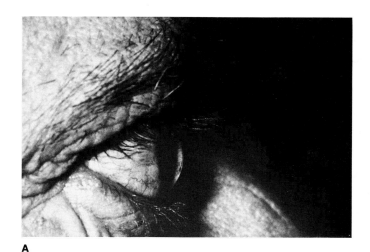

A

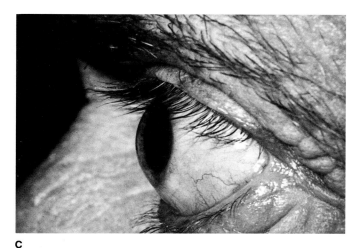

C

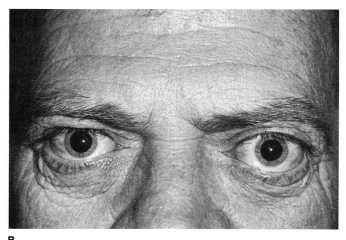

B

FIGURE 37–1. (*A*) Profile of right globe; (*B*) bilateral exophthalmos, greater in left eye: middle-aged man with Graves' eye disease. The exophthalmometry readings have increased 2 mm over the past 2 years; (*C*) profile of left globe. Note the very low position of the lower lid margin.

positioning of the globe vertically and horizontally within the orbit.[9] This instrument was called an ocular topometer. The rationale for measurements other than along an anteroposterior axis is based upon the fact that, depending upon the location of an orbital mass, the globe may be displaced only minimally forward and, more significantly, either laterally or vertically within the orbit. No instrument had previously been available that was designed to measure displacements in any direction other than along an anterior to posterior axis. However, Watson states that his topometer was no better than a Hertel for measurements of exophthalmos.[9]

Clinical Use

The basic clinical use of exophthalmometry is the detection, diagnosis, and monitoring of exophthalmos or, less frequently, enophthalmos. There are several possible causes of exophthalmos (Table 37–1) and enophthalmos (Table 37–2). Exophthalmometry can be very useful in monitoring the progression of exophthalmos to monitor the status of these disorders. For example, exophthalmometry is recommended as a routine for all patients with suspected or known Graves' eye disease. Graves' disease is the single most common cause of unilateral or bilateral exophthalmos.[10–12] The degree of exophthalmos may increase with time.

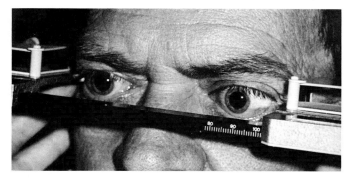

FIGURE 37–2. Hertel type (Marco) exophthalmometric examination of patient in Figure 37–1.

FIGURE 37–3. Luedde exophthalmometer.

Table 37–1
Causes of Bilateral Exophthalmos in Adults

Graves' eye disease
Orbital pseudotumor
Cavernous sinus thrombosis
Orbital infiltration from leukemia
Wagner's granulomatosis
Metastatic neuroblastoma

There are several conditions that mimic exophthalmos and can be termed pseudoexophthalmos. In *pseudoexophthalmos,* the globe is either displaced anteriorly with corresponding high exophthalmometry readings (however, there are none of the typical causes of true exophthalmos such as retrobulbar mass or Graves' disease) or the globe merely *appears* to protrude abnormally.

Those conditions that mimic true exophthalmos are listed in Table 37–3. The differential diagnosis of true exophthalmos from pseudoexophthalmos cannot be made on the basis of exophthalmometry alone.

There are also conditions that mimic enophthalmos. These include a contralateral lid retraction, ptosis, and microphthalmia. Often, close observation of the patient will reveal the presence of either pseudoexophthalmos or pseudoenophthalmos. Exophthalmometry can be used to detect and measure subtle presentations of exophthalmos and enophthalmos and to assist in differentiating some pseudoexophthalmos and pseudoenophthalmos from true exophthalmos and true enophthalmos.

The clinical uses of exophthalmometry are summarized in Table 37–4.

It is apparent that very careful observation of the facial symmetry, external eye, refractive error, globe and corneal size, lid position and function are prerequisites to the performance and accurate interpretation of exophthalmometry.

INSTRUMENTATION

Theory and Use

In exophthalmometry, a measurement of the distance between a point on the temporal orbital rim and the apex of the cornea is made. The point on the orbital rim is accepted, for greatest consistency in readings, to be the deepest palpable point on the angle of the lateral orbital margin in each eye.

A plane including this point on the temporal orbital rim for each orbit will generally be parallel to the frontal plane for that patient. However, there is much individual variation of the positioning of the globe within the orbit and volume of the orbit. This produces the wide range of "normal" exophthalmometric readings. There is also some asymmetry in some patients between the orbit and the globe, producing a normal intraocular asymmetry.

During exophthalmometry the patient's gaze should be directed straight ahead in primary gaze, whereas the examiner views the cornea in profile while measuring the distance from the point on the temporal orbital rim to the corneal apex.

Table 37–2
Causes of Enophthalmos

Orbital blow-out fracture
Age-related degeneration of orbital fat
Progressive hemifacial atrophy

Table 37–3
Causes of Pseudoexophthalmos

Long axial length of the globe
  High axial myopia
  Congenital glaucoma
Orbital asymmetry
  Congenital
  Traumatic
Asymmetry of the palpebral fissures
  Lid retraction
  Contralateral ptosis (Horner's syndrome, CN III palsy)
  Contralateral enophthalmos (orbital blow-out fracture)
  Entropion or ectropion
Loss of tonus in extraocular muscles
  Third nerve palsy

For greatest accuracy, the examiner must obtain a view from a position temporal to the patient's line of sight. The examiner must view along a line perpendicular to the patient's line of sight. The examiner's line of sight will, when properly performed, be parallel to the frontal plane of the patient and along a tangent to the corneal apex.

There are two basic types of exophthalmometers in widespread use today. These are the Luedde exophthalmometer and the Hertel exophthalmometer. Each of these utilizes a different approach for defining the frontal plane and positioning the examiner's line of sight.

COMMERCIALLY AVAILABLE INSTRUMENTS

Basic Design

Luedde Exophthalmometer

The Luedde exophthalmometer consists of a clear, square plastic rod that is about a centimeter in thickness. The rod is ruled in millimeters on both sides, with a scale from 0 to 40 mm. The zero point of the scale is at the tapered end of the rod (see Fig. 37–3). The tapered end of the rod is notched to fit firmly against the lateral orbital margin. The millimeter scale on each side of the rod when viewed from the proper position and coinciding with the corneal apex should be seen as superimposed to minimize parallax error.

Although this is a very simple instrument it incorporates some significant advances over ophthalmic millimeter rules, which have been used by many. First, the zero point of the measuring scale coincides with the end of the rod when it rests against the lateral orbital margin. Also the use of a scale on both sides of the rod to minimize parallax error is a substantial advantage.

The Luedde exophthalmometer is designed to be positioned parallel to a sagittal plane through the eye and perpendicular to

Table 37–4
Uses of Exophthalmometry

Detection of exophthalmos
Detection of enophthalmos
Monitoring by serial-reading the progression of exophthalmos
Detection and monitoring of Graves' eye disease
Differentiation of pseudoexophthalmos from true exophthalmos
Differentiation of pseudoenophthalmos from true enophthalmos

the facial plane. The facial plane will be parallel to the frontal plane passing through the deepest point on the lateral orbital margin of each eye. However, facial asymmetry is very common, such that the two lateral orbital margins are often not symmetric in position. This may cause significant error in Luedde exophthalmometry.

In Luedde exophthalmometry the instrument must be positioned parallel to a sagittal plane through the eye and roughly parallel to the line of sight when the eyes are in the primary position. When this is done, the examiner's line of sight should be perpendicular to the plane of the instrument and perpendicular to the sagittal plane. Failure to hold the instrument in this position produces substantial error. Davanger has analyzed this error and found that a 5° deviation from parallel to the sagittal plane produces a 1.7-mm error in the reading, and a 10° deviation produces approximately twice as much.[13] Deviation of the ruler temporally away from the sagittal plane produces a falsely low reading (Fig. 37–4). Obviously opposite 5° errors in each eye will produce an apparent interocular asymmetry in exophthalmometer readings of about 3.5 mm. This is a significant interocular asymmetry. Drew has suggested that a short ruler such as the regular Luedde exophthalmometer is more difficult to position parallel to the sagittal plane; a long ruler can more easily be aligned.[4]

Davanger has also found examples of the Luedde-type instrument on which the millimeter scales on each side of the instrument do not match. This produces an error in readings of 0.5 mm or greater.[13] If the Luedde exophthalmometer is manufactured such that the zero point does not fall at the very edge of the notched end of the scale, the readings will be erroneous.

Excessive or prolonged pressure on the lateral orbital rim with any exophthalmometer can compress the soft tissues at this location, producing an error of 0.5 to 1 mm.[4]

The common sources of error in Luedde exophthalmometry are summarized in Table 37–5.

Hertel Exophthalmometer

The Hertel exophthalmometer, originally described in 1905 by Hertel, is the most commonly used exophthalmometer in clinical practice today. The Hertel exophthalmometer is designed such that both lateral orbital margins and corneal apices are visible to

Table 37–5
Luedde Exophthalmometry: Sources of Error

Instrument not oriented to parallel to sagittal plane
Parallax error
Asymmetry in position of lateral orbital rim
Manufacturing error
Excessive or prolonged pressure on lateral orbital rim

the examiner in rapid succession (almost simultaneously). The examiner can thus take the measurements and compare that of the right eye with that of the left eye very rapidly. This enhances the recognition of interocular asymmetry.

The Hertel exophthalmometer may be constructed in either of two ways; that is, either a mirror or a prism may be used to view the lateral orbital rims and profile of the corneal apices as if the examiner is viewing from the temporal side.

In the mirror version (Bausch & Lomb) the mirror is inclined at about 45° from the sagittal plane (Fig. 37–5). A millimeter rule oriented roughly parallel to the sagittal plane is viewed similarly through a mirror inclined at 45° to its plane. The examiner thus sees the orbital rim and corneal profile in the bottom mirror, while a millimeter rule with the zero point at the lateral orbital rim is seen immediately above the corneal profile. The prism model (Marco, Rodenstock) produces a similar image (Fig. 37–6).

The most important difference between the two models of Hertel exophthalmometers lies in the design of the footplate that rests at the lateral orbital margin. Because the footplate design is

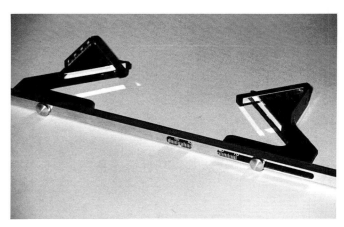

FIGURE 37–5. Hertel mirror-type exophthalmometer by Bausch & Lomb.

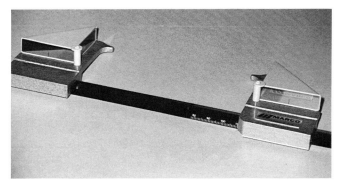

FIGURE 37–6. Hertel prism-type exophthalmometer by Marco.

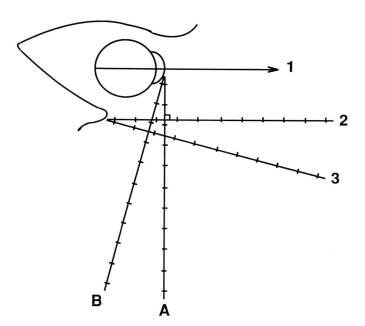

FIGURE 37–4. Effects of deviation from the sagittal plane with the Luedde exophthalmometer.

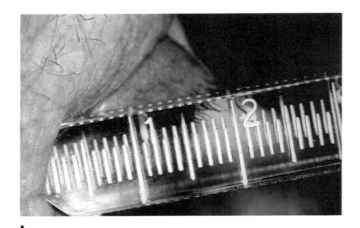

FIGURE 37–7. Marco exophthalmometer. Note parallax lines misaligned.

different, there can be slight differences in the positioning of the footplate (and zero point of the ruler), such that one instrument reads slightly different from the other.

Davanger has found that the footplate designs on both the prism and mirror Hertel exophthalmometers permit a range of different footplate positions and corresponding different readings. He found that a 2-mm medial displacement of the footplate resulted in 3.8-mm higher reading.[13] Although this will have little effect on the difference between the right eye and left eye or any given measurement, it is critical for serial exophthalmometry to use the same instrument, set at the same base, and with the footplate positioned in consistent location at the lateral orbital margin, so that measuring conditions are consistent.

Hertel's original description assumed a distance of 20 mm between the sagittal plane through the globe and the lateral orbital rim, based upon his measurements.[5] This is true, on the average, but there is much individual variation in facial and orbital symmetry. This is one reason in all forms of exophthalmometry for the substantial spread of "normal" exophthalmometry readings. If the distance is different from 20 mm, a parallax error will result. This error usually tends to be no greater than 1 mm, according to Davanger's calculations.[13] To further minimize parallax error, some Hertel exophthalmometers, such as the Marco and Rodenstock prism exophthalmometers, have parallax lines that the examiner superimposes by changing his sighting position before taking the reading (Fig. 37–7).

Table 37–6
Hertel Exophthalmometry: Sources of Error

Asymmetry in the position of the lateral orbital rim
Positioning of the footplate on the orbital rim
Parallax error due to sagittal plane to orbit margin distance ≠ 20 mm
Parallax error in reading the scale
Excessive or prolonged pressure on lateral orbital rim

The Hertel exophthalmometer is less subject to parallax error induced by failure to properly orient the measuring scale relative to the sagittal plane or visual axis. The common sources of error in Hertel exophthalmometry are listed in Table 37–6.

CLINICAL PROCEDURE

Luedde Exophthalmometer

The clinical procedure of taking exophthalmometer readings with the Luedde exophthalmometer is as follows:

1. Carefully observe the facial symmetry, symmetry of the globes and orbits, the external eye, globe and corneal size, lid position and function before taking the exophthalmometry readings. It is also advisable to be aware of the patient's refractive error.
2. Palpate the lateral orbital rim to locate the deepest angle of the rim.
3. Carefully place the notched end of the exophthalmometer firmly against the deepest point on the lateral orbital margin.
4. Tilt the exophthalmometer either medially or laterally to align the exophthalmometer with a sagittal plane through the patient's globe and parallel to the patient's visual axis.
5. From the patient's temporal side look through the exophthalmometer and sight the corneal apex.
6. Slightly adjust the position of your head to superimpose the markings on both sides of the ruler, specifically those that correspond to the corneal apex, to minimize parallax (Fig. 37–8).
7. Read the marking that is tangent to the corneal apex, while ensuring that the markings on each side are superimposed and the ruler is parallel to the sagittal plane.

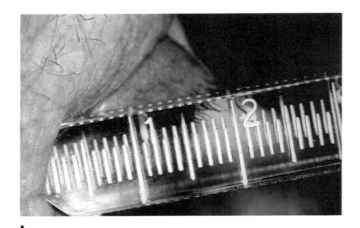

A

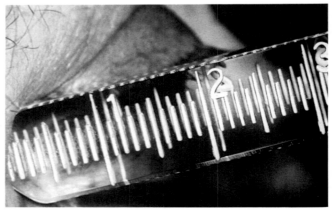

B

FIGURE 37–8. (*A*) Luedde exophthalmometry; reading is 17 mm. Note the markings are superimposed. (*B*) Luedde exophthalmometry; reading is 19 mm. Note that the markings are slightly out of superimposition.

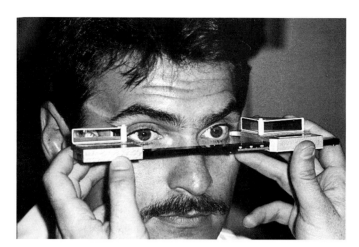

FIGURE 37–9. Performance of exophthalmometry with Marco exophthalmometer.

8. Repeat the reading and record the reading in millimeters as well as the name of the instrument used, for example:

$$\text{Luedde} < \frac{17,\ 18}{17,\ 17}$$

Hertel Exophthalmometer: Prism-Type (Marco, Rodenstock)

The clinical procedure of obtaining exophthalmometer readings with a prism-type Hertel exophthalmometer is as follows:

1. Carefully observe the facial symmetry, symmetry of the globes and orbits, the external eye, globe and corneal size, lid position and function before taking the exophthalmometry readings. It is also advisable to be aware of the patient's refractive error.
2. Palpate the lateral orbital rim of each eye to locate the deepest angle of the rim.
3. Slide the prisms along the horizontal bar to adjust location of the footplate to correspond to the location of the lateral orbital rim.
4. Place the footplates firmly against the deepest point on the lateral orbital rims and adjust the prisms to the proper location so that the footplates are positioned firmly on the deepest point and symmetrically (Fig. 37–9).

5. Note the reading on the crossbar, this is the base reading.
6. Position your head directly in front of the patient's. Adjust the position of your head to superimpose the two red lines (parallax lines) in the prism to minimize parallax (Fig. 37–10).
7. With the patient looking straight ahead note the marking on the ruler that is tangent in the corneal apex in the right eye (right prism).
8. Shift your head to again superimpose the red parallax lines in the left prism and note the marking on the ruler that is tangent to the corneal apex.
9. Note and record the reading for each eye, the base (crossbar) setting, and the instrument used. Record each of these as follows, for example:

$$\text{Marco} < \frac{18}{18}\quad 105\ \text{base}$$

Hertel Exophthalmometer: Mirror-Type (Bausch & Lomb)

The clinical procedure of obtaining exophthalmometry readings with a mirror-type (Bausch & Lomb) Hertel exophthalmometer is as follows:

1. Carefully observe the facial symmetry, symmetry of the globes and orbits, the external eye, globe and corneal size, and lid position and function before taking the exophthalmometry readings. It is also advisable to be aware of the patient's refractive error.
2. Palpate the lateral orbital rim to locate the deepest angle of the rim.
3. Loosen the setscrew to allow the mirrors to be adjusted farther or closer together.
4. Place the footplates firmly against the deepest point on the lateral orbital rims and adjust the mirror to the proper location so that the footplates are positioned firmly in the deepest point and symmetrically (Fig. 37–11).
5. Note the reading on the crossbar (base reading).
6. With the patient looking straight ahead, note the marking on the ruler that is tangent in the corneal apex in the right eye (right mirror) and in the left eye (left mirror).
7. Note and record the reading for each eye, the base (crossbar) setting, and the instrument used. Record each of these as follows, for example:

$$\text{Hertel (B \& L)} < \frac{18}{18}\quad 105\ \text{base}$$

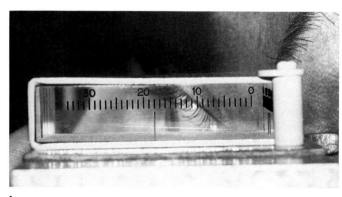

A

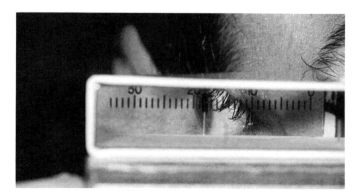

B

FIGURE 37–10. (*A*) Parallax lines superimposed during performance of Marco exophthalmometry. (*B*) Parallax lines out of alignment.

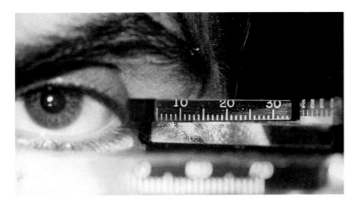

FIGURE 37–11. Performance of exophthalmometry with Bausch & Lomb exophthalmometer, examiners view: Note the corneal apex is not visible. The mirror should be tilted upward slightly.

CLINICAL IMPLICATIONS

Clinical Significance

The primary clinical value of exophthalmometry lies in its use to detect abnormally high readings, suggestive of exophthalmos, and to monitor the degree of exophthalmos over time. Exophthalmometry is much less frequently used to detect and measure enophthalmos.

Exophthalmos, as can be seen from Table 37–1, is an important clinical sign of orbital disease, most commonly Graves' disease. Space-taking orbital mass lesions also are a very common cause of unilateral exophthalmos.[14]

Exophthalmometry, although an important component of the diagnostic evaluation for orbital disease, is not, by itself, usually adequate for the detection or differential diagnosis as pointed out by Terry.[15] A careful case history; evaluation of neurovisual function, including ocular motility, lid position and function, visual acuity, color vision, and visual fields; physical evaluation of the eye, including palpation and auscultation of the globe; exophthalmometry and ophthalmoscopy constitute the minimal in-office evaluation for orbital disease. Recent advances in techniques of imaging the orbit, including ultrasonography and computed tomography (CT) scanning, have tremendously improved the detection and diagnosis of orbital disease.

The most common causes of enophthalmos are listed in Table 37–2. Exophthalmometry can be useful in monitoring the progressive degeneration of orbital fat, such as in progressive hemifacial atrophy or in age-related degeneration, and in evaluating the effects of orbital blow-out fracture. In blow-out fracture, orbital fat often herniates through the break in the orbital wall, usually the orbital floor, resulting in a settling of the globe more posteriorly into the orbit. This may be progressive in some cases.

Clinical Interpretation

It is useful to consider three types of exophthalmometry measurements and interpretations: absolute exophthalmometry, relative exophthalmometry, and comparative exophthalmometry.

Comparative exophthalmometry is the comparison of serial exophthalmometry measurements with previous measurements. This is a very commonly used technique, particularly in following patients with Graves' eye disease. Measurement variation and error will, of course, affect the interpretation of serial (comparative) exophthalmometry. Repeated exophthalmometry readings should vary by no more than 1 to 2 mm. Also, the Hertel exophthalmome-

ter is generally considered more accurate and repeatable than the Luedde exophthalmometer.[10] Regardless of the instrument used to enhance recognition of a change, the same instrument must be used by the same examiner on all readings. A change in exophthalmometric readings of greater than 2 mm is highly suggestive of active orbital disease.

Relative exophthalmometry is the comparison of exophthalmometry measurements between the two eyes at the same measurement to detect an interocular asymmetry. Since there is very often some interocular asymmetry between the globes or the orbits, there is a variation in the "normal" amount of interocular difference. In the normal population, it is very unusual to find more than 2 mm of interocular asymmetry.[2,4,16] Megliori found no patients with an asymmetry of equal to or greater than 2 mm in his study of 681 normal adults. About 98% of Megliori's subjects had an interocular asymmetry of 1.5 mm or less.[17]

Absolute exophthalmometry is the comparison of exophthalmometry readings to known, normal values. There is a wide range of normal values owing to the very common interocular asymmetry of the globe or orbit. Most normal patients have exophthalmometry readings in the range of about 10 mm to 21 or 22 mm, with the average adult measurement in the 15- to 17-mm range.[2,4,16,17] These are significantly affected by numerous other factors.

Other factors affecting exophthalmometry measurements include the following:

Race: Blacks tend to have higher exophthalmometry readings than whites. This difference has been shown in several clinical studies to be about 2 to 2.5 mm in both males and females.[17,18,19] This has been confirmed with a radiographic technique indicating a shallower orbit in blacks.[20] The upper limit of normal (mean plus 2 standard deviations) in blacks should be considered to be about 23 to 24 mm.

Sex: Males tend to have higher exophthalmometric readings than females by about 1 mm.[2,4,16–18] This has not been found to be true in patients with Graves' eye disease because of its propensity to affect females.[21]

Age: Children have an average exophthalmometric reading of about 14.5 mm.[2] From age 10 to 18, there is an increase in exophthalmometric readings by about 3 mm.[16] In the elderly, there appears to be a slight lowering of the normal exophthalmometric reading of about 1 mm.[21,22] This may be due to a degeneration of orbital fat.

Refractive error: There appears to be no relation between exophthalmometric findings and low to moderate refractive error.[16,17] High axial myopia, such as buphthalmos, however, may produce increased exophthalmometric readings.

Posture and head position: The normal globe will sink into the orbit approximately 1 to 3 mm when the patient is supine. It has been suggested that this does not occur, even in the apparently normal, nonproptotic eye of patients with Graves' disease.[23] This may be useful on the differentiation of Graves' eye disease from a retrobulbar mass lesion.

REFERENCES

1. Cohn H. Massungen der prominenz der Augen Mittelst eines neuen instrumentes des exophthalmometers. Klin Monatsbl Augenheilkd 1867;5:339–351.
2. Duke–Elder S. Textbook of ophthalmology, vol 5. St Louis: CV Mosby Co, 1952:5375.
3. Cline D, Hofstetter H, Griffin J. Dictionary of visual science, 4th ed. Radnor, Penn: Chilton Book Co, 1989.
4. Drews L. Exophthalmometry. Am J Ophthalmol 1957;43:37–58.
5. Hertel E. Ein einfaches exophthalmometer. Arch Ophthalmol 1905; 60:171–175.

6. Luedde W. An improved transparent exophthalmometer. Am J Ophthalmol 1938;21:426.
7. Copeland L, Villareal A, Gwinup G. A new simple exophthalmometer: comparison with existing instruments. JAMA 1976;235:1134–1136.
8. Cohen S, Rizzuti A. An illuminated Luedde exophthalmometer. Arch Ophthalmol 1980;98:747.
9. Watson P. An instrument for measuring ocular displacement: the ocular topometer. Trans Ophthal Soc UK 1967;87:409–430.
10. Wright JE. Proptosis. Ann R Coll Surg 1970;47:323–330.
11. Sisler HA, Jakobiec FA, Trokel SL. Ocular abnormalities and orbital changes of Graves' disease. In: Duane's Clinical ophthalmology, Chap 36, vol 2. Philadelphia: Harper & Row, 1988:1.
12. Jones IS, Jakobiec FA. Diseases of the orbit. Hagerstown: Harper & Row, 1979:15.
13. Davanger M. Principles and sources of error in exophthalmometry; a new exophthalmometer. Acta Ophthalmol 1970;48:625–633.
14. Palmer B. Unilateral exophthalmos. Arch Otolaryngol 1965;82:415–423.
15. Terry J. Ocular disease: detection, diagnosis and treatment. Stoneham, Mass: Butterworths, 1984.
16. Fledelius H, Stubgard M. Changes in eye position during growth and adult life. Acta Ophthalmol 1986;64:481–486.
17. Migliori M, Gladstone J. Determination of the normal range of exophthalmometric values for black and white adults. Am J Ophthalmol 1984;98:432–442.
18. Brown R, Douglas J. Exophthalmometry of blacks. Ann Intern Med 1975;83:835.
19. de Juan E, Hurley D, Sapira J. Racial differences in normal values of proptosis. Arch Intern Med 1980;140:1230–1231.
20. Bogren H, Schirmer M, Frantic R, Elfstrom G, Tengroth B. Radiographic exophthalmometry. Trans Am Acad Ophthalmol Otolaryngol 1976;81:298–304.
21. Frueh B, Musch D, Garber F. Exophthalmometer findings in patients with Graves' eye disease. Ophthal Surg 1986;17:37–40.
22. Nath K, Gogi R, Rao G, et al. Normal exophthalmometry. Indian J Ophthalmol 1977;25:47–52.
23. Hauer J. Additional clinical sign of "unilateral" endocrine exophthalmos. Br J Ophthalmol 1969;53:210–211.

Topical Ophthalmic Dyes

Diane P. Yolton

INTRODUCTION

Definition

Staining with topical dyes is a commonly used technique for assessing the integrity of the cornea and conjunctiva. Many agents have been used as vital dyes for this purpose: rose bengal,[1] Congo red,[2] methylene blue,[3] iodonitrotetrazolium,[4] trypan blue,[5] alcian blue,[4] lissamine green,[6] and fluorescein.[4] Of these, only fluorescein and rose bengal will be discussed in this chapter because they are the only ones that are commonly used topically.

History

Fluorescein was first synthesized by Baeyer in 1871.[7] Pfluger in 1882 and Straub in 1888 used fluorescein to detect epithelial defects[8] and Ehrlich described the entry of fluorescein into the anterior chamber after subcutaneous injection in 1882.[9] In 1910, Burk described the use of fluorescein for the detection of retinal disease.[10]

Rose bengal was synthesized in 1882 by Gnehm[11] and was first used as a vital stain of the cornea and conjunctiva in 1914 by Romer, Gebb, and Lohlein.[1] In 1933 Sjogren[12] described the use of rose bengal for revealing the conjunctival and corneal changes accompanying deficient tear formation in keratoconjunctivitis sicca.

Clinical Use

Fluorescein is topically applied to the eye for many purposes, including detecting breaks in the corneal epithelium (punctate epithelial erosions, abrasions, ulcers), locating foreign bodies, de-

termining tear breakup time, detecting posttraumatic or postsurgical aqueous leakage,[13] fitting and managing contact lenses, evaluating the lacrimal drainage system, and performing applanation tonometry. The first three applications will be discussed here, and the remaining uses of fluorescein will be presented in other chapters.

Although not used as extensively as fluorescein, many clinical studies have shown that rose bengal is a valuable diagnostic aid for disclosing degenerative tissue changes of the cornea and conjunctiva. Rose bengal selectively stains devitalized cells; thus, it is used primarily for the diagnosis of keratoconjunctivitis sicca and related forms of dry-eye. This stain is also useful for diagnosing other corneal diseases that involve devitalization of epithelial cells such as punctate epithelial keratitis, filamentary keratitis, exposure keratitis, and herpes simplex keratitis.

INSTRUMENTATION

Theory

Fluorescein

Fluorescein is a weak dibasic acid of the xanthene group with a molecular weight of 330. It is poorly soluble in water and, because of this, is generally used as its highly water-soluble sodium salt.* When viewed under white light, fluorescein appears yellow or orange, but under cobalt blue illumination it fluoresces to produce a green-yellow light.† For dilute concentrations of fluorescein in

---

* The term *fluorescein* as used in this chapter refers to the water-soluble sodium salt of fluorescein.

† *Fluorescence* is the ability of certain substances to absorb light of certain wavelengths (the excitation spectrum) and emit light at longer wavelengths (the emission spectrum).

aqueous solution, light of wavelength 490 nm produces maximum excitation, resulting in fluorescence at about 530 nm. Because long-wavelength light has little effect on fluorescein, optical devices, such as slit lamps, typically reduce overall light levels by filtering this portion of the spectrum out of the illumination beam. This is usually accomplished by use of a cobalt blue excitation filter that transmits light from about 320 to 500 nm (with a maximum at about 400 nm).

When an eye with fluorescein instilled is illuminated by blue light, an observer detects a mixture of reflected blue light and green-yellow light emitted by the fluorescein. In devices such as fundus cameras, the reflected blue excitation light is filtered out by a barrier filter, but barrier filters are usually not used in slit lamps because it is difficult to become oriented to the structures of the eye when only fluorescent light can be seen. To visualize subtle corneal staining, however, a barrier filter (e.g., Kodak Wratten No. 12 yellow gelatin) placed in the slit lamp viewing path has been suggested.[14] This filter absorbs most of the reflected blue light and allows only the fluorescence to be seen by the observer.

The concentration of fluorescein in a solution affects both the wavelength of the emitted light and its intensity.[15] At high concentrations, the emission spectrum of fluorescein shifts toward longer wavelengths so the emitted light appears more yellow; at lower concentrations, the emitted light spectrum is shifted toward shorter wavelengths and the light appears more green.

At concentrations higher than 0.001%, internal quenching causes the intensity of fluorescence to be decreased. Thus, when fluorescein is first instilled into the eye and the concentration is high, the fluorescence is weak and the emitted light is yellow. As the fluorescein is diluted by tears, and especially if it moves into the intercellular spaces of the epithelium due to a defect, the intensity of the fluorescence increases, and it becomes more apple-green.

Because of its ability to fluoresce at very low concentrations, fluorescein has many clinical uses. When used topically, it does not stain the corneal cells because it is an anionic, hydrophilic agent and cannot penetrate the cell membranes of the individual epithelial cells nor the zonula occludens (tight junctions between the surface epithelial cells). Rather, fluorescein discloses breaks in the continuity of the epithelial cells by accumulating in the intercellular spaces. When extensive epithelial loss is present, the dye can spread into the stromal tissue and even enter the anterior chamber, where it appears as a green aqueous flare.

Rose Bengal

Rose bengal (dichlorotetraiodofluorescein) is an iodine derivative of fluorescein; mixed with water, it forms a bluish red solution. When instilled into the eye, rose bengal stains mildly degenerated corneal and conjunctival cells a light bluish red, severely degenerated cells appear dark red, and dead cells become an intense red. Rose bengal is particularly useful because the intensity and color of the stain make it easy to identify devitalized cells of both the corneal and conjunctival epithelia.

COMMERCIALLY AVAILABLE INSTRUMENTS

Fluorescein

Fluorescein can be applied to the eye in the form of a solution or by use of fluorescein-impregnated paper strips (Table 38–1, and Fig. 38–1). Because of concerns that even preserved solutions of fluorescein can support the growth of bacteria, especially *Pseudomonas aeruginosa*,[16] sterile fluorescein-impregnated paper strips are most often used clinically.[17] There are some differences in the amount of fluorescein and other ingredients found in the strips

Table 38–1
Fluorescein and Rose Bengal Preparations For Topical Ocular Use

Preparations	Strength	Manufacturer
Solutions		
Fluorescein	2%; 1, 2, 15 mL	Various manufacturers
Rose Bengal	1%; 5 mL	Akorn
Strips		
Fluorescein		
Ful-Glo	0.6 mL; sterile	Sola/Barnes-Hind
Fluor-I-Strip	9 mg; with buffers, 0.5% chlorobutanol, polysorbate 80	Wyeth–Ayerst
Fluor-I-Strip-A.T.	1 mg; with buffers, 0.5% chlorobutanol, polysorbate 80	Wyeth–Ayerst
Fluorets	1 mg; sterile	Akorn
Rose Bengal		
Rose Bengal		
Ophthalmic Strips	1.3 mg; sterile	Sola/Barnes-Hind

produced by different companies, but these differences seem relatively unimportant clinically (see Table 38–1).

Rose Bengal

Rose bengal can also be applied either in the form of a solution or by use of impregnated paper strips (see Table 38–1 and Fig. 38–1). Instillation of rose bengal solution can cause discomfort for many patients, which is usually proportional to the degree of preexisting epithelial damage. To lessen this discomfort, a drop of anesthetic can be applied before staining, but the anesthetic can cause false

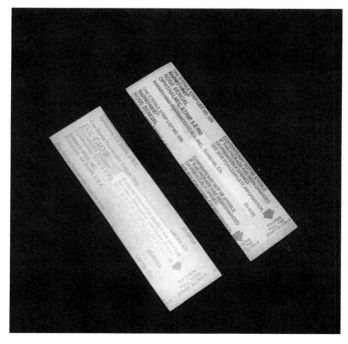

FIGURE 38–1. Drug-impregnated filter paper strips: fluorescein (*left*) and rose bengal (*right*).

staining. Use of the impregnated paper strips seems to greatly reduce patient discomfort and, for most patients, eliminates the need for anesthetic. Use of paper strips also helps to avoid accidental staining of lid tissues or the patient's clothing, which can occur if rose bengal solution is used.

CLINICAL PROCEDURE

To stain the cornea or conjunctiva with either fluorescein or rose bengal strips, the same basic procedure is used.

1. If the patient is wearing hydrogel contact lenses, they must be removed because both dyes can permanently stain these lenses. Opinions on the length of time that lenses must remain out of the eye after staining vary. However, if fluorescein is used, and the eye is irrigated so that no fluorescein is left in the tear meniscus, lenses can usually be reinserted immediately. For rose bengal staining, even if the eye is irrigated after instillation of the dye, lenses usually should not be reinserted for 6 hours.
2. After explaining the procedure to the patient, the paper strip impregnated with the dye is removed from its protective envelope. To avoid contamination, care should be taken to ensure the protective envelope is unbroken prior to use and the strip is not touched by the clinician in the area impregnated with dye.
3. The dye-impregnated part of the strip is moistened with a drop of sterile saline or irrigating solution. Care should be taken to ensure that the tip of the bottle does not contact the strip, since this would contaminate the bottle and require that it be discarded. Rose bengal strips are slightly more difficult to wet than fluorescein strips and may require the use of several drops of solution. Again, care should be taken not to allow dye to drip onto the patient's clothing.
4. With the patient's gaze directed downward, the superior lid is elevated and the wet strip is gently touched to the superior sclera (Fig. 38–2). Alternatively, and equally acceptable, the patient's gaze is directed up, the lower lid is pulled down and the strip is gently touched to the inferior bulbar conjunctiva or the inferior conjunctival sac (Fig. 38–3). The cornea should not be touched with the dye

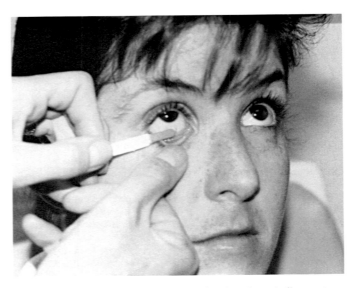

FIGURE 38–3. Application of rose bengal to the inferior bulbar conjunctiva with a paper strip.

strip. To avoid the risk of cross-contamination, separate strips should be used for each eye. An anesthetic should not be instilled before either dye is used because it may cause sufficient corneal surface damage to result in false-positive staining. Some anesthetics, such as proparacaine, also tend to quench the fluorescence of fluorescein.
5. The patient is asked to blink a few times to distribute the dye uniformly.
6. When using fluorescein, the patient's cornea is initially viewed with the slit lamp using the cobalt blue filter, maximally open slit width, and 16× (moderate) magnification. Epithelial defects will appear as brightly fluorescent green spots, areas, or lines on the cornea. Slit width and magnification can then be changed to best evaluate any defects found. With rose bengal, the patient's cornea and conjunctiva are initially viewed with white light, open slit width, and moderate magnification. Devitalized cells will appear as bluish red or red spots, areas, or lines on the cornea or conjunctiva. Again, changes in slit width and magnification may be needed to fully evaluate any stained areas.
7. Fluorescein can be used to determine the tear breakup time (TBUT). To measure TBUT, fluorescein is applied to the eye following the procedure outline above, the patient is asked to blink several times to distribute the fluorescein over the cornea and then to hold the eye open. Using the cobalt blue filter, maximally open slit width, and 16× magnification, the time until the appearance of the first black spot, indicating a dried area, is measured. The procedure is usually repeated several times to get an average measurement. Topical anesthetics can cause a spuriously rapid tear breakup time and should be avoided.[18] Fluorescein instillation itself reduces breakup time, compared with the time measured by noninvasive techniques,[19] but the use of fluorescein is the only practical way to measure this parameter clinically.

Sequential evaluation of the degree of fluorescein staining will maximize the diagnostic value of this procedure. Tissue staining usually cannot be assessed immediately after instillation of the dye because the intensely stained tear film will conceal modest staining of the epithelium. Gradually, as the coloring of the tear film fades, bright green fluorescent staining of any epithelial de-

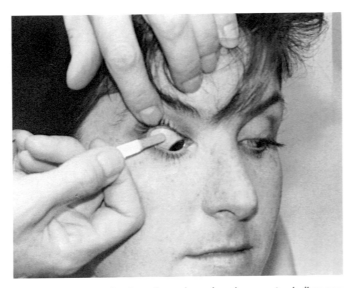

FIGURE 38–2. Application of rose bengal to the superior bulbar conjunctiva with a paper strip.

fects will be seen. After a few minutes, large defects will still be intensely stained, whereas the stain that accumulated in small defects will have diffused. In about 10 minutes, intercellular diffusion surrounding a lesion may mask its exact nature.

Staining from rose bengal is best assessed immediately after the excess dye in the tear film has disappeared, but observation of staining has diagnostic value up to 5 minutes after instillation of rose bengal.

CLINICAL IMPLICATIONS

Clinical Significance of Fluorescein Staining

The ability of fluorescein to accumulate in epithelial defects and around foreign bodies, along with its fluorescent properties, make it an ideal dye. When used following the foregoing procedure, significant fluorescein staining of the cornea is not usually observed in healthy eyes. However, if special examination techniques are employed, healthy corneas can demonstrate staining.[20-22] This suggests that subclinical epitheliopathy can occur in normal individuals, perhaps because of the normal desquamation of the epithelium or because of differences in the continuity of the epithelium between individuals. Any staining that is observed following routine fluorescein application indicates a disruption of the epithelium, which is usually associated with a disease process or trauma. When the causative disease or trauma is properly managed and an intact corneal epithelium is reestablished, staining will no longer be observed.

Clinical Interpretation of Fluorescein Staining

A wide range of diseases and traumas can affect the superficial cornea and cause fluorescein staining. Therefore, patients presenting with fluorescein staining can pose a major diagnostic challenge. To begin the diagnostic process, it is usually best to determine the type and pattern of the epithelial lesions revealed by the fluorescein. Punctate epithelial erosions are fine depressions or pits extending partially or completely through the epithelium.[23] Because of their transparency, these lesions are very difficult to see

with direct illumination, but the tiny pits stain brightly with fluorescein. Recognition of these defects, particularly the extent to which they are present, requires the use of topical fluorescein. The geographic pattern of punctate epithelial erosions can often be associated with certain diseases, and this can be a helpful diagnostic sign. Some of the most common patterns of superficial punctate erosions and their associated diseases are shown in Figure 38–4.

Traumas of various types cause epithelial abrasions that manifest as focal areas of cell loss and stain intensely with fluorescein. A common type of abrasion, which appears as a linear track, can be caused by a foreign body under the superior lid, scratching the cornea with each blink (see Fig. 38–4).

The use of fluorescein can help to detect foreign bodies on the cornea or conjunctiva. They will often appear as dark objects surrounded by a fluorescent green ring of pooled fluorescein, and, since the foreign bodies can break the epithelial continuity, fluorescein staining is helpful in determining the extent of associated tissue damage.

Use of fluorescein can be very valuable in detecting and assessing corneal ulcers. These lesions appear as white-based excavations that extend into the stromal tissue; fluorescein accumulates in the ulcer, staining its base intensely, and diffuses into the surrounding intercellular spaces, staining the epithelium.

Healing of the corneal epithelium after a break in continuity can also be monitored with fluorescein.[8] After a superficial trauma, regeneration is usually a rapid process with cover first reestablished by a cell-sliding mechanism. Once the epithelial defect is covered, the cells begin to multiply and develop tight junctions. As these changes are completed, an intact epithelial surface will be observed and the traumatized area will no longer stain with fluorescein.

A patient with a tear film deficiency may report symptoms of ocular itching, burning, or stinging. Such patients may have a reduced tear breakup time. Tear breakup is a natural phenomenon occurring when the mucin layer of the tears becomes contaminated with the lipid layer. Estimates of normal breakup time vary, but repeated low readings (10 seconds or less) suggest further and more definitive testing for dry-eye.[24] In normal eyes, tear breakup and resulting dry areas appear in a random pattern on the cornea (Fig. 38–5). Breakup occurring repeatedly in the same location suggests that the location wets poorly, possibly due to previous corneal insult.

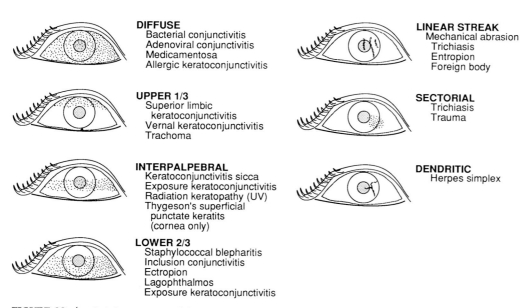

DIFFUSE
Bacterial conjunctivitis
Adenoviral conjunctivitis
Medicamentosa
Allergic keratoconjunctivitis

UPPER 1/3
Superior limbic
 keratoconjunctivitis
Vernal keratoconjunctivitis
Trachoma

INTERPALPEBRAL
Keratoconjunctivitis sicca
Exposure keratoconjunctivitis
Radiation keratopathy (UV)
Thygeson's superficial
 punctate keratits
 (cornea only)

LOWER 2/3
Staphylococcal blepharitis
Inclusion conjunctivitis
Ectropion
Lagophthalmos
Exposure keratoconjunctivitis

LINEAR STREAK
Mechanical abrasion
Trichiasis
Entropion
Foreign body

SECTORIAL
Trichiasis
Trauma

DENDRITIC
Herpes simplex

FIGURE 38–4. Staining patterns of the cornea and conjunctiva in various disease states.

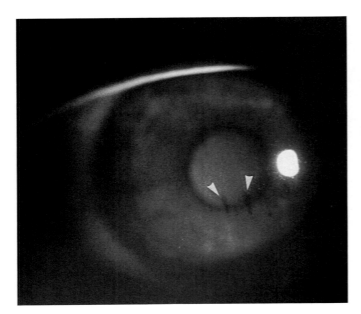

FIGURE 38-5. Tear breakup test showing dry spots (*arrowheads*).

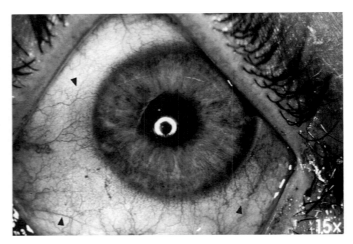

FIGURE 38-6. Rose bengal staining of interpalpebral bulbar conjunctiva and cornea in a patient with moderately severe dry-eye (*arrowheads*).

Clinical Significance of Rose Bengal Staining

Rose bengal selectively stains devitalized tissue and, consequently, normal eyes show no perceptible staining of the conjunctiva or cornea. In normal individuals, rose bengal does, however, stain a punctate line on the inferior and superior tarsal conjunctiva along the ciliary margin, the caruncle, and the plica semilunaris.

Clinical Interpretation of Rose Bengal Staining

In contrast with fluorescein, rose bengal does not accumulate in epithelial defects, but stains dead or degenerated cells and mucus. The main indication for rose bengal staining is, therefore, suspicion of dry-eye. In a patient with keratoconjunctivitis sicca, use of rose bengal produces a characteristic pattern of staining, with the bulbar conjunctiva stained intensely in the form of two base-in triangles on the medial and lateral sides of the cornea.[25] The lower two thirds of the cornea may also be stained (Fig. 38–6). A similar staining pattern is seen when the desiccation of the corneal and conjunctival epithelium is caused by lagophthalmos, neuroparalytic keratitis, facial nerve palsy, ectropion, pronounced exophthalmos, or ptosis surgery.

Rose bengal staining is also useful in the diagnosis of filamentary keratopathy, in which the dye stains filaments of desiccated epithelial cells and mucus that are attached to the corneal epithelium. Filamentary keratopathy can accompany any form of dry-eye and can also be seen with viral infection, corneal trauma, superior limbic keratoconjunctivitis, and following cataract or corneal surgery.

Assessment of punctate epithelial keratitis and herpes simplex epithelial keratitis are also facilitated by the use of rose bengal staining. Punctate epithelial keratitis presents as fine, grayish white opaque spots of intraepithelial edema and infiltration.[23] Because these lesions contain devitalized cells, they often stain more prominently with rose bengal than with fluorescein. Commonly, punctate epithelial keratitis and punctate epithelial erosions occur simultaneously in the same cornea, so the etiologic significance of the location of the lesions, as outlined in Figure 38–4, is similar when either or both types of lesions are present. In herpes sim-

plex epithelial keratitis, fluorescein stains the ulcer crater intensely where the loss of epithelium has occurred, whereas rose bengal brightly stains the damaged epithelial cells on the ulcer border.[26]

In some cases, rose bengal staining may still be seen in a keratitis that no longer stains with fluorescein because, although the epithelial defect has healed, the lesion still contains devitalized cells.

REFERENCES

1. Norn MS. Rose bengal vital staining. Staining of cornea and conjunctiva by 10% rose bengal, compared with 1%. Acta Ophthalmol 1970;48:546–559.
2. Norn MS. Congo red vital staining of cornea and conjunctiva. Acta Ophthalmol 1976;54:601–610.
3. Norn MS. Methylene blue (methylthionine) vital staining of the cornea and conjunctiva. Acta Ophthalmol 1967;45:347–358.
4. Norn MS. Vital staining of the cornea and conjunctiva. EENT Monthly 1971;50:294–299.
5. Norn MS. Trypan blue. Vital staining of cornea and conjunctiva. Acta Ophthalmol 1967;45:380–389.
6. Norn MS. Lissamine green. Vital staining of cornea and conjunctiva. Acta Ophthalmol 1973;51:483–491.
7. Baeyer A. Ueber eine neue klasse von farbstoffen. Ber Deutsch Chem Ges 1871;4:555–558.
8. Campbell FW, Boyd TAS. The use of sodium fluorescein in assessing the rate of healing in corneal ulcers. Br J Ophthalmol 1950;34:545–549.
9. Ehrlich P. Ueber provocirte fluorescenzerschei nungen am auge. Deutsch Med Wochenschr 1882;8:35–37.
10. Burke A. Die klinische physiologische und pathologische bedeutung der fluoreszenz in auge nach darreichung von uranin. Klin Monatsbl Augenheilkd 1910;48:445–454.
11. Marx E. Uber vitale farbungen am auge und an den liedern. I. Grafes Archiv Ophthalmol 1924;114:465–482.
12. Sjogren H. Zur kenntnis der keratoconjunctivitis sicca (keratitis filiformis bei hypofunktion der tranendrusen). Acta Ophthalmol 1933;11:1–151.
13. Romanchuk KG. Seidel's test using 10% fluorescein. Can J Ophthalmol 1979;14:253–256.
14. Justice J, Soper JW. An improved method of viewing topical fluorescein. Trans Am Acad Ophthalmol Otolaryngol 1976;81:927–928.
15. Romanchuk KG. Fluorescein. Physicochemical factors affecting its fluorescence. Surv Ophthalmol 1982;26:269–283.
16. Yolton DP, German CJ. Fluress, fluorescein and benoxinate: recovery from bacterial contamination. J Am Optom Assoc 1980;51:471–474.
17. Kimura SJ. Fluorescein paper. Am J Ophthalmol 1951;34:446–447.
18. Josephson JE, Caffery BE. Corneal staining after instillation of topical anesthetic (SSII). Invest Ophthalmol Vis Sci 1988;29:1096–1099.

19. Mengher LS, Bron AJ, Tonge SR, et al. Effects of fluorescein instillation on the pre-corneal tear film stability. Curr Eye Res 1985;4:9–12.
20. Korb DR, Herman JP. Corneal staining subsequent to sequential fluorescein instillations. J Am Optom Assoc 1979;50:361–367.
21. Korb DR, Korb JME. Corneal staining prior to contact lens wearing. J Am Optom Assoc 1970;41:228–232.
22. Norn MS. Micropunctate fluorescein vital staining of the cornea. Acta Ophthalmol 1970;48:108–118.
23. Jones BR. Differential diagnosis of punctate keratitis. Int Ophthalmol Clin 1962;2:591–611.
24. Lang MA, Hamill JR. Factors affecting TBUT. Arch Ophthalmol 1973;89:103–105.
25. Sjogren H, Bloch KJ. Keratoconjunctivitis sicca and the Sjogren syndrome. Surv Ophthalmol 1971;16:145–159.
26. Marsh RJ, Fraunfelder FT, McGill JI. Herpetic corneal epithelial disease. Arch Ophthalmol 1976;94:1899–1902.

Ocular Microbiology

Pierrette Dayhaw–Barker

BACTERIOLOGY AND CYTOLOGY

Definition

Bacteriology and cytology smears are procedures whereby a sampling of infected tissue is fixed on a glass slide, treated with varying stains, and inspected under the microscope. Differential staining allows identification of mainly epithelial cells, inflammatory cells, and cellular elements, such as inclusions and microorganisms.

Clinical Use

This procedure is a helpful adjunct in establishing or confirming the diagnosis of anterior segment bacterial infections, especially when the signs and symptoms are somewhat inconclusive. Furthermore, it is appropriate to harvest a specimen for culturing before instituting therapy, even though one must initially administer a broad-spectrum antibiotic.

Clinical Procedure

Swabbing

Although the technique will vary depending on the affected tissue, under all circumstances collection should occur from that area most affected by the bacterial contamination. For example, in infections of the tear ducts, purulent material should be extruded using pressure on or over the lacrimal sac. The sample is collected with a sterile swab or curette and is immediately placed on a glass slide to be fixed and stained (see later). In certain conditions, the use of an anesthetic may be required because additional pressure is needed and pain may ensue. In canaliculitis, Stenson[1] recom-

mends anesthetizing the inferior cul-de-sac initially, then with two sterile applicators, one that is soaked in the anesthetic is applied against the nasal inferior palpebral conjunctiva, while the second dry applicator is placed on the external lid in apposition to the first. During such procedures the patient is instructed to gaze away to prevent injury. Under all circumstances the material, once collected, is immediately spread on a glass slide, fixed with methanol for 5 minutes and stained.

When a cytologic specimen is required from the lid, a sterile cotton swab is run over the tightly held lid margin and the collected material is spread onto the slide. If an abscess is present, sampling is taken from the center of the abscess.

Sampling of the conjunctiva is a frequently used procedure. Specimen collected for smears must precede the anesthesia required for scraping, since this anesthesia may interfere with the microbes.[2] The palpebral conjunctiva is gently swabbed and the specimen is spread on the slide.

Scraping

Scraping requires administration of an anesthetic before collecting the specimen. A cooled sterile platinum spatula is then used to obtain the specimen. The motion should be repeated in the same direction to ensure the collection of sufficient material for analysis. Next, when spreading the material onto the slide, care should be taken to have an even distribution. Lastly, quick fixation should be followed by staining.

The most commonly utilized stains are the Giesma, Wright, Diff-Quik, and Papanicolaou. The staining procedures described herein are abbreviated methods from either Humason,[3] Stenson,[1] or from directions supplied in commercially available kits. The stain specific for bacteria is the gram stain, from which the gram-positive versus gram-negative classification evolved. Utilizing some of the physical and chemical properties of bacterial cell walls, the

Table 39–1
Gram-Staining Procedure

Procedure	Time
Dry and fix specimen	
Stain with crystal violet	1 min
Wash with tap water	
Stain with Gram's iodine	1 min
Wash with tap water	
Decolorize with 95% ethanol	30 sec
Wash with tap water	
Stain with 0.25% safranin	30 sec
Wash and dry	
Slide is then ready for identification.	

Table 39–3
Diff–Quik-Staining Procedure

Procedure	Time
Air-dry specimen on slide	
Dip five times in fixative	5–10 sec total
Dip five times in solution I	Same as above
Dip five times in solution II	Same as above
Rinse with tap water and dry	

staining procedure identifies the *gram-positive* organisms as those staining purple, whereas the *gram-negative* stain pink to red. The procedure is summarized in Table 39–1.

Additionally, it is often appropriate to identify some of the epithelial or blood cells found on slide preparations.[4] Some of the stains used for these purposes are the Giesma, Diff-Quik, and Wright stains. The Giesma stain is a widely used method composed of methylene blue, methylene violet, azure A and B, and eosin (Table 39–2). Upon microscopic evaluation, the stain allows identification of lymphocytes and monocytes (blue cytoplasm), of eosinophils (pink to orange granules), of neutrophils (pink to purple granules), and basophils (dark blue cytoplasmic granules). The red blood cells are pink. This stain is also effective in outlining the morphologic structures of bacteria.[5]

The Diff-Quik stain is a commercially available kit composed of fixative, solution I, and solution II, which are poured each into a screw top Coplin jar (Table 39–3). Since the solutions are stable for several weeks, this relatively easy method is highly advantageous in a private office. However, it should be noted that in some preparations the staining quality is not as good as Giesma's method. The polymorphonuclear leukocytes have a clear cytoplasm with lobular nuclei, the lymphocytes have a large round gray-blue nucleus, the monocytes are large vacuolated cells with bluish bean-shaped nuclei, plasma cells have a dark blue cytoplasm, and eosinophils have pink-staining granules.

The Wright stain may also be used (Table 39–4). Although this stain is widely available, the staining quality and shelf-life make it less useful than the Giesma or the Diff-Quik.

Clinical Implications

Clinical Significance

There are several instances for which culturing is very appropriate. In cases of neonatal conjunctivitis and hyperacute conjunctivitis, culturing should be performed so that the management of cases unresponsive to a broad-spectrum antibiotic can be effectively al-

tered. It must also be recognized that for situations in which the patient fails to respond to treatment, culturing will identify the agent and help to initiate appropriate management.

Clinical Interpretation

The role played by laboratory analysis of microbial samples, leading to the identification of pathogens and the prevalence of cell types is widely recognized as a useful adjunct in the differential diagnostic process of ocular infections and inflammations, especially when there is ambiguity in clinical signs or symptoms.[6,7] General considerations of laboratory procedures in infectious diseases are discussed by Goldstein and Joye.[8]

Bacterial infections may involve the lids, conjunctiva, lacrimal apparatus, orbit, and the cornea.[1,2,9] Table 39–5 lists organisms and their staining and morphologic characteristics as these relate to conjunctivitis. The laboratory staining procedures and findings are similar for diseases of other anterior segment structures. Table 39–6 summarizes various blood cell types with associated disorders and an abbreviated discussion of the appearance of the cells.

Scrapings are often utilized for culturing purposes. It is essential that as soon as gathered the specimen be spread onto the appropriate agar. Failure to do so often leads to negative results. Table 39–7 suggests the use of different agar media for identification of specific specimens.[10] Information on preparation of culture media may be found in Finegold and Martin.[6] Once the specimen has been collected, it is placed on the side of a Petri dish containing the appropriate medium. With a sterile wire loop, the specimen is then streaked across the surface of the medium, depositing one layer of cells onto the surface. Once incubated for the appropriate time at the appropriate temperature, the organism is identified and determination of sensitivity to antibiotics can be established.[7]

VIROLOGY AND HISTOLOGIC PROCEDURES

Definition

The procedures described in the following are used for the identification of viral agents. They consist of clinically collected specimens, stains, and microscopic evaluation.

Table 39–2
Geisma-Staining Procedure

Procedure	Time
Fix the specimen in methanol	5 min
Stain and incubate at 37°C	1 hr
Rinse twice in 95% ethyl alcohol	
Dry	

Table 39–4
Wright-Staining Procedure

Procedure	Time
Fix in methanol	5 min
Place a few drops of stain on slide	2–3 min
Pour off stain	
Cover specimen with phosphate-buffered saline (pH 7.0)	4–6 min
Dry specimen	

Table 39-5
Acute and Chronic Conjunctivitis

Condition	Organisms	Laboratory Test	Finding
Acute bacterial conjunctivitis Blepharitis Keratitis	Staphylococcus aureus	Smear and stain Gram stain Giemsa/Wright stain Culture	Gram-positive coccus; grapelike cluster; neutrophils; when needed use blood or chocolate agar for culturing
Acute blepharoconjunctivitis	S. epidermidis	Same as above	
Acute conjunctivitis especially in children	Streptococcus pneumoniae	Same as above	Gram-positive diplococcus
Acute pseudomembranous conjunctivitis	Strep. pyogenes	Same as above	Gram-positive coccus occurring in chains
Periorbital (preseptal) cellulitis	Haemophilus influenzae	Same as above	Gram-negative; range from coccobacilli to slender rods
Acute angular blepharoroconjunctivitis	Moraxella lacunata (S. aureus is now a common cause of angular)	Same as above	Gram-negative diplobacilli; range from coccobacilli to long and short broad rods
Acute purulent conjunctivitis	Neisseria	Same as above	Gram-negative diplococci
Chronic blepharoconjunctivitis	S. aureus	Same procedures as for acute conjunctivitis	
Chronic conjunctivitis	Proteus mirabilis Klebsiella pneumoniae Serratia marcescens Escherichia coli	Same as above	Gram-negative rods
Inclusion conjunctivitis	Chlamydia (TRIC)	Giemsa stain	Gram-negative; use Giemsa for inclusion bodies

Table 39-6
Differences in Cell Populations in Infectious and Inflammatory Disorders

Cell Type	Associated Disorders	Appearance of Cell	Role of Cell
Neutrophils (polymorphonuclear leukocytes)	Frequently seen in bacterial infections, membranous disease, chlamydial disorders, and drug toxicity	Blue cytoplasm with fine granules that stain lightly with neutral dyes. Nuclei have lobulation. This increases with age. Under toxic conditions hyper-segmentation also occurs.[1]	Phagocytosis
Basophils	Associated with allergic and chronic inflammatory disorders	Small, darkly staining cells with especially dark-blue staining granules. Small roundish nucleus, may be lobular.	Produce heparin and histamine, phagocytosis
Eosinophils	Acute and chronic allergic reactions	Fragile cells containing red-staining granules. Nucleus has two lobes.	Phagocytosis of foreign protein, release substance that counters the effect of histamine
Lymphocytes	Viral infections and chlamydial diseases	Cell size about 10 μm. Bluish cytoplasm that stains darkly around nucleus in which nucleoli are often observed.	Macrophagocytosis of invading micro-organisms
Blast cells	Occasionally seen in viral conjunctivitis	Immature, undifferentiated precursor cells	
Plasma cells	Immune-mediated reactions; chlamydial infections.	Rounded cells with abundant cytoplasm; eccentrically placed around nucleus	Cells are formed from B lymphocytes; produce and release antibodies.
Leber cells	Chlamydial infections, especially trachoma	Giant cells with pale blue cytoplasm with many vacuoles and cellular debris	Phagocytosis

(Modified from Snell RS. Clinical and functional histology for medical students. Boston: Little, Brown & Co, 1984; and Stenson S. The anterior segment cytopathology. In: Karciogliu Z, ed. Laboratory diagnosis in ophthalmology. New York: Macmillan Publishing Co, 1987)

Table 39–7
*Agar Media Use in Ocular Bacteriology**

Procedure	Bacteria
Blood agar	S. aureus
	Streptococcus
	Moraxella
	Pseudomonas
Chocolate agar	Neisseria
	Haemophilus
MacConkey agar	Moraxella (except M. lacunata)
	Proteus
Thayer–Martin	Neisseria gonorrhoeae
Mannitol–salt agar	S. aureus
Thioglycollate	Anaerobes

* Chlamydia cannot be cultured as such; it requires inoculation with McCoy cells.[5]

Clinical Use

The laboratory tests identified in the following are useful in the verification of the causative agent of a viral infection. Although several of the viruses produce systemic effects that help in the diagnostic process, some, such as herpes virus, cytomegalovirus, and the adenovirus infections, for example, manifest specific ocular involvement. The following procedures allow confirmation of the diagnosis through microscopic tests, but should be supported by serologic or isolation techniques.

Clinical Procedure

For routine microscopic evaluation, the specimen, obtained with scraping and collecting methods identified in the foregoing, is placed on a slide. It is fixed in Bouin's solution for no more than 1 hour and stained. Pavan–Langston[2] recommends the use of Giesma as a stain to detect intranuclear inclusion bodies, whereas others (Oh[11]) prefer hematoxylin and eosin or Papanicolaou stains. Upon examination, eosinophic or basophilic cytoplasmic or intranuclear inclusions may be observed. Table 39–8 lists viruses affecting the eye and describes the serologic tests; other isolation techniques are described in specific sections in this chapter.

Clinical Implications

Clinical Significance

The use of microscopic tests, by themselves, can be of limited application because the findings could be attributable to more than one virus. For example, the presence of intranuclear inclusions could be attributed to varicella, herpesvirus, cytomegalovirus, or adenovirus. Although specific staining and morphometric descriptions can be helpful in narrowing down the list of agents, the utilization of highly specific immunologic tests, such as the immune fluorescence or enzyme-linked immunosorbent assay (ELISA) tests allows much greater reliability. Therefore, it is not surprising to find their availability and use increasing, whereas the microscopic method is used by some as a quick "screening" test for determination of the viral nature of the infection.

Clinical Interpretation

Conventional histologic study provides limited information, which most often must be enhanced by other tests to confirm the identifi-

Table 39–8
Serologic Tests for Virus Isolation

Virus	Collection	Recommended Laboratory Tests
Herpesviruses		
Herpes simplex (HSV)	Scrapings; blood	• Direct examination using Bouin's fixative and H&E or Papanicolaou stain will identify giant cells and intranuclear inclusions
		• Use immunofluorescence or immunoperoxidase for definitive identification
		• Any of the serologic tests can also be used
Varicella–zoster (VZV)	Scraping/smears; blood	• Immunofluorescence specific for VZV
		• Complement fixation most widely utilized serologic test
Cytomegalovirus (CMV)	Blood	• Since cytology will not differentiate between HSV, VZV, and CMV, serologic tests, especially complement fixation
Poxviruses		
Molluscum contagiosum (MCU)	Scrapings	• Giemsa stain
Picornaviruses		
Picornavirus	Scrapings	• Immunofluorescence, isolation of enteroviruses, and rhinovirus in cell culture
Paramyxoviruses		
Paramyxovirus		
Measle virus	Scrapings and	• Immunofluorescence, hemagglutination
Mumps	serologic	• Indirect immunofluorescence, serologic tests
Newcastle disease virus		• Hemagglutination
Rubella		• Immunofluorescence serologic testing

cation of the pathogen. Certain features are nonetheless characteristic of a viral infection. Examples of these are the presence of large immature epithelial cells with several nucleoli or the presence of multinucleated cells. Giant cells with an aggregation of many nuclei surrounded by a thin layer of cytoplasm are characteristic of herpetic disease. In herpes simplex infection, there are a number of eosinophilic nuclear inclusions the identification of which should be verified with immunofluorescent techniques, since the inclusions could also result from infection with the varicella–zoster virus.[10,11]

VIROLOGY AND CULTURING

In a manner similar to that described in bacteriology, it is also possible to culture viruses. However, there are some important differences. Scrapings collected, preferably early on, from an active site of infection are deposited immediately in culturettes and should be transported at temperatures slightly above freezing to maintain virus infectivity.[12] Smolin et al.[10] recommends freezing if delays greater than 24 hours are anticipated.

To permit identification of the virus, inoculation of susceptible cells is followed by incubation of these cells at 37°C for varying lengths of time, depending on the virus. The cytopathic effects (CPE) indicating cell damage are then evaluated. This procedure sometimes permits identification of the virus. However, other techniques, such as immunologic or serologic analyses may be required.

VIROLOGY AND IMMUNOHISTOCHEMISTRY

These sensitive and comparatively rapid techniques are ones that utilize a dye or an enzyme marker coupled to antibodies to identify the distribution of a viral antigen in a tissue preparation. The more common fluorescent methods are indirect ones that utilize fluorescein isothiocyanate as a label. The antibody thus labeled has specificity against the primary antibody which, in turn, is specific for the viral antigen.[13,14]

For clinicians, the successful application of these techniques necessitates proper collection of the specimen. Selecting a swab of cotton or Dacron that does not bind or inactivate the virus is especially important.[10] Once the specimen has been collected and fixed, the antibodies are added and the whole sample is incubated. The cells are then viewed using a fluorescence microscope. The exciting wavelength used is about 480 nm and the emitting wavelength 520 nm.

The indirect peroxidase method is similar.[15,16] It utilizes a peroxidase-labeled antibody with specificity for the primary antibody, which is, in turn, specific for the viral antigen. A counterstain may also be used, allowing the identification of other cytologic markers in the preparation. It should be emphasized that errors can easily be introduced in these comparatively rigorous techniques.

There are a number of variations of these techniques that are based on antibody technology. Although commercially available kits are presently available and very attractive to the private practitioner, some caution must be exercised in using them, since not all have been appropriately standardized, nor have they undergone clinical trials for ophthalmic application.

Clinical Implications

Although the antibody-based histochemical techniques have already proved useful in the identification of various viruses,[17] their application to the diagnosis of ophthalmic conditions remains limited especially in the milieu of the private office. It is hoped that as new commercially available kits are directed toward ocular problems, these techniques may be used with greater confidence. Nonetheless, the necessary purchase of expensive equipment, such as a fluorescence microscope, may be a deterrent.

VIROLOGY AND BLOOD CHEMISTRY ANALYSIS

Definition

The diagnostic identification tests using blood specimens from acutely ill and convalescent patients are a combination of tests in which antibodies to specific viral components are used to identify the viral agent, or ones in which antibody titers to a viral agent are measured. The basis and methodology for the techniques can be found in a number of reviews and texts.[10,14,17,18]

Clinical Use

The serologic tests are of increasing importance in the identification of the viral agents. They are highly specific tests that are based on immunologic rationales and provide the clinician with a high degree of certainty.

Clinical Procedure

The procedures routinely test several serum samples from infected individuals. The tests available are complement fixation, neutralization, hemagglutination and hemagglutination inhibition, radioimmunoassays, and ELISA, as well as other immunologic-based tests.[14]

In *complement fixation,* antibody-sensitized antigens are bound by complement in a process called complement fixation. This method is widely utilized in diagnostic microbiology. When bound, complement is no longer capable of hemolyzing erythrocytes. Thus, if sensitized erythrocytes are added to a specific sample, the degree to which these are hemolyzed reflects the presence or absence of unbound complement.

In the *neutralization* test, the presence of highly specific antibodies to the virus is established. These are capable of interacting with viral antigens, thereby reducing the overall infectious ability of the virus. The method involves heating the test serum, followed by serial dilutions of serum to which are added constant amounts of virus. This is followed by inoculation of cell cultures with the viral suspensions, and establishing the presence or absence of antibody.[14]

In *hemagglutination* and *hemagglutination inhibition,* red blood cell agglutination reactions can occur as a result of specific viral infections.[14] Inhibition of these reactions occurs during the convalescent phase as a result of rise in antibody titer. Consequently, one advantage of this test lies in that isolation and identification of the virus are not absolutely necessary to determine the presence of the antibodies.[10]

Radioimmunoassays (RIA) are a way of measuring, as well as identifying, antigens.[18] They involve the tagging of a known quantity of ligand (antigen) with a radioactive label. This ligand and the naturally occurring unlabeled ligand then compete for the antibody. The greater the radioactivity, the lower is the concentration of naturally occurring ligand.

The *ELISA,* or enzyme-linked immunosorbent assay, test uses a principle similar to that of RIAs, but offers the advantage of an enzyme label rather than the expensive and comparatively more dangerous radioactive label.[14]

Table 39–9
Stains Used in Mycology

Stains	Diagnostic Characteristics
Giemsa	Yeast cells and pseudohyphae stain blue; filamentous fungi are blue.
Acridine orange (AO) (fluorochrome stain)	DA green RNA orange to red Yeast reddish orange with green nucleus; filamentous fungi, bright green (bacteria, cell wall-deficient organisms and chlamydial inclusion bodies stain orange to red) Nuclei of epithelial cells and leukocytes stain light to bright green, and cytoplasm does not stain. The nuclei of macrophages stain yellow-green, yellow-brown, or dark red, whereas granular cytoplasm is light green to yellow-orange.
Cellufluor	Stain similar to AO in that the fluorescent stain has an affinity for chiten and cellulase—used with fluorescent microscope and filter B612 and no. 44 and 47 barrier filters.
Periodic Acid–Schiff	Useful for filamentous and yeast forms. Fungal walls are bright magenta (phycomycetes do not stain).
Gomori's methenamine silver stain	Good for filamentous and yeast forms.

Clinical Implications

Each of these tests may significantly enhance the reliability of virus identification, especially in clinical situations for which, heretofore, clinicians have primarily relied on histologic procedures.[2,9–12]

MYCOLOGY CULTURING

Definition

Mycocytology culture includes procedures whereby clinical specimens are inoculated into a specific medium for organism identification.

Clinical Use

The diagnosis of a mycotic infection can be particularly frustrating. Confirmation can be made with certainty only after culturing.[19] The use of appropriate collection techniques and incubation procedures is paramount in the identification process.

Clinical Procedure

The scraping is collected from an area of active infection and is inoculated directly into the medium. Although numerous media can be used,[8] Sabouraud's dextrose agar medium is the more commonly chosen.[19] One should add gentamicin to the medium to prevent bacterial contamination, and the cultures are incubated at 30°C for several weeks.[8,19]

Clinical Implications

Clinical Significance

Microscopic evaluation based on differential staining (Table 39–9) is rather routinely performed. But culturing remains the important procedure in the identification process.

Clinical Interpretation

To properly identify some of the fungi, a pure culture is required. Even under ideal culturing conditions, additional information from microscopic examination may be necessary. A useful survey of the various fungi, their medical implications, and optimum techniques for identification may be found in Myrvik and Weiser.[7] Biochemical methods or fluorescent antibody techniques may be utilized, although the latter do not exhibit the highest specificity.[19]

MYCOLOGY AND CYTOLOGY

Definition

The specimen is stained and identified by standard fixation and paraffin methods or from freshly removed biopsy tissue. Recently, several commercial kits have been marketed and appear to be reliable.

Clinical Procedure

The specimen is fixed, embedded, and sectioned. A number of dyes are available for more specific identification. Although hematoxylin and eosin have been used, the stains listed in Table 39–9 are recommended.[19]

Clinical Implications

The choice of stain may be directed by the clinical presentation and the presumptive diagnosis.

REFERENCES

1. Stenson S. Cytologic diagnosis. In: Karciogliu Z, ed. Laboratory diagnosis in ophthalmology. New York: Macmillan Publishing Co, 1987: 90–107.
2. Pavan–Langston D. Manual of ocular diagnosis and therapy. Boston: Little, Brown & Co, 1985.

3. Humason G. Animal tissue techniques. San Francisco: Freeman & Co, 1967.
4. Snell RS. Clinical and functional histology for medical students. Boston: Little, Brown & Co, 1984.
5. Insler MS, Johnson MK. Microbiologic diagnosis: bacteriology. In: Karciogliu, Z, ed. Laboratory diagnosis in ophthalmology. New York: Macmillan Publishing Co, 1987:131–152.
6. Finegold S, Martin W. Diagnostic microbiology. St Louis: CV Mosby Co, 1982.
7. Myrvik ON, Weiser RS. Fundamentals of medical bacteriology and mycology. Philadelphia: Lea & Febiger, 1988.
8. Goldstein E, Joye N. Laboratory procedures in infectious diseases. In: Halsted JA, Halsted CH, eds. The laboratory in clinical medicine. Philadelphia: WB Saunders Co, 1981.
9. Catania LJ. Primary care of the anterior segment. Norwalk, Conn: Appleton–Lange, 1988.
10. Smolin G, Tabbara K, Whitacher J. Infectious diseases of the eye. Baltimore: Williams & Wilkins, 1984.
11. Oh JO. Microbiologic diagnosis: virology. In: Karciogliu Z, ed. Laboratory diagnosis in ophthalmology. New York: Macmillan Publishing Co, 1987:153–170.
12. Darrell RW. Viral diseases of the eye. Philadelphia: Lea & Febiger, 1985.
13. Emmons RW, Riggs JL. Application of immunofluorescence to diagnosis of viral infections. Methods Virol 1977;6:1–28.
14. Halsted CC. Viral and rickettsial infections. In: Halsted JA, Halsted CH, eds. The laboratory in clinical medicine. Philadelphia: WB Saunders, 1981.
15. Sternberger LA. Immunocytochemistry. New York: John Wiley & Sons, 1979.
16. Wordinger RJ, Miller GW, Nicodemus DS. Manual of immunoperoxidase techniques. Chicago: American Society of Clinical Pathologists, 1983.
17. Voller A, Bidwell DE. Enzyme immunoassay and their potential in diagnostic virology. In: Kurstak E, Kurstak C, eds. Comparative diagnosis of viral diseases. New York: Academic Press, 1977.
18. Dougherty H, Ziegler DW. Radioimmunoassay in viral diagnosis. In: Kurstak E, Kurstak C, eds. Comparative diagnosis of viral diseases. New York: Academic Press, 1977.
19. Margo CE, Brinser JH. Microbiologic diagnosis: mycology. In: Karciogliu Z, ed. Laboratory diagnosis in ophthalmology. New York: Macmillan Publishing Co, 1987.

Corneal Esthesiometry

Michel Millodot

INTRODUCTION

Definition

Corneal sensitivity is the capability of the cornea to respond to stimulation. The aspect of corneal sensitivity to touch, as distinct from heat, cold, or pain stimulation, is assessed by an *esthesiometer* which measures the *corneal touch threshold* (CTT). The CTT is the reciprocal of corneal sensitivity.

History

The first measurements of corneal sensitivity were conducted by von Frey in 1894. He used horse hairs of different lengths attached with wax to the tip of a glass rod. These hairs had different tip configurations, thus evoking touch as well as pain, but the calibration left much to be desired. Nevertheless, he used a set of eight hairs which could exert 2, 5, 10, 20, 50, 100, 150, and 250 mg/area[2]. Sterilization of the hairs was not easily achieved, and the rigidity of such a hair was affected by the humidity in the air.

In their review paper, Cochet and Bonnet[1] reported that, in 1900, Toulouse and Vachide used small aluminum rods of different weights, but noted that this was a difficult method to use. They also gave an account of another esthesiometer designed by Franceschetti which resembled that of von Frey. Instead of using hairs, Nafe and Wagoner[2] used metal rods. However, it was not until Boberg-Ans[3] made his own instrument that radical improvements were made. Boberg-Ans[3] replaced the horse hairs by a single nylon thread 11/100 mm in diameter, the length of which could be varied, thus allowing it to exert pressures between 15 mg and 1800 mg/area[2]. In 1960, Cochet and Bonnet[1] devised an instrument that was based on the same principle as that of Boberg-Ans, with some

mechanical improvements (Fig. 40–1). This new instrument made it possible to use one hand only, made it easier to read the length and, in particular, it provided better and more even rigidity of the nylon thread throughout its length. Cochet and Bonnet's instrument has become, since its introduction in 1960, the most widely used esthesiometer in the world. Other instruments have been proposed in the last 20 years.[4,5] Some are more accurate than that of Cochet and Bonnet, but in corneal esthesiometry, unlike in keratometry or biomicroscopy, the results obtained are not directly proportional to the sophistication of the instrument. The response is more dependent on the subject's attitude and apprehension. To obtain reliable results various precautions must be taken.

Clinical Use

The cornea is probably the most sensitive tissue of the body. For example, a small speck of dust, which would remain unnoticed on the tip of the finger, can cause a significant amount of discomfort. Such extraordinary response is obviously related to the alarm system of the cornea that warns one that something destructive is happening to that tissue and may jeopardize its ultimate raison d'être (i.e., transparency). Consequently, the palpebral reflex mechanism, which closes the eyelids and protects the eye against potential trauma, is triggered. However, many eye diseases, mainly of the cornea and conjunctiva, as well as contact lens wear, interfere with the mechanism of corneal sensitivity.

The main clinical uses of esthesiometry are the following:

1. A test of the functioning integrity of the cornea, as any condition affecting the cornea from whatever source (see later) gives rise to a change in its sensitivity, almost always lowering it.

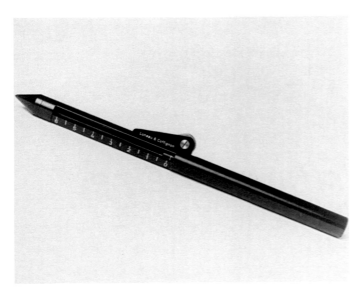

FIGURE 40–1. Hand-held esthesiometer (Cochet–Bonnet).

2. It is a useful test for monitoring the recovery from a condition that has affected the cornea by observing the return of corneal sensitivity to its baseline.
3. To ensure that corneal anesthesia with a given topical anesthetic agent is of sufficient depth to perform the appropriate procedure.
4. To assess the baseline corneal sensitivity of each eye before contact lens fitting and, thus, allow better management of the patient.

INSTRUMENTATION

Theory

The esthesiometer consists of a means of exerting a given pressure on a specific area of the cornea or the skin. The most common method is by use of a nylon thread. However, metal rods have been used.[2,6] The nylon monofilament, as used in the Cochet–Bonnet instrument, has a constant diameter, and the pressure that it exerts on a surface is dependent on its length, which can be varied by retracting the thread into the body of the instrument. The longer the monofilament, the smaller the pressure, and the smaller the monofilament, the larger the pressure. The calibration between length of the nylon thread and force is easily accomplished using a scale with a precision better than 0.5 mg.[7] The esthesiometer is placed vertically and with the tip of the nylon thread resting on one of two trays of the scale. On the other tray one places known small weights until the minimum angle of bending of the monofilament is visible and the scale is in balance. Thus, the force exerted by the nylon thread of a given length is easily obtained (Fig. 40–2). The area of cornea tested is small, covering at most a dozen epithelial cells, and the instrument can be used to test any area of the cornea.

There are two models of the Cochet–Bonnet esthesiometer. One equipped with a nylon monofilament, 0.08 mm in diameter, which produces pressures ranging from 2 to 90 mg/0.005 mm,[2] and the other with a nylon monofilament, 0.12 mm in diameter, which produces pressures ranging from 11 to 200 mg/0.0113 mm[2].

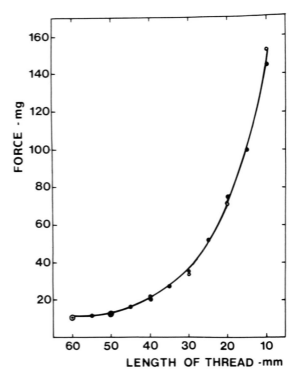

FIGURE 40–2. Calibration of the Cochet–Bonnet esthesiometer. *Closed circles,* Cochet and Bonnet (1960); *open circles,* Millodot and Larson (1967).

Use

The instrument can be held by hand and brought to the cornea (Fig. 40–3). This procedure, however, demands great dexterity. It is better to mount the esthesiometer on a slit lamp or similar type of table so that the esthesiometer can be moved in three directions. The nylon monofilament must touch the cornea at right angles to its surface (see Fig. 40–3). The criterion of a touch is the minimum angle of bending of the nylon thread. It is often convenient to use the arm with the magnifying optical device to assess the

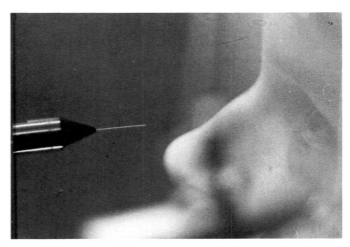

FIGURE 40–3. Nylon monofilament of the Cochet–Bonnet esthesiometer moving toward the eye.

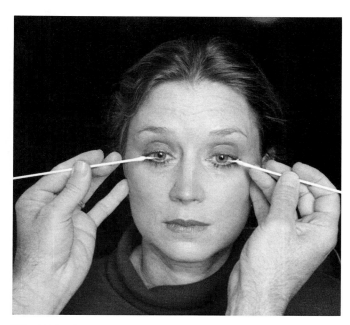

FIGURE 40–4. Comparative testing of corneal sensitivity with use of bilateral cotton wisps.

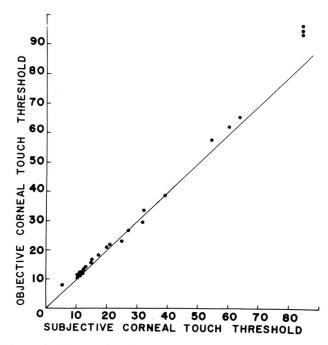

FIGURE 40–5. Correlation between subjective and objective CTT measured near the limbus at 6 o'clock. (From Millodot M. Objective measurement of corneal sensitivity. Acta Ophthalmol 1973;51:325–334, with permission)

angle of contact of the nylon thread of the esthesiometer and the minimum angle of bending.

There are other precautions to take when using the Cochet–Bonnet esthesiometer.

1. The humidity in the room should not exceed 60%, as the nylon thread would otherwise be affected and calibration would be inappropriate, thus giving a false reading.[7]
2. The mounting of the instrument should also incorporate a concealment of the instrument from the patient to minimize apprehension effects.

Clinically one can also use cotton-tipped applicators in which the cotton has been pulled into a thin thread or wisp. In this manner when performed bilaterally the clinician makes a relative judgment of one eye versus its fellow (Fig. 40–4). Although this technique does not permit precise measurement, it may be quite useful.

Method of Measurement

Whichever instrument one uses, it is important to start from a low pressure and increase it by small increments. Otherwise, if one starts with a high pressure, it leaves an "after-glow" that persists for some time[8] and tends to elevate the corneal touch threshold or CTT.[9] Moreover starting with a high pressure can present a serious risk to the cornea of the patient.

At each length of the nylon thread (i.e., for a given pressure), four to eight measurements are conducted, and the patient is requested to indicate when the probe is felt by pressing a buzzer or any other hand signal. This is preferable, because if it is verbalized the head moves and this alters the adjustment. A few blanks (i.e., the nylon thread is brought close to the cornea without touching it) are also made to test the reliability of the patient. The length of the monofilament is then decreased (in 0.5-cm steps) until the threshold is encompassed. The CTT is usually defined as the length of the nylon thread at which the subject responds to 50% of the number of stimulations. This length is converted into pressure

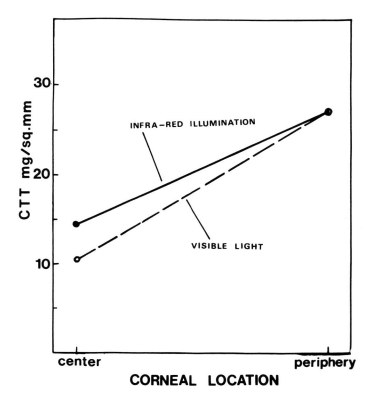

FIGURE 40–6. CTT measured in the center and periphery of the cornea under infrared and visible illumination. Each data point represents the mean of nine subjects. (From Bonnet R, Millodot M. Corneal esthesiometry, its measurement in the dark. Am J Optom 1966;43:238–243)

using the table given with the esthesiometer or a curve relating the length of the monofilament to pressure (see Fig. 40–2). *Corneal sensitivity* is defined as the reciprocal of the CTT.

Alternatively, data can be obtained objectively by monitoring the eye blinks in response to stimulation. Many measurements have to be made with this technique because of the confusion with the physiologic eye blinks. Nonetheless, the results are highly correlated with the subjective measurements (Fig. 40–5). The objective technique is very useful with infants, malingerers, and other people on whom an examination is difficult.

Reproducibility of measurement has been shown to be excellent ($r = +0.99$) on the same subject, and the variation in results do not usually exceed ±5% from one time to another.[9]

Apprehension Factors

The determination of CTT creates a certain amount of fear on the part of the patient, especially when testing the center of the cornea. Indeed, the sight of the esthesiometer moving along the visual axis toward one's eye is distressing. Thus, it is not surprising that this apprehension factor affects the evaluation of the threshold. Bonnet and Millodot[10] measured CTT centrally and peripherally (near the limbus at the 6-o'clock position) under normal room lighting and under infrared illumination with an infrared image converter to allow the investigator to see in the dark. The results showed that the threshold measured in the center of the cornea was significantly lower (mean 18%) in visible light than in complete darkness when the subject was not able to see the esthesiometer (Fig. 40–6). In the periphery of the cornea, the CTT was approximately the same under both conditions, presumably because even in daylight the esthesiometer appears blurred and does not frighten the patient. It is unfortunately not possible to adopt a correction factor of 18% for central measurements, because apprehension affects people to very different extents. In some cases, there was no difference between the two conditions and, in others, the difference was twice as great.

COMMERCIALLY AVAILABLE INSTRUMENTS

There are two instruments available commercially. The simple and well-established instrument of Cochet and Bonnet, manufactured in Paris by Luneau and Coffignon since 1960, and the newer and much more expensive instrument devised by Draeger[11] and manufactured by his own company. The latter is an electro-optical device built as a portable instrument using a metallic thread to touch the eye and some optical system to facilitate the measurement.

CLINICAL PROCEDURE

The procedure for only the most common instrument, the Cochet–Bonnet esthesiometer, will be described.

1. The patient is instructed to press on a buzzer when he or she feels that the eye has been touched, but must not move the head, as this alters the adjustment. Subjective measurements are preferable to objective ones, as the latter are not easily differentiated from physiologic blinks. As described earlier, many stimulations are made at various pressures, always going from low to high pressure.
2. The patient is asked to fixate a point or a letter of a test chart projected on the wall in front. The fixation target is either straight in front or well above the horizontal plane, depending upon which corneal area is to be tested. To test near the limbus at the 6-o'clock position, the patient fixates a target well above the horizontal plane of the patient's eye.
3. After having placed the instrument in a mounting device

such as a slit lamp the patient is asked to place his or her head on the chin rest and against the forehead holder.
4. The clinician is seated at right angles to the patient's median plane.
5. The clinician then adjusts the mounting device in three directions so that the esthesiometer monofilament comes into contact with the cornea at the desired spot and at right angles.
6. The instrument is moved forward by turning one of the knobs, always at the same speed and contact with the cornea is recorded when the clinician can see the minimum angle of bending of the nylon monofilament. The clinician should avoid touching the lids or the eyelashes.

CLINICAL IMPLICATIONS

Clinical Significance

The demonstration of a loss of corneal sensitivity and the quantification of that loss is what esthesiometry is used for. There are many conditions that lead to a reduction in sensitivity (hypoesthesia). Keratoconus leads to a decrease in sensitivity of the central part of the cornea and only a slight diminution in the peripheral cornea. The severity of the conical area in keratoconus is not correlated with the amount of loss of corneal sensitivity.[12] Following corneal keratoplasty corneal sensitivity decreases markedly, but new nerve fibers eventually regenerate and penetrate the graft, and corneal sensitivity returns partially and only in a small proportion of cases. The process is very slow and takes several years.[13] Draeger[4] found that the younger the patient, the more rapid the recovery. Esthesiometry is valuable as an additional test in evaluating corneal graft integrity. Other factors or tests are corneal transparency, pachometry, and corneal endothelial examination.

On the other hand, keratoplasty performed after herpes simplex infection is not accompanied by a return of corneal sensitivity, unlike keratoplasty after corneal dystrophy. This, of course, depends on the compatibility between host and donor, and the best recovery occurs when the tissues have been matched for human leukocyte antigen (HLA). The recovery of corneal sensitivity gives a good indication of the reinnervation occurring in the graft.

In general, any disease of the cornea gives rise to hypoesthesia. In corneal ulcers, the hypoesthesia is located on or near the ulcer. The loss of sensitivity depends on the condition and also the type of keratitis. Esthesiometry is useful in monitoring the recovery from corneal disease. Norn[14] believes that esthesiometry is an important diagnostic and prognostic tool. He felt that the greater the reduction in sensitivity the greater the chance of recurrent infections.

Chronic open-angle glaucoma, in which the glaucomatous cup is evident, usually leads to a small reduction in corneal sensitivity, although in this condition esthesiometry is not correlated with intraocular pressure.[4]

Herpetic keratitis is usually accompanied by a large diminution of corneal sensitivity. It is not limited to the area of the dendritic lesion, but is depressed across the entire cornea, unlike some other types of keratitis (e.g., bacterial keratitis). Esthesiometry is thus very valuable in the differential diagnosis of these diseases. Some investigators have also found a relationship between the severity of the herpetic disease and the loss of corneal sensitivity.[4] Moreover, the recovery of sensitivity following the cure of superficial herpetic keratitis is much more rapid (about 2 years) compared with the almost permanent loss occurring after the treatment of herpetic interstitial keratitis.

Trachoma also produces a depression of corneal sensitivity, although the extent depends upon the amount of neovascularization of the cornea.[15]

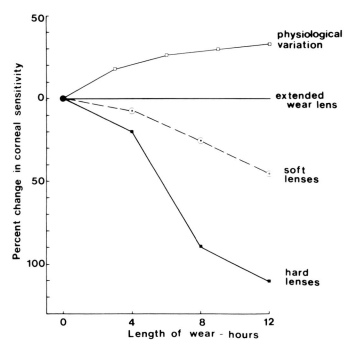

FIGURE 40–7. Loss of corneal sensitivity as a function of the number of hours of wear, for several types of contact lenses. Soft was HEMA and hard was PMMA. The physiologic variation of corneal sensitivity is also shown. (From Millodot M. Effect of the length of wear of contact lenses on corneal sensitivity. Acta Ophthalmol 1976;54:721–730)

Lattice corneal dystrophy produces a reduction in corneal sensitivity,[16] as does hereditary fleck dystrophy of the cornea.[17]

In trigeminal neuralgia, corneal sensitivity is usually normal unless the corneal reflex is diminished or lost.[3] In this case, corneal sensitivity will also be reduced, and corneal sensitivity will always be decreased after severing the ophthalmic branch of the trigeminal nerve, as would be expected.[4]

Diabetes

Diabetes mellitus also leads to corneal hypoesthesia, and the longer the duration of the disease, the greater the decrease in sensitivity.[4,18–20] Those with diabetic retinopathy showed a greater loss than those without retinopathy. The decrease in corneal sensitivity is believed to be due to a diffuse neuropathy affecting the peripheral sensory–motor nervous system. Neilsen and Lund,[21] found in 100 diabetic patients alterations not only in corneal sensation, but also in vibratory perception of the index finger and big toe, and in the Achilles tendon reflex.

Treatment of the disease by insulin was accompanied by a higher sensitivity, similar to that found in a group of persons with recent diabetes. Esthesiometry appears to be of value in the management of diabetes.

β-Blockers, such as timolol, which are used in the treatment of glaucoma, have sometimes been thought to cause a corneal hypoesthesia. This claim has been difficult to assess, since the depression may be due to the underlying disease or to the age of the patient. In an investigation on rabbits, Millodot and Vogel[22] found no long-term effect of the β-blocker timolol. In men the results vary, but generally it appears that they have no prolonged

effect. Some diminution of sensitivity in older persons occurs for a short time after instillation of the drop.[4,23]

Contact Lenses

The wearing of contact lenses is almost always accompanied by an attenuation of corneal sensitivity, albeit to different degrees, depending on the type of lens and the fit of the lens. Lenses with greater oxygen transmissibility produce the least decrease in sensitivity, and for a given type of material a tighter fit usually leads to a greater reduction in sensitivity (Fig. 40–7). Also shown in Figure 40–7 is the normal diurnal variation in corneal sensitivity against which the changes induced by contact lenses must be compared.[24]

The diminution of corneal sensitivity with contact lens wear is not totally unwelcome, as the contact lenses feel more comfortable. Eventually there is the risk that a corneal lesion could begin without the patient being aware of it, at least for some time, and infection, therefore, would spread more rapidly. The loss of corneal sensitivity for a given material is directly dependent on the length of time that the lens has been worn. With polymethylmethacrylate (PMMA) lenses worn for up to 22 years, Millodot[25] has noted a progressive loss of sensitivity (Fig. 40–8).

However, after the lenses were removed, sensitivity began to return. If lenses had been worn for only 2 to 3 years, sensitivity was usually back to normal within a few hours, but with more years of wear, this recovery was much slower. After more than 10 years of wear, it may take some months to recover from PMMA wear (Fig. 40–9). These figures would be greatly reduced with gas-permeable lenses or any other lens with high oxygen transmissibility. There is, indeed, a clear relationship between oxygen pressure at the epithelial level and loss of corneal sensitivity.[26]

Formerly it was thought that measurement of corneal sensitivity would aid in the prediction of tolerance and success of contact lenses.[27,28] However, this view was never tested systematically, and it now seems that the correlation would be low, as many other

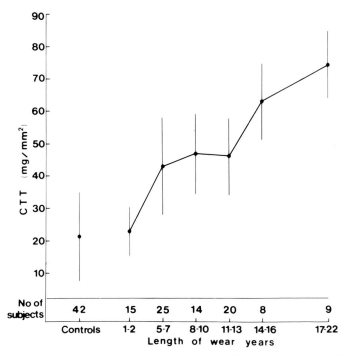

FIGURE 40–8. Increase in CTT as a function of the number of years of wear of PMMA lenses: N, number of subjects. (From Millodot M. Effect of long term wear of hard contact lenses on corneal sensitivity. Arch Ophthalmol 1978; 96:1225–1227, with permission)

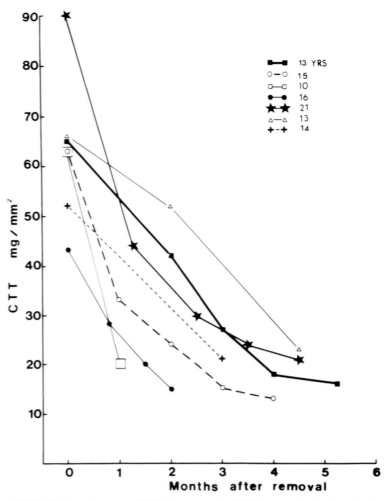

FIGURE 40–9. Recovery of CTT after removal of PMMA lenses that had previously been worn for the number of years indicated in the right-hand corner. (From Millodot M. Effect of long term wear of hard contact lenses on corneal sensitivity. Arch Ophthalmol 1978;96:1225–1227)

factors (e.g., motivation, oxygen requirement of each patient's cornea, or others) are more decisive in determining the success of contact lens wear. However, in cases of hypoesthesia, especially unilateral, esthesiometry is valuable in management, as the patient may be warned to heed the slightest discomfort and abide more rigidly to the wearing schedule because failing to do so could lead to a corneal infection being unnoticed until quite advanced. Nevertheless, the principal benefit of testing corneal sensitivity in contact lens practice is to assess the state of corneal integrity. It is important to ensure that the hypoesthesia does not go beyond a given amount such as, for example, half its initial value. Otherwise, the contact lens fit and material should be altered.

Clinical Interpretation

The results of corneal esthesiometry are dependent on several factors that must be understood by the clinician to fully appreciate its clinical implications.

Corneal Area

Corneal sensitivity varies from a maximum at the center of the cornea to a minimum at the periphery, with least sensitivity at the superior region, which is frequently covered by the upper lid (Fig. 40–10). Average central CTT varies between 8 and 14 mg/mm². The average CTT in the periphery ranges between 20 and 40 mg/mm², whereas in the superior periphery it ranges between 30 and 50 mg/mm². This corneal area of reduced sensitivity is actually useful in contact lens wear, as this is where the contact lens often rests most heavily because of the pressure produced by the upper lid. A considerable drop in sensitivity is found beyond the limbus.

Age

Corneal sensitivity remains practically the same from about the age of 10 years to 50 years. Beyond that age it diminishes, reducing to half after 65 years (Fig. 40–11).

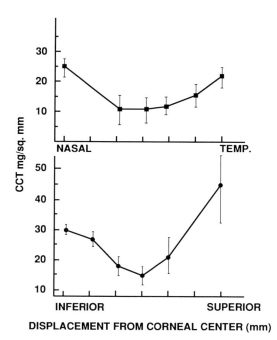

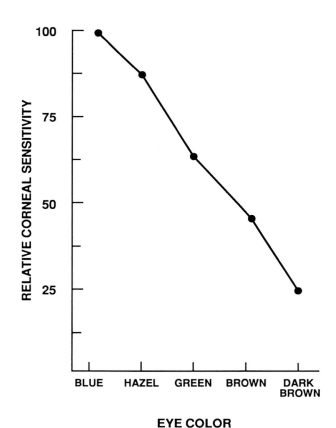

FIGURE 40–10. CTT across the cornea. (From Millodot M, Larson W. New measurements of corneal sensitivity: a preliminary report. Am J Optom 1969;46:261–265)

Iris Color

Another important consideration that affects results is iris color. Persons with blue eyes have, on average, much more sensitive corneas than people with brown eyes. And nonwhite persons with dark brown irides usually have less sensitive corneas than Caucasians.[29] There are large variations among subjects of each group, and the data points shown in Figure 40–12 are mean values. The reason for the different results among differently colored eyes remains an enigma.

FIGURE 40–12. Relative corneal sensitivity as a function of eye color. (From Millodot M. Do blue eyed people have more sensitive corneas than brown eyed people? Nature 1975;255:151–152)

Miscellaneous

Corneal sensitivity should be about the same in the two eyes. Cases of asymmetry have usually resulted from trauma to the head or from eye disease. Corneal sensitivity is also about the same between males and females, although at premenstruation time (if no contraceptive pill is used) and in the last few weeks of pregnancy, corneal sensitivity in women is reduced.[30–32] Ambient temperatures also affect corneal sensitivity. Kolstrad[33] observed a ninefold reduction as the outside temperature varied between 22° and −14°C. This may explain the relative comfort of contact lens wearers outside when it is cold.

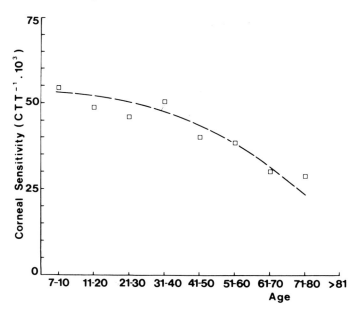

FIGURE 40–11. Corneal sensitivity as a function of age. (From Millodot M. Influence of age on the sensitivity of the cornea. Invest Ophthalmol 1977;16:540–542)

REFERENCES

1. Cochet P, Bonnet R. L'esthésie cornéenne. Clin Ophthalmol 1960;4:3–27.
2. Nafe J, Wagoner K. Insensitivity of cornea to heat and pain derived from high temperature. Am J Psychol 1973;49:631–635.
3. Boberg-Ans J. Experience in clinical examination of corneal sensitivity. Br J Ophthalmol 1955;39:709–726.
4. Draeger J. Corneal sensitivity, measurement and clinical importance. New York: Springer-Verlag, 1984.
5. Millodot M. A review of research on the sensitivity of the cornea. Ophthal Physiol Opt 1984;4:305–318.
6. Larson WL. Electro-mechanical corneal aesthesiometer. Br J Ophthalmol 1970;54:342–347.
7. Millodot M, Larson W. Effect of bending of the nylon thread of the

Cochet–Bonnet aesthesiometer upon recorded pressure. Contact Lens 1967;1:5–28.

8. Millodot M. The sensitivity of the cornea. Atti Fond G Ronchi Ist Ottica 1974;29:889–901.

9. Millodot M, O'Leary DJ. Corneal fragility and its relationship to sensitivity. Acta Ophthalmol 1981;59:820–826.

10. Bonnet R, Millodot M. Corneal esthesiometry, its measurement in the dark. Am J Optom 1966;43:238–243.

11. Draeger J. Modern aethesiometry. Trans Ophthalmol Soc UK 1979; 99:247–250.

12. Millodot M, Owens H. Sensitivity and fragility in keratoconus. Acta Ophthalmol 1983;61:908–917.

13. Ruben M, Colebrook E. Keratoplasty sensitivity. Br J Ophthalmol 1979;63:265–267.

14. Norn MS. Dendritic (herpetic) keratitis. IV. Follow-up examination of corneal sensitivity. Acta Ophthalmol 1970;48:383–395.

15. Sedan J. Recherches et reflexions sur la sensibilité de la cornée trachomateuse. Acta 16th Concil Ophthalmol 1951;2:1411–1418.

16. Petursson GJ. Corneal sensitivity in lattice dystrophy. Am J Ophthalmol 1967;64:880–885.

17. Birndorf LA, Ginsberg SP. Hereditary fleck dystrophy associated with decreased corneal sensitivity. Am J Ophthalmol 1972;73:670–672.

18. Schwartz DE. Corneal sensitivity in diabetics. Arch Ophthalmol 1974; 91:174–178.

19. Rogell GD. Corneal hypoesthesia and retinopathy in diabetes mellitus. Ophthalmology 1980;87:229–233.

20. O'Leary DJ, Millodot M. Abnormal epithelial fragility in diabetes and contact lens wear. Acta Ophthalmol 1981;59:827–833.

21. Neilsen NV, Lund FS. Diabetic polyneuropathy. Corneal sensitivity, vibratory perception and Achilles tendon reflex in diabetics. Acta Neurol Scand 1979;59:15–22.

22. Millodot M, Vogel R. The effect of timolol eye drops on corneal sensitivity in pigmented rabbits. Res Clin Forums 1981;3:79–83.

23. Kitazawa Y, Tsuchisaka H. Effects of timolol on corneal sensitivity and tear production. Int Ophthalmol 1980;3:25–29.

24. Millodot M. Diurnal variation of corneal sensitivity. Br J Ophthalmol 1972;56:844–847.

25. Millodot M. Effect of long term wear of hard contact lenses on corneal sensitivity. Arch Ophthalmol 1978;96:1225–1227.

26. Millodot M, O'Leary DJ. Effect of oxygen deprivation on corneal sensitivity. Acta Ophthalmol 1980;58:434–439.

27. Hamano H. Topical and systemic influences of wearing contact lenses. Contacto 1960;4:41–48.

28. Kraar RS, Cummings CM. Lacrimation, corneal sensitivity and corneal abrasive resistance in contact lens wearability. Optom Weekly 1965;56:25–32.

29. Millodot M. Do blue eyed people have more sensitive corneas than brown eyed people? Nature 1975;255:151–152.

30. Millodot M, Lamont A. Influence of menstruation on corneal sensitivity. Br J Ophthalmol 1974;58:49–51.

31. Millodot M. The influence of pregnancy on the sensitivity of the cornea. Br J Ophthalmol 1977;61:646–649.

32. Riss B, Riss P. Corneal sensitivity in pregnancy. Ophthalmologica 1981;183:57–62.

33. Kolstrad A. Corneal sensitivity by low temperatures. Acta Ophthalmol 1970;48:789–793.

Keratoscopy

David A. Goss

INTRODUCTION

Definition

Keratoscopy is the examination of the curvature and topography of the anterior surface of the cornea.[1] A *keratoscope* generally consists of an alternating pattern of black and white concentric rings, which is reflected from the cornea, and some type of viewing system. The viewing system may be as simple as a hole in the center of the target, or it may involve an imaging and photographic system. In the latter, the instrument is referred to as a *photokeratoscope*.

History

The invention of the keratoscope is credited to the English physician Henry Goode, in 1847.[2] Goode studied astigmatic eyes with his keratoscope. The inventor of the photokeratoscope was the Portuguese oculist, Placido.[2] Placido described the instrument in 1880. Additional early contributions to photokeratoscopy were made by Javal, Schiotz, Nordenson, and Gullstrand.[2,3] Javal was apparently the first to describe the use of photokeratoscopy to observe an ocular disease, specifically, keratoconus.[2] In the second half of this century, there have been a number of investigators[4-10] who have made contributions to the development of photokeratoscope instrumentation.

Clinical Use

The primary clinical applications of keratoscopy and photokeratoscopy (Table 41–1) are the following:

1. Photokeratoscopy has been used by contact lens fitters to aid in the prescription of contact lens measurements for an optimum contact lens–cornea relationship.[11-15]
2. In orthokeratology, the central cornea undergoes flattening and the peripheral cornea steepens.[16,17] Greater refractive changes from orthokeratology might be expected in patients with greater peripheral corneal flattening before the orthokeratology program.
3. Photokeratoscopy can be used for differential diagnosis, monitoring, and contact lens fitting in keratoconus.[18]
4. Photokeratoscopy can be utilized by the ophthalmic surgeon in cases of ocular trauma affecting the cornea[19] or to monitor corneal changes in other ophthalmic surgical procedures, including cataract surgery.[15,20]
5. Photokeratoscopy has revealed that corneal refractive surgery, such as radial keratotomy, induces changes in corneal topography.[21-26] The corneal changes correlate with the amount of refractive error change.

INSTRUMENTATION

Theory and Use

Keratoscopy uses the image (usually of concentric rings) reflected from the cornea to evaluate the curvature and topography. It is based upon the principle that the size of a reflected image is directly proportional to the radius of curvature of the reflecting surface. Therefore, the farther a given point on one of the imaged rings is from the center of the image pattern, the greater the radius of curvature at the point on the cornea from which reflection occurred.

Table 41–1
Clinical Applications of Photokeratoscopy

Contact lens fitting
Orthokeratology
Diagnosis and management of keratoconus
Ocular trauma and ophthalmic surgery
Keratorefractive surgery

Potential sources of inaccuracy in photokeratoscopy include precise alignment of the system with the cornea; design of the object pattern and optical system, such that the image will be formed in a single plane, coincident with that of the camera film; ability to cover a significant portion of the cornea, without obstruction by the nose and brow; and film-processing instabilities.[6,9,10,27–30] Developers of modern photokeratoscopy systems have attempted to minimize these problems.

The average cornea shows flattening (i.e., an increase in radius of curvature) going peripherally from central cornea.[10,27,31–34] There is great variability in the amount and rate of peripheral flattening, and the rate of peripheral flattening does not appear to be correlated with the radius of curvature at the corneal apex.[10] Furthermore, as much as 10% of the population may exhibit peripheral corneal steepening.[31,33]

COMMERCIALLY AVAILABLE INSTRUMENTS

Placido Disc

Basic Design

The Placido disc consists simply of a flat plate with black and white concentric rings on one side, and with a handle attached (Fig. 41–1). In the center of the plate there is a viewing hole for the examiner. On the examiner's side of the plate there is a lens well into which a plus lens of 5 to 20 diopters can be placed to increase magnification.

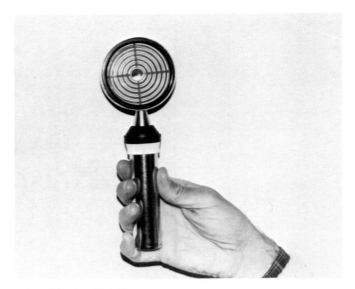

FIGURE 41–2. Klein keratoscope.

Klein Keratoscope

Basic Design

A Klein keratoscope is simply a transilluminated Placido disc with a battery handle (Fig. 41–2).

Kera Corneascope

Basic Design

The Kera Corneascope[20,35,36] (Figs. 41–3 and 41–4) available with either 9 rings (Model 900) or 12 rings (Model 1200). These transilluminated rings are on a hemispherical faceplate (see Fig. 41–3). The instrument was designed so that with proper alignment the center of curvature of the faceplate will be approximately coincident with the center of curvature of the anterior corneal surface. The light reflected from the cornea is imaged by an imaging system and a Polaroid camera. The camera uses Polaroid type 669 or 108 color film, providing a color photograph of the anterior segment of the eye and the reflected keratoscope rings.

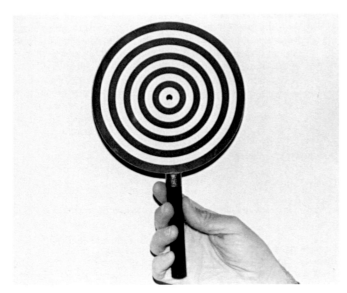

FIGURE 41–1. Placido disc.

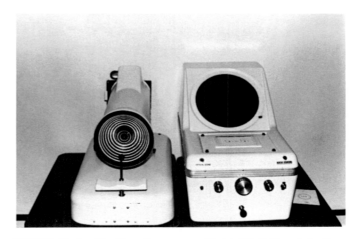

FIGURE 41–3. The Kera Corneascope Model 900 (*left*) and the Comparator.

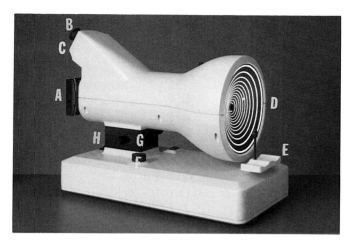

FIGURE 41–4. Labeled photograph of the Kera Corneascope: (*A*) camera; (*B*) magnifier; (*C*) viewing screen; (*D*) placido disc; (*E*) chin rest; (*F*) chin rest knob; (*G*) focus knob; (*H*) master switch.

Nidek Photokeratoscope PKS-1000

Basic Design

The Nidek photokeratoscope[37,38] (Figs. 41–5 and 41–6) was formerly called the Sun photokeratoscope, having once been marketed by the Sun Optical Company in Japan. It has a head- and chin rest for the patient. The target is 11 transilluminated concentric rings. The attached camera uses Polaroid type 667 or type 107 film, with both eyes being photographed in one frame.

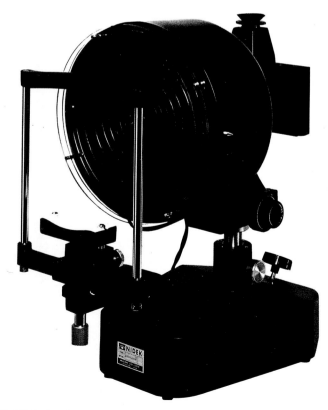

FIGURE 41–5. Nidek Photokeratoscope.

CLINICAL PROCEDURE

Placido Disc

The procedures to be followed to use the Placido disc are the following:

1. The patient should be comfortably seated and wearing no ophthalmic lenses or contact lenses.
2. The Placido disc needs to be illuminated by a lamp or some other similar light source.
3. The Placido disc is held about 20 cm from the patient's eye and perpendicular to the patient's line of sight. The patient is requested to look at the center of the Placido disc (Fig. 41–7).
4. The clinician views the patient's cornea through the hole in the center of the Placido disc with a plus lens added for magnification if desired, and observes the reflected rings to determine if there is any change in the rings from a circular form.
5. If the rings are not circular, a drawing should be made of the shape of the rings (Fig. 41–8).

Klein Keratoscope

The Klein keratoscope is used in essentially the same fashion as the Placido disc, with the exception that a lamp is not necessary because the Klein keratoscope is self-luminous.

Kera Corneascope

To operate the Kera Corneascope, these steps should be followed (Table 41–2):

1. Turn the master switch on. A few seconds after the master switch is turned on, the red indicator light will begin to flash, indicating that the corneascope is ready for use.
2. Position the patient so that the chin is on the left side of the chin rest to photograph the right eye, or on the right side to photograph the left eye. The patient's cheek should be placed up against the cheek rest. Adjust the chin rest up or down by using the chin rest knob until the outer canthus of the eye to be photographed is even with the middle ridge of the metal band running along the side of the instrument casing.
3. With the horizontal positioning knob, turn the instrument so that it is pointed toward the patient's eye. Direct the patient to look at the green fixation light inside the center of the inside ring.
4. While looking through the viewing screen, adjust the alignment of the instrument. Use the horizontal-positioning knob and the chin rest knob until the eye and the reflected rings are in the center of the screen. There are cross hairs on the viewing screen to aid in this adjustment.

Table 41–2
Steps for Taking Photokeratograms with Commercially Available Photokeratoscopes

---

1. Turn the instrument on.
2. Position the patient and adjust the head and chin rest.
3. Direct the patient to look at the fixation target.
4. Adjust the alignment of the instrument.
5. Focus the instrument.
6. Take the picture.

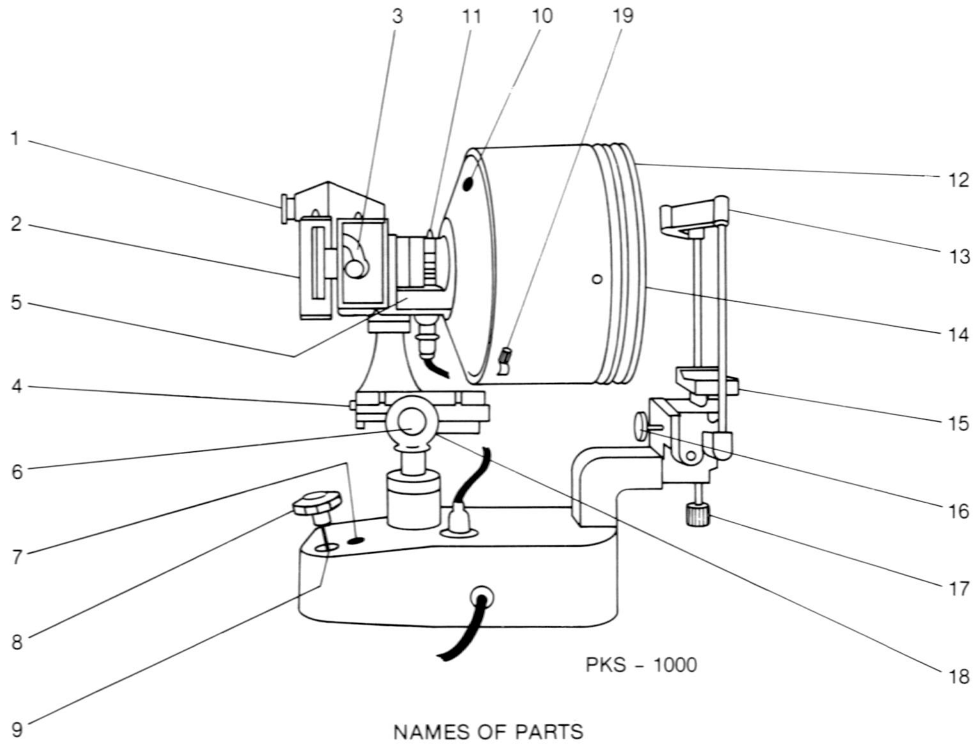

PKS – 1000

NAMES OF PARTS

1. Finder
2. Film magazine
3. Crank
4. Focus adjustment knob
5. Shutter button
6. Rotation adjustment knob (tremor)
7. Pilot lamp
8. Elevation knob
9. Main switch
10. Charge lamp

11. Iris adjustment pin
12. Placido plate
13. Brow fixation
14. Level pin
15. Chinrest
16. Brow fixation elevation knob
17. Chinrest elevation knob
18. Crank knob
19. Cord fastener

FIGURE 41–6. Labeled diagram of the Nidek Photokeratoscope.

5. With the focus knob, bring the inner ring and the small cross next to the inner ring into best focus. It may be necessary at this time to make an additional alignment adjustment.
6. When the cross and the innermost ring are centered in the viewing screen and the cross is sharply focused, press the flash button to take a picture.

Analysis of photokeratograms can be made by either the Kera Comparator or the Kera Scan keratographic autoanalyzer. The Comparator is an optical magnifier, which compares the rings on the Corneascope photokeratogram to a calibrated set of concentric rings. The variable magnification used in making this comparison is calibrated with radius of curvature. Radii of curvature from 6.35 to 9.60 mm can be determined at various points on the photographed rings. A guide for using the Comparator is provided as an aid to contact lens fitting.

The keratographic autoanalyzer is a computer system that optically scans and digitizes information from corneascope photokeratograms. It consists of a television camera and monitor and computer with keyboard, monitor, and printer. It can be used with either the 9-ring or the 12-ring corneascope. It will print out diop-

tric values or radii of curvature at points on the cornea corresponding to points on the rings reflected from the cornea.

Nidek Photokeratoscope

To take a photokeratogram with the Nidek Photokeratoscope PKS-1000, the clinician should follow this procedure:

1. Turn on the main switch. Bring the crank next to the film magazine down.
2. Position the patient using the chin rest elevation control knob and the brow control knob.
3. Slide the film magazine all the way to the left to photograph the right eye, and later, all the way to the right to photograph the left eye.
4. Loosen the crank knob and turn the photokeratoscope target toward the eye to be photographed. Adjust the height of the instrument by the elevation knob. When the photokeratoscope is in position, tighten the crank knob. Viewing through the finder, the clinician should center the ring images in the center of the sight, using the elevation knob

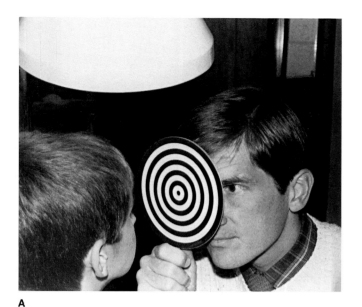

A

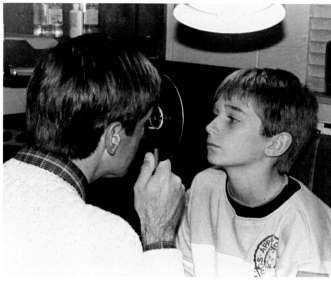

B

FIGURE 41–7. Examination with the Placido disc. (*A*) The examiner holds the Placido disc with the plane of the disc perpendicular to the patient's visual axis. The concentric ring pattern is illuminated by a lamp. (*B*) The examiner views through the hole in the center of the disc using a plus lens of about 5 diopters for magnification.

and the rotation knob. The patient should be instructed to look at the cross mark for proper fixation.

5. Bring the inside ring into best focus with the focus adjustment knob.
6. Once proper alignment and focus have been achieved, release the shutter to take the picture.

Although the photokeratogram itself can be used for qualitative evaluation and photodocumentation, the Nidek Kerato Analyzer system is available for quantitative evaluation. This system consists of a television camera and monitor, computer with keyboard and monitor, and a printer. This system will print out corneal profile, radii of curvature, or dioptric power values at various points on the cornea, and three-dimensional representations of the cornea.

CLINICAL IMPLICATIONS

Clinical Significance

The information obtained from the Placido disk and the Klein keratoscope is qualitative, rather than quantitative. They aid the clinician in observing gross irregularities of the anterior corneal surface. Photokeratoscopy can be used to provide photographic documentation of corneal conditions. Analysis of photokeratograms can be employed to design contact lenses, to monitor cor-

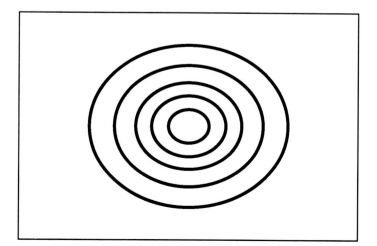

FIGURE 41–8. A drawing following examination with the Placido disc: The appearance of the reflected rings indicates with-the-rule astigmatism.

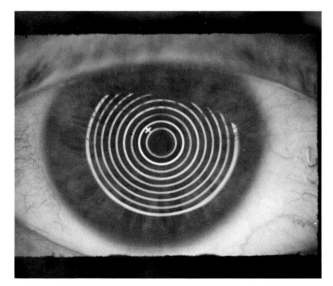

FIGURE 41–9. A keratogram taken of a relatively flat but otherwise normal cornea. (Keratometer readings: 41.25 @ 180; 41.62 @ 90.) Compare this photo to that of a relatively steep cornea in Figure 41–10.

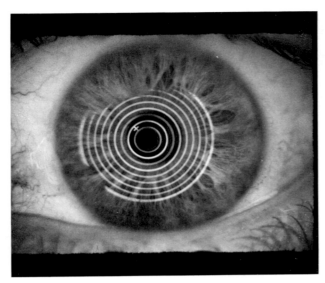

FIGURE 41–10. A keratogram taken of a relatively steep, but otherwise normal, cornea. The rings have a slightly greater diameter horizontally than vertically owing to with-the-rule astigmatism. (Keratometer readings: 45.50 @ 180; 47.00 @ 90.) Compare this photo to that of a relatively flat cornea in Figure 41–9.

neal changes in disease or trauma, and to assess corneal alterations in orthokeratology, keratorefractive surgery, or cataract surgery.

Detailed analysis of photokeratograms can yield information about corneal topography for a variety of specialized clinical uses, as mentioned earlier. One way that the topographical data has been presented is in terms of a power plot, in which dioptric powers are given at various locations on each of the visible reflected rings.[15,20,39,40]

Clinical Interpretation

The closer the reflected rings are to each other, the steeper the cornea, while widely separated rings indicate flatter corneal curvatures (Figs. 41–9 and 41–10). In regular astigmatism, the rings will

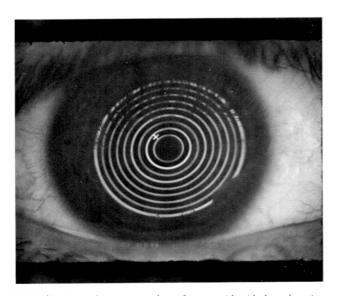

FIGURE 41–11. A keratogram taken of an eye with with-the-rule astigmatism. (Keratometer readings: 42.12 @ 27; 46.75 @ 117.)

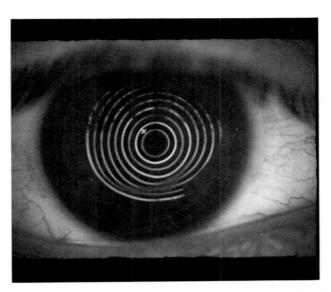

FIGURE 41–12. A keratogram from a patient with keratoconus. Note the distortion of the fifth through eighth rings in the inferior aspect.

be oval, with the long axis horizontal in with-the-rule astigmatism and long axis vertical in against-the-rule astigmatism. An example of with-the-rule astigmatism is shown in Figure 41–11. Waviness or distortion of the rings indicates irregular astigmatism or some type of corneal anomaly or disease, as, for instance, keratoconus (Fig. 41–12).

Corneal topography has also been described in various mathematical terms, such as eccentricity or shape factor, which estimate the degree of asphericity of the cornea in given meridians.[10,33,41] Such quantitative analyses of photokeratograms are now primarily used in specialty practices or for research. Analyses of nonpathologic corneas show a great deal of individual variability in corneal topography. Most, but by no means all, corneas show flattening in the corneal periphery, compared with the center of the cornea.[10,33,40,41] The interested reader should consult the literature for additional information on the power analysis or mathematical analysis of photokeratograms.[10,15,20,33,39,40]

REFERENCES

1. Cline H, Hofstetter HW, Griffin JR. Dictionary of visual science, 3rd ed. Philadelphia: Chilton Book Co, 1980:330.
2. Levene JR. The true inventors of the keratoscope and photokeratoscope. Br J Hist Sci 1965;2:324–342.
3. Duke–Elder S, Abrams D. Ophthalmic optics and refraction. In: Duke–Elder S, ed. System of ophthalmology, vol 5. St Louis: CV Mosby Co, 1970:127–128.
4. Knoll HA, Stimson R, Weeks CL. New photokeratoscope utilizing a hemispherical object surface. J Opt Soc Am 1957;47:221–222.
5. Reynolds AE, Kratt HJ. The photo-electronic keratoscope. Contacto 1959;3(3):53–59.
6. Stone J. The validity of some existing methods of measuring corneal contour compared with suggested new methods. Br J Physiol Opt 1962;19:205–230.
7. Townsley MG. New equipment and methods for determining the contour of the human cornea. Contacto 1967;11(4):72–81.
8. El Hage SG. Suggested new methods for photokeratoscopy—a comparison of their validities. Part I. Am J Optom Arch Am Acad Optom 1971; 48:897–912.
9. Clark BAJ. Conventional keratoscopy—a critical review. Aust J Optom 1973;56:140–155.
10. Mandell RB. Corneal topography. In: Mandell RB, ed. Contact lens practice, 4th ed. Springfield, Ill: Charles C Thomas, 1988:107–135.
11. Carey SM. Comparison of fitting results with the keratometer and PEK. Contacto 1974;18(6):36–38.

12. Feldman GL. Photokeratoscopy in the fitting of soft contact lenses. Ann Ophthalmol 1975;7:517–529.

13. Bibby MW, Townsley MG. Corneal contour: the things to know. Contact Lens Forum 1977;2:45–53.

14. Rich GE. Fitting hydrogel lenses with photokeratology. Int Contact Lens Clin 1977;4:36–47.

15. Rowsey JJ. Corneal topography. In: Dabezies OH Jr, ed. Contact lenses—the CLAO guide to basic science and clinical practice, vol 1, Chap. 4. New York: Grune & Stratton, 1984.

16. Kerns RL. Research in orthokeratology. Part III: results and observations. J Am Optom Assoc 1976;47:1505–1515.

17. Coon LJ. The Pacific study—research in orthokeratology. Orthokeratology 1981;5:11–83.

18. Rich GE. The geometry of keratoconus: alternative approaches to fitting. Rev Optom 1979;116(4):88–91.

19. Rowsey JJ, Hays JC. Refractive reconstruction for acute eye injuries. Ophthal Surg 1984;15:569–574.

20. Rowsey JJ, Reynolds AE, Brown R. Corneal topography—corneascope. Arch Ophthalmol 1981;99:1093–1100.

21. Rowsey JJ. Ten caveats in keratorefractive surgery. Ophthalmology 1983;90:148–155.

22. Rowsey JJ, Isaac MS. Corneoscopy in keratorefractive surgery. Cornea 1983;2:133–142.

23. Henslee SL, Rowsey JJ. New corneal shapes in keratorefractive surgery. Ophthalmology 1983;90:245–250.

24. Terry MA, Rowsey JJ. Dynamic shifts in corneal topography during the modified Ruiz procedure for astigmatism. Arch Ophthalmol 1986;104:1611–1616.

25. Fleming JF. Corneal topography and radial keratotomy. J Refract Surg 1986;2:149–254.

26. Rowsey JJ, Balyeat HD, Monlux R, et al. Prospective evaluation of radial keratotomy—photokeratoscope corneal topography. Ophthalmology 1988;95:322–334.

27. Knoll HA. Corneal contours in the general population as revealed by the photokeratoscope. Am J Optom Arch Am Acad Optom 1961;38:389–397.

28. Ludlam WM, Wittenberg S. Measurements of the ocular dioptric elements utilizing photographic methods. Part II. Cornea—theoretical considerations. Am J Optom Arch Am Acad Optom 1966;43:249–267.

29. Ludlam WM, Wittenberg S, Rosenthal J, Harris G. Photographic analysis of the ocular dioptric components. Part III. The acquisition, storage, retrieval and utilization of primary data in photokeratoscopy. Am J Optom Arch Am Acad Optom 1967;44:276–296.

30. Mandell RB, York MA. A new calibration system for photokeratoscopy. Am J Optom Arch Am Acad Optom 1969;49:410–417.

31. Kiely PM, Smith G, Carney LG. Meridional variations of corneal shape. Am J Optom Physiol Opt 1984;61:619–626.

32. Edmund C, Sjontoft E. The central–peripheral radius of the normal corneal curvature—a photokeratoscopic study. Acta Ophthalmol 1985;63:670–677.

33. Guillon M, Lydon DPM, Wilson C. Corneal topography: A clinical model. Ophthal Physiol Opt 1986;6:47–56.

34. Bibby MM. The Wesley–Jessen System 2000 photokeratoscope. Contact Lens Forum 1976;1(7):37–45.

35. Doss JD, Hutson RL, Rowsey JJ, Brown R. Method for calculation of corneal profile and power distribution. Arch Ophthalmol 1981;99:1261–1265.

36. Roddy KC, Goss DA. Reliability of corneal topography measurements with the Corneascope and Comparator. Int Contact Lens Clin 1988;15:287–290.

37. Kuyama H, Kenji S, Setsuro M, Itoi M. A new photokeratometer for contact lens in clinic. J Jpn Contact Lens Soc 1979;21:80–84.

38. Villasenor RA, Motokazu I, Harris DF, Robin JB. Corneal topography and refractive surgery. Cornea 1983;2:323–331.

39. Maguire LJ, Singer DE, Klyce SD. Graphic presentation of computer-analyzed keratoscope photographs. Arch Ophthalmol 1987;105:223–230.

40. Dingeldein SA, Klyce SD. The topography of normal corneas. Arch Ophthalmol 1989;107:512–518.

41. Bibby MM, Townsley MG. Analysis and description of corneal shape. Contact Lens Forum 1976;1(8):27–35.

Ophthalmic Lasers

Linda J. Bass

INTRODUCTION

Definition

Laser is an acronym for *l*ight *a*mplification by *s*timulated *e*mission of *r*adiation. It is a source of coherent, monochromatic light that can be precisely focused and used to vaporize and cut tissue, with minimal bleeding, scarring, or patient morbidity. These features make the laser a useful clinical tool for ophthalmic surgery.

History

The first laser was produced by Dr. Theodore Maiman at Hughes Aircraft Company in 1960. This was a ruby crystal laser that produced a red light, with a wavelength of 694.3 nm. Ophthalmic experimentation of retinal photocoagulation began with animals in 1961. In 1962, Campbell and Zweng were the first to use a ruby laser for ophthalmic purposes on a human.[1]

The argon laser was first used for ophthalmic purposes by L'Esperance in 1965, and the first argon photocoagulation was performed on a human in February 1968. Ophthalmic argon lasers became commercially available in 1971. L'Esperance introduced the frequency-doubled neodymium:yttrium–aluminum–garnet (Nd:YAG) laser clinically, in 1971, and the krypton laser in 1972. Beckman introduced the continuous-wave neodymium:yttrium–aluminum–garnett (CW Nd:YAG) laser in 1973. Tunable dye lasers were introduced in the laboratory by L'Esperance in 1981. Also, in 1981, the Q-switched Nd:YAG laser was introduced by Frunkhauser and mode-locked Nd:YAG laser was introduced by Aron–Rosa.[1]

Excimer, the newest addition to clinical lasers, became commercially available in 1979, but was not used clinically until 1985. Its development continues, and it is presently under investigation in humans for ophthalmic use.[1]

A number of other lasers are currently undergoing laboratory investigation. These include helium–cadmium, helium–selenium, helium–neon, xenon, copper vapor, and gold vapor. It is hoped that these might lend themselves to clinical use in the future.

Clinical Use

Lasers are used clinically for a variety of conditions from treatment of external lid papillomas and age-related keratosis to photocoagulation of the retina and photovaporization of choroidal tumors. Certain lasers are better suited for specific procedures, depending upon the wavelength of the laser and the absorption characteristics of the target tissue. The desired tissue effect is also a factor.

Some common clinical ophthalmic uses of lasers are:

- *Posterior capsulotomies.* This procedure is performed to create an opening in the posterior lens capsule when secondary cataract formation occurs following extracapsular cataract extraction.
- *Photocoagulation of the retina.* Photocoagulation, the first ophthalmic use of lasers, continues to be a frequent procedure. Lasers are used to treat peripheral retinal disorders, such as retinal breaks, retinal detachments, as well as retinal and choroidal tumors. Lasers are also used to treat ocular vascular disease, in the cauterization of vessels in branch retinal vein and artery occlusion; sickle cell retinopathy; or for the treatment of choroidal neovascular membrane. Photocoagulation is also used extensively in the treatment of both proliferative and background diabetic retinopathy, specifically diabetic maculopathy.
- *Laser trabeculoplasty.* Laser trabeculoplasty is performed on open-angle glaucoma patients who are not controlled with maximum medical therapy. This is performed prior to filtration surgery.

- *Laser iridotomy.* Lasers are also used to create an opening in the iris when acute angle closure glaucoma appears imminent, is present, or has occurred in one eye, or when chronic angle closure glaucoma is present.

INSTRUMENTATION

Theory

A brief overview of the electromagnetic spectrum is necessary before discussing the principles of lasers. Electromagnetic waves exist in a wide range of wavelengths and contain both an electrical and a magnetic component. This range of wavelengths is called the *electromagnetic spectrum* (Fig. 42–1). Visible light, which is the most familiar part of the spectrum, ranges in wavelength from approximately 400 to 700 nm. Visible light, however, constitutes only a small portion of the entire electromagnetic spectrum, which extends from the very long wavelengths of radio, television, and radar waves, through microwaves, far and near infrared waves, visible light, the short-ultraviolet wavelengths and x-rays, to the very short wavelengths of gamma and cosmic rays. To date, clinical lasers use only a limited portion of the spectrum, from 10,600 nm (infrared) for the carbon dioxide (CO_2) laser to approximately 200 nm (ultraviolet) for the excimer laser.[2]

There is an inverse relationship between wavelength and frequency. Radiation of higher frequencies and shorter wavelengths have the most energy. Conversely, the lower frequencies or longer wavelengths have the least energy.

The activity within an atom is important in the production of light. Each atom comprises a positively charged nucleus that is orbited by negatively charged electrons. Each orbit is a different distance from the nucleus and has a fixed energy level. Supplying energy to the material, in the form of heat, can excite an atom. Increasing the temperature increases the kinetic energy of the electrons and boosts them to a higher energy level. Therefore, the orbital location of the electrons determines the energy level of the atoms.

Transition, which is the movement of electrons from orbit to orbit, changes the internal energy of the atom. According to quantum theory, the amounts of energy involved in these transitions are

considered as finite bundles or packets of energy called *quanta.* The quantum of light is termed a *photon.*[3]

Figure 42–2 represents a simplified energy level diagram of a hypothetical atom. This atom contains five distinct energy levels. E_0 designates the lowest energy level and is called the ground state. A ground-state atom cannot lose energy, but only absorb it. To move from the ground state to an excited state, say E_3, a photon, the energy of which is equal to ($E_3 - E_0$), must be absorbed by the atom. In this excited state, this unstable atom will spontaneously emit a photon of energy ($E_3 - E_0$) and return to the ground state. Each atom emits its photon on its own accord and independent of the other atoms. This results in spontaneous emission, producing energy or light that is neither coherent (in phase), directional, nor monochromatic (one wavelength).

The difference between spontaneous and stimulated emission of light was explained by Einstein, in 1917. He predicted that photon emission could be stimulated to occur before its natural time if the excited atom is struck by a photon of the same energy as the photon to be emitted. This would cause the atom to decay to a lower state, emitting a photon in the process. The emitted photon would have the same phase and wavelengths as the photon striking the atom. This original photon, instead of being absorbed, would continue on its path with the emitted photon adding to it. As this process is repeated over and over an amplified beam of photons is produced, all of which have the same wavelength and are in phase with each other. The light produced in this manner is both coherent and monochromatic, and the emission process is called *stimulated emission.*[2,4,5]

The system of atoms must contain an excess of atoms in high-energy states for this process to be sustained, because atoms in the low-energy states are more likely to absorb a striking photon than to stimulate the emission of one. When more atoms are in higher-energy levels than in the ground state, this is called a *population inversion.*[2,4] This situation is so alien from the normal state of atoms that the practical problems of producing a population inversion were not overcome until 1960, when Dr. Theodore Maiman produced the ruby laser at Hughes Aircraft Company.

A population inversion may be achieved by external excitation of the atoms by "pumping" them to higher orbits. Various sources, such as a flash lamp, electricity, or another laser may provide the energy for this. Atoms will begin to decay to lower excited levels,

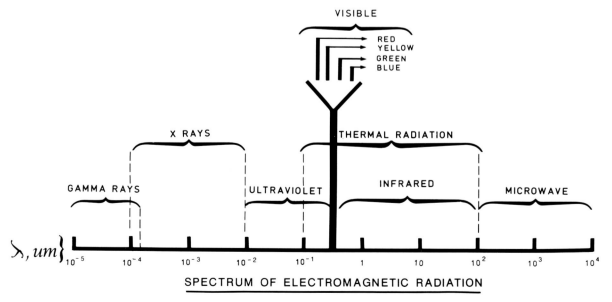

FIGURE 42–1. Diagrammatic representation of the electromagnetic spectrum. (From Bass LJ, Miller RG. Lasers: their function and clinical applications—Part I. South J Optom 1987;5(4):12, with permission)

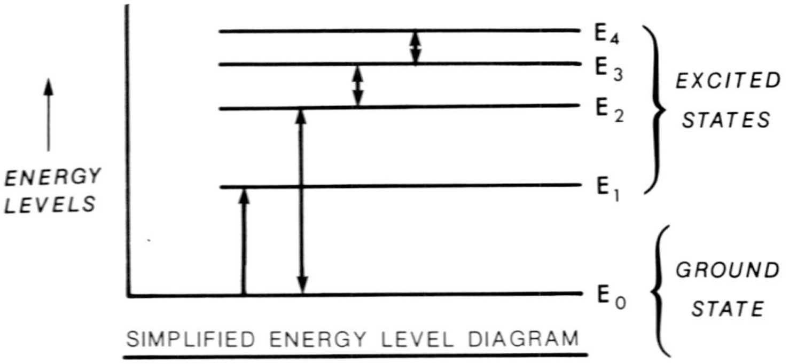

ENERGY
LEVELS

E_4
E_3 } *EXCITED*
E_2 } *STATES*

E_1

E_0 } *GROUND*
STATE

SIMPLIFIED ENERGY LEVEL DIAGRAM

FIGURE 42–2. Electron energy level diagram. (From Bass LJ, Miller RG. Lasers: their function and clinical applications—Part I. South J Optom 1987;5(4):12, with permission)

assuming a transitional state, once the population inversion is achieved. Some atoms will spontaneously emit photons and return to the ground state during these transitional states. These spontaneously emitted photons will collide with atoms in the transitional state, stimulating them to emit photons. A chain reaction of stimulation emission begins as these photons strike other atoms in the transitional state.

The basic components of a laser system are shown in Figure 42–3. To produce the population inversion and, thus, the lasing effect of stimulated emission, a lasing medium is used. The medium may be a liquid dye, a gas, a semiconductor material, or a synthetic crystal. Each medium produces its own unique wavelength. A ruby crystal was first used as a laser medium in 1960. Gaseous lasing mediums are frequently used and include carbon dioxide, helium–neon, and argon. Liquid dye lasers have the flexibility of being able to vary their wavelength output being "tunable" to a specific wavelength.

An excitation mechanism, or power source, provides the energy that "pumps" or excites the lasing medium into the population inversion. The type of power source depends upon the lasing medium. Electrical power is usually used for gas and semiconductor lasers. Optical power sources such as a flash lamp or another laser may be used with solid and liquid dye lasers.

The optical resonator or laser cavity consists of a hollow tube with mirrors at each end. The resonator contains the lasing medium. The lasing effect is amplified by reflecting the laser light back and forth through the lasing medium which stimulates additional photons. One of the mirrors is partially transmitting and allows a small amount of laser light to be transmitted at the wavelength of the laser.

When the power source is activated, power is introduced into the lasing medium, causing a population inversion. Some of the atoms in higher-energy levels spontaneously emit photons and drop to lower-energy states. These are incoherent photons, traveling in random directions, although at the laser wavelength. Those that move along the axis of the lasing medium strike other atoms, which stimulate emission of photons that are monochromatic and coherent. This beam is reflected back and forth through the lasing medium, stimulating emission of additional photons and amplifying the beam. Part of the beam is transmitted through the partly transmitting end-mirror, producing a bright, coherent, monochromatic laser beam that is easily focused with collimating lenses.

Duration of Laser Emission

There are four different modes of laser operation that affect the duration and power of laser emission.

A *continuous wave* (CW) laser is one in which the laser medium is continuously pumped, and laser light is continually emitted. Exposure is controlled by a shutter.

In a *pulsed* laser, the medium is pulse pumped, and the duration of emission corresponds to the duration of the pump pulse. This provides higher powers than continuous wave. Both continuous wave and pulsed lasers are free-running, meaning that the emission duration is controlled by the pump source only.

Q-switched lasers have an optical switch that provides a very

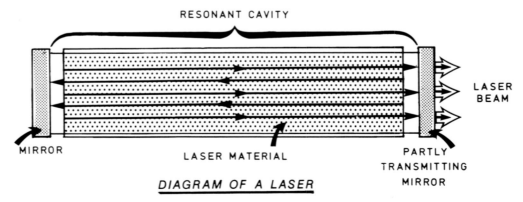

RESONANT CAVITY

LASER BEAM

MIRROR   LASER MATERIAL   PARTLY TRANSMITTING MIRROR

DIAGRAM OF A LASER

FIGURE 42–3. Basic components of a laser. (From Bass LJ, Miller RG. Lasers: their function and clinical applications—Part I. South J Optom 1987;5(4):13, with permission)

short pulse of emission at a high power. The pulse durations are shorter than 1 microsecond. An optical gate in the laser resonator prohibits laser action for a certain time. The active medium is pumped and stored during this time. When the switch is open, the stored energy is released at a higher peak power. This optical switch is called a quality switch and, thus, these lasers are referred to as Q-switched.

A *mode-locked* laser has an output of very short pulses of less than 1 nanosecond. A dye that is opaque for low irradiances prevents laser action. The longitudinal modes are brought into phase and added constructively until the dye is bleached. An intense short pulse is then released.[3,6]

Biologic Tissue Changes

Lasers produce permanent changes in the cells of biologic tissue. The types of changes that laser photons cause varies with the wavelength of the photon and the absorption characteristics of the target tissue. Lasers affect biologic tissues in five different ways: photodynamic changes, photocoagulation, photovaporization, photodisruption, and photoablation.[7–9]

Photodynamic changes occur when the tissue temperature is raised from 37°C (98.6°F) to 38°C (100.4°F).[8] This is used in conjunction with prior treatment of the tissue with a photosensitizing agent and is used primarily to treat tumors.[9,10]

Photocoagulation occurs when tissue temperature is raised from 37°C (98.6°F) to 65°C (149°F).[8,9] This results in thermal damage that causes denaturization of protein, which results in enzyme deactivation.[11] Photocoagulation causes four therapeutic changes in tissues: (1) scars, which cause tissue to bind or adhere; (2) tissue atrophy; (3) collagen or smooth-muscle contraction; and (4) blockage of blood vessels.

Photovaporization occurs when the tissue temperature is raised from 37°C (98.6°F) to over 100°C (212 F).[9,12] This results in the target tissue being converted to water vapor and smoke. This process is used to hemostatically incise tissue.[8]

Photodisruption occurs with an extremely high increase in tissue temperature from 37°C (98.6°F) to 20,000°C (36,032°F). This results from very high laser energy, which causes a transient shock wave. This causes a controlled microexplosion that results in torn tissue due to mechanical stress.[9,12]

Photoablative decomposition takes place when intramolecular bonds are broken by high-energy photons. The affected tissue disappears from the treated area without charring or heat production.[9,12]

COMMERCIALLY AVAILABLE INSTRUMENTS

Basic Design

Clinical lasers consist of an exciting medium, a laser medium, and a delivery system. Most generate large amounts of heat and require a cooling system of either air or water. The delivery system is the manner in which laser light is introduced to the patient. Types of delivery systems include free-hand surgery, slit lamp with a contact lens, fiberoptic, endoscopic, and endoscopic with mirrors.[2,11] Figure 42–4 shows the position of ophthalmic lasers in the electromagnetic spectrum. Clinical lasers are discussed in order of their clinical introduction.

Argon Laser

The argon laser is one of the most commonly used lasers in the United States today. This laser was first used clinically in 1968. It emits light from 457.9 to 524.7 nm in wavelength that is a blue-green light, although monochromatic green (514 nm) is usually used clinically. A choice in power density and spot sizes is available, which makes this a flexible laser that can be used to treat anterior as well as posterior structures of the eye. There are several delivery systems used for the argon laser. They include monocular indirect ophthalmoscopy, biomicroscopy (with or without a contact lens), and endophotocoagulation, which uses an intraocular probe to deliver laser light. Biomicroscopy is the most frequently used delivery system. An argon laser is shown in Figure 42–5.

The main advantage of argon laser photocoagulation over xenon-arc photocoagulation is that the surgeon is able to move the

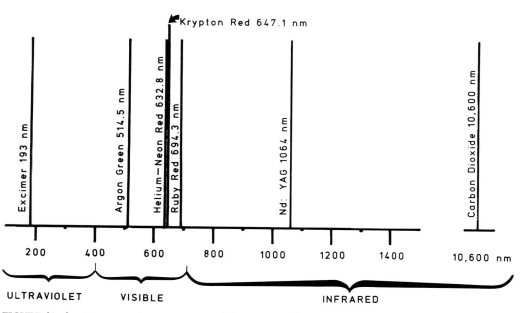

FIGURE 42–4. Diagrammatic representation of the position of laser wavelengths in the electromagnetic spectrum. (From Bass LJ. Lasers: their function and clinical applications—Part II. South J Optom 1988;6(1): 18, with permission)

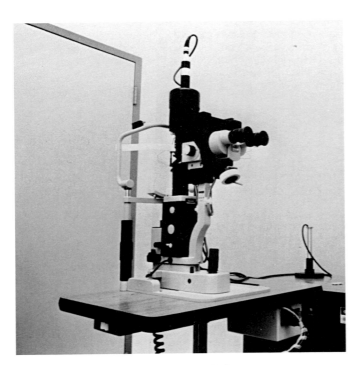

FIGURE 42–5. Coherent Argon Innova 920 laser.

light beam closer to the macula because of the much smaller spot size.[13]

The main disadvantage of the argon laser is that the presence of diffuse extensive hemorrhage in the superficial retinal layers or vitreous prevents its use. Since the argon wavelength is so well absorbed by the hemoglobin in the hemorrhage there is potential for thermal damage to the nerve fiber layer. The blue component of argon is also absorbed by xanthophyll pigment, which precludes its use in the macular area, as this would result in damage to the inner retina as well as the intentional damage to pigment epithelium and subretina. A large portion of the argon laser wavelength is also absorbed by the yellowing of an aging crystalline lens, preventing adequate retinal photocoagulation in the presence of dense cataracts.

As long as there is minimal superficial retinal hemorrhage, the argon laser may be routinely used clinically to treat diabetic retinopathy; sickle cell retinopathy; retinal breaks, tears, and detachments; choroidal neovascular membrane near the macula; central retinal vein occlusions; and branch retinal vein occlusions. It is also used to perform trabeculoplasties,[14] iris sphincterotomies, iridotomies, synechiotomies,[15] secondary membranectomies, and posterior capsulotomies.[16]

Krypton Laser

First used in 1972, the krypton laser produces beams of three different wavelengths: 521 nm, 568 nm, and 647 nm. Clinically, the last two are most frequently used. Krypton lasers use a slit lamp delivery system.

The yellow krypton laser beam (568.2 nm) is easily transmitted through nuclear sclerotic cataracts. It is highly absorbed by pigment epithelium and hemoglobin. Because of the high hemoglobin absorption, the yellow krypton laser is not useful in patients with vitreal and preretinal hemorrhage. This instrument is rarely used clinically.

Passing through the inner retina, the red krypton laser beam (647.1 nm) is absorbed primarily by the retinal pigment epithelium and choroid. Photocoagulation occurs at the level of the retinal pigment epithelium, Bruch's membrane, and the choroid. The tissue burns created with the krypton laser occur deeper in the choroid than those created with the argon beam. Because there is little absorption by hemoglobin, the red krypton laser is used successfully in the presence of retinal or vitreal hemorrhage.

The primary disadvantage of red krypton is the small amount of absorption occurring in the inner retinal layers. Therefore, it is not useful in the treatment of partial-thickness retinal tears and cysts, as the beam would be transmitted through these structures. Vitreoretinal disorders, such as proliferative diabetic retinopathy, with fibrous proliferation or neovascularization into the vitreous, are also treatable with red krypton.

Both yellow and red krypton are useful in areas around the foveola for the treatment of choroidal neovascular membrane, as there is little xanthophyll absorption.

Both yellow and red krypton lasers require a greater amount of electrical power than the argon laser to produce enough energy for clinically useful burns. This problem is being improved with advancing laser technology.[17]

Carbon Dioxide Laser

First used clinically in 1972, the carbon dioxide (CO_2) laser has a very long wavelength in the far infrared (10,600 nm) portion of the spectrum. Since this beam is out of the visible spectrum, it reacts differently with ocular tissues than other lasers. Photovaporization occurs in biologic tissues as a result of this laser, as opposed to photocoagulation with the visible spectrum lasers. Considered the best in operative surgery, the CO_2 laser is used primarily on soft tissue for excision and cutting. The CO_2 laser is quite useful in surgical procedures for which a large amount of bleeding is expected, as it is highly hemostatic and lymphostatic. These properties make it particularly useful in treating neovascular disorders and tumors.[12,18] Vaporization can be controlled; hence, tissue can be treated at selected depths, and wound healing is excellent with little scarring.

The CO_2 laser is used successfully in the treatment of such lid lesions as tumors and papilloma. It is also used to treat corneal neovascularization, pterygia, and conjunctival tumors.

Compared with visible spectrum lasers, the CO_2 laser is highly absorbed by the cornea. This limits intraocular use to the use of an intraocular probe.[19]

Neodymium: YAG Laser

The first Nd:YAG laser was in the free-running mode and was introduced in 1973. It was not until the high-powered Q-switched and mode-locked Nd:YAG lasers were introduced in 1980 and 1981, respectively, that a more widespread ophthalmic use was provided.

The Nd:YAG laser beam falls in the infrared portion of the electromagnetic spectrum with a wavelength of 1064 nm. This laser produces very short pulses of very high power light energy. YAG stands for yttrium–aluminum–garnet which is the crystal laser medium. As opposed to conventional lasers that depend upon absorption of the beam by a pigmented target tissue, the Nd:YAG functions differently in that it is used primarily on relatively transparent tissue. The intense power produced by the laser beam over a relatively small area ionizes the medium by stripping electrons from their nuclei. The medium is changed to a gaseous state of matter, called plasma, when the electrons are stripped. This causes a microexplosion within the tissue, causing vaporization and a transient shock wave, which can affect adjacent tissue. Surrounding ocular tissue is protected, since little energy transmits beyond the area of breakdown.[20–22]

This process of vaporization, plasma formation, and shock

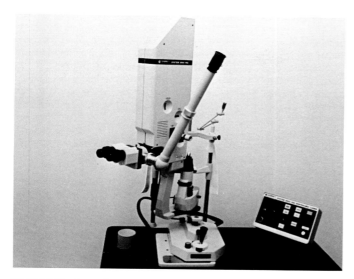

FIGURE 42–6. Coherent YAG 9900 laser.

waves causes photodisruption of biologic tissues and is responsible for the cutting action of the YAG laser.[20–22] This cutting process produces a popping sound and a bluish spark.[23]

The YAG laser uses primarily a slit lamp delivery system, although it sometimes is used with a hand-held contact lens. Since the wavelength of the Nd:YAG laser is out of the visible spectrum, a helium–neon (HeNe) laser, which produces a red beam (632.3 nm) is used in conjunction with the Nd:YAG laser to allow focusing.[20,24,25] Figure 42–6 shows a YAG laser mounted for use on a slit lamp.

The Nd:YAG laser is most commonly used to perform posterior capsulotomies when a secondary cataract forms on the posterior lens capsule after extracapsular cataract extraction. It is also used for numerous other procedures including iridotomies,* synechiotomies, anterior capsulotomies, and trabecular surgery.[24,25]

It has also been used to lyse vitreous strands trapped in postsurgical wounds and to lyse vitreous adhesions. It is felt that this reduces the severity and incidence of postsurgical cystoid macular edema.[26]

Compared with the argon laser, a much smaller percentage of radiation is absorbed by the retina. This causes more painful, deeper photocoagulation burns, and increases the chance of hemorrhage. The current sentiment is that there is little advantage in the use of the YAG over the argon laser for retinal photocoagulation.[27]

Dye Laser

The dye laser was developed by L'Esperance in 1979. This versatile laser is referred to as "tunable" because the surgeon can select the wavelength desired over a broad spectral range of 360 nm to 960 nm depending upon the dye used.[20,28]

The dyes, which are organic compounds dissolved in a solvent, are pumped optically by either a flash lamp or another laser to produce a population inversion. Currently, the most commonly used dyes are rhodamine 6G and DCM dyes. An argon laser is generally used to pump the dyes. The particular dye is squirted across the argon laser beam to produce the population inversion. The laser output is not very energy efficient, as only 25% to 30% of

---

* Although technically the suffix -*otomy* means to make an opening and -*ectomy* means to excise tissue the term irid*ectomy* has been used in the literature to describe this procedure.

the pumping power is produced. The selection of wavelength, or "tuning" is precisely accomplished with the use of a birefringent mirror. This mirror is rotated to allow only the desired wavelength of photons to resonate in the laser tube.[28]

Currently, three main wavelengths are being used. The yellow wavelength (560 nm) is used to treat discrete vascular lesions. The orange wavelength (590 to 600 nm) is used to treat choroidal neovascularization. The red wavelength (630 nm) is used to photocoagulate hemorrhagic choroid and retina, as the absorption by hemoglobin is negligible, and primary absorption takes place by the choroidal pigment and the retinal pigment epithelium.[28,29]

The dye laser is also being used to treat ocular tumors. Referred to as *photodynamic therapy,* in this procedure a tumor is treated with a photosensitizing agent, dihematoporphyrin. This agent is tumor-specific in that it is absorbed more by the tumor than by surrounding tissue. The photosensitizing agent will selectively absorb the laser light at a wavelength of about 630 nm.[20,28]

The slit lamp delivery system is used with a dye laser. The main disadvantage is that it is difficult to maintain laser alignment and the fluid level of the dyes. The versatility of this laser can allow it to take the place of all other lasers currently used for photocoagulation.[28]

Excimer Laser

First used on the cornea by Trokel in 1983, the excimer laser is currently investigational. The name excimer is a contraction of "excited dimer."[3] This term indicates any diatomic molecule in which the atoms are not bound in the ground state, but are bound in the excited state. The two excited atoms are drawn together to form a stable molecule. A population inversion occurs as soon as the excited molecules are formed. The most popular excimer lasers are produced by combining a noble gas, such as argon, krypton, or xenon, with a halogen, such as fluoride or chloride. These lasers yield a beam of very short wavelength (157 to 351 nm) and extremely high energy. The pulses from the excimer are of extremely short duration and last between 12 and 15 nanoseconds. Because of this short duration there is limited time for heat transfer to the surrounding tissue.[30] The target tissue disappears by a process called photoablative decomposition or ablative photodecomposition.[12,20,31] It is so precise that a single human cell can be divided. There is no charring or heat dispersion, nor is there a microexplosion.

The excimer laser is currently being investigated for use in a new technique called "photorefractive keratectomy." Also referred to as "corneal sculpting," this technique reshapes the cornea to eliminate myopia, hyperopia, or astigmatism.[30,32,33] It is also being investigated for trephination in penetrating keratoplasty,[34] for lamellar keratoplasty,[35] epikeratophakia,[36] and trabeculoplasty.

The argon–fluoride excimer laser, which produces a far-ultraviolet wavelength of 193 nm, has been found to be the most suitable for corneal incisions. The exact mechanism that occurs to ablate the target tissue is controversial and not clearly understood. One theory is that there are very fast thermal events taking place. The second theory is that the high-energy photons fracture molecules into smaller pieces that are expelled at supersonic speeds as gaseous ablation plumes, leaving a crater. It is also felt that there might be a combination of heat and the ablation process occurring.[34,37]

One disadvantage of the excimer laser is that special delivery systems must be used. The invisible nature of the far-ultraviolet light does not lend itself to use with fiberoptics. A beam delivery system is used in which different types of optical masks are used to control the amounts and location of tissue to be ablated. The most promising delivery system is a recent development by Taunton Technologies, Inc., which consists of rotating aperture wheels depicted diagrammatically in Figures 42–7 and 42–8.[30,32] A computer

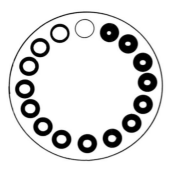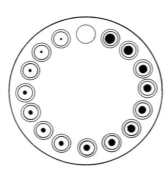

FIGURE 42–7. Diagram of the aperture wheels used to correct spherical refractive error with the excimer laser. The wheel on the left would enable the cornea to be ablated more deeply centrally than peripherally, thus correcting for myopia. The wheel on the right would enable more ablation of the peripheral cornea to correct for hyperopia. (From L'Esperance FA. Ophthalmic lasers, 3rd ed. St Louis: CV Mosby Co, 1989:898–899, with permission)

aids the clinician in determining the amount of tissue to be ablated and provides feedback on the quality of the beam during the procedure. A digital keratoscope measures corneal topography before and after the procedure. A HeNe laser is incorporated into the beam for focusing, since the excimer is out of the visible spectrum.[32]

Investigational trials have produced results far superior to those obtained with a diamond knife or trephine. Very precise cuts are produced, with minimal damage to neighboring tissue.[30,32,38] After laser keratotomy, the cornea has been shown to remain transparent with reepithelialization occurring within 60 to 72 hours.[32] The excimer has a limited penetration depth, which prevents complications from penetrating to the deeper corneal stroma, Descemet's, or endothelium.

Disadvantages, however, remain with this investigational instrument. The eye must be totally stabilized for uniform corneal incisions. Even eye movements from respiration and choroidal pulsation must be taken into account.[30,32] Systems are being developed to couple these eye movements with the delivery system. Additionally, it is common knowledge that ultraviolet light can be carcinogenic or mutagenic. It is as yet unknown what long-term effects the excimer laser light will have on the DNA of corneal cells.[39]

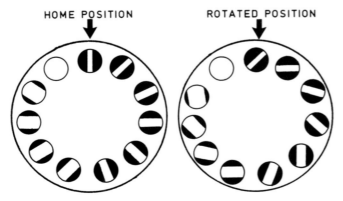

HOME POSITION   ROTATED POSITION

FIGURE 42–8. Diagram of the aperture wheel used to correct for astigmatism. (From L'Esperance FA. Ophthalmic lasers, 3rd ed. St Louis: CV Mosby Co, 1989;899, with permission)

CLINICAL PROCEDURE

For ophthalmic procedures in which the laser is used with a slit lamp delivery system, topical anesthesia is usually adequate. The clinician and the patient should be seated comfortably.

Four common clinical procedures will be discussed. They are argon laser trabeculoplasty, laser iridotomy, YAG laser posterior capsulotomy, and retinal photocoagulation.

Argon Laser Trabeculoplasty

Since introduced by Wise and Wittner in 1976,[40] argon laser trabeculoplasty (ALT) or laser trabeculoplasty (LTP) has become an accepted stage of open-angle glaucoma therapy for patients whose pressure cannot be controlled by maximum medical therapy. It is considered to be the next step before filtration surgery.[41,42] The mechanism by which this procedure lowers intraocular pressure is uncertain, although it is postulated that the thermal burns shrink the tissue of the trabecular meshwork and, thereby, open trabecular spaces.[41,42]

Patients are given apraclonidine (Iopidine) topically 1 hour before the procedure. This has been found to help decrease the postlaser rise in intraocular pressure (IOP) associated with laser treatment of the iris or trabecular area,[41] although some clinicians still use a β-blocker or carbonic anhydrase inhibitor instead. A topical anesthetic, such as proparacaine, is applied to both eyes at the time of the procedure. The argon laser, with a slit lamp delivery system, is used in conjunction with a Goldmann three-mirror contact lens that has an antireflection coating. The clinical protocol used is a 50-μm spot size of 0.1-second duration, with about 1000 milliwatts (mW) of power. The operator will start at approximately 800 mW and gradually increase power until blanching is observed. The desired end point is blanching or small bubble formation in the trabecular meshwork. If a large bubble is seen or if rupture of the trabecular meshwork is observed, then the power is too high. The objective of this procedure is to leave small superficial scars, not to penetrate the meshwork. Generally, 100 burns are made 360° around the trabeculum. Currently, it is recommended the clinician perform two 180° sessions of 50 burns each. It is felt that this decreases the acute rise in IOP.[41–43]

Laser trabeculoplasty can be used on patients with primary or secondary open-angle glaucoma who are not controlled with maximum medical therapy. It is most effective in patients with exfoliative glaucoma and least effective in young glaucoma patients. It is not as effective following cataract extraction and, therefore, should be performed before any incipient cataract surgery.[42] Although some doctors are resorting to LTP before reaching maximum medical therapy, such as before administration of carbonic anhydrase inhibitors or before any medical therapy at all, caution is advised because the long-term effects of LTP are still unknown. This procedure has been reported to have a 70% to 75% success rate of clinically significant improvement.[43,44] Postoperatively lowering of IOP between 6 and 10 mmHg is not necessarily immediate, but occurs within 4 to 5 weeks. The results of lower IOP tend to continue for several years in most patients, although some will develop an increase in IOP in 6 months. After 5 years, 30% to 60% of those treated continue to have well-controlled IOP.[43,44]

Mild complications are associated with LTP. The acute rise in IOP is the most common development. It is recommended that IOP be monitored closely for several hours after LTP and also for several weeks following the procedure. A rise in pressure is usually controllable with medical therapy. The use of apraclonidine (Iopidine) and splitting the laser treatment into two sessions have significantly decreased the incidence of IOP rise. Less common complications include uveitis, peripheral anterior synechiae, corneal burns, and hyphema.[2,42]

Laser Iridotomy

Laser iridotomies are currently the treatment of choice for all forms of angle closure glaucoma in which pupillary block is suspected to be the cause. It should also be used prophylactically when narrow occludable angles exist or when a fellow eye has undergone an acute angle closure attack.[42] As in argon laser trabeculoplasty, apraclonidine or a β-blocker is administered topically 1 hour before the procedure. A carbonic anhydrase inhibitor may also be used before treatment. To thin the iris stroma, pilocarpine, 4%, is instilled topically to induce miosis. A topical ocular anesthetic (proparacaine; 0.5%) is instilled, and an antireflective-coated contact lens, such as the Abraham lens, is inserted in the eye. A slit lamp delivery system is employed. A spot is chosen approximately 3 mm away from the iris root; an iris crypt is preferable, as the stroma will be thinner and easier to penetrate in the crypt area. The 11-o'clock or 1-o'clock position under the superior lid is usually chosen, since these sites are normally hidden by the lid. Some procedures employ the use of contraction burns or stretch burns surrounding the area to be penetrated. These are lower-power, larger–spot-sized burns that will stretch the tissue. Power, spot size, and duration will vary, depending upon the color of the iris. The spot size used is generally 50 μm of a 0.1- or 0.2-second duration, with between 600 and 1200 mW of power. Consecutive short blasts are delivered to the exact same location while the depression gradually increases. When the posterior pigment epithelial layer is reached, a release of pigment, referred to as a "smoke signal," will be noted. This indicates that penetration is nearly complete. Iris transillumination and careful slit lamp examination allow the surgeon to determine when penetration is achieved.[41-43] An example of argon laser iridotomy is seen in Figure 42–9.

As with LTP, an acute rise in IOP may occur following the procedure. A second drop of apraclonidine is given to help decrease the IOP.

Pressure should be checked 1 to 2 hours after the iridotomy, and increased pressure should be treated medically. Baseline IOPs usually return within 24 hours. Ocular steroids, such as fluoromethalone, may be used for several days following the procedure. Patency of the iridotomy is monitored and, occasionally, retreat-

ment is necessary if the opening becomes blocked with pigment.[41-43]

Other complications of the procedure include pupillary distortion, monocular diplopia and glare, iritis, hemorrhage, and lenticular opacities.

Frequently, argon iridotomy is difficult in patients with blue irides due to the lack of pigment to absorb the laser light. In the event that argon iridotomy is not successful, Nd:YAG laser, which is nonthermal may be used. Frequently, only one dose of YAG laser energy is necessary to penetrate the iris. There is a disadvantage in the use of the YAG laser, in that there is no hemostasis, since there is no thermal coagulation. A self-limiting hemorrhage from the iridotomy site is noted in about one-third of the cases. There is also an increased chance of damage to the crystalline lens. Little is currently known about the long-term effects of YAG iridotomies. For these reasons, it has historically been recommended that YAG laser treatment be reserved for situations for which argon has failed.[43,45] However, it appears that the YAG has gained favor as the instrument of first choice in recent years.[46-48] Laser iridotomies have the advantage of being simple, quick, and noninvasive, when compared with intraocular surgical iridotomies.

Nd:YAG Posterior Capsulotomy

With the rise in popularity of extracapsular cataract extraction with "in-the-bag" placement of posterior chamber intraocular lenses, YAG posterior capsulotomy (YPC) has become a commonplace procedure. As illustrated in Figure 42–10, secondary opacification of the posterior capsule following extracapsular cataract extraction occurs frequently, causing a gradual decrease in vision and an increase in glare. Before the advent of YAG laser, surgical discission of the capsule was performed.[23-45] The YAG laser permits a noninvasive means of performing a capsulotomy without the risks of endophthalmitis or other vision-threatening complications. Figure 42–11 shows an area of opacification after a YAG laser capsulotomy. Capsulotomies are indicated when significant blurred vision or glare is affecting the patient's life-style or if the opacification precludes an imperative view of the fundus, such as in diabetic retinopathy, age-related maculopathy, and other retinal disease. The YAG laser is preferable over visible spectrum laser

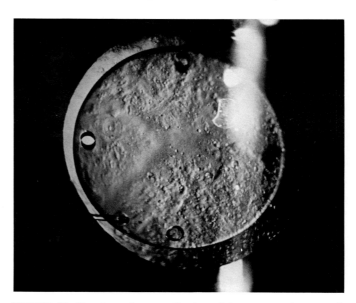

FIGURE 42–10. Secondary opacification of the posterior lens capsule following an extracapsular cataract extraction.

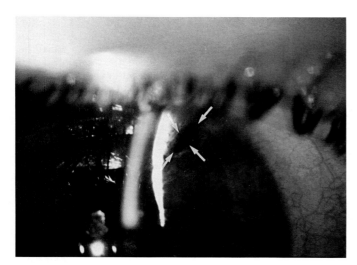

FIGURE 42–9. Argon laser iridectomy.

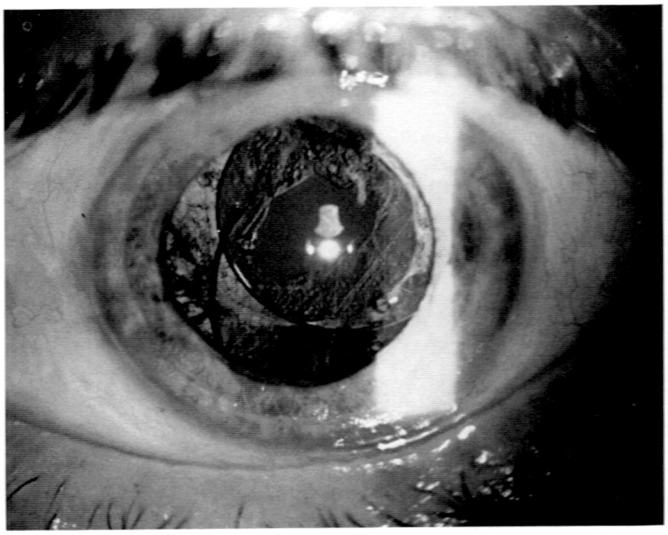

FIGURE 42–11. YAG laser posterior capsulotomy.

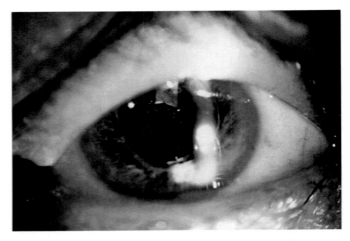

FIGURE 42–12. Nicks in the intraocular lens implant, following YAG laser posterior capsulotomy.

because the opacified area is relatively unpigmented and does not adequately absorb thermal lasers.

A slit lamp delivery system is used in conjunction with a contact lens. A topical anesthetic, such as proparacaine, is used preceding the procedure. Apraclonidine is also being used 1 hour before YPC surgery to decrease the posttreatment increase in IOP.[49] A Q-switched Nd:YAG laser is used, with a pulse energy starting at about 0.5 millijoules (mJ) to 4 mJ, not to exceed 5 mJ. The laser energy will be scattered by any opacities in the media, making a clear view necessary.[41,45]

Two procedures may be used to create capsule rupture. They are the small-pupil or the large-pupil procedure. The small-pupil procedure is performed on an undilated pupil. The illumination arm of the slit lamp is placed at an oblique angle, with decreased illumination intensity to prevent pupillary constriction. Generally, laser blasts are made in a linear configuration, starting vertically and then proceeding horizontally. This procedure has the advantage of requiring fewer laser blasts while preserving the hyaloid face. The disadvantage is that, although visual acuity will be improved, fundus examination will not be enhanced. Also, focusing is more difficult, and nicking of the intraocular lens is more likely to occur.[45]

In the large-pupil procedure, the pupil is maximally dilated. The linear method of blasts may also be used, but frequently a circular pattern is used starting superiorly and continuing for 360°. This procedure has the advantage of a larger opening, which makes fundus examination easier. The disadvantages are that it takes longer, the hyaloid face is frequently disturbed, and, since more capsule material is released, theoretically, the chance of postsurgical increase in IOP will be greater.[45]

Increase in IOP, the major postsurgical complication with YPC, reaches its peak within the first 4 postsurgical hours. The average increase is about 15 mmHg. This pressure rise can be treated medically and should be monitored closely following YPC.[20,41,45,49]

As shown in Figure 42–12, nicks will occur in the intraocular lens. The denser the membrane and the closer the membrane to the intraocular lens, the more likely damage is to occur. This is generally of no consequence, as long as there are not excessive nicks in the central part of the lens. Although no longer implanted, glass intraocular lenses may fracture due to laser irradiation, and YPC should not be attempted in their presence.[20,41]

Commonly, transient uveitis will occur after YPC surgery, but this usually resolves within 24 hours. Retinal detachment has been reported related to YPC, with a 1% incidence, but a causal relationship has not been proved.[41,50]

Retinal Photocoagulation

Laser photocoagulation is used to treat a wide range of retinal conditions. The effect of the laser depends upon the wavelength of laser being used and the part of the retina being targeted. Laser wavelengths can be chosen to match the absorptive characteristics of a particular part of the retina. A wavelength must be selected that transmits well through the ocular media, but is absorbed by the appropriate retinal tissue.

Melanin, contained within the retinal pigment epithelium (RPE), has good absorption properties and absorbs wavelengths from 400 to 700 nm. Therefore, visible light affects the RPE fairly equally, although photocoagulation is deeper in the retina as the wavelength increases. The xanthophyll pigment of the macula absorbs blue light well, but absorbs little yellow and red light; therefore, the red and yellow wavelengths are best suited to treat a choroidal neovascular membrane around the fovea. Hemoglobin absorbs all but red light, which makes this wavelength useful in the presence of hemorrhage, whereas yellow light passes well through cataracts and is preferable in their presence.[2,7,9]

The amount of heat produced by a laser burn is affected by three factors: spot size, power, and duration of the beam. A diverging lens in front of the beam is used to increase the spot size.[51] This results in the same amount of energy being applied over a larger area. Therefore, to achieve the same thermal effects, the power of the laser must be increased as the spot size is increased. The clinician will start with a low-power setting and gradually increase the power until test spots have the proper appearance.[51,52]

Laser photocoagulation can treat many ocular conditions, including retinal tears, retinal detachment, and rubeosis irides. The National Eye Institute sponsored Senile Macular Degeneration Study (SMDS) and Ocular Histoplasmosis Study (OHS) demonstrate that the risk of severe visual loss from choroidal neovascular membrane is reduced with argon photocoagulation if the membrane is symptomatic and greater than 200 μm from the center of the foveal avascular zone.[53,54] One of the most important uses of laser photocoagulation is in the treatment of diabetic retinopathy. Since the Diabetic Retinopathy Study (DRS) of the 1970s, pan-

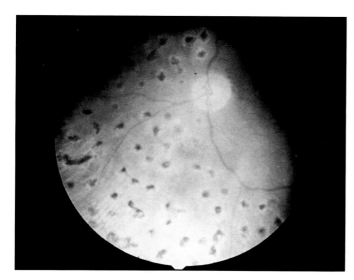

FIGURE 42–13. Panretinal photocoagulation of the retina.

retinal photocoagulation has become accepted as the standard treatment of proliferative diabetic retinopathy, which is characterized by neovascularization of the disc (NVD) or neovascularization elsewhere in the retina (NVE).[55]

Panretinal photocoagulation (PRP), as seen in Figure 42–13, uses a slit lamp delivery system with argon laser and a Goldmann three-mirror contact lens. Topical anesthetic is used in both eyes before treatment. The procedure is carried out in three to six stages. Each stage is separated by 2 to 7 days. Stages I and II are performed in the posterior pole. Spot sizes are 100 to 200 μm in diameter, with exposures of 0.05 to 0.2 second, with power from 100 to 400 mW. Coagulation sites are gradually increased in size to 500 μm as burns become more peripheral. The burns are about 0.5 coagulation diameter away from each other in the posterior pole. Stages III through VI treat the midperipheral and peripheral zones of the retina. The diameter of the burns is 200 to 500 μm with 400 to 800 mW of power, at 0.05 to 0.2 second exposure. They are made 0.5 to 0.75 coagulation diameter apart and are made as far peripheral as possible. Approximately 1500 to 2500 burns are made with a 20% to 30% destruction of retinal surface.[56]

The National Eye Institute sponsored Early Treatment Diabetic Retinopathy Study (ETDRS) has shown that risk of vision loss from "clinically significant" macular edema can be significantly decreased with focal laser treatment.[42,57,58] The following criteria are used to define *clinically significant macular edema:* (1) retinal thickening at or within 500 μm from the center of macula; (2) hard exudates at or within 500 μm from the center of the macula, if adjacent retinal thickening is present; and (3) a zone of retinal thickening 1-disc area or larger situated within 1-disc diameter of the center of the macula.[56–58]

Direct focal laser is performed on treatable lesions, which include microaneurysms, focal leaks, intraretinal microvascular abnormalities (IRMA), or a thickened vascular zone. The objective of treatment is the closure of the leak. Spot sizes of 50 to 100 μm are usually used, with exposure time of less than 0.1 second at power intensities of 200 to 300 mW.[57,58]

Diffuse macular edema, where no discrete treatable lesions are identified, is treated with grid-pattern photocoagulation. The area of macular edema is burned with a pattern of spots 50 to 200 μm in size with one-burn width between burns. The grid is not placed within 500 μm of the macula or disc margin. Medium laser intensity is used. Treatment is more successful before vision loss is

too great, obtaining better results if laser is done early even in 20/20 eyes.[57,58]

Proper explanation to the patient about retinal laser surgery is important. False expectations about the outcome of laser surgery often result in disappointed patients. They must be prepared that, at best, current visual acuity will be maintained, but normally not improved. In spite of laser surgery, their disease may progress and vision may continue to decrease. Pain may be experienced for several hours after the procedure. Scotomas, constricted visual fields, delayed dark adaptation, and color vision defects may also result.[52]

CLINICAL IMPLICATIONS

The use of ophthalmic lasers is opening many new avenues of treatment of ocular abnormalities. The clinician should be familiar with the use of lasers to ensure "state-of-the-art" care for his or her patients. This is a rapidly changing field, and many new lasers are currently under investigation for ophthalmic use, including metal vapor lasers, such as gold and copper.[12]

Lasers are not without their risks. Accidental injury by the laser beam may occur to the patient or clinician. The wrong tissue may be radiated or the correct tissue may be overradiated. As a result of the high electrical voltages needed to power lasers an electrical hazard also exists.

Most hospitals establish strict guidelines by a laser safety committee to prevent inadvertent injury. It is recommended that the operator and any observer wear safety glasses. Reflective surgical instruments and shiny objects should be removed from the area and windows should be blackened to protect passersby.[59]

REFERENCES

1. L'Esperance FA. Historical aspects of ophthalmic lasers. In: L'Esperance FA, ed. Ophthalmic lasers, 3rd ed. St Louis: CV Mosby Co, 1989:13–32.
2. Bass LJ, Miller RG. Lasers: their function and clinical applications—Part I. South J Optom 1987;5(4):11–14.
3. Vassiliadis A. Laser sources and ocular effects. In: L'Esperance FA, ed. Ophthalmic lasers, 3rd ed. St Louis: CV Mosby Co, 1989:33–60.
4. Huether SE. How lasers work. AORN J 1983;38:207–216.
5. Burroughs W. A new form of light. In: Burroughs W. Understanding science—lasers. New York: Warwick Press, 1982:11–18.
6. Loertscher H, Rol P. Basic physics of neodymium:YAG laser. In: Klapper RM, ed. Neodymium:YAG laser microsurgery: fundamental principles and clinical applications. Boston: Little, Brown & Co, 1985:1–14.
7. Mainster MA. Laser light, interactions, and clinical systems. IN: L'Esperance FA, ed. Ophthalmic lasers, 3rd ed. St Louis: CV Mosby Co, 1989:61–77.
8. Boraiko AA, ed. The laser: "a splendid light." Nat Geogr 1984;165:335–363.
9. Mainster MA. Finding your way in the photoforest: laser effects for clinicians. Ophthalmology 1984;91:886–888.
10. Goth PR, Fry SM. The Nd:YAG laser in ophthalmology. In: Joffe SN, ed. Neodymium:YAG laser in medicine and surgery. New York: Elsevier, 1983:150–162.
11. Schawlow AL. Lasers and their light. In: Zweng HC, Little HL, Peabody RR. Laser photocoagulation and retinal angiography. St Louis: CV Mosby Co, 1969:3–14.
12. L'Esperance FA. Introduction. In: L'Esperance FA, ed. Ophthalmic lasers, 3rd ed. St Louis: CV Mosby Co, 1989:1–10.
13. Morse PH. Photocoagulation. In: Duane TD, Jaeger EA, eds. Clinical ophthalmology. Philadelphia: JB Lippincott, 1989;5:1–9.
14. Yablonski ME, Cook DJ, Gray J. A fluorophotometric study of the effect of argon laser trabeculoplasty on aqueous humor dynamics. Am J Ophthalmol 1985;99:579–582.
15. Wise JB. Iris spincterotomy, iridotomy, and synechiotomy by linear incision with the argon laser. Ophthalmology 1985;92:641–645.
16. Lunde MW. Capsulectomy and membranectomy with the argon laser. Am J Ophthalmol 1983;95:94–97.

17. L'Esperance FA. Krypton laser. In: L'Esperance FA, ed. Ophthalmic lasers, 3rd ed. St Louis: CV Mosby Co, 1989:225–248.
18. Qin J. Medical laser instrumentation—from a medical doctor's point of view. In: Atsumi K, ed. New frontiers in laser medicine and surgery. New York: Elsevier, 1983:59–67.
19. L'Esperance FA. Carbon dioxide laser. In: L'Esperance FA, ed. Ophthalmic lasers, 3rd ed. St Louis: CV Mosby Co, 1989:751–780.
20. Bass LJ. Lasers: their function and clinical applications—Part II. South J Optom 1988;6(1):17–21.
21. Goth PR. The Nd:YAG laser in ophthalmology—a review. In: Joffe SN, ed. Neodymium:YAG laser in medicine and surgery. New York: Elsevier, 1983:150–162.
22. Reese BL. Uses of Nd:YAG laser in the anterior segment. South J Optom 1984;2:32–34.
23. Axt JC. Nd:YAG laser posterior capsulotomy: a clinical study. Am J Optom Physiol Opt 1985;62:173–187.
24. Belcher CD, Mainster MA, Buzney SM. Current status of neodymium:YAG laser photodisruptors in ophthalmology–Part II. Ann Opthalmol 1983;15:1097–1099.
25. Katzen LE, Fleischman JA, Trokel SL. The YAG laser: an American experience. J Am Intraocul Implant Soc 1983;9:151–156.
26. Katzen LE, Fleischman JA, Trokel SL. YAG laser treatment of cystoid macular edema. Am J Ophthalmol 1983;95:589–592.
27. Mainster MA, Sliney DH, Belcher CD, et al. Laser photodisruptors—damage mechanisms, instrument design and safety. Ophthalmology 1983;90:973–991.
28. L'Esperance FA. Tunable organic dye laser. In: L'Esperance FA, ed. Ophthalmic lasers, 3rd ed. St Louis: CV Mosby Co, 1989:249–287.
29. Smiddy WE, Patz A, Quigley HA, et al. Histopathology of the effects of tunable dye laser on monkey retina. Ophthalmology 1988;95:956–963.
30. L'Esperance FA, Warner JW, Telfair WB, et al. Excimer laser instrumentation and technique for human corneal surgery. Arch Ophthalmol 1989;107:131–139.
31. Puliafito CA, Stern D, Krueger RR, et al. High-speed photography of excimer laser ablation of the cornea. Arch Ophthalmol 1987;105:1255–1259.
32. L'Esperance RA. Excimer laser. In: L'Esperance FA, ed. Ophthalmic lasers, 3rd ed. St Louis: CV Mosby Co, 1989:887–918.
33. Aron-Rosa DS, Boerner CF, Bath P, et al. Corneal wound after excimer laser keratotomy in a human eye. Am J Ophthalmol 1987;103:454–464.
34. Serdarevic ON, Khalil H, Gribomont A, et al. Excimer laser trephination in penetrating keratoplasty. Ophthalmology 1988;95:493–505.
35. Shimon G, Slomovic A, Jares T. Excimer laser—processed donor corneal lenticles for lamellar keratoplasty. Am J Ophthalmol 1989;107:45–51.
36. Lieurance R, Patel AC, Wan WL, et al. Excimer laser cut lenticules for eipikeratophakia. Am J Ophthalmol 1987;103:475–476.
37. Bende T, Seiler T, Wollensak J. Side effects in excimer corneal surgery. Graefe's Arch Clin Exp Ophthalmol 1988;266:277–280.
38. Kerr–Muir MG, Trokel SL, Marshall J, et al. Ultrastructural comparison of conventional surgical and argon fluoride excimer laser keratectomy. Am J Ophthalmol 1987;103:448–453.
39. Seiler T, Bende T, Winkler K, et al. Side effects in excimer corneal surgery. Graefe's Arch Clin Exp Ophthalmol 1988;226:273–276.
40. Wise JB, Wittner SL. Argon laser therapy for open angle glaucoma: a pilot study. Arch Ophthalmol 1976;94:61–64.
41. Ritch R, Solomon IS. Laser treatment of glaucoma. In: L'Esperance FA, ed. Ophthalmic lasers, 3rd ed. St Louis: CV Mosby Co, 1989:650–748.
42. Epstein DL. Chandler and Grant's glaucoma, 3rd ed. Philadelphia: Lea & Febiger, 1986:104–125.
43. Spaeth GL. Ophthalmic surgery—principles and practice. Philadelphia: WB Saunders Co, 1982:215–357.
44. Shingleton PF, Richter CU, Bellows AR, et al. Long-term efficacy of argon laser trabeculoplasty. Ophthalmology 1987;94:1513–1518.
45. Deutsch TA, Goldbery MF. Neodymium:YAG laser capsulotomy. In: Klapper RM, ed. Neodymium:YAG laser microsurgery: fundamental principles and clinical applications. Boston: Little, Brown & Co, 1985:87–100.
46. Robin AL, Pollack IP. Q-switched neodymium-YAG laser iridotomy in patients in whom the argon laser fails. Arch Ophthalmol 1986;104:531–535.
47. Master MR, Schwartz LW, Spaeth Gal, et al. Laser iridectomy. A controlled study comparing argon and neodymium:YAG ophthalmology 1986;93:20–24.
48. Priore LVD, Robin AL, Pollack IP. Neodymium:YAG and argon laser iridotomy. Long-term follow-up in a prospective, randomized clinical trial. Ophthalmology 1988;95:1207–1211.
49. Pollak IP, Brown RH, Crandall AS, et al. Prevention of the rise in intraocular pressure following neodymium:YAG posterior capsulotomy using topical 1% apraclonidine. Arch Ophthalmol 1988;106:754–757.
50. Leff SR, Welch JC, Tasman W. Rhegmatogenous retinal detachment YAG laser posterior capsulotomy. Ophthalmology 1987;94:1222–1225.
51. L'Esperance FA. Technical considerations for ocular photocoagulation. In: L'Esperance FA, ed. Ophthalmic lasers, 3rd ed. St Louis: CV Mosby Co, 1989:78–112.
52. Constable IJ, Ming AI. Laser—its clinical uses in eye diseases. New York: Churchill–Livingstone, 1981:28–37.
53. Macular Photocoagulation Study Group. Argon laser photocoagulation for senile macular degeneration: results of a randomized clinical trial. Arch Ophthalmol 1982;100:912–918.
54. Macular Photocoagulation Study Group. Argon laser photocoagulation for ocular histoplasmosis: results of a randomized clinical trial. Arch Ophthalmol 1983;101:1347–1357.
55. Cavallerano J. Clinical considerations in the management of diabetic retinopathy. J Am Optom Assoc 1988;59:855–861.
56. L'Esperance FA. Diabetic retinopathy. In: L'Esperance FA, ed. Ophthalmic lasers, 3rd ed. St Louis: CV Mosby Co, 1989:347–424.
57. Early Treatment Diabetic Retinopathy Study Research Group. Photocoagulation for diabetic macular edema. Early Treatment Diabetic Retinopathy Study report Number 1. Arch Ophthalmol 1985;103:1796–1806.
58. Early Treatment Diabetic Retinopathy Study Research Group. Treatment techniques and clinical guidelines for photocoagulation of diabetic macular edema. Early Treatment Diabetic Retinopathy Study report Number 2. Ophthalmology 1987;94:761–774.
59. Polanyi TG. The physics and basic instrumentation of surgery with lasers. In: Atsumi K, ed. New frontiers in laser medicine and surgery. New York: Elsevier, 1983:49–58.

Eyelid Procedures

Jimmy D. Bartlett

INTRODUCTION

Definition

The care of eyelid disease by the optometrist often entails use of several procedures that are easily mastered. Techniques used to evaluate the lid structure are discussed in Chapters 7 and 22; this chapter emphasizes three procedures: (1) epilation, or eyelash removal in cases of trichiasis; (2) eyelid scrubs used to treat blepharitis; and (3) meibomian gland expression or massage, used to manage meibomianitis and other forms of meibomian gland dysfunction. Epilation involves the simple removal of one or more eyelashes with commercially available cilia forceps. Eyelid scrubs entail commercially available packaged materials for gently debriding the eyelash margin of debris and other inflammatory products associated with blepharitis. Meibomian gland massage involves the manual expression of meibomian gland contents, either as an office procedure or as a home remedy.

History

The primary care of eyelid disease has often included home remedies such as boric acid soaks. It is difficult, therefore, to ascribe a definitive date to the development of eyelid procedures performed by the primary care clinician. The treatment of blepharitis, for example, has, for many years, involved scrubbing of the eyelid margin using commercially available baby shampoos, recommended because of their mildness on eyelid tissues. In 1987, however, I-Scrub became the first commercially available eyelid cleanser for use directly on eyelid tissue.[1] The advent of such eyelid cleansers has improved the efficiency of blepharitis treatment by combining commercial availability with an effective mode of administration.

Clinical Use

Epilation is used to manually remove eyelashes that impinge on the ocular surface, creating irritation and sometimes substantial ocular injury. Although some patients can self-administer the procedure for offending lashes, the technique is usually best performed by the clinician in the office to reduce the risk of ocular injury.

Lid scrubs, on the other hand, are nearly always performed by the patient at home with use of nonspecific cleansers such as baby shampoo or the commercially available products. When infection is problematic, antibiotic eyelid scrubs with agents effective against *Staphylococcus* species are prescribed. The procedure is usually performed twice daily during the acute phase of blepharitis, but can often be reduced in frequency to once daily or less often according to the response to therapy.

Meibomian gland massage (expression) can be performed either by the practitioner in the office or by the patient at home by using different methods. Meibomian gland massage is usually prescribed for patients with meibomianitis or for patients with meibomian seborrhea. The purpose of the procedure is to "milk" the meibomian glands of inspissated contents so that meibomian gland function can return to normal, thus reducing associated symptoms of eyelid irritation, burning, stinging, and itching. The techniques are usually performed twice daily, but can be reduced in frequency according to the patient's response to therapy.

INSTRUMENTATION

Theory

The theoretical basis of eyelid epilation is simply the manual removal of an inturned eyelash. This is easily accomplished by using specially designed instruments termed *cilia forceps*.

The clinical effectiveness of eyelid scrubs is based on their abrasive action to loosen and remove eyelid debris and inflammatory products. This abrasive and cleaning activity is an important component of routine eyelid hygiene in the treatment of seborrheic blepharitis, and when the technique employs antibacterial agents, it becomes an important part of the treatment of infectious blepharitis.

The efficacy of meibomian gland massage is based on the "milking" action of the maneuver, whereby the blocked contents of the meibomian glands are physically extruded from the affected glands. The procedure is made somewhat more effective by the prior application of heat, in the form of warm compresses, which serve to liquify the meibomian gland contents, thus making them more easily removed.[2]

Use

Cilia forceps are used with the aid of magnification provided by the slit lamp or a binocular loupe. Eyelid scrubs, in contrast, are performed by the patient at home. Meibomian gland procedures are performed without additional magnification and are executed using a commercially available meibomian gland expressor, cotton-tipped applicators, or the practitioner's index finger.

COMMERCIALLY AVAILABLE INSTRUMENTS

Cilia forceps are available in a variety of forms (Fig. 43–1). The most popular have a curved, smooth tip that is tapered. Although household tweezers can be used for this purpose, the commercially available forceps are usually more effective because the tapered tip can more easily isolate and engage individual cilia. The most popular cilia forceps are manufactured and distributed by Storz.

Although baby shampoos can be applied to the eyelid margin using the abrasive action of a cotton-tipped applicator, various mild eyelid cleansers are now commercially available and are formulated specifically for use on eyelid tissue (Table 43–1). These solutions are usually packaged together with gauze pads for use in applying the solution directly to the eyelid margin. The gauze pads supply the abrasive action to loosen and clean away crusting and other eyelid debris (Fig. 43–2).

Although most practitioners use cotton-tipped applicators or the index finger for meibomian gland massage, Storz Instruments manufactures and distributes a commercially available meibomian gland expressor designed specifically for this purpose. The device

Table 43–1
Eyelid Cleansers

EV Lid Cleanser (Eagle Vision)
I-Scrub (Spectra Pharmaceutical)
OcuSoft Lid Scrub (OcuSoft)
Ultra-Mild Eyelid Cleanser (Medmoor)

is placed in the inferior cul-de-sac, and pressure is supplied through the eyelid from its anterior surface to "milk" the meibomian glands of their inspissated contents (Fig. 43–3).

CLINICAL PROCEDURE

Epilation of Eyelashes

1. Epilation of eyelashes is most easily accomplished with the patient comfortably positioned at the slit lamp.
2. Topical anesthesia may make the procedure more comfortable, but it is not essential.
3. For epilation of offending eyelashes in the lower eyelid the patient should be instructed to look upward and, with the index finger of the practitioner's nondominant hand stabilizing the lower lid, the base of the offending eyelash should be grasped with the cilia forceps and the entire eyelash removed in one motion.
4. If more than one eyelash is involved, repeated isolation and removal of each individual eyelash are required.
5. For lashes involving the upper eyelid, the patient should be instructed to look downward to move the cornea away from the action of the cilia forceps.
6. Once the offending lashes have been removed, the cornea should be carefully inspected for compromise induced by the trichiasis, and treatment should be offered depending on the amount of ocular damage. This may include simple ocular lubricants or prophylactic anti-infective agents.

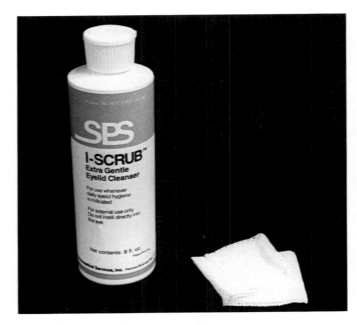

FIGURE 43–2. I-Scrub with gauze pads.

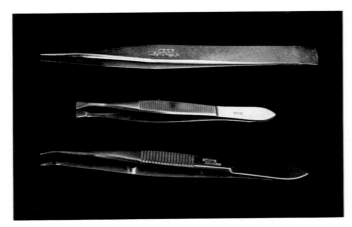

FIGURE 43–1. Cilia forceps.

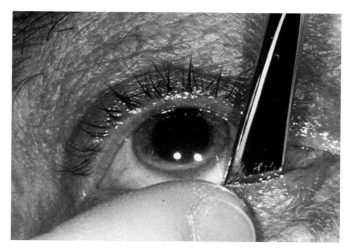

FIGURE 43–3. Meibomian gland expressor (Storz).

Lid Scrubs

1. Lid scrubs are performed by applying several drops of baby shampoo or other commercially available cleanser directly to a cotton-tipped applicator or gauze pad and then applying the applicator or pad to the lid margin in a gentle circular or oscillating fashion to clean the lid margin of debris and inflammatory products.
2. Anti-infective agents for infectious blepharitis are applied either in solution or ointment form using a cotton-tipped applicator in the same way.
3. Drug application to the lid margin is accomplished with the cotton swab applied to the opened or closed eyelids (Fig. 43–4).
4. So that the treatment is as effective as possible, it is usually best not to remove the antibiotic from the eyelid margin once the drug has been applied.
5. Depending on the severity of blepharitis, the procedure is usually performed twice daily by the patient at home.
6. Patients whose manual dexterity is poor because of arthritis or other physical impairment may require assistance from an attendant or family member.

Meibomian Gland Massage

The technique of meibomian gland massage is performed by the practitioner in the office using two cotton-tipped applicators.

1. Following topical anesthesia, one applicator is placed deep within the conjunctival sac and parallel to the eyelid margin while the other applicator is placed outside the eyelid on level with the other applicator.
2. In one continuous motion the applicators are rolled together toward the lid margin, thus extruding the meibomian gland contents (Fig. 43–5).
3. The procedure is initiated near the medial or lateral canthal region and then performed on adjacent meibomian glands until the entire eyelid has been treated.
4. Both upper and lower eyelids can be treated in this fashion, and for patients with secondary meibomianitis, in which only a small cluster of glands is involved,[3] it is satisfactory to treat only the affected glands.
5. When properly performed, the procedure may be somewhat uncomfortable for the patient, but it is usually well tolerated.
6. The desired end point of the technique is the production of a quantity of thick, white meibomian gland secretion, indicative of true meibomianitis. In fact, the procedure can be employed diagnostically to aid in evaluating patients with suspected meibomian gland dysfunction.

Meibomian gland expression can also be performed by the patient.

1. Following 10 to 15 minutes of hot compress application, the patient can be instructed to exert firm pressure with the index finger near the eyelid margin for about 5 seconds, beginning near the medial or lateral canthal region and progressively moving across the eyelid until the entire lower eyelid is treated (Fig. 43–6).
2. Care should be taken to avoid injuring the globe with the fingertip or fingernail, and it is helpful to instruct the patient in the office using a mirror, so that the patient fully understands the procedures to be followed.
3. It is important to stress to the patient that pressure be applied near the eyelid margin; if placed too low on the eyelid, the applied pressure will serve simply to evert the

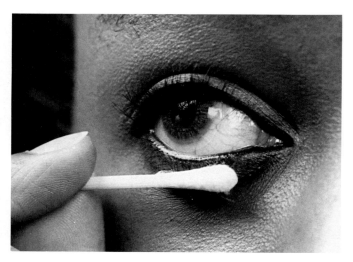

FIGURE 43–4. Lid scrub procedure with cotton swab applied to lid margin.

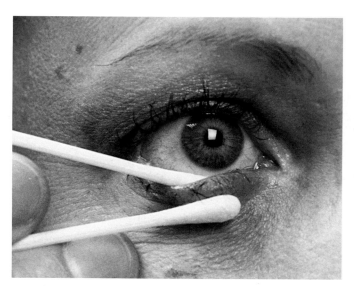

FIGURE 43–5. Meibomian gland massage using cotton-tipped applicators positioned on both sides of lower lid.

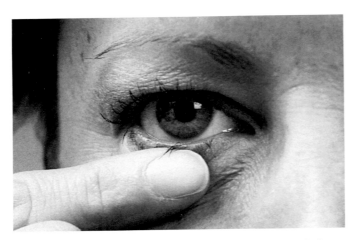

FIGURE 43–6. Meibomian gland massage using fingertip applied near lid margin.

lower eyelid, without providing pressure over the meibomian glands.

4. Because of inherent difficulty in performing the technique on the upper eyelid, it is usually sufficient to limit the procedure to the lower lid.
5. This technique can also be performed diagnostically by the optometrist. With the patient at the slit lamp and looking upward, the clinician places firm pressure with the index finger near the eyelid margin. The quality and quantity of meibomian gland fluid expressed reflects the presence or absence of meibomian gland dysfunction. A scant amount of clear, oily fluid is normal, whereas a thick white or yellow-white pasty material is indicative of true meibomianitis.

CLINICAL IMPLICATIONS

Trichiasis is a common clinical problem characterized by the presence of one or more inturning lashes of the upper or lower lid. When the condition is severe, it may lead to blindness, especially in areas of the world where trachoma is endemic. In most cases, however, trichiasis is the result of aging changes of the lid, and there is no underlying disease process. Other causes include trachoma, Stevens–Johnson syndrome, ocular pemphigoid, and trauma. These conditions can produce deformity of the eyelid and

conjunctiva. In some cases, simple epilation of offending eyelashes, together with attention to the compromised conjunctiva or cornea, can be vision-saving because these maneuvers may prevent corneal injury with resultant loss of vision. When only a few lashes are involved, manual epilation is effective, but often must be repeated every few weeks or months because it fails to destroy the lash follicle. When the condition is chronic or involves many lashes, further care may be required, including electrolysis, cryosurgery, or argon laser thermal ablation.[4]

Since staphylococcal blepharitis can become chronic and more difficult to treat, the condition must be treated aggressively to be successful. It is important to stress to the patient that treatment is usually intended to control the condition, rather than to cure it. Following each session of hot compresses and hygienic scrubs, antibiotics should be applied, in the form of a lid scrub, directly to the lid margin. Preferred anti-infective agents include erythromycin, bacitracin, or an aminoglycoside, such as gentamicin or tobramycin.[5] Whichever antibacterial agent is chosen as initial therapy, it is important to alternate treatment using a different antibiotic on consecutive weeks to avoid or minimize the development of resistant organisms. It is also important to impress upon the patient the necessity of complying with the recommended therapy. Because of complications associated with chronic staphylococcal blepharitis, the importance of early and effective treatment cannot be overemphasized. It is extremely helpful for the practitioner to observe the patient performing lid scrubs, to be sure the patient is able to properly administer the therapy at home.

In addition to the use of hot compresses and meibomian gland expression several times daily in cases of meibomianitis, antibiotic ointment can be applied to the lid margin twice daily. Although no pathogen is implicated in meibomianitis, the use of eyelid scrubs to deliver bacitracin or erythromycin ointment to the lid margin is recommended and often allows significant clinical improvement within 2 to 4 weeks.[5,6]

REFERENCES

1. Polack FM, Goodman DF. Experience with a new detergent lid scrub in the management of chronic blepharitis. Arch Ophthalmol 1988;106:719–720.
2. Dougherty JM, McCulley JP. Analysis of the free fatty acid component of meibomian secretions in chronic blepharitis. Invest Ophthalmol Vis Sci 1986;27:52–56.
3. McCulley JP, Dougherty JM, Deneau DG. Classification of chronic blepharitis. Ophthalmology 1982;89:1173–1180.
4. Bartley GB, Bullock JD, Olsen TG, et al. An experimental study to compare methods of eyelash ablation. Ophthalmology 1987;94:1286–1289.
5. McCulley JP. Blepharoconjunctivitis. Int Ophthalmol Clin 1984;24:65–77.
6. Flora MR. Meibomianitis and meibomian hypersecretion. South J Optom 1979;21:46–48.

Ocular Foreign Body Removal

Richard J. Clompus

INTRODUCTION

Definition

Accidents or injuries can result in foreign material becoming superficially embedded in the ocular surfaces and adnexa or, in some cases, it can penetrate and perforate the globe. *Foreign body removal* is the procedure for properly removing a foreign body from the involved surface.

History

Much of the early history of eye disease and its treatment were recorded after the birth of Christ by Galen, Demosthenes, and Archigenes in the first and second centuries AD. This early ophthalmic history has been passed along in separate works by a variety of authors. Paullus of Aëtius[1] (AD 502–575) mentions from the book by Demosthenes, foreign bodies in the conjunctival sac and those firmly embedded in the ocular tissues. He described removal of small foreign bodies, such as gnats by opening and closing the eyes or plant materials, or sand grains, by oneself, or if attached to the conjunctiva, by irrigation with water, milk, or honey; or using a ring or sticky substance such as honey to remove the foreign body. Firmly embedded foreign bodies such as fine splinters or small bones were to be removed by forceps. Blood of a pigeon or egg white should then be applied to the eye after removal.

In some cases, irrigation or removal by a loop or forceps are still appropriate methods for foreign body removal. Of course, the introduction of the biomicroscope in the early part of this century and such hand instruments as spuds, disposable needles, and rust ring removers, along with quick-acting topical anesthetics have greatly enhanced the removal of ocular foreign bodies.

Clinical Use

Foreign bodies seen in clinical practice vary widely from wind-blown debris, insect parts, fibers, to glass or metal particles. Magnetic foreign bodies are more common during industrial injuries due to the frequent use of iron and its alloys in manufacturing processes.[2,3] The use and development of the slit lamp biomicroscope has permitted precise methods of identifying and determining the specific location of the foreign material in the eye and adnexa.

A foreign body in the cornea is one of the most common injuries caused by accidents.[4] Prompt assessment and treatment is needed to preserve vision for patients with ocular foreign bodies.[5] Optometry is a primary health care profession with the education, clinical experience, and necessary diagnostic equipment to provide prompt care for these patients. This chapter will describe techniques for identifying, removing, and treating patients with ocular foreign bodies. The use and care of specialized hand instruments will also be discussed.

INSTRUMENTATION

The careful removal of an ocular foreign body requires the clinician to be proficient with the slit lamp biomicroscope and a variety of hand instruments. The biomicroscope is used to locate and identify the foreign body and to specifically identify the depth of penetration into the ocular tissues. The biomicroscope should have variable magnification to permit both a wide view of the ocular structures under low magnification (4 to 10×) and a highly magnified view, using higher power objectives (16 to 25×). Illumination should be adjustable to permit a wide direct beam for general examination techniques, a small conical beam to examine

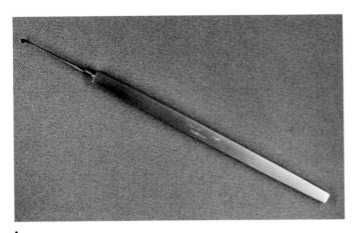

A

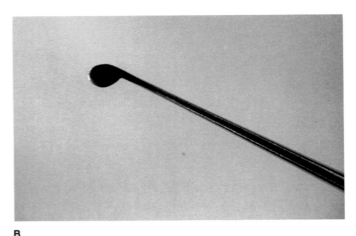

B

FIGURE 44–1. (*A*) Golf club spud for removal of ocular foreign bodies; (*B*) close-up view of the head of the spud.

for cells and flare in the anterior chamber, and a fine slit beam to observe the depth of penetration of the foreign body. A cobalt blue filter is also necessary to assess loss of epithelial tissue using sodium fluorescein dye or perform a Seidel's or percolation test.

Stainless steel hand instruments are also necessary for the removal of superficial or embedded ocular foreign bodies. Instruments commonly used include: foreign body spud, foreign body loop, jeweler's forceps, disposable hypodermic needles, and a corneal rust ring remover. There are also a number of additional innovative hand instruments designed by practitioners that have been described in the ophthalmic literature, but are not widely available.[6–8]

COMMERCIALLY AVAILABLE INSTRUMENTS

Hand Instruments

One of the most common foreign body spuds is the "golf club" spud because it resembles the tip of a golf putter (Fig. 44–1*A,B*). It is made from a single piece of stainless steel, 15 cm in length, and has a sharp edge to remove foreign bodies from the cornea, bulbar, or palpebral conjunctiva. Foreign body spuds also come in a variety of other tip shapes that may be preferred by some clinicians.

The foreign body loop, or Bailey loop, is a metal holder with a tip that consists of a plastic monofilament loop (Fig. 44–2). This monofilament loop, similar to fishing line, is used to snag the foreign body and lift it off the cornea. If an edge of the foreign body is exposed above the level of the epithelium, the loop will catch the edge and help dislodge it. The shorter the loop, the less flexible it will be when pulled across the cornea. Although not as effective as a spud for removing embedded debris from the cornea, the Bailey loop is much safer when the patient is a young child or uncooperative.

As an alternative to spuds or loops, sterile disposable hypodermic needles are useful for removing ocular foreign bodies. They are available as sterile individually packaged instruments that are disposable and cost-effective. Some clinicians prefer the larger handle of the foreign body spud to the small plastic base of the disposable needle. If a longer "handle" is desired for use with sterile needles, the needle can be mounted onto a stainless steel Maumenee goniotomy knife handle* for improved control during

*The Maumenee goniotomy knife handle is available from Storz Ophthalmic Instruments, 3365 Tree Court Industrial Boulevard, St. Louis, MO 63122.

foreign body removal (Fig. 44–3*A*). Although designed for goniotomy surgery, this stainless steel instrument can also be used to improve handling of the small base of sterile hypodermic needles. This instrument is 11.5-cm long with a round knurled surface. It has a standard Luer-Lok tip that permits the clinician to secure the needle base firmly to the end of the handle with a simple twist. The sterile needle can be mounted onto the stainless steel handle with the protective plastic cover over the end of the needle so the tip is not exposed until ready for use. Once the ocular foreign body has been removed, the plastic protective cover is replaced over the needle, twisted off the handle, and disposed of properly. The goniotomy knife handle does not require sterilization before use, since it does not come into contact with ocular tissues or adnexa.

Needles are described by their diameter (gauge) and length. A commonly used needle for foreign body removal is the 18-gauge, 1-1/2-in. size (see Fig. 44–3*B,C*). It is large enough to hold comfortably by its base and can be thrown away after use. Sterility is guaranteed by the manufacturer as long as the package's hermetic seal is intact. Disposable needles are always stored sealed and are opened one at a time, as needed. After use, the needle should be broken and disposed of properly to prevent abuse if found in office waste.

Jeweler's forceps are made from stainless steel and have fine sharp tips that come together without grooves or teeth (Fig. 44–4). Light pressure must be exerted by the clinician to bring the tips together. With the forceps closed, the sharp tip can be used to pry a foreign body loose, which can then be grasped with the forceps and removed from the eye. If the edge of a foreign body is ex-

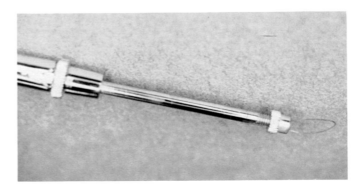

FIGURE 44–2. Bailey loop for removing a foreign body that protrudes above the surface of the epithelium.

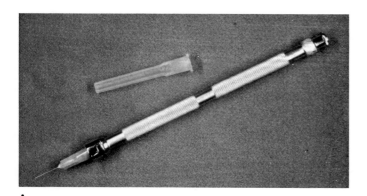

A

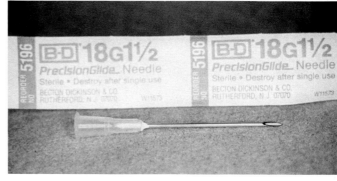

B

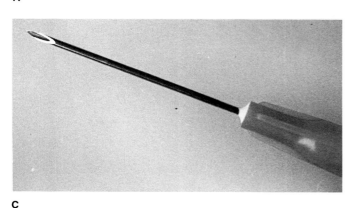

C

FIGURE 44–3. (*A*) Goniotomy knife handle with 27-gauge needle attached; (*B*) an 18-gauge needle; (*C*) close-up view of the needle, illustrating the contour of the tip.

posed, the forceps can be used to pull it from the eye, with minimal disturbance to the surrounding ocular tissues.

Rust Ring Remover

A motorized corneal rust ring remover is useful to efficiently clean away areas of damaged corneal epithelium that have been stained with iron.[9] Siderosis is the oxidizing of the metallic foreign body in the corneal epithelium and can occur within 2 hours after embedding. The rust is very irritating to the cornea, and healing will be delayed if it is not removed.[10]

A recommended corneal rust ring remover is the Alger Brush (Fig. 44–5). This hand-held instrument consists of a weak battery-operated motor that spins a small metal burr (brush) with chisel-like edges. The motor is purposely weak to prevent damage to the deeper layers of the cornea. Power is supplied by one AA-sized battery. It is started by the clinician, with the index finger, spinning a collar around the tip, and it is weak enough that damage to Bowman's layer is unlikely with proper removal technique. Motor noise is minimal and is less likely to cause an increase in patient anxiety than stronger and louder rust ring removers. Other higher-powered corneal rust ring removers are available, but they are not recommended because of their more powerful motors and high cost. The tungsten burr is available in two sizes: 0.5-mm and 1.0-mm diameter. The 0.5-mm diameter burr is recommended and will appear quite large under 16× magnification of the biomicroscope. The tungsten burr should be removed for sterilization between uses. [A kit containing an Alger Brush, spud, tweezers, loop, lid speculum and taper for punctal dilation (Fig. 44–6) is available from Spectrum Scientific Pharmaceuticals Inc., 9626 Baseline Rd., Rancho Cucamonga, CA 91701. A similar kit including a stainless steel tray is available from Eagle Vision, 6263 Popular Ave., Suite 650, Memphis, TN 38119.]

Eye Shields

Additional items are also needed when caring for patients with ocular foreign bodies. The Fox eye shield is necessary for patients who have sustained a penetrating or perforating ocular injury (Fig. 44–7). It is used to protect the eye during patient transport to a secondary or tertiary care site. The aluminum shield prevents pressure from being applied to the eye, thereby protecting the contents from prolapsing or being further damaged.[11]

Instrument Tray

A stainless steel instrument tray with cover is also necessary to carefully store hand instruments and provide a container for disinfection (Fig. 44–8). It is recommended that each treatment room have a complete set of sterile hand instruments in a tray, so efficient treatment may be initiated. The instruments should be stored in a disinfecting solution when not being used for patient care.

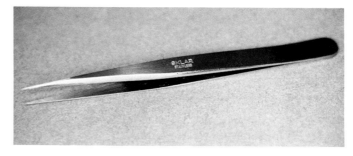

FIGURE 44–4. Stainless steel jewelers forceps. (Sklar).

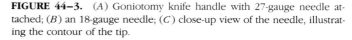

Sterilization of stainless steel hand instruments is best accomplished using a steam autoclave or by exposure to ethylene oxide gas. Unfortunately, most private practices do not employ either of these techniques. In-office disinfection of hand instruments can be accomplished by using a chemical germicide. Disinfection will destroy most bacteria and viruses, but will not necessarily eliminate all spores. Since these instruments will not be used for intraocular surgery, disinfection, rather than sterilization, is adequate.

An example of a potent and effective chemical disinfectant agent is Cetylcide (Manufactured by Cetylite Industries, Pennsauken, NJ 08110). This is a mixture of a quaternary ammonium compound with isopropyl alcohol and a rust inhibitor. Even when greatly diluted, it has a potent and rapid bactericidal action against a wide variety of microorganisms. It has been shown by standard microbiologic tests to be effective against the following organisms: *Staphylococcus aureus, Escherichia coli, Pseudomonas aeruginosa, Salmonella choleraesuis, Streptococcus pyogenes, Candida albicans, Haemophilus parainfluenzae,* and herpes simplex virus type I.[13–15]

Cetylcide, when diluted with distilled water according to instructions, makes a highly stable, rust-proof, colorless, and odorless solution. It will not harm metal, rubber, or plastic, whereas excessive heat may deteriorate the material or dull fine edges. The working solution is made by adding 1 or 2 oz (30 or 60 ml) of concentrate to 1 gal (3.78 L) of distilled water. This diluted solution can also be used for environmental cleaning and disinfecting of countertops and other exposed surfaces.

Another disinfecting solution that is reasonable in cost can be made by a local pharmacist. It consists of benzalkonium chloride (Zephiran hydrochloride), 1 : 750, with antirust tablets added. This solution can also be used for instrument disinfection.

The instrument tray should be filled about half way, so that the solution completely covers the instruments. After soaking for 20 to 30 minutes, the instruments will be disinfected. The instruments may remain in the disinfecting solution until their use is required. The disinfecting solution in the instrument tray should be discarded and refilled with new disinfectant at least every 2 weeks, depending upon how many times one uses the hand instruments.

The disinfecting solution should *not* come into contact with the cornea or any of the conjunctival mucosa of the eye or lid, since it would be very irritating to these delicate ocular structures. Disinfecting solution should be vigorously rinsed from each instrument with sterile saline before use. The most efficient method of rinsing is to use the sterile nonpreserved aerosol saline to rinse the instrument over the sink or paper towel. The pressurized spray is very effective in rinsing off disinfectant and will not contaminate instruments before patient use.

The steel tip of the Alger Brush can be safely soaked in the disinfectant solution or flamed with a butane lighter before each use. Allow ample time for the burr to cool before applying it to the cornea. The package insert that is provided with the Alger Brush carefully explains the flame-sterilization technique.

CLINICAL PROCEDURE

General Comments

The typical patient presenting with an acute corneal foreign body will report pain, lacrimation, and photophobia, often associated with a recent history of ocular injury. If the patient's first contact with the clinician's office is by phone, it is important that the receptionist be able to identify the problem from a layman's description and schedule the patient for an office visit that same morning or afternoon. Many patients who have sustained their first foreign body or abrasion may feel relatively comfortable during the first few hours after the incident. These patients may also obtain and use over-the-counter topical decongestants or lubricants, thinking that their symptoms will soon clear. Four to six hours later, as a painful secondary anterior uveitis develops, patients call the office for help, realizing the condition was more serious than they had originally thought. In other cases, superficial ocular foreign bodies that have gone unnoticed by the patient can be discovered during biomicroscopy on a routine eye examination. If these foreign bodies are inert, such as gold, silver, or glass, and do not cause an inflammatory response, they should be left intact. Removing them may cause unnecessary trauma and scarring, with a potential decrease in visual acuity if they are located along the visual axis.

Specific Procedure

1. Once the patient has arrived in the office, a careful history should be obtained that includes the time of onset of the initial foreign body symptoms, a description of the activity or machinery used at the time of the incident, and any emergency treatment rendered. A penetrating ocular foreign body must always be considered when the patient was hammering metal to metal or using high-speed machinery, such as a grinding wheel. A small high-speed projectile can penetrate the eye with the patient reporting only an irritation or no symptoms at all.[16] Iron, copper, and zinc particles are toxic to the retina and must be identified and removed as soon as possible.[17–19] If the patient works with strands of metal wire, the tip of the wire can partially penetrate the corneal layers and exit the epithelium without perforating the endothelium. A resulting scar will later develop showing the path of the wire through the layers of the cornea.

2. The next step in evaluating the patient requires the assessment of the patient's best corrected visual acuity. If the patient's glasses were broken or left behind, a pinhole or multiple pinhole occluder can be used. If the patient is experiencing photophobia or blepharospasm and cannot comfortably open the lids, a topical anesthetic, such as proparacaine HCl, 0.5%, can be instilled in the eye to facilitate visual acuity assessment. The topical anesthetic will permit a more comfortable examination with a duration of about 30 minutes. This initial visual acuity measurement is important for medicolegal reasons and for charting the patient's progress during follow-up visits. Central corneal foreign bodies will have the greatest blurring effect, whereas peripheral ones may not show any substantial compromise in visual acuity. If treatment is delayed, the vision may be worse, due to a secondary anterior uveitis. The protein content of the aqueous will increase as the blood–brain barrier begins to break down causing an identifiable flare in the anterior chamber.

3. External examination of the lids and adnexa should be performed with a penlight or transilluminator. The lids should be gently examined externally and then everted to carefully investigate any superficial damage from foreign matter. If significant debris was present, the lid should be double everted to fully investigate particles carried far under the lid.

4. Biomicroscopy should be performed next, using low magnification (4 to 10×) to examine the cornea, conjunctiva, and adnexa for the location of the foreign body. Broad-beam direct illumination, with white light, can be used for an overview of these ocular structures, followed by a narrow slit-beam or optic section to localize the penetration depth of the foreign body into the ocular tissues (Fig. 44–9). Many superficial corneal foreign bodies will stop at Bowman's layer and not leave a scar, if skillfully removed. Corneal epithelium does not scar when damaged by a foreign body. It heals by neighboring healthy epithelial cells sliding into the vacant space left after the foreign body has been removed.[20] After 24 hours, cell mitosis and replication thicken the layers of the corneal epithelium and fill in the compromised area.

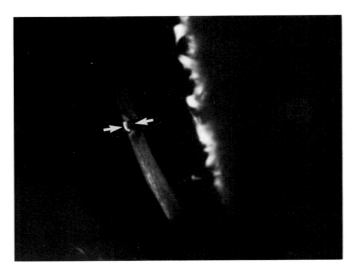

FIGURE 44–9. Optic section of the cornea illustrating the depth of penetration of a metallic foreign body into the midstroma (Courtesy of J. R. Pederson, OD)

Bowman's layer and stroma will scar when damaged by a foreign body or by poor removal techniques. If the area involved is located along the visual axis of the central cornea, the patient's visual acuity will be decreased, regardless of the clinician's skill in removing it. For this reason, referral of deep central corneal foreign bodies to a corneal specialist may be advisable.

5. Once the corneal foreign body has been identified and localized, a small circular beam (1- to 2-mm diameter) is focused in the anterior chamber to detect the presence of cells and flare. It is best to darken room illumination to a minimum for visualization of any anterior chamber inflammatory response. Flare will present as a foggy or smoky appearance within the confines of the circular beam in the anterior chamber between the corneal endothelium and the anterior surface of the crystalline lens. Inflammatory cells or leukocytes will appear as small white dots or particles that slowly float past and through the beam, as the convection currents move within the aqueous humor of the anterior chamber. Both cells and flare should be graded separately on the following scale:

    0   None present
    1+   Trace amount
    2+   Mild amount
    3+   Moderate amount
    4+   Severe amount

Flare and cells in the anterior chamber indicate a secondary anterior uveitis involving the iris and ciliary body. This is an inflammatory response that may also cause ciliary spasm, inducing deep ocular pain. Externally, the uveitis will appear as a ciliary flush owing to dilation of the deep circumlimbal vessels. Flare and cells can usually be found within a few hours after corneal compromise. It is important that the anterior chamber be evaluated *before* sodium fluorescein is instilled in the external cul-de-sac. Subtle amounts of flare and cells can be overlooked when viewing through a tear layer stained with sodium fluorescein. If the foreign body has also caused a large corneal abrasion, with loss of epithelium, the fluorescein can be found to enter the anterior chamber and will appear as green flare due to loss of the tight cellular junctions of the corneal epithelium. Sodium fluorescein will help delineate areas of the corneal surface from which epithelial cells have been lost or damaged. If the foreign body is located on the surface of the superior tarsus of the lid, vertical stripes of stained corneal epithelium may be found during biomicroscopy. If these foreign bodies are embedded in the tarsal conjunctiva, it will be

necessary to evert the upper lid and remove them in the same manner as corneal foreign bodies.

Sodium fluorescein does not actually stain tissue, but is most useful as an indicator dye. The tear film is mildly acidic and will appear as a yellowish color when fluorescein is instilled. If the corneal epithelium is damaged, the fluorescein will color Bowman's layer and the stroma a greenish color, due to the influence of the anterior chamber's alkalinity. It is this pH change that determines the bright green color of damaged corneal tissue.

6. Once identified and localized, the foreign body should be drawn and described in the patient's record. It should also be noted if a rust ring is present, indicating the iron-containing nature of the foreign body (Fig. 44–10). The slow diffusion of iron molecules into the neighboring epithelial cells will complicate and inhibit the healing process. In patients, usually those with a recurrent history of metallic foreign bodies, such as automobile mechanics, a small white circle or ring at the level of Bowman's layer may be found. This is a Coat's ring which is the result of a rust ring that has become sclerotic.

7. The level of penetration must be identified before treatment may be initiated. If the corneal foreign body has penetrated beyond the midstroma and it appears that manipulation may push it into the anterior chamber, the patient should be referred to a corneal specialist or other experienced clinician for removal in the operating room.[21] If perforation occurs there, it is much easier to provide the proper treatment for the patient. If a corneal foreign body has penetrated through the entire thickness of the cornea, a path of tissue disturbance should be visible through Bowman's layer, stroma, and the endothelium.

8. The percolation or Seidel's test should be performed if penetration is suspected, to discover if the ocular integrity has been violated. Sodium fluorescein is instilled in the tear film. The patient is instructed to blink and then to hold the lids open wide. If

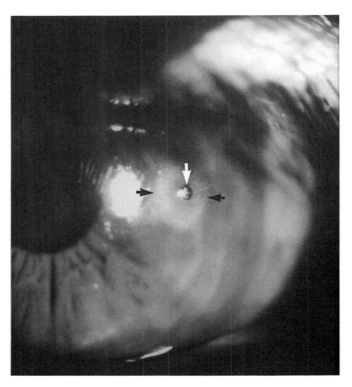

FIGURE 44–10. Corneal metallic foreign body with fluorescein stain, adjacent rust ring (*white arrow*) and surrounding leukocytic infiltrate (*black arrows*). (Courtesy of J. R. Pederson, OD)

there is a small entrance wound through the entire corneal thickness, the clear aqueous will percolate through the cornea and rinse the fluorescein away leaving a small clear spot over the wound site without fluorescence. The small circular clear area will continue to increase in size until the next blink when the process starts over again. This is an indication of a true penetrating foreign body and represents a positive Seidel's sign. When this occurs, the patient's eye should be protected by covering with a Fox shield and immediate arrangements made for referral to a corneal specialist. Do not perform gonioscopy or put any pressure on the eye that may cause further internal damage. It is also advisable to view the posterior segment of each eye with the direct ophthalmoscope as another method of ruling out an intraocular foreign body. Further testing may include x-rays, computed tomography (CT) scan, and B-scan ultrasonography.[3,21,22]

9. Once it has been determined that the foreign body does not penetrate or perforate the eye, it must be removed, causing the least amount of ocular trauma. Additional topical anesthesia can be provided with 2 drops of 0.5% proparacaine HCl for most foreign body removal techniques. For those foreign bodies located deeper within the corneal layers or at the sensitive limbus, 2 drops of tetracaine (Pontocaine) or a 4% cocaine ophthalmic solution will provide additional deeper anesthesia.

10. If the foreign body is superficial and not embedded, a steady stream of sterile ophthalmic irrigating solution can be directed adjacent to or on the area of the foreign body. This may dislodge the foreign body if it is relatively loose. This is done with the patient's head against the headrest. Following irrigation, biomicroscopic examination of the anterior segment is recommended to make sure the foreign body does not become lodged into the superior or inferior fornix. Fiberglass material can be removed with irrigation and then swabbing of the superior and inferior cul-de-sac with a moistened sterile cotton-tipped applicator. Repeated swabbing of the ocular adnexa may be necessary to remove all of the foreign material. A cotton-tipped applicator may also be used to remove foreign matter from the palpebral and bulbar conjunctiva. However cotton-tipped swabs are *not* recommended to remove an embedded corneal foreign body. This may push the particle into the deeper layers of the cornea and disturb large areas of corneal epithelium surrounding it.

11. A stainless steel foreign body spud or sterile disposable hypodermic needle are the recommended instruments for removing embedded corneal, conjunctival, and tarsal foreign bodies. The patient is instructed to place his or her chin firmly in the chin rest with the head against the forehead rest of the biomicroscope and to stare at the fixation device of the biomicroscope with the eyes open wide.

It is much easier to remove a foreign body from a stable target than one that is constantly moving. If the patient cannot open the eye with the foreign body, the clinician or assistant should hold the lids open. The spud or needle should be kept out of sight of the patient until ready for use. It is then brought in from the side anterior to the patient's cornea *without* using the biomicroscope (Fig. 44–11). Next, the clinician should locate the tip of the spud or needle through the broad beam of the biomicroscope. It is always held tangential to the cornea and never pointed directly at the cornea along an anteroposterior axis. The tip is then brought closer to the cornea until contact is made with the foreign body. If the patient jerks the head forward, the spud or needle will not cause a stab wound and will simply be pushed away. The foreign body should be removed by sliding the edge of the spud or needle under the edge of the foreign body and lifting outward. The procedure is very similar to removing a hubcap from an automobile wheel. The edges of the foreign body are manipulated until it is loose enough to be lifted off the cornea. The foreign body may be removed in one piece or, occasionally, removal of several pieces may become necessary. Never try to push the foreign body or it

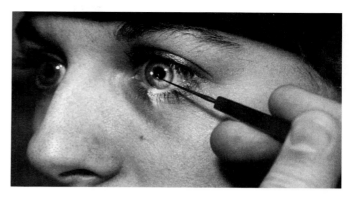

FIGURE 44–11. Positioning of the hand-held instrument in front of the cornea is performed without use of the biomicroscope.

may become embedded further. The clinician may also notice an area of damaged epithelial cells immediately surrounding the foreign body. These cells will have the consistency of soft gelatin, whereas healthy epithelial tissue will be more like firm gelatin. If one probes deep enough and pushes against Bowman's layer, the entire cornea will be dragged and move with the hand instrument. This tissue is a very tenacious layer, but will scar if compromised, even though nonscarring epithelium will eventually cover the area. Removing a conjunctival foreign body is accomplished in the same manner as a corneal one, except reduction in visual acuity does not occur.

If the patient is a young child or an adult who cannot keep the head in the biomicroscope, the Bailey loop can be repeatedly drawn across the cornea in an attempt to snag and remove the foreign body. It is less likely to damage surrounding healthy tissue when trying to remove a foreign body with poor patient cooperation.

Embedded foreign bodies can also be removed with jeweler's forceps. The forceps are brought in from the side with the patient's head in the biomicroscope. When the tips are kept closed together, they act as a large foreign body spud. Once the edges of the foreign body are exposed, the forceps can be opened and the foreign body grasped and removed from the eye. Jeweler's forceps can also be used to remove foreign bodies attached to the superior tarsus. The superior lid is everted and held stable so the forceps are used to lift off the foreign body.

12. If a rust ring is present, efforts must be made to remove the ring as much as possible during the patient's first visit, with the least amount of trauma to the surrounding corneal tissues. In some cases, when the rust ring is small, the foreign body spud or needle can be used to gently scrape away the stained and loosely adherent epithelium. If the rust ring is larger, the rust ring remover will remove the damaged epithelium more efficiently. The Alger Brush should be started with the flick of the thumb and brought in from the side with patient maintaining proper fixation (Fig. 44–12).

The lids may also be held open if necessary. The spinning tip is brought gently in contact with the rust-stained epithelium. The damaged epithelium can be wiped away and, occasionally, when loosely attached, it will appear to spray off the cornea, leaving a clean undisturbed Bowman's layer underneath. The spinning burr of the Alger Brush is not to be pushed hard against the cornea, but is gently brought in contact with the stained cells and lifted off again. It is not necessary to remove all signs of rust from the corneal epithelium. Some of the remaining rust will eventually slough off as epithelial cells mature and move from deeper to more superficial layers of the cornea. If the iron has been in contact with Bowman's layer for an extended period, it may also become stained. It is recommended that Bowman's layer not be

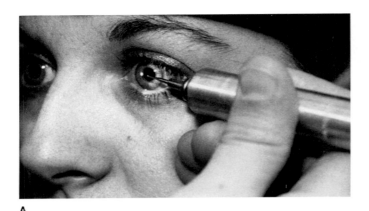

A

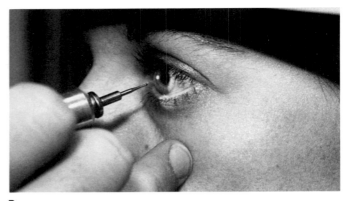

B

FIGURE 44–12. (*A*) Correct position of Alger Brush relative to the cornea; (*B*) incorrect position of Alger Brush.

disturbed to remove the rust stain. If left intact, the stained area will gradually fade to white and then gray. If Bowman's layer is disturbed further in an attempt to remove the rust stain, increased scarring will occur.

13. Once the corneal foreign body and rust ring are removed, it is necessary to treat the compromised cornea to prevent secondary infection and establish patient comfort. If the foreign body was very small, with little epithelial disturbance and no anterior chamber reaction, broad-spectrum ophthalmic antibiotic drops, such as tobramycin or gentamicin should be instilled every 4 hours (q4h) for 5 days. Both of these aminoglycosides inhibit growth of gram-positive and gram-negative bacteria including *Pseudomonas aeruginosa*. The cornea will reepithelialize within 24 hours, and the patient should be seen for an office visit the next day. The topical antibiotic drops may be continued for 2 or 3 days after epithelialization, as much for their lubricant effect as for their antibacterial effect. If corneal edema persists after epithelialization has been completed, a hyperosmotic agent such as 2% or 5% sodium chloride solution can be used four times a day. If the cornea has not completed its epithelialization, topical hyperosmotic drops will be ineffective, since a semipermeable membrane is not present over the corneal surface.

14. In patients for whom the foreign body and its subsequent removal have caused more extensive damage to the surrounding corneal epithelium and, in the presence of an anterior uveitis, cycloplegia is recommended. Anticholinergic agents, such as 1% cyclopentolate HCl or 5% homatropine hydrobromide is suggested. The duration of action for a single drop instillation will be less than 24 hours for 1% cyclopentolate and about 48 hours for 5% homatropine. The purpose of these anticholinergics is to reduce ciliary spasm and to help maintain the blood–aqueous barrier, with a reduction in cells and flare in the anterior chamber.

Ocular pain usually accompanies a foreign body and abrasion of the cornea. Pain control is an important aspect of patient care and should not be overlooked. A topical anesthetic should *never* be dispensed to the patient for ocular pain caused by a foreign body or corneal abrasion. It will retard the healing process and is toxic to epithelium with repeated doses.[23] Ocular pain can be effectively treated with therapeutic doses of aspirin, acetaminophen, ibuprofin, or narcotic analgesics, when indicated, taken orally about every 4 to 6 hours. Always check with the patient to determine if medication hypersensitivities exist or for pregnancy potential before recommending oral medications.

Larger or multiple corneal foreign bodies involving greater losses of epithelium will require pressure patching to facilitate prompt healing and decrease patient discomfort. Pressure patching may also decrease the patient's chances of developing a recur-

rent corneal erosion over the site of the injury.[11,24] Pressure patching involves the application of two or three sterile cotton eye pads held firmly in place with hypoallergenic adhesive tape to prevent the superior lid from blinking across the cornea (see Chap. 45).

CLINICAL IMPLICATIONS

Clinical Significance

The ability to provide timely first aid and treatment to patients suffering from an ocular foreign body can mean the difference of saving or losing vision permanently. It is no longer adequate to remove ocular foreign bodies with a cotton-tipped applicator without a biomicroscope for close examination of the eye and adnexa. Ignoring or failing to diagnose an intraocular foreign body can be devastating for the eye.

Clinical Interpretation

Careful observation of the patient's progress and recovery from an ocular injury is very important. In most cases, epithelialization of a damaged cornea from a foreign body or abrasion occurs without serious complications of infection or inflammation. Careful observation and clinical notations in the patient's record will help determine if healing is proceeding normally. Each day that the clinician is treating a compromised cornea, it should appear improved over the preceding day. Biomicroscopic examination should include assessment of corneal edema, staining with sodium fluorescein, presence and grading of anterior chamber reaction, and visual acuity measurement. All of these factors should be improving if healing is occurring. In some patients, the anterior chamber reaction may be worse the second day if a weak anticholinergic was used. The presence of corneal infiltrates surrounding an otherwise normal-appearing foreign body may indicate a prolonged delay from the time the injury occurred and a more guarded prognosis. Although topical steroids may provide earlier symptomatic relief and reduce conjunctival injection, they are not indicated for early treatment of ocular foreign bodies. Visual acuity should slowly improve and is also an indicator of normal recovery.

Careful patient education is also very important so that the patient can actively participate in his or her own care and recovery. The patient should be instructed concerning care and the reasonable course of healing. If a cycloplegic is used to control ocular inflammation, light sensitivity and blurred vision should be further explained.

Most corneal foreign bodies can be treated successfully without complications by optometrists. When in doubt of globe penetration or when specialized diagnostic imaging is indicated, referral to another health care provider is indicated. The best form of treatment is prevention by educating patients about safety eye wear and polycarbonate spectacle lenses. It is especially important to spend a few extra minutes with patients who have sustained an ocular injury to prevent future occurrences.

REFERENCES

1. Aëtius of Amida, *Actii medici Graeci Contractae ex veteribus sermones XVI,* sermo septimus: "De morbis oculorum," Cap. XIX: De hisquaoculo infiguntur" (Venetiis: Ex officina Farrea, 1543) l. 330–331, Cited in Hirshberg J. History of ophthalmology. trans by Blodi FC. Bonn: Wagenborgh, 1982;1:337–338.
2. Terry JE. Ocular disease: detection, diagnosis and treatment. Boston: Butterworths, 1985:680.
3. Ittyerah TP. Magnetic intraocular foreign bodies in the posterior segment. Ind J Ophthalmol 1987;35:129.
4. Gombos GM. Handbook of ophthalmologic emergencies, 2nd ed. Garden City, NY: Medical Examination Publishing Co, 1977:99–101.
5. Stein HA, Slatt BJ. The ophthalmic assistant, 3rd ed. St Louis: CV Mosby Co, 1976:296.
6. Weiss J, Kachadoorian H. Removal of corneal foreign bodies with ocular magnet. [Letters to the Editor]. Ophthal Surg 1989;20:378–379.
7. Arnold RW, Erie JC. Magnetized forceps for metallic corneal foreign bodies [Letters to the Editor]. Arch Ophthalmol 1988;106:1502.
8. Lobel D, Blumenthal M, Belkin M. A new instrument for removing corneal foreign bodies [Letters to Journal]. Am J Ophthalmol 1983;95:715–716.
9. Sigurdsson M, Hanna I, Lockwood AJ, et al. Removal of rust rings, comparing electric drill and hypodermic needle. Eye 1987;1:430.
10. Deutch TA, Feller DB. Paton and Goldberg's management of ocular injuries, 2nd ed. Philadelphia: WB Saunders Co, 1985:1–8.
11. Catania LJ. Primary care of the anterior segment. Norwalk, Conn: Appleton and Lange, 1988;148–158.
12. Storz surgical instrument catalogue. St Louis: Storz Instrument Company, 1979:455–456.
13. Use-Dilution Tests. Hill Top Research Inc, Reference no 82-05235-11, 4-30-82 (unpublished).
14. Virucidal activity of cetylcide germicidal solution vs. influenza A2 and herpes simplex type 1. Testing conducted by Morton Klien, Ph.D., Department of Microbiology, Temple University School of Medicine, 9-10-80, (unpublished).
15. Cetylcide use-dilution test on *Streptococcus pyogenes, Actinomyces israelii, Candida albicans, Haemophilus parainfluenzae* and *Streptococcus mutans.* Testing conducted at Hill Top Research, Inc., Miamiville, Ohio, 5-5-81 (unpublished).
16. Potts AM, Distler JA. Shape factor in the penetration of intraocular foreign bodies. Am J Ophthalmol 1985;100:183–197.
17. Schmidt JGH. Intravitreal cupriferous foreign bodies: electroretinograms and inflammatory responses. Doc Ophthalmol 1988;67:253–261.
18. Schmidt JGH, Mansfeld–Nies R, Nies C. On the recovery of the electroretinogram of the intravitreal copper particles, Doc Ophthalmol 1987;65:135–142.
19. Schmidt JGH, Nies C, Mansfeld–Nies R. On the recovery of the electroretinogram after removal of the intravitreal zinc particles. Doc Ophthalmol 1987;65:471–480.
20. Friedenwald JS, Buschke W. Mitotic and wound healing activities of the corneal epithelium. Arch Ophthalmol 1944;32:410–413.
21. Duke–Elder SW, MacFaul PA. Injuries, part 1: mechanical injuries. In: Duke–Elder SW, ed. System of ophthalmology. St Louis: CV Mosby Co, 1965:477–500.
22. Eagling EM, Roper-Hall MJ. Eye injuries—an illustrated guide. Philadelphia: JB Lippincott Co, 1986:14–16.
23. Pavan–Langston D. Manual of ocular diagnosis and therapy. Boston: Little, Brown & Co, 1980:36–38.
24. Weene LE. Recurrent corneal erosion after trauma: a statistical study. Ann Ophthalmol 1985;17:521–522, 524.

Ocular Pressure Patching

Richard J. Clompus

INTRODUCTION

Definition

Pressure patching involves the use of sterile eye pads, therapeutic ophthalmic ointments, and adhesive tape to hold the superior lid in apposition to the globe and prevent blinking of the patched eye.

After the pressure patch has been applied, the patient should not be able to blink or significantly move the superior lid when the fellow eyelid is moved. If significant lid movement under the patch is possible, the patch should be removed and reapplied.

History

Applying a patch to the eye for treatment of a removed ocular foreign body or abrasion has been practiced since antiquity. Paullus of Aëtius (AD 502–575) passed along writings of the Greek physician Demosthenes from the first century AD. Demosthenes described the application of patches (compresses) soaked in anti-inflammatory solutions applied to the eye. Here, the compresses were used before removal of the foreign body so that when the injury became purulent the foreign body would be extruded spontaneously. He also described the use of anti-inflammatory compresses using poppy, clover, saffron, and bread as one of several methods for treating deep or large injuries of the eye.[1]

Oval eye pads, paper tape, and special types of patches are recent or relatively recent additions to the application of pressure patches to the eye.

Clinical Use

Corneal foreign bodies involving significant losses of epithelium require pressure patching to facilitate normal healing and decrease patient discomfort. The larger the loss of corneal epithelium, the greater the possibility of secondary infections, ocular inflammation, and recurrent erosions. Pressure patching can significantly reduce the risk of recurrent erosion over the site of the injury[2,3] and improve corneal healing.

Neighboring epithelial cells slide to cover over the denuded area before significant cellular mitosis takes place.[4] The sliding epithelial cells will provide protection for the exposed deeper layers of the cornea until cellular mitosis occurs. A pressure patch is recommended whenever more than 30% of the corneal epithelium has been lost to trauma.

INSTRUMENTATION

Pressure patching of the eye requires the following materials: broad-spectrum antibiotic ointment, alcohol swabs, individually packaged sterile cotton eye pads, and hypoallergenic 1-in. wide adhesive tape. The adhesive tapes used in pressure patching can be made from either paper, such as with Micropore, or from plastic, such as with Transpore.

COMMERCIALLY AVAILABLE INSTRUMENTS

The essential materials necessary for pressure patching of the eye, the sterile eye pads, and hypoallergenic tape, are available in most

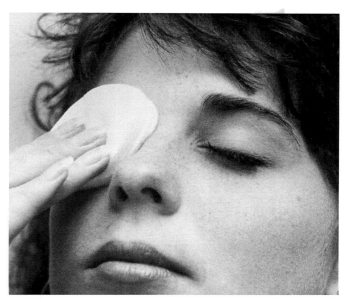

FIGURE 45–1. Single eye pad held by the patient over the closed eyelid.

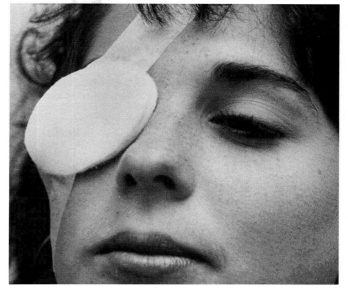

FIGURE 45–2. Eye patch held in place by a single piece of adhesive tape.

pharmacies. Specialized patches such as the Presspatch* or the Donaldson Natural Eyepatch* are available from specific manufacturers.

CLINICAL PROCEDURE

Pressure Patching

1. Alcohol swabs are used to clean and remove oil from the patient's forehead and cheek area to help the tape adhere to the skin. This also aids the reapplication of a patch if it must be removed at night for instillation of medication.
2. A strip of antibiotic ophthalmic ointment, such as tobramycin, gentamicin, or polymyxin B–bacitracin combination is placed in the inferior cul-de-sac. Topical ophthalmic ointment will not delay corneal healing.[5] Antibiotic ointment will permit longer drug contact time with the damaged ocular tissues than a single-drop instillation used before patching.
3. After the antibiotic ointment has been instilled in the eye, the patient is instructed to close both eyes and relax. A single sterile eye pad is placed over the closed eyelid and the patient is requested to hold the patch in place over the lid (Fig. 45–1). This occupies the patient and permits the clinician to tear off six to eight 1-in. strips of adhesive tape.
4. A second sterile cotton eye pad is now placed over the first one and a single piece of adhesive tape is placed over both pads with one end stuck to the middle of the patient's forehead and the other to the cheek to temporarily secure the eye pads (Fig. 45–2).
5. If the patient's eye is anatomically deep set or enophthalmic, a third or fourth eye pad may be necessary to prevent the lid from blinking under the patch. Additional strips of adhesive tape are applied from the middle of the forehead, across the eye pads, and then firmly attached to

the mandible or jaw. The tape should be curved or contoured across the nasal and temporal edges of the eye pads to exert enough force to prevent lid blinking. Additional strips of tape are then applied to the patch so that it is completely covered (Fig. 45–3). If the lower end of the tape is attached to the chin instead of the jaw, normal eating and speaking will be interfered with and will become a further source of discomfort for the patient.

6. After having successfully placed the adhesive tape strips over the patch, ask the patient to blink. If the lid does not move under the patch, the pressure patch has been successfully applied and the patient may now be discharged. An excessively tight patch may compress the cornea and result in temporarily decreased visual acuity when the patch is removed. If the patient feels excessive lid move-

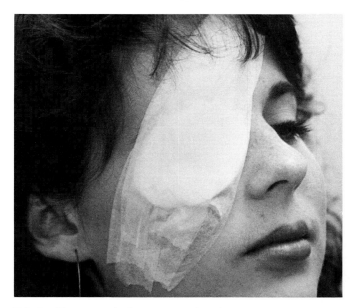

FIGURE 45–3. Finished pressure patch with contoured tape.

* Presspatch is available from Akorn, Inc., 100 Akorn Drive, Abita Springs, LA 70920; and the Donaldson Natural Eyepatch from Keeler Instruments, 456 Parkway, Broomall, PA 19008.

ment under the patch, the patch should be removed and a new one reapplied.

Direct Lid Taping

An alternative to pressure patching has been suggested by Winski and Stephens.[6] This new procedure has been termed direct lid patching. These authors noted that in some patients excessive pressure is necessary to immobilize the lid, thereby creating added discomfort, or that for a variety of reasons the patch may gradually work loose. In the latter event, excessive lid movement may delay healing and prolong patient discomfort.

With this technique, the lid is taped directly without pressure (Fig. 45–4). The procedure used is as follows:

1. The lids, brow, and cheek area are cleaned with an alcohol-saturated pad to promote adherence of the tape.
2. The pupil may be dilated with a cycloplegic agent, depending upon the patient discomfort and degree of secondary anterior chamber reaction.
3. A 1-in. ribbon of antibiotic ointment is applied to the inferior cul-de-sac (see Fig. 45–4A).
4. A strip of tape is placed horizontally along the upper lid of the involved eye, exerting outward pressure as the tape is applied. A tab may be created at the outer edge of the tape by folding the end of the tape over (see Fig. 45–4B).
5. A second piece of tape is placed vertically from the upper aspect of the lid to the cheek (see Fig. 45–4C). The clinician may ask the patient to attempt to gently open the eye to ensure the lid is taped correctly.
6. A single or double gauze pad is placed over the lid and three or four strips of adhesive tape are applied from the lower cheek to the upper brow area with a minimal amount of pressure (see Fig. 45–4D). This latter step is to protect the eye and prevent the patient from removing the tape.

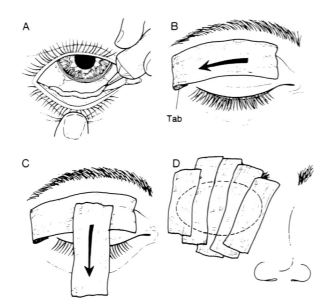

FIGURE 45–4. Direct lid-taping procedure: (A) instillation of broad-spectrum antibiotic; (B) apply the horizontal tab strip with lateral and downward force; (C) apply the vertical strip from the upper lid down to the cheek; (D) completely cover the gauze to protect against outside moisture. (From Winski F, Stephens P. Direct lid taping: an alternative to pressure patching. Clin Eye Vision Care 1989;1:226–227, with permission)

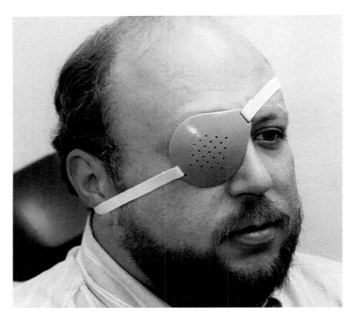

FIGURE 45–5. Akorn Presspatch is particularly convenient for patients with beards.

Pressure patches are easily applied to clean skin with little body hair. However, it is difficult, even under the best circumstances, to successfully apply a pressure patch on patients with a beard. The hypoallergenic adhesive tapes do not stick well to hair and are a constant source of frustration for the clinician. A new sterile disposable compressive dressing, called Presspatch, is available from Akorn that consists of a sterile foam pad attached to a firm plastic eye shield, with an elastic and Velcro fastener (Fig. 45–5). To use the pressure patch, drops and ointment are applied to the eye and the eyelid is closed. The patch is then removed from its sterile wrapper and placed over the eyelid. The elastic strap is placed around the head and secured with the Velcro fastener, with enough pressure to prevent the lid from blinking.

Adhesive tape is not necessary for the patch to remain in place overnight. The patch is removed by simply lifting it off the eyelid and discarding. If pressure patching is to be continued for another day, a new sterile foam pad can be placed in the firm plastic shield. This new method is effective and decreases the amount of time needed to apply a pressure dressing to the eye. Its only disadvantage is that it can also be removed by the patient when instructed not to do so. It may also be used as an effective eye shield to safely transport patients, with penetrating or perforating injuries, by removing the foam pad so that pressure is not applied to the globe.

One other form of patching can be accomplished by using the Donaldson Natural Eyepatch from Keeler Instruments. It consists of a T-shaped patch and a Velcro dot made from polyethylene surgical tape (Fig. 45–6).

This patch will not apply significant pressure to the eye, but is very useful in cases of lagophthalmos in which corneal exposure remains a problem after the initial trauma has been cared for. Its main advantage is that additional medications can be easily applied to the eye and the patch reattached using the Velcro dot fastener.

Once the pressure dressing or patch is applied, the patient is discharged after scheduling an office visit for the next day. The patient should be instructed to go home and rest. Driving is not recommended because of the newly acquired monocularity. Showering is also not recommended in an effort to keep the pressure patch dry; however, warm compresses may be used to increase patient comfort if necessary following trauma.

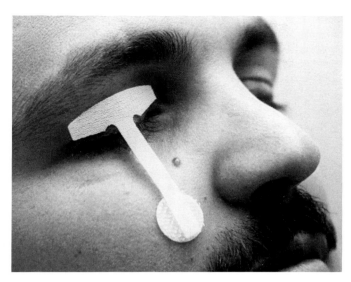

FIGURE 45–6. Donaldson Natural Eyepatch is particularly effective when medication must be repeatedly instilled.

The patch should be removed by the clinician on the patient's follow-up visit the next day. Patching an eye creates a warm, moist, and dark environment that is well suited for bacterial growth. It is necessary to examine the patient the following day to prevent complications from patching the eye. Patient history, visual acuity, external examination, and biomicroscopy should be performed. Vision may continue to be blurred due to corneal edema or cycloplegia. If the corneal epithelium is observed under high magnification immediately after the pressure patch is removed, the epithelial surface may appear rough and uneven. This will smooth out within a short time, once the pressure patch has been removed. If a large area of the cornea has not yet epithelialized, additional cycloplegia, antibiotic ointment, and a new pressure patch should be applied for another 24-hour period. Patients with diabetes mellitus may heal slowly, and this must be taken into account with their follow-up care. It has also been reported that peripheral corneal abrasions closer to the limbus heal faster than those located centrally.[7,8] Once the cornea has epithelialized, antibiotic drops should be continued every 4 hours for another 3 to 5 days. If an anterior uveitis persists, topical steroids can be prescribed, along with the antibiotic, to decrease inflammation. In general, topical steroids are not necessary to treat superficial corneal foreign bodies. Table 45–1 presents a summary for treating ocular foreign bodies.

CLINICAL IMPLICATIONS

Clinical Significance

Pressure patching is a necessary method of treatment for patients sustaining an ocular injury that results in loss of corneal epithelium. It will also permit greater patient comfort while the cornea heals.

Table 45–1
Outline for Removal and Treatment of Ocular Foreign Bodies

1. Obtain a careful history of the incident as well as a patient history.
2. Measure best-corrected visual acuity in each eye.
3. Perform external evaluation of the eye and adnexa.
4. Perform biomicroscopy of the eye with sodium fluorescein. May perform the percolation test to rule out corneal penetration.
5. Lavage the cornea with sterile saline or use a foreign body spud or 20-gauge sterile needle to remove object(s) depending on the size and depth of the foreign body.
6. Cycloplegia may be instilled, if necessary, with 1% cyclopentolate or 5% homatropine.
7. If epithelial compromise is small, prescribe topical broad-spectrum antibiotic drops q4h.
   If a large area of the cornea is compromised, apply a broad-spectrum antibiotic ointment and pressure patch overnight.
   Control pain with oral aspirin, acetaminophen, or ibuprofen. Always question patient for any previous medication sensitivities.
8. Review the patient's progress in 24 hours with patient history, visual acuity, and biomicroscopy. If the epithelium is healed with edema, topical hyperosmotic drops may be prescribed. If the cornea is not healed, patching can be repeated. Continue topical antibiotic therapy for at least 3 days after reepithelialization.

Clinical Interpretation

The pressure patch must prevent the superior lid from moving across the surface of the corneal epithelium. If the patch does not perform this function, healing may be delayed. It is important for the clinician to evaluate the patch before the patient leaves the office. If the patch is not performing this function, remove it and reapply.

REFERENCES

1. Aëtuis of Amida, *Actii medici Graeci Contractae ex veteribus medicinae sermones XVI,* sermo septimus: "De morbis oculorum," Cap. XIX: De hisquae oculo infiguntur" (Venetiis: Ex officina Farrea, 1543), 1. 330–331, Cited in Hirschberg J. History of ophthalmology. Trans by Blodi FC. Bonn: Wayenbourgh, 1982;1:338.
2. Catania LJ. Primary care of the anterior segment. Norwalk, Conn: Appleton and Lange, 1988:156–158.
3. Weene LE. Recurrent corneal erosion after trauma: a statistical study. Ann Ophthalmol 1985;17:521–522, 524.
4. Friedenald JS, Buschke W. Mitotic and wound healing activities of the corneal epithelium. Arch Ophthalmol 1944;32:410–413.
5. Hanna C, Fraunfelder FT, Cable M, et al. The effects of ophthalmic ointments on corneal wound healing. Am J Ophthalmol 1973;76:193–200.
6. Winski F, Stephens P. Direct lid taping: an alternative to pressure patching. Clin Eye Vision Care 1989;1:26–27.
7. Dua HS, Forester JV. Clinical patterns of corneal epithelial wound healing. Am J Ophthalmol 1987;104:481–489.
8. Danjo S, Friend J, Thoft RA. Conjunctival epithelium in healing of corneal epithelial wounds. Invest Ophthalmol Vis Sci 1987;28:1445–1449.

Anisocoria Evaluation

Richard London
Jimmy D. Bartlett

INTRODUCTION

Definition

Many clinical conditions can exhibit anisocoria as a primary or secondary feature (Table 46–1). Most of these conditions have in common that only one pupil is abnormal, demonstrating an inability either to dilate or to constrict. In most persons, either the sympathetic or the parasympathetic nervous system can be implicated, and various autonomic drugs may thus be used to pharmacologically differentiate the site of physical impairment. Routine pupillary testing, as discussed in Chapter 6, is the foundation of anisocoria evaluation, but, occasionally, photography of the pupils can be helpful, as can pharmacologic testing with topically applied eyedrops. This chapter emphasizes the clinical and pharmacologic procedures most useful for the diagnosis of the underlying causes of anisocoria.

History

The history of routine pupillary testing is described in Chapter 6. Perhaps the most evolutionary historical accounts of pharmacologic pupillary testing are those associated with Horner's syndrome and Adie's syndrome.

Topically applied cocaine and epinephrine have been used for almost 100 years for the pupillary drug testing of patients with suspected Horner's syndrome. Langley,[1] in 1901, discovered the physiologic properties of epinephrine and found that this drug seemed to have the same effect on the eye as does stimulation of the cervical sympathetic nerves. In 1910, Cords[2] described a patient with traumatic Horner's syndrome in which the pupil on the affected side dilated to extremely low concentrations of epinephrine. This observation led to epinephrine's use as an adjunct to cocaine in the diagnosis of Horner's syndrome. Later, however, Morone and Andreani[3] and Jaffe[4] demonstrated that the hypersensitivity response to epinephrine is unreliable in differentiating the location of the lesion causing Horner's syndrome. This fact, along with the individual differences in sensitivity to epinephrine, make the epinephrine test unreliable in the pharmacologic evaluation of Horner's syndrome. Since 1971,[5] hydroxyamphetamine has been used in conjunction with cocaine to evaluate the location of the lesion causing Horner's syndrome. Thus, cocaine is now used to establish the initial diagnosis of Horner's syndrome, whereas hydroxyamphetamine is used to help determine location of the lesion.

Denervation hypersensitivity of the cholinergic nervous system has been known to be associated with Adie's syndrome almost since the syndrome was first described in 1932.[6] In 1940, Scheie[7] demonstrated that most Adie's pupils would constrict to 2.5% methacholine but that normal pupils required as strong as 20% methacholine for miosis to occur. It was soon recognized, however, that numerous Adie's pupils failed to constrict to 2.5% methacholine, and it became apparent that there were large interindividual variations in sensitivity to this drug when low concentrations were used. Although methacholine became popular to elicit the cholinergic denervation hypersensitivity in Adie's pupil, this drug test became supplanted by the use of topically applied pilocarpine. This drug has been shown to be more useful and more reliable for the diagnosis of Adie's syndrome.

Table 46–1
Conditions That Exhibit Anisocoria

Physiologic anisocoria	Adrenergic mydriasis
Claude Bernard syndrome	Anticholinergic mydriasis
Horner's syndrome	Argyll Robertson pupils
Episodic unilateral mydriasis	Iris sphincter atrophy
Adie's syndrome	Angle-closure glaucoma
Third nerve palsy	

Clinical Use

Pupillary drug testing is used to help establish the diagnosis of the cause of anisocoria when routine pupillary testing (see Chap. 6) fails to reveal the diagnosis. The simple instillation of topically applied autonomic agents often obviates further neuroradiologic or laboratory investigation.

INSTRUMENTATION

Theory

The theoretical basis of pupillary drug testing in patients with anisocoria lies in the fact that topically instilled drugs that affect the autonomic nervous system will produce asymmetric responses between the two eyes depending on the degree of parasympathetic or sympathetic abnormality. Nearly every condition leading to anisocoria will affect only one pupil and will be manifest as an inability of the affected pupil either to dilate or to constrict. Usually either the sympathetic or parasympathetic nervous system can be implicated and will allow the topically instilled drug to reveal the abnormal pupillary response. It is important, therefore, that the drug be instilled into both eyes so that a comparison can be made of the pupillary response in each eye.

In the pupillary drug testing of patients suspected to have Horner's syndrome or Adie's syndrome, the evaluation makes use of the principle of denervation hypersensitivity. This condition frequently follows lesions affecting autonomic neurons and is manifested by a greater than normal end-organ response to the endogenous neurotransmitter.[6] In clinical practice, this phenomenon can be demonstrated using exogenously administered neurochemicals. In Horner's syndrome, there is denervation of the adrenergic nervous system, which gives rise to hypersensitivity to applied catecholamines such as epinephrine or phenylephrine. Although denervation hypersensitivity tests are not commonly used for the diagnosis of Horner's syndrome, epinephrine or phenylephrine, nevertheless, will often cause a greater than normal dilatation of the affected pupil.

In contrast with the adrenergic hypersensitivity shown in patients with Horner's syndrome, patients with Adie's syndrome have hypersensitivity in the cholinergic system and thus will demonstrate pupillary constriction, which is greater than in normal eyes, to low concentrations of miotics. Cholinergic hypersensitivity of the denervated iris sphincter in Adie's pupil has been known for many years and can be quite useful in the diagnosis of this syndrome. It should be recognized, however, that the hypersensitivity does not seem to be correlated with the amount of sphincter denervation, the duration of the Adie's pupil, or the amount of light-near dissociation. Occasionally, an acute Adie's pupil will demonstrate very little hypersensitivity during the first several weeks after onset, but will gradually become more hypersensitive several months following the initial episode. Low concentrations of pilocarpine are now commonly used to show this hypersensitivity response in the affected pupil.

Use

The practitioner should proceed with pupillary drug testing when the patient's history is incomplete or noncontributory, or when the clinical signs and symptoms are too ambiguous to enable a definitive diagnosis. The following general guidelines will facilitate pupillary drug testing and improve the accuracy with which the drugs allow a definitive diagnosis.[8]

1. One drop of the indicated drug should be instilled into each eye and repeated after several minutes.
2. The indicated drug should always be instilled into both eyes so that the response of the affected pupil can be compared with that of the normal pupil. If the condition is bilateral, however, as in anticholinergic mydriasis caused by systemic agents, the topical drop should be placed into only one eye so that the response of each pupil can be compared.
3. The amount of ambient illumination before and after drug instillation must be constant.
4. Accommodation should be carefully controlled during the "before" and "after" evaluations so that it can be eliminated as a factor producing the pupillary size change.
5. Photography of the pupils is strongly recommended to enable a more accurate evaluation of pupil size both before and after instillation of the indicated drug. Since appropriate patient management depends on accurate diagnosis, the clinician should not simply estimate the differences in pupil size.

COMMERCIALLY AVAILABLE INSTRUMENTS

Routine clinical assessment of the pupils (see Chap. 6) is indicated before evaluation procedures specific for anisocoria are initiated. Pupillary drug testing requires only the commercially available pharmaceuticals. Contemporary pupillary drug testing of patients with anisocoria involves the use of topically applied cocaine, hydroxyamphetamine, or pilocarpine. The most satisfactory results with cocaine are obtained with the 10% concentration. Although a suitable preparation is not available specifically for ophthalmic use, good results can be obtained with commercially prepared 10% cocaine formulated for topical use in otolaryngology. Hydroxyamphetamine is used in a 1% concentration, and pilocarpine should be available in 0.125%, 0.5%, and 1.0% concentrations. The 0.125% pilocarpine can be prepared from the commercially available 1.0% formulation by simply diluting the latter concentration in a ratio of 7 drops of normal saline or extraocular irrigating solution to 1 drop of 1.0% pilocarpine. This can be extemporaneously prepared in a clean and dry artificial tear bottle for application directly into the eye.

CLINICAL PROCEDURE

Clinical Evaluation

1. The routine examination of pupillary function, as described in Chapter 6, should precede the evaluation procedures specific for anisocoria. The existence of anisocoria must be documented by careful measurement of the pupillary size difference. This can be accomplished using external photography, or it can be accurately estimated by pupillary area.
2. When evaluating the responses of the pupils to direct light, if one pupil responds poorly, this indicates that the sluggish pupil has been affected by abnormal parasympathetic innervation or by a physical or mechanical impediment to

its constriction. On the other hand, if the light reaction is good in both eyes, the anisocoria is probably due to abnormal sympathetic innervation. Physiologic anisocoria is also commonly associated with normally responsive pupils.

3. A comparison of the anisocoria in bright and dim ambient illuminations may be helpful in determining the diagnosis. A darkened examination room, or the use of an ultraviolet light in a completely darkened room to allow lenticular fluorescence, will be adequate to reveal the status of the anisocoria in dim illumination. A Burton lamp can be held 8 to 12 in. from the patient to illuminate the pupils. If the anisocoria increases in darkness, the differential diagnosis includes Horner's syndrome or physiologic anisocoria (Fig. 46–1). If the anisocoria is greater in the light than in darkness, this generally indicates an abnormal parasympathetic innervation to the iris sphincter, and the differential diagnosis includes Adie's pupil, iris sphincter atrophy, or any of the disorders implicated as a "unilateral fixed and dilated" pupil.

4. Careful slit lamp examination is necessary to reveal evidence of mechanical restrictions of the pupil. Iris damage from previous ocular inflammation or trauma is a common cause of anisocoria and a poorly responsive pupil. Slit lamp evaluation may uncover areas of posterior synechiae or iris sphincter atrophy.

5. It is important to inspect recent and old personal photographs of the patient to help reveal the possible onset of the condition. Patients are often quite insistent that their newly discovered condition is of recent onset, but upon inspection of old photographs it may be discovered that the condition is indeed long-standing. This fact can be extremely important in the differential diagnosis and prognosis of the condition.

6. The observed anisocoria may often have associated diagnostic physical findings. The existence of ipsilateral ptosis

and anhydrosis, for example, is highly suggestive of Horner's syndrome. The patient with a unilateral sluggish pupil, with associated accommodative insufficiency and diminished deep tendon reflexes, may be suspected of having Adie's syndrome. Thus, careful pupillary examination, with special attention given to the patient's history as well as to other ocular or systemic physical findings, may allow the clinician to determine the diagnosis, without need for pharmacologic or other more sophisticated examination methods.

Pharmacologic Evaluation

Patients with suspected Horner's syndrome should be initially evaluated with topically instilled cocaine. The pharmacologic properties of cocaine permit the initial diagnosis of Horner's syndrome by revealing dilatation of the normal pupil, whereas the Horner's pupil exhibits reduced or absent dilatation.[9] This is true regardless of the site of the lesion causing Horner's syndrome. To perform the test, 1 drop of 10% cocaine solution should be instilled into each eye and repeated after several minutes. The pupils should be evaluated after 30 to 45 minutes (Fig. 46–2). A positive cocaine test should be followed several days later by testing with hydroxyamphetamine. The site of the lesion can be predicted with the hydroxyamphetamine test, in which 1 drop of the 1% concentration is instilled into each eye and repeated after several minutes. The indirect pharmacologic action of hydroxyamphetamine is useful to distinguish between central or preganglionic and postganglionic lesions. The normal pupil will be seen to dilate, whereas the Horner's pupil will dilate normally if the lesion is central or preganglionic, but will dilate poorly if the lesion is postganglionic (see Fig. 46–2).

Patients with suspected Adie's pupil should be evaluated by instilling topical pilocarpine 0.125% into each eye and repeated

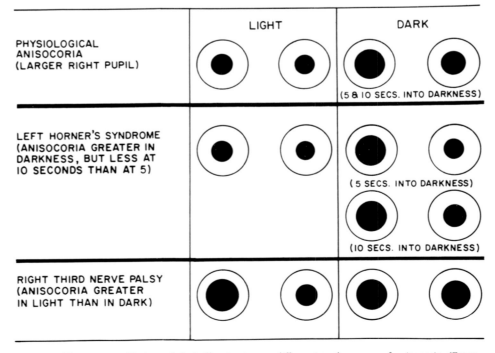

FIGURE 46–1. Use of light and dark illumination to differentiate the cause of anisocoria. (From Bartlett JD. Abnormalities of the pupil. In: Bartlett JD, Jaanus SD, eds. Clinical ocular pharmacology, 2nd ed. Boston: Butterworth, 1989:431–454, with permission)

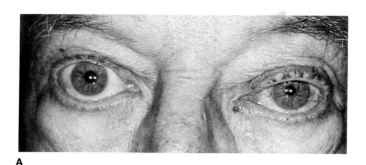

A

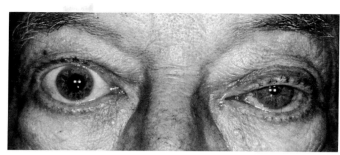

B

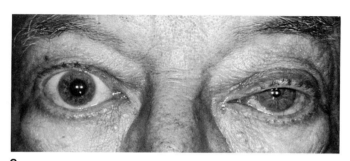

C

FIGURE 46–2. Patient with Horner's syndrome affecting left eye: (*A*) normal ambient illumination; (*B*) following instillation of 10% cocaine into each eye there is dilatation of the normal right pupil, but absence of dilatation of the left Horner's pupil; (*C*) following instillation of 1% hydroxyamphetamine into each eye, there is dilatation of the normal right pupil, but absence of dilatation of the left Horner's pupil, indicating a postganglionic lesion. (From Bartlett JD. Abnormalities of the pupil. In: Bartlett JD, Jaanus SD, eds. Clinical ocular pharmacology, 2nd ed. Boston: Butterworth, 1989:431–454, with permission)

after several minutes. Since the usefulness of the pilocarpine test in eliciting cholinergic hypersensitivity depends on the presence of a standardized concentration of pilocarpine at the iris sphincter, any clinical procedure that compromises the corneal epithelium may result in false-positive findings. Thus, tonometry, gonioscopy, use of anesthetics, or other procedures that enhance corneal penetration should be avoided before initiation of pupillary drug testing for Adie's syndrome. If Adie's pupil is present, the pilocarpine will, after 30 minutes, slightly constrict the normal pupil, but will cause significant constriction of the Adie's pupil (Fig. 46–3).

Patients suspected of having intracranial third nerve palsy, without other obvious signs, such as exotropia and ptosis, should be evaluated by first using 0.125% pilocarpine to reveal any cholinergic hypersensitivity as evidence for Adie's pupil. If no cholinergic hypersensitivity is demonstrated to 0.125% pilocarpine, the clinician should subsequently instill pilocarpine in a concentration of 0.5% or 1.0%. If third nerve palsy is the cause of the dilated pupil, the affected pupil should promptly constrict (Fig. 46–4).

The diagnostic procedure of choice in patients suspected of having anticholinergic mydriasis is 0.5% or 1.0% pilocarpine instilled into each eye and repeated after several minutes. If the muscarinic receptor sites on the affected iris sphincter are occu-

pied by an anticholinergic drug, the pilocarpine will be unable to activate the receptors and constrict the pupil. Thus, if the pupil has been inadvertently dilated with an anticholinergic agent or substance, the pilocarpine will be unable to constrict the pupil (Fig. 46–5), whereas if the pupil is dilated because of intracranial third nerve palsy, the 0.5% or 1.0% pilocarpine will promptly constrict the affected pupil.

CLINICAL IMPLICATIONS

Clinical Significance

Almost all patients with anisocoria have no evidence of debilitating neurologic disease; therefore, these patients can be appropriately evaluated and managed in the optometric practice without neurologic consultation. By performing routine pupillary testing as described in Chapter 6 and by evaluating pupils pharmacologically using topically applied autonomic agents, the optometrist can often quickly and easily differentiate the site of impairment. Accordingly, pupillary drug testing serves as an invaluable adjunct to routine testing of pupillary function.[10]

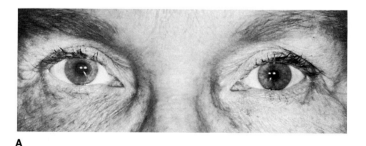

A

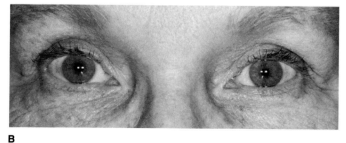

B

FIGURE 46–3. Pilocarpine test in 57-year-old woman with right Adie's pupil: (*A*) before drug instillation; (*B*) following instillation of 0.125% pilocarpine into each eye the normal left pupil constricts slightly, whereas the right Adie's pupil constricts significantly. (From Bartlett JD. Abnormalities of the pupil. In: Bartlett JD, Jaanus SD, eds. Clinical ocular pharmacology, 2nd ed. Boston: Butterworth, 1989:431–454, with permission)

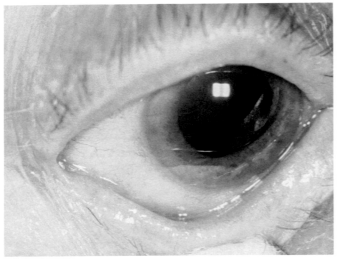

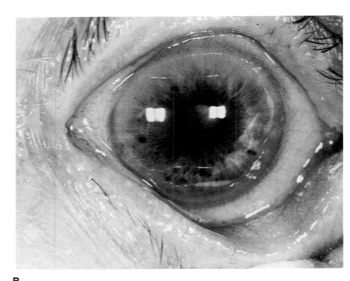

A   **B**

FIGURE 46–4. Pilocarpine test in third nerve palsy: (*A*) before drug instillation; (*B*) following instillation of 1.0% pilocarpine, the pupil promptly constricts. (From Bartlett JD. Abnormalities of the pupil. In: Bartlett JD, Jaanus SD, eds. Clinical ocular pharmacology, 2nd ed. Boston: Butterworths, 1989:431–454, with permission)

Clinical Interpretation

The most common condition characterized by unequal pupils is physiologic (essential) anisocoria. The condition is found in from 1% to more than 50% of the general population,[11] but it is seldom greater than 1 mm and can be variable, changing from day to day or hour to hour. Both pupils constrict normally to light and will dilate normally with cocaine. When the degree of anisocoria is compared in darkness and in light, there is greater anisocoria in darkness. Patients with physiologic anisocoria can thus be reassured about their condition, and no further evaluation is necessary.

Findings typical of Horner's syndrome include unilateral ptosis, ipsilateral miosis, conjunctival hyperemia in acute cases, facial or body anhydrosis depending on the site of the lesion, and heterochromia iridis (if congenital). The cocaine test will confirm the clinical diagnosis, and the hydroxyamphetamine test will help to localize the site of the lesion causing the Horner's pupil. A useful mnemonic for the hydroxyamphetamine test is "fail-safe."[12] This phrase suggests that failure of the pupil to dilate with hydroxyamphetamine indicates a good prognosis because it indicates a postganglionic lesion. Such lesions are frequently associated with typical cluster headache—a benign disorder—whereas patients with central or preganglionic lesions must receive further evaluation by an internist or neurologist to exclude the possibility of neoplastic or vascular disease.

Adie's syndrome is characterized by relative mydriasis in bright illumination, absent or poor light response, slow contraction to prolonged near effort, sector palsies of the iris sphincter, paresis of accommodation, and diminished deep tendon reflexes. These findings usually occur in women, with an onset in the third to fifth decade of life. Although most cases of Adie's syndrome can be confirmed clinically without pupillary drug testing, evaluation with topically instilled pilocarpine 0.125% can be helpful to confirm the diagnosis in questionable cases. Once the diagnosis is confirmed, the patient can be reassured that the condition is a benign disorder with a favorable prognosis. Pilocarpine should generally not be prescribed to overcome the mydriasis or to stimulate accommodation. Symptomatic patients, however, may sometimes benefit from the prescription of unequal spectacle additions or from the instillation of pilocarpine several times daily.

The patient in whom pilocarpine confirms the diagnosis of third nerve palsy should generally receive neurologic consultation, especially if the lesion is of recent onset. The numerous neoplastic and vascular etiologies of intracranial third nerve palsy necessitate complete neurologic, radiologic, and laboratory investigation for definitive diagnosis and management.

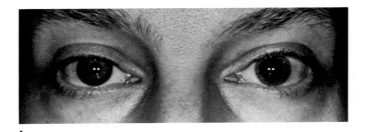

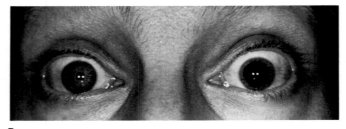

A   **B**

FIGURE 46–5. Pilocarpine test in anticholinergic mydriasis: (*A*) 27-year-old man with fixed and dilated left pupil; (*B*) following instillation of 1.0% pilocarpine into each eye, the right pupil constricts, whereas the left pupil does not. (From Bartlett JD. Abnormalities of the pupil. In: Bartlett JD, Jaanus SD, eds. Clinical ocular pharmacology, 2nd ed. Boston: Butterworth, 1989:431–454, with permission)

Anticholinergic mydriasis, also known as pharmacologic blockade or "atropine" mydriasis, refers to the fixed and dilated pupil resulting from the accidental inoculation into the eye of drugs or substances with anticholinergic properties. These substances can include cycloplegic agents, jimson weed dust, medication for motion sickness, and cosmetics and perfumes. Thus, a careful history is especially important before initiating pupillary drug testing. A history of a drug or substance accidentally instilled into the eye will often lead the practitioner quickly to perform the pilocarpine test, which readily confirms the diagnosis. Once the diagnosis of anticholinergic mydriasis has been confirmed, the patient can simply be reassured that the pupil will spontaneously return to its original size, and accommodation will improve as the effects of the inoculated substance subside.

REFERENCES

1. Langley JN. Observations on the physiological action of extracts of the supra-renal bodies. J Physiol 1901;27:237–256.
2. Cords R. Ein fall von schlafenschuss mit lahmung des Augen sympathicus. Arch Klin Exp Ophthalmol 1910;75:113–128.
3. Morone G, Andreani F. Richerche pupillografiche nella sindrome di Bernard-Horner sotto l'azione di alcuni medicamenti. Riv Oto-Neuro-Oftal 1949;24:180–194.
4. Jaffe NS. Localization of lesions causing Horner's syndrome. Arch Ophthalmol 1950;44:710–728.
5. Thompson HS, Mensher JH. Adrenergic mydriasis in Horner's syndrome. Hydroxyamphetamine test for diagnosis of postganglionic defects. Am J Ophthalmol 1971;72:472–480.
6. Adie WJ. Tonic pupils and absent tendon reflexes: a benign disorder sui generis; its complete and incomplete forms. Brain 1932;55:98–113.
7. Scheie HG. Site of disturbance in Adie's syndrome. Arch Ophthalmol 1940;24:225–237.
8. Bartlett JD. Abnormalities of the pupil. In: Bartlett JD, Jaanus SD, eds. Clinical ocular pharmacology, 2nd ed. Boston: Butterworths, 1989:431–454.
9. Thompson HS. Diagnosing Horner's syndrome. Trans Am Acad Ophthalmol Otolaryngol 1977;83:840–842.
10. Thompson HS, Pilley SFJ. Unequal pupils. A flow chart for sorting out the anisocorias. Surv Ophthalmol 1976;21:45–48.
11. Lam BL, Thompson HS, Corbett JJ. The prevalence of simple anisocoria. Am J Ophthalmol 1987;104:69–73.
12. Brumberg JB. Horner's syndrome and the ultraviolet light as an aid in its detection. J Am Optom Assoc 1981;52:641–646.

Fundus Biomicroscopy

Felix M. Barker

INTRODUCTION

Definition

Fundus biomicroscopy is the procedure for examination of the vitreoretinal cavity by using the slit lamp biomicroscope.[1-4] Since the biomicroscope is a focal instrument, an auxiliary lens is required to bring the more posterior structures of the eye into view.

History

It was during the early part of this century that the slit lamp biomicroscope was first used in examination of the internal eye.[2-4] In 1918, Koeppe used a −54-diopter (D) contact lens to neutralize the power of the eye so that the vitreous and retina could be visualized.[4,5]

In 1923, Lemoine and Valois demonstrated that this high-minus lens need not be placed in contact with the eye.[6] The use of a minus lens in air was brought to practical usage in 1941 by Hruby,[5] who demonstrated that a −58-D lens held in front of the eye was a less invasive method for fundus biomicroscopy. The Hruby lens is found today on virtually every modern biomicroscope.

In 1937, Goldmann[3,5] introduced a Plexiglas contact lens that contained a mirror to allow a more peripheral fundus view. Eisner,[4,7] in 1967, added the use of a scleral indentation attachment to the Goldmann mirror contact lens to include the ora serrata in this peripheral view.

Although the use of a condensing lens had been described a century earlier by Ruete[8] in the technique of indirect ophthalmoscopy, it was not until 1953 that El Bayadi suggested using such a lens (+55 D) with the biomicroscope.[5] El Bayadi claimed that this method was superior to the Hruby technique because of its much wider field of view and its improved capability for the examination of the retinal periphery. He also commented that it was more convenient than contact lens procedures because it required no eye contact. Termed indirect biomicroscopy or micro-ophthalmoscopy, this method had been used for both routine and specialized examination[9-15] as well as photography,[15-21] but primarily in countries outside the United States. It has, however, recently been reintroduced in the United States and abroad by Volk as first the +60-D lens[12] and later as the more popular +90-D and +78-D lens.[22] Most clinicians in the United States were introduced to the +90-D lens first. Since the introduction of the +90-D lens, many authors have reported the technique of indirect biomicroscopy and its varied uses.[15-17,22-25] More recently, holders for the Volk +90-D lens have been described[26-28] that provide a more stable image and better ease of use, especially for the novice clinician.

The contact lens approach has also been combined with the convex condensing lens in the form of the "panfunduscope" introduced by Schlegel in 1969.[29-31] The panfunduscope system was designed for both diagnostic evaluation and for panretinal photocoagulation. Volk[32,33] has also recently introduced an indirect fundus contact lens with a very wide field of view (~125°). This lens is named the quadraspheric lens because of its four aspheric surfaces.

Clinical Use

Fundus biomicroscopy is frequently advantageous in comparison with direct ophthalmoscopy because it is a binocular technique that allows the use of variable magnification, access to the periphery, and can give a very wide field of view.[2,3,5,9,15,24] Fundus biomicroscopy also provides the clinician with slit beam illumination of the retina, which is often critical to proper assessment.[4] The use of the biomicroscope does not eliminate the need for binocular indi-

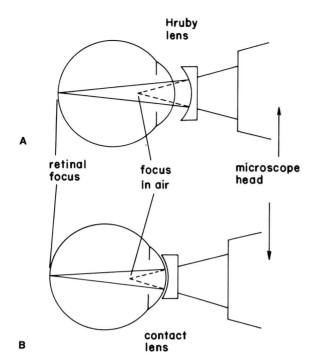

Hruby lens

A

retinal focus

focus in air

microscope head

contact lens

B

FIGURE 47–1. Direct fundus biomicroscopy: (*A*) use of a minus lens in air (Hruby method); (*B*) use of a minus lens in contact with the eye (Koeppe/Goldmann method). (From Barker FM. Vitreoretinal biomicroscopy: a comparison of techniques. J Am Optom Assoc 1987;58:985–992, with permission)

rect ophthalmoscopy (BIO), but rather, complements BIO by giving the clinician the opportunity to examine and photograph vitreoretinal lesions binocularly under high magnification after they have been detected during the ophthalmoscopic survey. Fundus biomicroscopy is also important because it is the principal method of delivery for laser photocoagulation of the fundus cavity.[34–43]

INSTRUMENTATION

Theory

The slit lamp biomicroscope has an objective focal distance that enables it to be most easily used for examination of the anterior segment to just beyond the posterior lens capsule. However, to

view the retina or the vitreous requires the use of one of the many available auxiliary lenses. The principal purpose of an auxiliary lens is to neutralize the optical power of the eye, so the fundus can be brought into focus. Another, equally important purpose of some lenses is to expand the available field of view.

Direct Fundus Biomicroscopy

Like direct ophthalmoscopy, the direct auxiliary lens serves mainly to neutralize the optical power of the eye so the microscope can be used to "focus back" to the vitreous humor and the retina (Fig. 47–1). The patient's pupil remains the field stop in this system and restricts the field of view to about 5° to 15°. This method can be performed with the neutralizing lens held in air (Hruby method; see Fig. 47–1*A*) or with the lens in contact with the eye (Koeppe/ Goldmann method; see Fig. 47–1*B*).

The optical principle of the fundus contact lens is much the same as the Hruby lens, but its closer proximity to the pupil gives a wider field of view. Mirrors are a common feature in the design of this type of lens and may possess various angles to view different areas of the peripheral fundus (Fig. 47–2). Fundus contact lenses differ primarily in the angle of the mirror and, therefore, the area of the fundus available to view. In general, the mirrors of fundus contact lenses are angled at varying degrees depending upon their use. The angle stated for any given mirror refers to the angle between the mirror and the front surface of the lens.[44] The larger the angle of the mirror, the more steeply inclined will that mirror be away from the observer and the farther posterior will be its viewing region within the eye.

Indirect Fundus Biomicroscopy

In contrast, the method of indirect biomicroscopy uses a high plus auxiliary lens, such as the Volk +60-D, +78-D, or +90-D lens. This type of lens focuses the light coming from the eye into a plane between the lens and the clinician's microscope (Fig. 47–3). As with BIO, the fundus is seen as an aerial image that is inverted and reversed. Although this may seem inconvenient to some at first, there is a significant advantage to learning this method in that field of view is much larger than the direct method (up to 60°). This is because the high-plus condensing lens optically eliminates the patient's pupil as a field stop in the system. It does so by focusing an image of the pupil around the clinician's biomicroscope (Fig. 47–4). This field stop condition has been effectively illustrated for indirect ophthalmoscopy by Rubin[45] in a cartoon showing the doctor to be focused in the plane of the pupil (Fig. 47–5). From this "internal" vantage point, the clinician, using an indirect-viewing technique, has complete access to vitreal and retinal structures up to the limit of the diameter of the condensing lens.

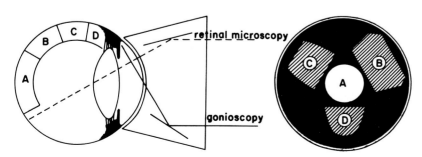

retinal microscopy

gonioscopy

FIGURE 47–2. Direct fundus biomicroscopy using a Goldmann three-mirror contact lens. (From Barker FM. Vitreoretinal biomicroscopy: a comparison of techniques. J Am Optom Assoc 1987;58:985–992, with permission)

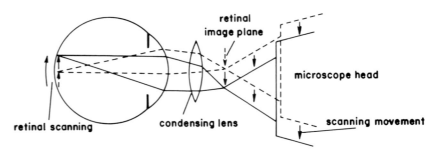

FIGURE 47–3. Indirect fundus biomicroscopy using a Volk +90-D lens in air, demonstrating image formation. (From Barker FM. Vitreoretinal biomicroscopy: a comparison of techniques. J Am Optom Assoc 1987;58:985–992, with permission)

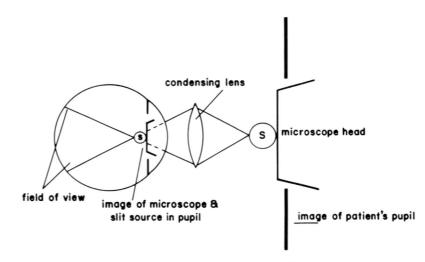

FIGURE 47–4. Indirect fundus biomicroscopy using a +90-D lens in air, demonstrating field stop considerations. (From Barker FM. Vitreoretinal biomicroscopy: a comparison of techniques. J Am Optom Assoc 1987;58:985–992, with permission)

Use

The Hruby method has the advantage of being easy to learn and can be used clinically with a minimum of inconvenience to the patient. The field of view, however, is very limited in this technique, and precise alignment with any given point on the retina requires exact control of the patient's gaze by use of the fixation light. The requirement for precise patient gaze control, coupled with the rather small field of view, make it difficult to conduct a thorough evaluation of the entire posterior pole. Rather, the most useful approach with the Hruby lens is to use it to carefully examine the macula, optic nerve head, or a specific lesion that has been previously noted in the posterior pole with the BIO.

The Goldmann contact lens method has fewer reflections, gives a slightly larger field of view, and permits greater control of eye position and fundus position. The use of mirrors gives this technique the advantage when a peripheral area must be viewed microscopically. Goldmann examination, however, is somewhat less convenient in that it requires contact of the lens with the corneal surface. This is easily accomplished, when necessary, but does involve the additional steps of corneal anesthesia, patient explanation, placement of the lens, and irrigation of the cul-de-sac upon removal. To a large degree, these steps have been an impediment to the establishment of the Goldmann technique as a routine examination procedure.

Indirect biomicroscopy with the Volk +90-D lens makes access to the central retinal surface relatively easy to control by simple slit lamp joystick movements. Peripheral examination and photography are also possible for the skilled clinician. However, the attainment of the ideal field of view condition in this technique is achieved only with precise alignment and distance placement of the condensing lens in relationship to the eye. This requires some practice, but is well worth the effort for the conscientious clinician.

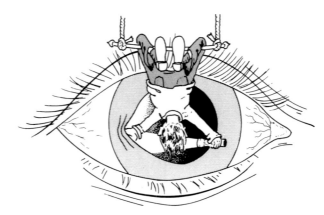

FIGURE 47–5. Cartoon depicting the indirect ophthalmoscopy examiner hanging upside down in the patient's pupil. (Adapted from Rubin M. The optics of indirect ophthalmoscopy. Surv Ophthalmol 1964;9:449–464, with permission)

COMMERCIALLY AVAILABLE INSTRUMENTS

In general, there are a wide variety of fundus biomicroscopy lenses designed for differing purposes (Tables 47–1 to 47–3) that can be obtained from various manufacturers. They currently range in cost from $150 to $550. The following discussion will cover these lenses listed by category of design.

Noncontact Lenses

Noncontact fundus lenses (see Table 47–1) have the distinct advantage of convenience for both clinician and patient. Their lack of eye contact makes them inherently less invasive and, as a result, the procedures take less time to perform. These features make them ideal for routine examination purposes. Their noncontact approach, however, also somewhat limits their image stability and eye movement control.

Hruby Lens

The first lens to consider is the −58-D Hruby lens[14,46] (see Figs. 47–1 and 47–6), which is perhaps the most commonly available lens because it has been supplied as a standard feature on most slit lamp microscopes currently in use. There are two basic mounting methods used, and these were originally found on the Zeiss and the Haag–Streit biomicroscope designs. Other manufacturers of biomicroscopes have used one of these two designs.

Table 47–1
Noncontact Fundus Lenses

Lens	Power	Optics	Field of View
Hruby	−58 D	Direct	Small
Volk +60 D	+60 D	Indirect	Large
Volk +78 D	+78 D	Indirect	Larger
Volk +90 D	+90 D	Indirect	Larger
Nikon +90 D	+90 D	Indirect	Larger

Table 47–2
Nonmirrored Fundus Contact Lenses

Lens	Front Curve	Scleral Contact	Comments
O'Malley	Plano	No	Soft contact lens
Krieger	Concave	Yes	Wide-field lens
Ruiz	Plano	Yes	Lid control lens
Peyman capsule	Convex	Yes	YAG capsulotomy lens
Peyman wide-field	Convex	Yes	Three front curves for various depths of penetration in vitreous
Abraham YAG	Convex	Yes	Capsulotomy button lens
Yannuzzi	Plano	Yes	Allows eye movement control
McLean prism	Plano	Yes	25-D prism
Layden infant	Convex	No	Gonio and fundus lens
Panfunduscope	Convex	Yes	Very wide field
Mainster	Convex	Yes	Very wide field
Volk Quadraspheric	Convex	Yes	Very wide field

Table 47–3
Mirrored Fundus Contact Lenses

Lens	Mirror Angles (degrees)	Uses (zones*)	Comments
Goldmann universal	59, 67, 73	I, II, III, IV	Most common four sizes
Hart pediatric	59, 67, 73	I, II, III, IV	Like Goldmann
Karickhoff	62, 67, 76, 80	I, II, III, IV	More field overlap than Goldmann
Thorpe	64 (2), 70 (2)	I, III, IV	Duplicate mirrors reduce lens rotation
Wilson	73 (3)	IV	Strictly peripheral
Boys–Smith	59, 67, 73	I, II, III, IV	Like Goldmann with pigment grading capability for gonioscopy
Urrets–Ferrer	70 (4)	I, II, III, IV	Has handle; scans zones by movement of lens on cornea

* Zones refer to the areas visible in the retina by each portion of lens in question. Refer to Fig. 47–2 for zones.

ZEISS HRUBY LENS. The Zeiss method mounts the Hruby lens permanently above the microscope on a swing-down holder that is retractable (see Fig. 47–6). The lens moves laterally in constant alignment with the movement of the microscope system during the examination. The distance of the lens from the eye is held constant by the use of a "fender" attached to the headrest above the patient's eye. This design is supposed to enable the clinician to examine the eye with hands free for lens control. Problems associated with this method are that lateral movement of the biomicroscope may cause alignment of the lens to move off-center, causing a need for maintenance alignment, and depending upon the patient, the "fender" may or may not position the lens at the optimal distance from the eye.

THE HAAG–STREIT HRUBY. The Haag–Streit Hruby lens mount is adjustable and sits at the top of a removable vertical rod that fits

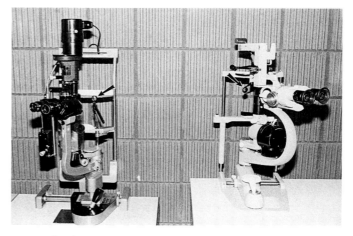

FIGURE 47–6. Hruby lens attachments (*arrows*) for the Zeiss (*right*) and the Haag-Streit (*left*) slit lamp biomicroscopes. (From Barker FM. Vitreoretinal biomicroscopy: a comparison of techniques. J Am Optom Assoc 1987;58:985–992, with permission)

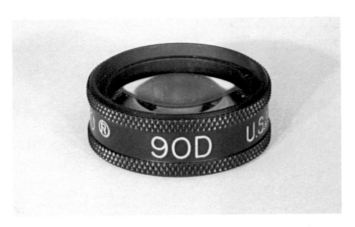

FIGURE 47–7. Volk +90-D lens. (Courtesy of Volk Optics, Inc.)

into a sliding track in front of the microscope (see Fig. 47–6). This design keeps the lens in lateral alignment with the biomicroscope and at a constant distance from the eye, but is more versatile than the Zeiss design by its ability to allow the specific adjustment of that distance for each patient.

Volk Lenses

VOLK +90-D LENS. The Volk +90-D lens (see Figs. 47–3 and 47–7) is a symmetrically double-aspheric biomicroscopic condensing lens that may be used with either surface toward the eye.[15]

Properly used, this lens can provide up to a 60° field of view, with excellent image resolution. Working distances with this lens are shorter than with the earlier designed +60-D lens and, therefore, are more natural. Volk lenses are available clear or tinted yellow to reduce the patient's light sensitivity.

Volk makes a lens holder called the "Steady Mount" that attaches to the headrest of the biomicroscope (Fig. 47–8) and has improved the steadiness of the fundus view with this lens, especially for the novice clinician.

Volk also has recently introduced a "snap-on" rim adapter (Fig. 47–9), which can help the novice user to maintain lens distance and position as well as to control lid action.

VOLK +60-D LENS. The Volk +60-D lens is an asymmetric double-aspheric convex fundus lens for slit lamp biomicroscopy.[12] As with the +20-D lens in indirect ophthalmoscopy, the steeper curve of the lens should be toward the clinician to maximize the image clarity. This is indicated by a cutout on the patient side of the lens rim for nasal clearance of this relatively large lens. The +60-D power of the lens provides a high magnification, but requires a relatively longer working distance.

VOLK +78-D LENS. The most recently introduced lens design from Volk of this design is the +78-D lens (see Fig. 47–9). Although lower in power than the +90-D version, this lens has a much larger diameter and, therefore, has the same, or slightly larger, field of view than the +90-D. The principal value of the lens is supposed to be its slightly larger magnification, without loss of field.

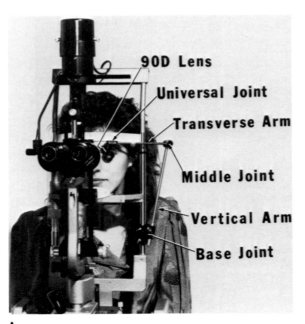
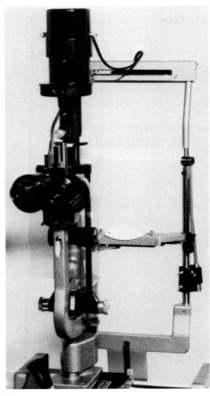

FIGURE 47–8. Volk +90-D lens in the Volk "Steady Mount": (A) in position for fundus biomicroscopy; (B) in storage position. (From Barker FM. The Volk steady mount holder for the +90 D lens. J Am Optom Assoc 1988;59:558–560, with permission)

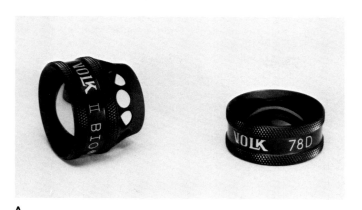
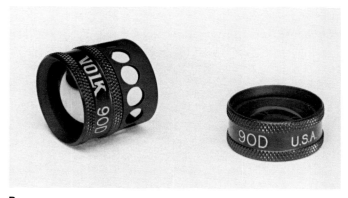

A   **B**

FIGURE 47–9. Volk +78-D (*A*) and +90-D (*B*) lenses with detachable lid control rim. (Courtesy of Volk Optics, Inc.)

Nikon +90-D Lens

The Nikon +90-D lens is patterned after the Volk +90-D lens and differs primarily in that Nikon offers a yellow filter that is threaded to fit over their basic clear lens (Fig. 47–10).

Nonmirror Fundus Contact Lenses

Fundus contact lenses without mirrors are available in a wide variety of designs (see Table 47–2).

Corneosclero Lenses

The corneosclero lenses were developed to improve control of the lens on the cornea during the examination. They accomplish this in a number of ways. First, there is a much larger diameter to these lenses, which allows them to cover a larger area of the cornea and sclera. Second, they often have a scleral flange that helps prevent lid tension from dislodging a lens and may even allow the lids to help hold the lens on the eye, thereby allowing some patients to be examined with both hands free. Third, these lenses are thicker and frequently have a knurled grasping ring at their anterior margin. Not only can the lens be held with more stability, but the patient's eye is held relatively immobile by the lens. The lens can also be moved to an off-center position to better view a paracentral area.

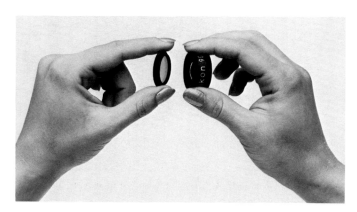

FIGURE 47–10. Nikon +90-D lens, with detachable yellow filter. (Courtesy of Nikon, Inc.)

RUIZ FUNDUS CONTACT LENS. The Ruiz lens is designed with a large scleral flange and is primarily intended for hands-free examination after insertion.[47] It stays on the eye by virtue of lid overlap of the haptic lens rim.

KRIEGER FUNDUS CONTACT LENS. The Krieger lens (Fig. 47–11*A*) is similar in its scleral design to the Ruiz lens, but has an opaque plastic ring extending forward for hand holding and manipulation of the lens.[36,43] The anterior surface also has a slight negative curve to which the lens owes its designation as a "wide-field" lens (40°).

YANNUZZI FUNDUS CONTACT LENS. The Yannuzzi lens (see Fig. 47–11*B*) has a design physically similar to the Krieger lens.[43] However, it has a plane front surface that provides a smaller field of view, but a correspondingly larger magnification, which the designer claims provides better control when photocoagulating near the macula. Also, the corneal surface of the lens has a steeper curvature to allow more direct pressure on the scleral contact area, without distorting the cornea. This is supposed to help maintain eye position and control subretinal hemorrhage during photocoagulation.

PEYMAN WIDE-FIELD YAG LENS. The Peyman wide-field lens (see Fig. 47–11*C*) is similar to the two previously described lenses, but has a smaller scleral flange and a positively curved front surface.[39] This front curve is available in three different curvatures (12.5 mm, 18 mm, and 25 mm), which are designed to provide focal access to the vitreous at various depths.

PEYMAN CAPSULOTOMY YAG LASER LENS. Another Peyman lens is designed to place the clinician's focus at the posterior capsule for capsulotomy using the Neodymium : YAG (yttrium–aluminum–garnett) laser (see Fig. 47–11*D*).

ABRAHAM YAG LASER LENS. The Abraham lens (see Fig. 47–11*E*) is much the same as the Peyman capsulotomy lens, except that the optical zone is steeper and is in the form of a centrally located lens button.[36]

PANFUNDUSCOPE. The Rodenstock Panfunduscope lens features a high-plus condensing lens, mounted in a tubular ring with a haptic contact lens surface for application to the eye.[29–31] It was designed for both examination and photocoagulation treatment for which its wide field of view would eliminate the need for excessive lens movement. It does, however, have some rather severe distortions in certain parts of the field that can limit its usefulness.

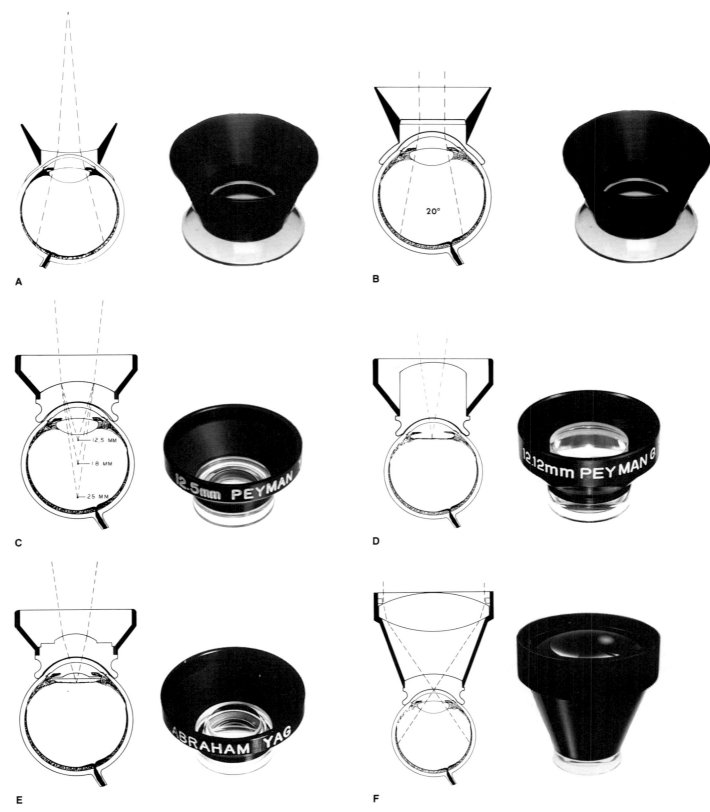

FIGURE 47–11. Nonmirrored fundus contact lenses (corresponding schematic diagrams are pictured adjacent to each type of lens): (*A*) Krieger fundus lens; (*B*) Yannuzzi fundus lens; (*C*) Peyman wide-field YAG lens; (*D*) Peyman capsulotomy YAG lens; (*E*) Abraham YAG lens; (*F*) Mainster fundus lens; (*G*) McLean prism lens; (*H*) Layden infant lens (Courtesy of Ocular Instruments, Inc.); (*I*) Volk Quadraspheric lens. (Courtesy of Volk Optical)

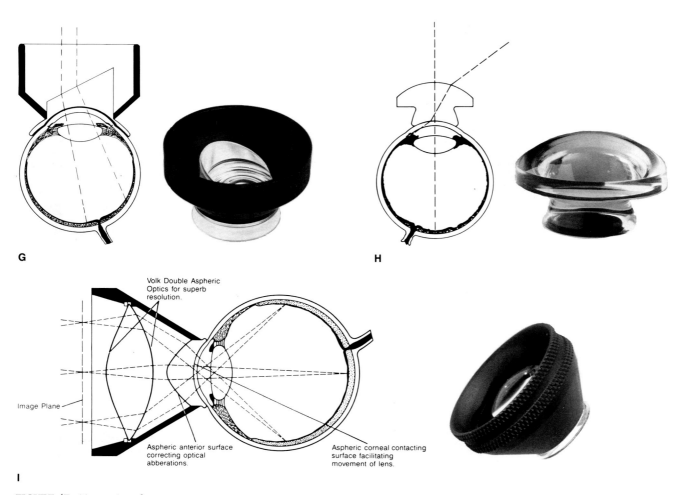

G

H

Volk Double Aspheric
Optics for superb
resolution.

Image Plane

Aspheric anterior surface
correcting optical
abberations.

Aspheric corneal contacting
surface facilitating
movement of lens.

I

FIGURE 47–11, *continued*

MAINSTER LENS. The Mainster lens is a convex condensing lens that has a corneal contact surface. It is similar in design and use to the panfunduscope (see Fig. 47–11*f*).

VOLK QUADRASPHERIC FUNDUS CONTACT LENS. The Volk quadraspheric fundus contact lens (see Fig. 47–11*I*) incorporates an approximately +120-D aspheric condensing element together with a contact lens to give a field of 125° or more.[32,33]

MCLEAN PRISMATIC FUNDUS CONTACT LENS. The McLean prismatic lens (see Fig. 47–11*G*) is different from the previously mentioned lenses in that it allows a paracentral view by the 25° prismatic deviation of its slanted plane front surface.

VACUUM-STYLE FUNDUS CONTACT LENS. Worst[48] described the use of a vacuum to help hold the fundus lens in place. This lens is available in a central fundus design, with a flat central optic zone, as well as for peripheral fundus viewing with a prismatically slanted front surface similar to the McLean lens.

LAYDEN INFANT LENS. The Layden lens (see Fig. 47–11*H*) is also unique in its design. It has a large-diameter convex front surface, but rests on the eye by use of a smaller-diameter pedestal with a concave corneal surface. It is recommended for premature infants requiring either gonioscopy or fundus evaluation.

Mirrored Fundus Contact Lenses

There are a number of designs available that provide the clinician a wide variety of options for use (see Table 47–3).

Goldmann Three-Mirror Lens

The most common, and perhaps the most generally useful, is the Goldmann three-mirror lens.[3] This lens is often referred to as the "universal" lens because it is literally useful for most purposes. This lens (Fig. 47–12*A*) can be used to view the posterior pole through the central optical zone or the periphery can be conveniently viewed through each of three differently angled mirrors (59°, 67°, and 75°). Also, the mirror that is most perpendicular (59°) to the examiner not only permits a view of the far periphery, but also permits gonioscopy to be performed.[49] The Goldmann three-mirror lens is available in regular, small, pediatric, and infant sizes and can be obtained with a scleral flange to aid stability on the eye.

Hart Pediatric Lens

The Hart pediatric lens is basically similar to the pediatric-sized Goldmann three-mirror lens. It is useful for small children and other patients having smaller eye sizes.

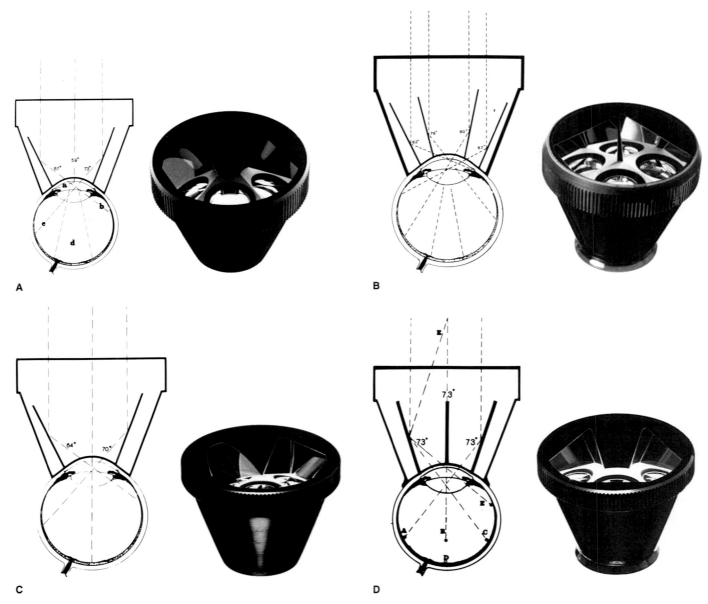

FIGURE 47–12. Mirrored fundus contact lenses (corresponding schematic diagrams are pictured adjacent to each lens type): (*A*) Goldmann "universal" three-mirror lens; (*B*) Karickhoff four-mirror lens; (*C*) Thorpe four-mirror vitreous–fundus lens; (*D*) Wilson three-mirror fundus lens. (Courtesy of Ocular Instruments, Inc.)

Karickhoff Four-Mirror Lens

The Karickhoff lens (see Fig. 47–12*B*) has four differently angled mirrors at 62°, 67°, 76°, and 80°.[36] It is similar in design and purpose to the Goldmann Universal three-mirror lens, except that the four viewing angles of the Karickhoff lens better overlap in their fields of view. This helps eliminate the need to manipulate the lens on the eye during examination.

Thorpe Four-Mirror Fundus Lens

A more specialized design is the Thorpe four-mirror[36,44] (see Fig. 47–12*C*). This lens is intended for use primarily with the mid- to far-periphery and, therefore, has no mirror for viewing the paracentral retina. Instead, two sets of peripheral mirrors angled at 64°

and 70° are used that reduce the amount of rotation of the lens required during examination.

Wilson Three-Mirror Fundus Lens

The Wilson lens (see Fig. 47–12*D*) further reduces the need to rotate the fundus lens in peripheral examination by providing the clinician three identical mirrors, each angled at 73°.[36] The use of this lens is correspondingly restricted to only that part of the fundus that is visible by mirrors at this angle.

Urrets–Ferrer Four-Mirror Lens

The Urrets–Ferrer lens has four identical mirrors of 70° inclination. The angle of these mirrors is ordinarily best for paramacular viewing only. However, the Urrets–Ferrer lens can be used to view the entire fundus periphery because its small corneal diameter and lack of a scleral flange permit it to be angled significantly while on the surface of the cornea. It is also distinctive from other lenses discussed thus far in that it has a handle for ease of control while on the eye.

Boys–Smith Pigment Gradation Lens

Although it is somewhat off the subject of fundus evaluation, it is perhaps important to point out that the Goldmann three-mirror has been adapted by Boys–Smith through the addition of a colored scale for grading pigment of the angle during gonioscopy. This feature makes this very popular design even more attractive as a single multipurpose lens for the primary care clinician.

Laser Lens Features

When reviewing the various fundus lenses that are available, the reader will often see the designation "laser lens" as an option. Laser lenses generally have antireflection-coated glass anterior front surfaces, instead of the usual plastic. This is to minimize reflection of the beam, which might be hazardous to the clinician or a technician in the room. Depending upon the application, these lenses may have convex "button lenses" bonded to their front surfaces to help focus the energy of the laser beam that is being used.[36]

The standard Goldmann three-mirror, the Thorpe four-mirror, and the Karickoff four-mirror lenses are available in laser quality, as are the more specialized designs such as the Abraham YAG capsulotomy lens. In the pseudophakic patient, to effectively cut an opening in the posterior capsule, the clinician must rely upon a concentration of laser energy, rather than upon energy absorption alone. This is accomplished by using the neodymium:YAG laser which concentrates its energy in both time and space so that the transparent tissue of the lens capsule is photo-disrupted by the formation of a "plasma."[34] The Abraham YAG laser lens (see Fig. 47–11E) aids this concentration process with a +66-D button lens that is glued to the central front surface of the fundus lens.

CLINICAL PROCEDURE

General Guidelines

When starting the biomicroscopic fundus examination, the clinician should explain to the patient why the procedure is necessary and what may be the potential side effects. If a contact lens procedure is being performed, this should include the fact that there can be associated irritation.

For all procedures, patients should be comfortably seated at a height that enables them to maintain good position in the biomicroscope headrest without undo stretching or straining of their necks. They should be directed to place and keep their foreheads and chins in contact with the headrest, and the clinician should be sure to adjust the patient's height in the headrest so their eyes are level with the "hashmark" located on the upright pole of the headrest.

The beam of the biomicroscope should be slightly shorter, but wider, than that used for corneal examination. The slit beam should be projected in the straight-ahead position at the outset of the procedure.

Hruby Lens

The use of the Hruby lens is described in a step-by-step procedure as follows:

1. The pupil is dilated with tropicamide HCl (0.5% or 1%) alone or combined with 2.5% phenylephrine HCl or 1% hydroxyamphetamine.

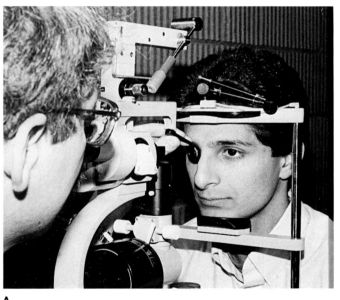

A

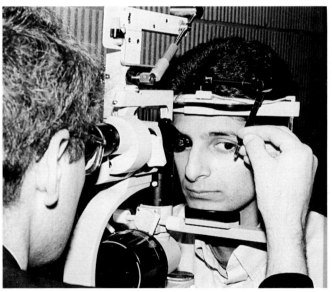

B

FIGURE 47–13. Clinical Hruby technique (Zeiss microscope). (A) With slit beam and microscope aligned, Hruby lens is swung down and released to touch the headrest "fender"; (B) microscope is moved inwardly to attain retinal focus while the patient fixates on the pointer light to control eye position. (From Barker FM. Vitreoretinal biomicroscopy: a comparison of techniques. J Am Optom Assoc 1987;58:985–992, with permission)

2. The patient is comfortably adjusted so he or she is centered in the headrest and the eyes are level with the headrest hashmark.
3. The patient is instructed to fixate straight ahead.
4. The slit beam is aligned with the microscope and is centered and focused upon the corneal surface.[15]
5. When using the Zeiss type Hruby, the lens is swung down (Fig. 47–13A) between the eye and the microscope, with the concave side toward the eye. The lens is released and allowed to travel forward until in contact with the headrest "fender."
6. The biomicroscope is then moved toward the patient under joystick control until the retina comes into focus.
7. When using the Haag–Streit Hruby lens, the lens is moved from the storage position into alignment with the beam.
8. The mounting rod is then fitted into the sliding track immediately above the slit beam–microscope axle.
9. The biomicroscope is moved inward until the fundus becomes focused (see Fig. 47–13B).
10. The Hruby lens can then be further adjusted to attain a distance from the eye that will yield a maximum field of view.
11. With either type of Hruby lens, scanning between retinal landmarks is accomplished by directing the patient's gaze precisely with the fixation pointer (see Fig. 47–13B) while maintaining focus and optical alignment with the joystick.

Angling the beam slightly allows the attainment of optical section illumination and helps to control reflections. The retinal periphery can be viewed, to a limited extent, by asking the patient to redirect his or her gaze to an extreme position and then by realignment of the system in the normal fashion with the now oblique pupil.

Volk Lenses

Hand-Held Procedure

1. The pupil is dilated with tropicamide HCl (0.5% or 1%) alone or combined with 2.5% phenylephrine HCl or 1% hydroxyamphetamine.
2. The patient is comfortably adjusted so he or she is centered in the headrest and the eyes are level with the headrest hashmark.
3. The patient is instructed to fixate straight ahead.
4. The slit beam is aligned with the microscope and is centered and focused upon the corneal surface[15] (Fig. 47–14A).
5. The Volk +90-D lens is held between the thumb and index finger, with either side toward the eye because the surfaces are symmetrically ground.
6. With the hand steadied against the patient's cheek or the headrest, the lens is then introduced at approximately 1 cm from the cornea, so that it is visually centered in the beam (see Figs. 47–14B and 47–15).
7. With the hand-held technique, the proximity of the lens to the eye may, in some patients, require physically separating the lids. This is easily accomplished with the lens held between the thumb and index finger, while the middle finger and ring finger open the upper and lower lids, respectively, in a scissorlike manner (Fig. 47–16).
8. Once the lens is in position, the microscope is withdrawn straight back from the eye until the red glow in the pupil becomes a focused image of the retina.
9. It is now possible to scan the posterior pole by simple joystick movements (Fig. 47–17).

A wide-open beam can be used to view the posterior pole all at once, but this produces excess reflections, is very dazzling to the patient, and should be kept to a minimum. The use of a somewhat

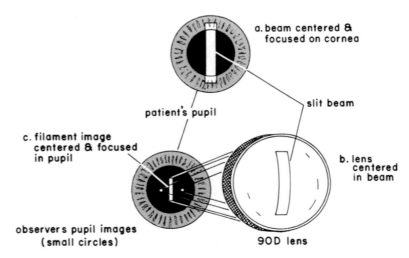

FIGURE 47–14. Alignment steps with the +90-D lens. (*A*) With the slit beam and microscope aligned, the slit is focused and exactly centered on the corneal surface; (*B*) while holding the slit still, the lens is centered in the beam about 1 cm from the cornea; (*C*) while observing the pupil, the lens is adjusted to precisely center and focus the coiled slit beam filament in the pupil (steady-mount only). (From Barker FM. The Volk steady mount holder for the +90 D lens. J Am Optom Assoc 1988;59:558–560, with permission)

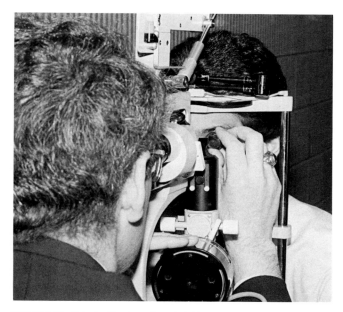

FIGURE 47–15. Volk +90-D lens held by hand during routine examination. (From Barker FM. Vitreoretinal biomicroscopy: a comparison of techniques. J Am Optom Assoc 1987;58:985–992, with permission)

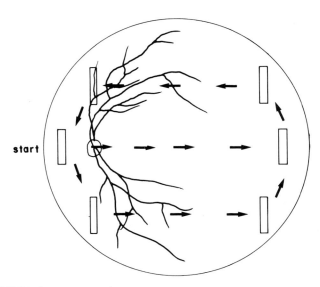

FIGURE 47–17. Retinal scanning procedure with the Volk +90-D lens. (From Barker FM. Vitreoretinal biomicroscopy: a comparison of techniques. J Am Optom Assoc 1987;58:985–992, with permission)

vertically shortened, yet widened, beam for scanning reduces the total illumination and is a very tolerable procedure for the patient, especially if a yellow-tinted lens is used.

When using lower powers, such as the +60-D or +78-D lens, a slightly longer 13-mm lens distance is preferred. It is important to remember that the +60-D or +78-D lens are not symmetrically aspheric; hence, the steeper curvature of these lenses should be held away from the eye. This is easily determined by holding the lens so the lettering on the lens rim is upright. In this position, the "bottom" of the lens is then held toward the patient's eye. Proper

positioning of the lens is also ensured when the cutout for nasal clearance is in position.

"Steady-Mount" Technique

The +90-D lens and the lower powers available can be mounted on the slit lamp headrest by using the Volk "Steady Mount."[27]

1. The Steady Mount is attached to the biomicroscope headrest upright so that its middle joint is just above the eye level hashmark (see Fig. 47–8).
2. The base of the mount should be radially oriented on the upright bar so that the transverse arm of the mount can be easily placed in front of either eye for examination. This is usually with the transverse arm projecting slightly forward from the headrest at its distal end (Fig. 47–18).
3. In using the Steady Mount, the slit beam is aligned and directed into the dilated pupil (see Fig. 47–14A–C).
4. The lens, in the mount, is then introduced into the center of the beam and close to the eye (1 cm).
5. With the beam position fixed, the lens is then adjusted so that the image of the coiled slit beam filament is seen behind the lens and is centered and focused to its minimum size in the pupil. This condition constitutes excellent alignment of the system and will be affected only if the patient substantially moves their head or eyes.
6. Retinal focus is then obtained by pulling the joystick of the biomicroscope back toward the clinician.
7. The Steady Mount allows easy storage of the Volk lens by simply dropping the lens to its lowest position beside the upright bar (see Fig. 47–8).

With either method, vitreous examination is accomplished by moving the microscope back a bit farther than for retinal examination. Peripheral viewing of the retina can be reliably obtained out to the equator by redirecting the patient's gaze and then repeating the basic alignment procedure through the obliquely oriented pupil. Views of the ora serrata are sometimes possible in some patients depending on the degree of pupil dilation and fixation control. Reflections and backscatter by the patient's crystalline lens can be virtually eliminated by angling the slit beam in relation to

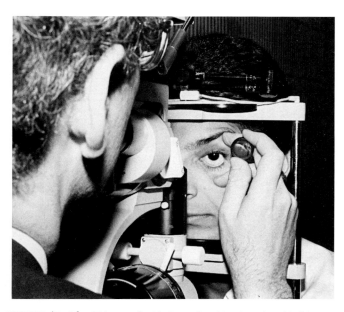

FIGURE 47–16. Lid control with the Volk +90-D lens: hand-held procedure. (From Barker FM. Vitreoretinal biomicroscopy: a comparison of techniques. J Am Optom Assoc 1987;58:985–992, with permission)

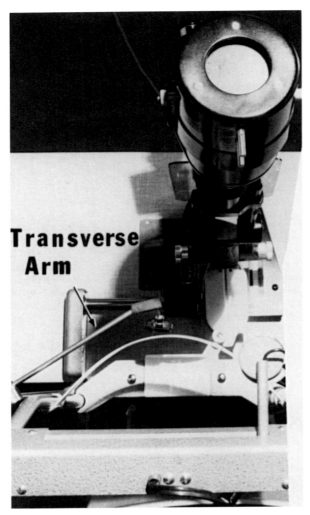

FIGURE 47–18. Proper Volk Steady Mount mounting angle as seen from above the biomicroscope headrest. (From Barker FM. The Volk steady mount holder for the +90 D lens. J Am Optom Assoc 1988;59:558–560, with permission)

the microscope head after the retinal image is obtained. Angling the slit beam before attaining retinal focus, however, tends to make lens alignment more difficult. Slight tilting of the lens itself is also helpful in controlling small surface reflections in the condensing lens, but care should be taken not to disrupt the central alignment and lens distance.

Contact Lenses

Hygiene and Disinfection

Contact lenses made from polymethyl methacrylate (PMMA) such as the Krieger or Goldmann lens should be disinfected by a 10 minute soak in 500 to 800 parts per million (PPM) sodium hypochlorite.[50] This solution can be prepared by mixing approximately 1/4 cup (60 ml) of bleach in 1 gal (3.78 L) of distilled water and has a shelf-life of 2 weeks. Latex gloves have been recommended whenever the clinician may come into contact with the tear layer during such procedures.

Corneal Lens Techniques

The Goldmann three-mirror retinal examination[3,15,24,49] is a procedure similar to other contact and contact mirror lenses and, therefore, is the only insertion and examination technique described here. The step-by-step procedure is as follows:

1. The pupil is dilated with tropicamide HCl (0.5% or 1%) alone or combined with 2.5% phenylephrine HCl or 1% hydroxyamphetamine.
2. The cornea is anesthetized with topical 0.5% proparacaine HCl.
3. The concave surface of the disinfected lens is filled with optical bonding gel (Fig. 47–19) (gonioscopic prism bonding gel, Alcon/Burton-Parsons, or similar solution). Care should be taken to eliminate bubbles from this solution, which can interfere with the view if trapped under the lens. This can be achieved by tapping the capped end of the bottle on the table or by shaking the capped bottle downward sharply with the top pointing toward the floor. Storing the bottle of prism bonding solution upside down can also help to control bubble formation.
4. The patient is comfortably adjusted so that he or she is centered in the headrest and the eyes are level with the headrest hashmark.
5. The slit beam is adjusted so that it is aligned and centered in the patient's pupil, and then, the slit lamp is positioned in front of the nonexamined eye for insertion of the lens.
6. To begin the insertion procedure, the patient is instructed to direct his or her gaze in a fully upward direction (Fig. 47–20), which gives better lid opening than the instruction to "open the eyes." The lower edge of the lens is gently pressed against the junction of the lower lid margin and inferior bulbar conjunctiva and is pushed downward to fully retract the lower lid to the inferior orbital rim. The lens is then rocked upward onto the corneal surface and

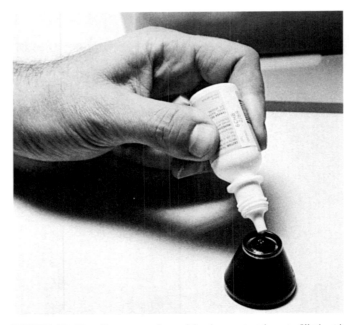

FIGURE 47–19. Concave surface of fundus contact lens is filled with optical bonding gel. (From Barker FM. Vitreoretinal biomicroscopy: a comparison of techniques. J Am Optom Assoc 1987;58:985–992, with permission)

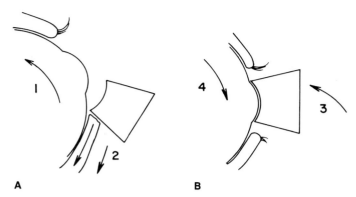

A   **B**

FIGURE 47–20. Insertion of fundus contact lens. (*A*) Patient looks up and lower lid is retracted by downward pressure from lens; (*B*) lens is rocked up onto the corneal surface, and the patient looks straight ahead. (From Barker FM. Vitreoretinal biomicroscopy: a comparison of techniques. J Am Optom Assoc 1987;58:985–992, with permission)

the patient is instructed to fixate straight ahead so that the internal examination can commence. Lenses that have a scleral flange are similarly inserted, making sure that the haptic portion of the lens is fitted under the lids.

7. The retinal view is obtained by focusing the biomicroscope inward (Fig. 47–21). The available retina is less dependent on patient fixation than with the Hruby technique; consequently, the posterior pole can be easily examined by movements of the biomicroscope or by minor fixational changes of the patient, or by both procedures. Peripheral retinal viewing is obtained by using the three mirrors that are located around the central optical zone (see Fig. 47–2).

8. In practice, the proper mirror is rotated to a position opposite the desired meridian of view. The slit beam is aligned with the microscope and focused inward until the retina becomes focused. If the precise retinal location is not im-

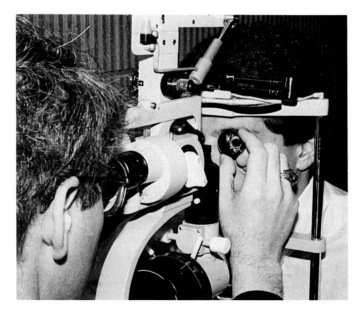

FIGURE 47–21. Fundus biomicroscopy with the Goldmann three-mirror lens. (From Barker FM. Vitreoretinal biomicroscopy: a comparison of techniques. J Am Optom Assoc 1987;58:985–992, with permission)

mediately visible, continued scanning of that meridian, coupled with gentle rocking or rotating of the lens on the cornea will usually bring the area of interest into view (Fig. 47–22). Scleral indentation is also possible in a technique called cycloscopy.[7]

9. After completion of the examination, the lens is removed and the cul-de-sac is rinsed out with sterile irrigation solution. If the lens has become adherent to the globe due to suction, gently rocking the lens will usually release the seal. A more difficult-to-remove lens can be freed easily by application of gentle finger pressure through the lid against the lens–sclera junction to release the suction.

Photography

It is also possible to take excellent retinal photographs using the biomicroscope.[15–17] The +90-D lens is an excellent tool for this purpose. Discrete areas such as the macula or optic nerve head can be photographed with a small beam diameter. Larger areas of retina will require a wider illumination beam, which may be distressing to the patient. Therefore, it is best to keep the beam size and total illumination to a minimum during focusing and alignment and then to increase only the beam size just before discharging the flash. Reflections are also a major problem in internal slit lamp photography and are best controlled by angling the beam entering the eye and tilting the lens to control any reflection before releasing the shutter.

The Goldmann three-mirror lens is also good for slit lamp photography, but reflection control is again very important.

In contrast, Hruby lens photography is less effective because of the severe field of view restrictions imposed by this technique. The reflections are also quite significant and are more difficult to control due to the limited amount that the slit beam can be angled with the Hruby lens.

CLINICAL IMPLICATIONS

Clinical Significance

Fundus biomicroscopy provides the optometrist a binocular, magnified view of the entire vitreoretinal cavity. Furthermore, this procedure has the advantage of slit beam illumination, which gives the clinician an optical section of the vitreous and the neural retina. These features of fundus biomicroscopy make it an important tool for both routine examination and for the more specialized evaluation of specific retinal lesions that have been noted by indirect ophthalmoscopy.

Fundus biomicroscopy requires the use of an auxiliary lens and, since no one lens is best for all circumstances, the competent clinician must be familiar with the use of several lens designs.

The Volk +90-D lens is currently the most useful auxiliary lens for routine posterior pole examination. It is superior to the classically used direct ophthalmoscope and Hruby lens biomicroscopy, mainly because of its much wider field of view. It is also a very convenient procedure for both patient and clinician because it requires no corneal contact. The principal drawback to the +90-D lens is that it requires more practice for the clinician to develop proficiency. This problem has been aided a great deal by the recent introduction of a slit lamp-mounted +90-D lens holder.[27] The +90-D lens is also helpful in the study of the peripheral retina, but it may not always provide the necessary view, thus, necessitating the use of the Goldmann three-mirror lens.

Another critical component of the optometrist's armamentarium is the mirrored contact lens. As discussed, there are many designs (see Table 47–3) that can be used, but the Goldmann Universal three-mirror remains the most practical for the primary care practitioner. With this basic tool, it is possible to reliably view almost any part of the vitreoretinal cavity. The use of a scleral indentation adapter with the lens makes it even more useful in the examination of the ora serrata. The mirror contact fundus lens is also important as the principal auxiliary lens that is used in retinal photocoagulation.

Other contact lenses, without mirrors, can be very useful for central retinal examination, but they are limited to that area. Exceptions to this rule include the McLean prism lens, the Mainster wide-angle lens, the panfunduscope, and the Volk quadraspheric lens.

Also convenient, although less powerful for fundus evaluation, is the Hruby lens. The noncontact approach is an attractive feature of the technique, but the field of view is much smaller than either the +90-D or the Goldmann lenses.

Clinical Interpretation

Fundus findings of significance for biomicroscopic evaluation are divided mainly into the central and peripheral retinal areas.

Centrally, the biomicroscope is the best tool for assessment of the optic nerve head, the peripapillary arcades, and the macula. Because of its binocularity and high resolution, no other technique provides a better view of the optic nerve head cupping in glaucoma evaluation. Furthermore, the view obtained is relatively good, even in the presence of a moderate cataract. Examination of the retinal vasculature is also very important, especially in hypertension and diabetes, which may manifest hemorrhagic or ischemic phenomena. Finally, the macula can be affected in numerous ways, including central serous chorioretinopathy, age-related maculopathy, and cystoid macular edema. The presence of these can be most effectively detected and evaluated by microscopic examination. Maculopathies involving subretinal fluid are especially important to evaluate microscopically to take advantage of the depth determination that is afforded by slit beam illumination.

Peripherally, areas of retinal degeneration change should also be carefully evaluated to ensure that retinal breaks are not present. Conditions such as lattice degeneration, peripheral cystoid degeneration, retinoschisis, or white without pressure may manifest vitreoretinal interface changes with associated small holes or larger tears that can ultimately lead to detachment if not prophylactically repaired. Many of these small holes can also be safely monitored without intervention by the competent primary eye care practitioner.

REFERENCES

1. Berliner ML. Biomicroscopy of the eye. New York: PB Hoeber, 1949: 1375–1400.
2. Goldmann H. Slit-lamp examination of the vitreous and the fundus. Br J Ophthalmol 1949;33:242–247.
3. Goldmann H. The diagnostic value of biomicroscopy of the posterior parts of the eye. Br J Ophthalmol 1961;45:449–460.
4. Goldmann H. Biomicroscopy of the eye. Am J Ophthalmol 1968;66: 789–804.
5. El Bayadi G. New method of slit lamp microophthalmoscopy. Br J Ophthalmol 1953;37:625–628.
6. Lemoine P, Valois G. Ophthalmoscopie microscopique du fond d'oeil vivant. Bull Soc Ophtal Fr 1923;36:366–373.
7. Eisner G. Attachment for Goldmann three mirror contact glass. Am J Ophthalmol 1967;64:467–468.
8. Jacklin HN. 125 years of indirect ophthalmoscopy. Ann Ophthalmol 1979;11:643–650.
9. Kajiura M. Biomicroscopy of the fundus: its theory and applications. Acta Soc Ophthalmol Jpn 1977;81:1581–1631.

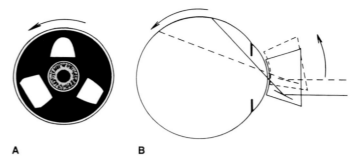

FIGURE 47–22. Rotation (*A*) and rocking (*B*) of the Goldmann three-mirror lens to alter retinal direction of view. (From Barker FM. Vitreoretinal biomicroscopy: a comparison of techniques. J Am Optom Assoc 1987;58:985–992, with permission)

10. Kajiura M, Hashimoto H, Takahashi F, et al. An aspheric plus preset lens for slit-lamp fundus microscopy. Jpn J Ophthalmol 1974;28:1161–1162.
11. Kajiura M, Takahashi M, Takahashi F, et al. Use of aspherical convex lens for slit-lamp fundoscopy. Jpn J Clin Ophthalmol 1977;31:1399–1403.
12. Lundberg C. Biomicroscopic examination of the ocular fundus with a +60 D lens. Am J Ophthalmol 1985;99:490–491.
13. Rosen E. Biomicroscopic examination of the fundus with a +55 D lens. Am J Ophthalmol 1959;48:782–787.
14. Rotter H. Technique of biomicroscopy of the eye. Am J Ophthalmol 1956;42:409–415.
15. Barker FM. Vitreoretinal biomicroscopy: a comparison of techniques. J Am Optom Assoc 1987;58:985–992.
16. Houston G. Fundus photography using the Volk 90 diopter lens. South J Optom 1988;6(1):23–26.
17. Houston G. Peripheral fundus photography using the Volk 90 diopter lens. South J Optom 1988;6(2):13–15.
18. Kajiura M. Slit lamp photography of the fundus by use of aspherical convex preset lens. Jpn J Ophthalmol 1978;22:214–228.
19. Takahashi M, Jalkh A, Hoskins J, et al. Biomicroscopic evaluation and photography of liquified vitreous in some vitreoretinal disorders. Arch Ophthalmol 1981;99:1555–1559.
20. Takahashi M, Kajiura M. Fundus photography through the slit-lamp microscope. Jpn J Clin Ophthalmol 1975;29:1319–1323.
21. Takahashi M, Trempe CL, Schepens CL. Biomicroscopic evaluation and photography of posterior vitreous detachment. Arch Ophthalmol 1980;98:665–668.
22. Eger AR. 90 D Volk fundus lens. J Am Optom Assoc 1986;57:784–785.
23. Cavallerano A, Gutner R, Garston M. Indirect biomicroscopy techniques. J Am Optom Assoc 1986;57:755–758.
24. Gutner R, Cavallerano A, Wong D. Fundus biomicroscopy: a comparison of four methods. J Am Optom Assoc 1988;59:388–390.
25. Jackson JE, Fisher M. Evaluation of the posterior pole with a 90 D lens and the slit-lamp biomicroscope. South J Optom 1987;5(1):80–83.
26. Abraham FA. A device for easy slit lamp fundoscopy with a +90-diopter lens. Ophthalmologica 1988;196:40–42.
27. Barker FM. The Volk steady mount holder for the +90D lens. J Am Optom Assoc 1988;59:558–560.
28. Rosenwasser GOD, Tiedeman JS. A stable slit lamp mounting device for 90 D lens use in non-contact ophthalmoscopy. Ophthal Surg 1988; 17:525.
29. Blankenship GE. Panretinal laser photocoagulation with a wide-angle fundus contact lens. Ann Ophthalmol 1982;14:362–363.
30. Lobes LA, Benson W, Grand MG. Panfunduscope contact lens for argon laser therapy. Ann Ophthalmol 1981;13:713–714.
31. Schlegel HJ. Eine einfache weitwinkeloptik zur spaltlampenmikroskopischen untersuchung des augenhintergrundes (Panfunduskop). Doc Ophthalmol 1969;26:300–308.
32. Barker FM, Wing J. The Volk quadraspheric lens—a new ultra-wide field fundus contact lens. J Am Optom Assoc 1990;61:573–575.
33. Wing J, Barker FM. Wide field fundus biomicroscopy lenses—a comparative study. J Am Optom Assoc 1990;61:544–547.
34. Aron–Rosa D, Aron JJ, Grieseman N, et al. Use of neodymium YAG laser

to open the posterior capsule after lens implant surgery: a preliminary report. Am Intraocul Implant Soc J 1980;6:352–354.

35. Comberg D. La photocoagulation avec un verre de contact a miroir. Bull Soc Fr Ophthalmol 1964;77:545–547.

36. Diekert JP, Mainster MA, Ho PC. Contact lenses for laser applications. Ophthalmology 1984;91(suppl):79–87.

37. Fankhauser F, Lotmar W. Photocoagulation through the Goldmann contact glass. Arch Ophthalmol 1967;77:320–330.

38. Peyman G. Contact lenses for Nd:YAG application in the vitreous. Retina 1984;4:129–131.

39. Riquin D, Fankhauser F, Lortscher H. Contact glasses for use with high power lasers. Int Ophthalmol 1983;6:191–200.

40. Rol P, Fankhauser F, Kwasniewska S. A new contact lens for posterior vitreous photodisruption. Invest Ophthalmol Vis Sci 1986;27:946–950.

41. Rol P, Fankhauser F, Kwasniewska S. Evaluation of contact lenses for laser therapy: Part I. Lasers Ophthalmol 1986;1:1–20.

42. Roussel P, Fankhauser F. Contact glass for use with high power lasers—geometrical and optical aspects. Int Ophthalmol 1983;6:183–190.

43. Yanuzzi LA, Slakter JS. Macula photocoagulation lens. Am J Ophthalmol 1986;101:619–620.

44. Thorpe HE. A new four-mirror contact lens for biomicroscopy of the posterior segment. Trans Am Acad Ophthalmol Otolaryngol 1966;70:853–854.

45. Rubin, M. The optics of indirect ophthalmoscopy. Surv Ophthalmol 1964;9:449–464.

46. Tolentino FI, Schepens CL, Freeman H. In: Vitreoretinal disorders: diagnosis and management. Philadelphia: WB Saunders Co, 1976:60–63.

47. Ruiz RS. A contact lens for biomicroscopy of the posterior segment. Trans Am Acad Ophthalmol Otolaryngol 1963;67:747–748.

48. Worst JGF, Otter K. Low vacuum diagnostic contact lenses. Am J Ophthalmol 1961;51:410–424.

49. Thurschwell L. How to perform gonioscopy and peripheral retinal examination with the Goldmann three-mirror contact lens. South J Optom 1983;1(1):18–24.

50. Center for Disease Control. Recommendations for prevention of HIV transmission in health care settings. MMWR 1987;36(suppl):2S–51S.

Amsler Charts

Charles J. Patorgis

INTRODUCTION

Definition

The Amsler Charts Manual comprises seven charts, each with a slightly different pattern and purpose. All charts are in the shape of squares, covering an area of 100 cm² (10 cm × 10 cm). When they are held 30 cm (~12 in.) from the eye, they allow assessment of the central 20° of visual field, which correlates anatomically with the area just inside the temporal vascular arcades, but not including the optic disc.

History

By developing a series of unique charts in the 1920s, Marc Amsler, a noted Swiss ophthalmologist, hoped to provide the clinician with a means of making better distinctions between quantitative and qualitative vision, the former being that which is measured with standard visual acuity charts and the latter representing the perception of the world as seen through the eyes of the patient.[1] Amsler envisioned his charts as "nets" that would catch any disturbances in the central field of vision. These disturbances would generally appear as missing areas or distortions within the limits of a particular chart. The first formal publication of his work in this area appeared in 1947, after more than 25 years of routinely using the test on his own patients and carefully documenting the results.[2] Since introduction of the manual, the charts and their clinical applications have been subject to some innovative modifications, all in an attempt to provide a more valid correlation between subjective visual response and the degree of physical insult to various vision-related structures.

Clinical Use

The Amsler charts have become commonplace in contemporary clinical practice because of their ease of administration and accessibility. They have greatly enhanced the ability of the clinician to evaluate the extent of functional damage caused by various disease processes of the retina, choroid, optic nerve, orbit, anterior visual system, visual pathways, and cortex.

INSTRUMENTATION

Conventional Charts

Chart 1

The most familiar and widely used of the charts is the first in the manual, the standard Amsler grid (Fig. 48–1A). This is merely a grid pattern consisting of 0.5-cm white squares, each corresponding to 1° of visual field, set against a black background and arranged in 20 horizontal (or vertical) rows of 20 squares each. This grid is the most versatile of the charts, enabling the clinician to identify various forms of distortion as well as relative and absolute scotomas.

Chart 2

The patient with a central scotoma may respond best if chart 2 is used (see Fig. 48–1B). The only difference between this and the standard grid is that diagonal lines intersect at the center of the grid to form an *X*, thus giving the patient a better idea of where the fixation point is located. A larger white central spot may be applied

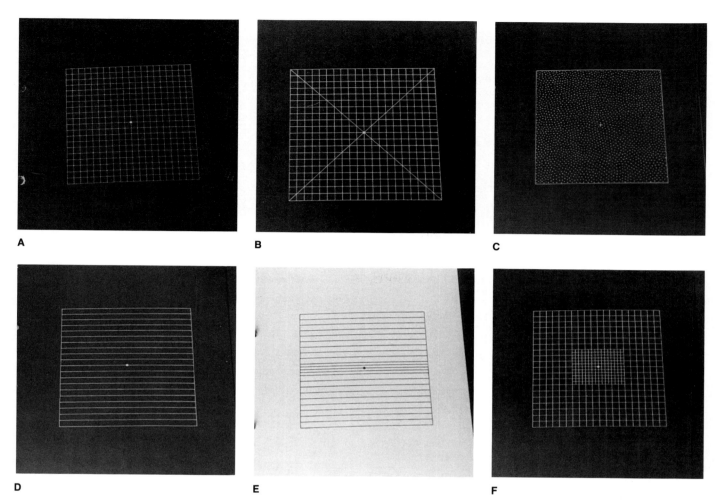

FIGURE 48–1. Amsler charts: (*A*) chart 1, (*B*) chart 2, (*C*) chart 4, (*D*) chart 5, (*E*) chart 6, (*F*) chart 7.

with tape to the center of the grid if the patient is still unable to achieve or maintain central fixation.

Chart 3

The patient suspected of having a central or cecocentral scotoma associated with nutritional amblyopia, as from alcohol-related thiamine deficiency, or toxic maculopathy, as from quinine and its derivatives, should be tested with chart 3. This has an identical configuration with that of the standard grid, but consists of red squares instead of white ones.

Another application of this chart relates to the patient with functional vision loss, as from malingering. If used in conjunction with red–green lenses, the red grid may allow detection of artificial monocular field loss.[3] Under normal circumstances, the grid will disappear when viewed through the green lens; conversely, it will remain visible when viewed through the red lens. In the patient claiming unilateral field loss, monocular viewing of the grid without red–green lenses will yield a field defect for the involved eye that disappears when the grid is viewed binocularly. With the green lens over the uninvolved eye and the red lens over the involved eye, the patient with true field loss will report persistence of the defect because of the simulated monocular viewing conditions created by the red–green lenses; the malingerer, having been deceived by the apparent use of both eyes, will report disappearance of the defect.

Chart 4

The patient with one or more paracentral scotomas may be able to delineate the area(s) of involvement more easily with chart 4 (see Fig. 48–1*C*). This chart has no lines to distort; instead it consists of small white dots randomly distributed over a black background like stars in the sky.

Chart 5

The patient with central or paracentral metamorphopsia resulting from various retinal and choroidal disorders may be especially sensitive to chart 5 (see Fig. 48–1*D*). This consists of 20 evenly spaced white horizontal lines on a black background. The chart may also be rotated to any other meridian to check for irregularities in a particular area.

Chart 6

Metamorphopsia along the reading level may be more easily observed with chart 6 (see Fig. 48–1*E*). This chart varies slightly from chart 5 in that it contains black lines against a white background and the areas 1° above and below the fixation dot are bisected by additional horizontal lines.

Chart 7

Subtle visual disturbance from macular disease, especially early in the course of the disease, may easily be overlooked unless chart 7 is used (see Fig. 48–1*F*). This chart breaks the horizontally oriented 6° × 8° central area, which corresponds anatomically to the normal macula, into 0.5° squares, rather than 1° squares, thus making it a more sensitive detector of insidious macular compromise.

Modified Amsler Charts (summarized in Table 48–1)

Yannuzzi Card

The Yannuzzi card is a minified version of the standard Amsler grid that assumes the shape of a credit card (Fig. 48–2).[4] It is composed of 16 × 10 0.5-cm squares that correspond to 16° × 10° of visual angle when held approximately 30 cm from the eye. The card may be positioned either vertically or horizontally to cover a larger overall area of visual field. A study of 84 patients [37 with central serous chorioretinopathy (CSC) and 47 with age-related macular degeneration (ARMD)] who used both the standard and credit-card grids revealed that 74 patients perceived no difference between the grids, 7 patients (3 with CSC and 4 with ARMD) preferred the standard grid over the credit-card grid because their defects were more easily observed, and three patients noticed a defect on the standard grid that was not seen with the modified grid. The main advantages of the Yannuzzi card are its convenience, portability, and relatively high sensitivity to macular disturbance.

Diamond Chart

The diamond chart was developed as an alternative to the standard Amsler grid to obtain more consistent and reliable responses in patients with age-related macular degeneration.[5] It is essentially a hybrid of Amsler charts 5 and 6, with two notable distinctions. It resembles chart 5 because of its evenly spaced bold horizontal lines and chart 6 because the lines are black on a white background. The differences are the central red 0.5-cm fixation dot and the red diamond situated 10 cm to one side of the dot (Fig. 48–3). The red dot is intended to hold the attention of the patient and the red diamond to ensure central fixation and monocular viewing. If the patient views the red dot while holding the chart at a distance of approximately 40 cm, the diamond should vanish within the normal blind spot; if the patient looks away from the red dot or inadvertently uses both eyes during self-assessment, appearance of all or part of the diamond will act as a reminder that fixation has become misdirected or that both eyes are open. After one eye has been tested, the chart may be rotated 180° to test the fellow eye. The reverse side of the chart consists of evenly spaced bold vertical lines along with the red dot and diamond.

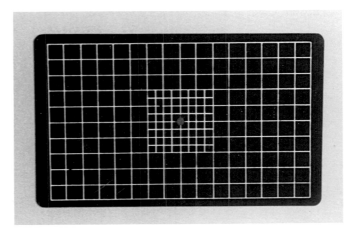

FIGURE 48–2. Yannuzzi card.

Transilluminated Grid

The transilluminated Amsler grid was developed to assess macular integrity in patients who were otherwise unable to see a standard Amsler grid or whose fundi were not ophthalmoscopically visible because of prominent corneal or lenticular opacities. It may be constructed by fitting a thin sheet of steel over an x-ray viewbox and punching 20 horizontal (or vertical) rows of 1-mm holes, placed 5-mm apart from each other, into the steel. This is identical to a standard grid in size and relies on points of light to simulate the grid pattern. Missing or distorted areas are considered abnormal, whereas blurry or faint areas are still regarded as normal.

One study of 25 patients with significant media opacities reported that 3 of 13 patients who could not see the standard grid had either a central or paracentral field defect with the transilluminated grid that was confirmed after surgery.[6] Another study of 80 patients with dense cataracts demonstrated that the transilluminated grid was superior to red–green color discrimination in evaluating macular integrity.[7] The grid accurately identified 90% of normal maculae, whereas the two-point discrimination method was only 81% accurate. Likewise, the grid had 68% accuracy in identifying diseased maculae, whereas the two-point method had only 42% accuracy. The transilluminated grid, therefore, may be a suitable option for testing macular function in patients who are being considered for either keratoplasty or dense cataract removal.

Table 48–1
Modified Amsler Charts and Testing Methods

Modified Amsler Charts
- Yannuzzi card
- Diamond chart
- Transilluminated grid

Modified Testing Methods
- Threshold testing
- Dynamic testing
- Binocular testing

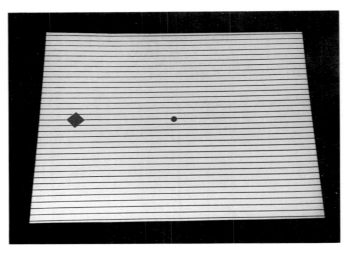

FIGURE 48–3. Diamond chart.

Modified Testing Methods (see Table 48–1)

Threshold Testing

Threshold Amsler grid testing may be employed to identify relative scotomas that may otherwise remain undetected by standard suprathreshold Amsler grid testing. With this method, a threshold is obtained for the patient by careful adjustment of two cross-polarizing filters before each eye. This creates a low-luminance situation that reduces the contrast of the grid against its black background until it is barely discernible. The patient is then asked to document the scotomatous area(s) on a tear-off chart.

Normal patients tested with this method may state that one or more corners are missing but nothing more. Patients with retinal or neuro-ophthalmic disease, on the other hand, may respond quite differently. A study of ten patients with optic nerve disease revealed 23 field defects with threshold testing, but only 5 defects with suprathreshold testing.[8] In fact, the standard grid was the least sensitive of all field tests employed in the study. Also, the total area of the defect was greater with threshold testing. Another study involving 15 eyes of 10 patients with macular disease uncovered 12 eyes with field defects during threshold testing.[9] None of these defects were observable on the standard grid, yet 10 were confirmed with tangent screen testing. The advantages of this method are that it is relatively inexpensive, may be administered in less than 1 minute for each eye, and is extremely sensitive to shallow field defects. It may be indicated in patients with visible macular disease and no apparent defect on the standard grid, or in patients at risk of developing toxic maculopathy or choroidal neovascularization.

Dynamic Testing

Dynamic visual field testing is a screening procedure that utilizes the standard Amsler grid along with a 1- or 2-mm white target on the tip of a wand, in much the same fashion as tangent screen testing. A red target may also be used with the red grid. In performing the technique, the clinician should initially plot the blind spot outside the limits of the grid to guarantee patient reliability. The target should then be moved slowly from invisibility to visibility to provide accurate limits of a particular field defect and to avoid overlooking smaller defects. The technique has been effective in identifying neuro-ophthalmic and glaucomatous field defects that are verifiable with more sophisticated field testing.

The only study employing this technique reported that it had 100% sensitivity and specificity, when compared with Autoplot or Goldmann perimetry, in detecting 61 neuro-ophthalmic defects, such as homonymous and bitemporal hemianopsias, constricted and hysterical fields, altitudinal defects, enlarged blind spots, and central scotomas.[10] It was also 97% sensitive and 93.4% specific for screening field defects in 212 glaucomatous eyes. The authors suggested that simultaneous presentation of two equally sized test targets on separate wands in opposite parts of the field could also be used to elicit subtle field defects. In this situation, the patient would not see the target in a less-sensitive region of the field because of an extinction phenomenon induced by target rivalry.

The advantages of this method are that it may be administered to bedridden patients, will enable the seated patient to remain in one chair, and will save time for the busy clinician. It may also be useful in monitoring the advancement or resolution of certain scotomas.

Binocular Testing

Binocular testing with the Amsler grid has been used to distinguish between anisometropic amblyopia and microstrabismic amblyopia.[11] This method employs polarized projection in such a way that the amblyopic eye sees an intact Amsler grid, whereas the normal eye sees only the central fixation dot and the four lines making up the large square. The anisometropic amblyopic patient will exhibit a central scotoma. The microstrabismic patient with mild amblyopia will demonstrate a temporal paracentral scotoma, with possible extension beyond midline, whereas the patient with deep amblyopia will suppress the grid altogether. The field defects will be larger and more easily seen with this technique than with monocular testing. Their visibility may be even greater with the red grid.

COMMERCIALLY AVAILABLE INSTRUMENTS

The Amsler Charts Manual may be obtained from Theodore Hamblin Instruments, Ltd., 1 Langham Place, London, England W1N 8HS or from a local ophthalmic equipment distributor. The standard Amsler grid may also be found on the inside front cover of the *Physician's Desk Reference (PDR) for Ophthalmology.*

The Yannuzzi card may be acquired through the Biomedical Information Corporation, 800 Second Avenue, New York, NY 10021. The diamond chart may be purchased through MIRA, Inc., 87 Rumford Avenue, Waltham, MA 02154.

CLINICAL PROCEDURE

Before the test is administered, the patient should be wearing the most appropriate correction for the test distance. This is especially true for the presbyopic or highly myopic patient. No lights should be shone in the eyes immediately before the test, and the pupils should not be dilated. The chart itself should be uniformly illuminated.

Amsler included in his manual a series of six questions that were to be asked as the patient viewed the grid. All the questions are very logical and should be introduced in a sequence that enables the clinician to separate one diagnostic possibility from another. Their only drawback is that they are somewhat wordy and the sixth question is improperly placed. For these reasons, the six questions in the manual may be streamlined and modified into the following five questions (Table 48–2):

Question 1. Can you see the central white dot?

The purpose of this question is to rule out a central scotoma.

1. If the answer is "Yes," a central scotoma is unlikely unless the clinician is obtaining a false-negative response due to poor patient compliance. If the patient is at risk of developing a central or paracentral scotoma, but has poor fixation or an inadequate understanding of the test, one method of improving future compliance is by demonstrating a scotoma to the patient.[12] This is achieved by asking the patient to look directly at or slightly to the side of a penlight for

---

Table 48–2

Sequence of Questions for In-Office Testing with the Standard Amsler Grid

Question 1. Can you see the central white dot?
Question 2. Can you see all four sides of the large square as well as all four of its corners?
Question 3. Are any of the small squares blurry or missing on any part of the grid?
Question 4. Do any of the horizontal or vertical lines that make up the squares appear wavy or bent?
Question 5. Is any part of the grid shimmering, flickering, or colored?

several seconds. The afterimage, which simulates a scotoma, may allow the patient to more easily identify an actual scotoma if and when it does appear. If the patient is reliable and answers "Yes" to this first question, the clinician may then proceed to question 2.

2. If the answer is "It looks washed out" or "It seems slightly blurry," a relative central scotoma may be indicated. The clinician should ask the patient to outline the limits of the scotomatous area on the grid with a finger. The patient may then be asked to describe the defect as accurately as possible and draw the limits of the disturbance with a pencil onto one of the tear-off charts provided with the manual. These are reversed in contrast from the actual test chart, appearing as black squares against a white background. Comments made by the patient concerning the appearance of the defect may be written outside the borders of the grid for future reference.

3. If the answer is "No," a central scotoma may be present. This type of defect may arise from several retinal, choroidal, and optic nerve disorders, as well as lesions of the anterior visual system. The patient should again outline the borders of the defect with a finger and document it on a tear-off chart. If a central scotoma is suspected but not evident because of poor patient compliance, the clinician may ask the patient to place an index finger on the central dot to receive proprioceptive feedback. If this technique is not effective, the clinician should then consider presenting chart 2.

Question 2. Continue looking at the white dot. Can you see all four sides of the large square as well as all four of its corners?

The purpose of this question is to rule out arcuate, altitudinal, quadrantic, or hemianopic field defects, as well as overall field constriction.

1. If the answer is "Yes," the clinician may then proceed to Question 3.
2. If the answer is "No," the patient should be asked to localize the involved area(s) and describe the defect(s) as accurately as possible. This information may greatly assist the clinician in establishing a diagnosis. For example, a superior arcuate scotoma, associated with glaucoma, may "clip off" one or both corners at the top of the square; an inferior altitudinal defect, associated with anterior ischemic optic neuropathy, may wipe out a considerable portion of the inferior grid; a right homonymous hemianopic defect, associated with an optic tract lesion, will prevent visualization of the right half of the grid for each eye; an inferior retinal detachment secondarily involving the posterior pole may disturb much of the superior grid; advanced retinitis pigmentosa may reveal an absence of all sides of the large square, with only a few small central squares remaining. If a cecocentral scotoma from nutritional amblyopia is suspected, the clinician should consider presenting chart 3.

Question 3. While concentrating on the white dot, are any of the small squares blurry or missing on any part of the grid?

The purpose of this question is to rule out relative or absolute paracentral, cecocentral, or altitudinal scotomas.

1. If the answer is "No," the clinician may then proceed to question 4.
2. If the answer is "Yes," the clinician must initially rule out false-positive responses that may occur if the patient is not

properly corrected for the test distance or if media opacities create a blurriness or a doubling of the horizontal or vertical lines (monocular diplopia). Elicitation of a true scotoma warrants investigation of its relative density. An area inside which the squares are missing indicates an absolute scotoma, whereas an area inside which the squares are visible but indistinct implies a relative scotoma. Their presence, whether absolute or relative, typically suggests disease of the optic nerve or anterior visual system, but rarely retinal disease (see *Clinical Implications* section). The patient must once again locate these areas and document them on a tear-off chart. To enhance their appearance, the clinician should consider presenting chart 4.

Question 4. Look directly at the white dot. Do any of the horizontal (going across) or vertical (going up-and-down) lines that make up the squares appear wavy or bent?

The purpose of this question is to rule out metamorphopsia.

1. If the answer is "No," the clinician may then proceed to question 5.
2. If the answer is "Yes," the clinician must initially rule out false-positive responses that may occur if the patient is looking through the line of a multifocal segment or noticing the peripheral distortions of a progressive addition lens. True metamorphopsia may assume a variety of configurations. The waviness of the lines may range from minimal to severe; some of the distorted lines may actually appear discontinuous, or broken; some squares may have barrel distortion (macropsia) due to an increase in photoreceptors per unit area, whereas others may have pincushion distortion (micropsia) because of a decrease in photoreceptors per unit area; sometimes the vertical lines will be affected more than the horizontal lines, and vice versa. Regardless of appearance, however, these disturbances are invariably associated with retinal or choroidal disease (see *Clinical Implications* section). Such distortions may be embellished to some degree by charts 5 and 6.

Question 5. Again, look only at the central white dot. Is any part of the grid shimmering, flickering, or colored?

The purpose of this question is to rule out scintillating scotomas.

1. If the answer is "No," the series of questions is complete.
2. If the answer is "Yes," this may herald the onset of a scotoma of retinal origin, particularly if early serous or hemorrhagic detachment is disrupting retinal topography. More often, however, such a response from the patient necessitates eliminating the presence of visual auras associated with migraine, arteriovenous malformation, transient ischemic attack, or visual pathway lesions.

CLINICAL IMPLICATIONS

Clinical Significance

Disturbances that appear on the Amsler grid should alert the clinician to the possibility of either acute or long-standing disease of the retina, choroid, optic nerve, orbit, anterior visual system, visual pathways and cortex. These disturbances are not, of themselves, diagnostic, but may contribute an important piece to the total diagnostic puzzle created by the results of additional clinical testing.

The clinician should consider dispensing an Amsler grid complete with instructions for self-assessment to three categories of

(*Text continues on page 445*)

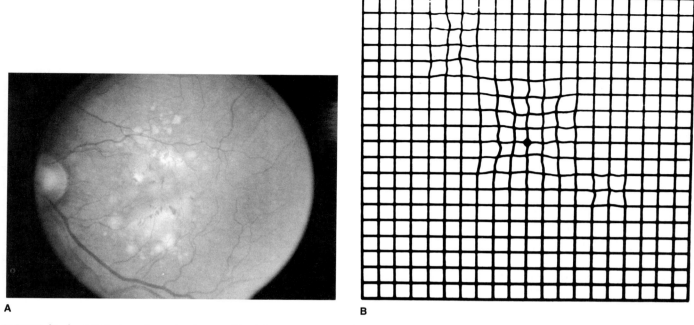

A   B

FIGURE 48–4. (*A*) Coalesced macular drusen of the left eye creating visual acuity of 20/30; (*B*) Amsler grid testing reveals several areas of metamorphopsia.

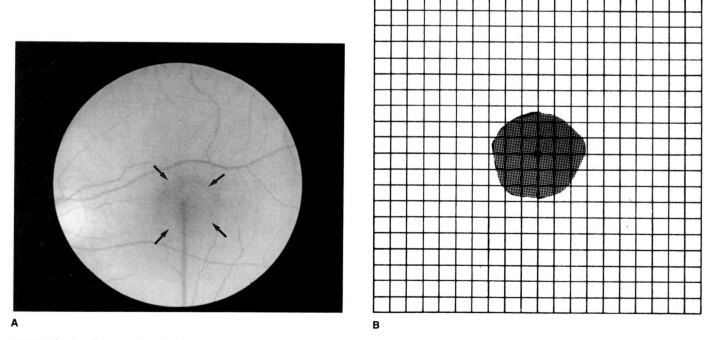

A   B

FIGURE 48–5. (*A*) Idiopathic detachment of the neurosensory retina (central serous chorioretinopathy) of the right eye creating visual acuity of 20/20-; (*B*) Amsler grid testing reveals circular relative central scotoma.

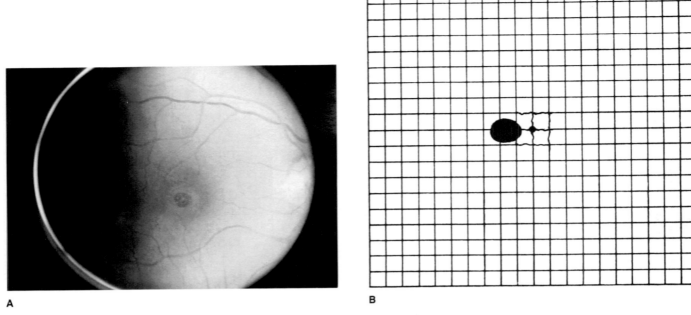

A   **B**

FIGURE 48–6. (*A*) Full-thickness macular hole slightly temporal to the fovea of the right eye creating visual acuity of 20/60; (*B*) Amsler grid testing reveals central metamorphopsia and an absolute paracentral scotoma to the left of fixation.

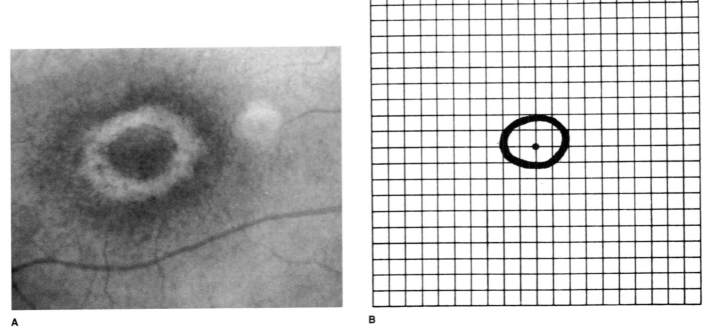

A   **B**

FIGURE 48–7. (*A*) Chloroquine-induced bull's-eye maculopathy of the right eye creating visual acuity of 20/40; (*B*) Amsler grid testing reveals an absolute annular scotoma around fixation with the center of the grid intact.

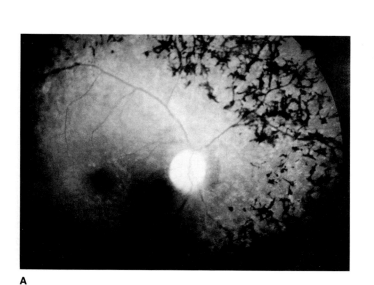

A

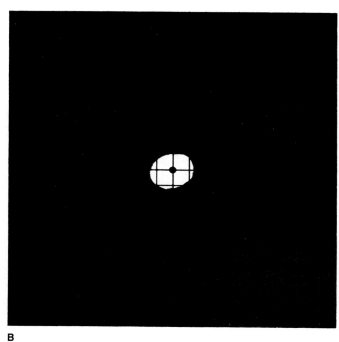

B

FIGURE 48–8. (*A*) Advanced retinitis pigmentosa in the left eye creating visual acuity of 20/60; (*B*) Amsler grid testing reveals the presence of only four squares around the fixation dot.

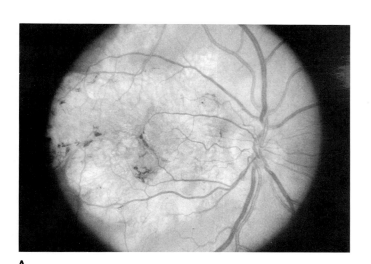

A

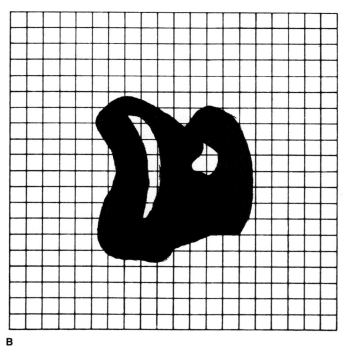

B

FIGURE 48–9. (*A*) Serpiginous choroiditis involving the posterior pole of the right eye and creating visual acuity of 20/50; (*B*) Amsler grid testing reveals intact islands of vision within a dense central scotoma.

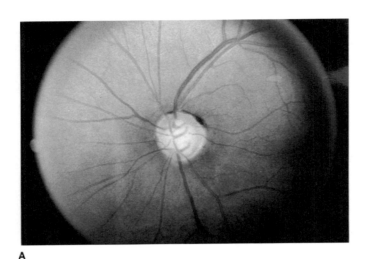

A

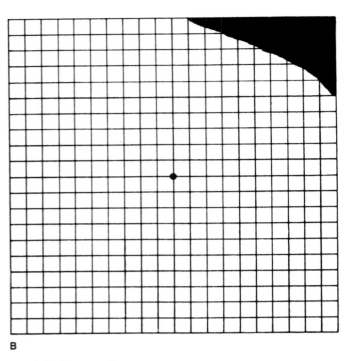

B

FIGURE 48–10. (*A*) Glaucomatous optic disc secondary to pseudoexfoliation of the lens capsule; (*B*) Amsler grid testing reveals an absence of the upper corner of the grid associated with a superior arcuate scotoma.

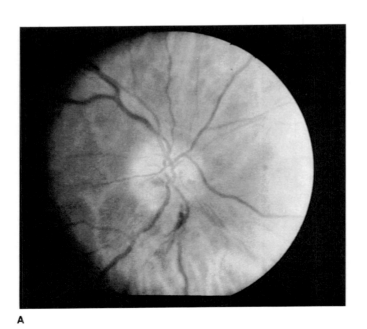

A

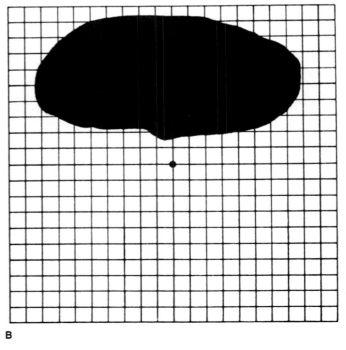

B

FIGURE 48–11. (*A*) Nonarteritic anterior ischemic optic neuropathy in the right eye creating visual acuity of 20/60; (*B*) Amsler grid testing reveals a superior altitudinal defect.

Table 48–3
*Instructions for Amsler Grid Self-Assessment**

1. Hold the grid 12-in. away from your eyes while wearing your reading glasses.
2. Cover your uninvolved eye (right or left).
3. Look directly at the central white dot at all times.
4. If you notice any (new) missing or distorted areas, mark them with a pencil.
5. Call the office as soon as possible to report your new symptoms. Bring your marked-up grid when you come to the office.

* Instructions should be in large print for visually impaired patient.

patients (Table 48–3). The first is the patient with progressive disease, such as toxic maculopathy or retinitis pigmentosa, who is predisposed to developing significant alterations over time. The second is the patient with active disease, such as acute macular neuroretinopathy or optic neuritis, whose visual quality may improve or worsen within a relatively short time span. The third is the patient with recurrent disease, such as central serous chorioretinopathy or toxoplasmic retinochoroiditis, who may have already suffered vision loss, but is at risk of experiencing a reactivation of the disease process.

A perfect example of a disorder that fits each of these categories (i.e., progressive, active, and recurrent) is age-related macular degeneration. The Amsler grid may be helpful in signaling when new complications arise at various stages of this disease. Patients with focal areas of macular hyperpigmentation or drusen that have *progressed* to the point of coalescence should be especially mindful of grid appearance, since they are more likely to develop neovascular maculopathy.[13] Because they may notice distortions on the grid before a choroidal neovascular membrane forms, how-

ever, these patients should carefully watch for new disturbances of sudden onset. Fine and coworkers[14] found that the most common symptoms of their patients with neovascular maculopathy were visual distortions, blurry or fuzzy vision, reading difficulty, or a spot in the field of vision. The genesis of such symptoms suggests an *active* process and warrants prompt consultation with a retinal specialist. Discovery and treatment of neovascular maculopathy before the foveal avascular zone is involved may improve visual outcome and prognosis considerably.[15] Patients who have been successfully treated with laser, however, have a good chance of experiencing *recurrent* neovascular complexes.[16] For this reason, such patients must perform Amsler grid self-assessment and undergo periodic follow-up clinical evaluations indefinitely.

Patients at risk of developing neovascular maculopathy should be asked to tape a grid next to their medicine cabinet or bedroom dresser and examine it periodically. The frequency with which they inspect it depends on the nature and severity of their disease. Unfortunately, the biggest drawback of self-assessment is poor patient compliance. In evaluating 103 patients with neovascular maculopathy, Fine et al.[14] discovered that only 5 of 49 patients supposedly performing regular self-assessment noticed an Amsler grid defect as their initial symptom. When examined clinically, however, 44 of these patients became aware of grid disturbances. Consequently, patients performing self-assessment with the grid should also monitor the straight edges and lines of telephone wires, the sides of buildings, window panes, or floor tiles. This "real world" approach may be an easier and more effective means of recognizing early visual distortions.[14,15]

One way of improving patient compliance involves using a different-colored pencil each day of the week to document findings on the grid.[17] This routine enables both patient and clinician to gauge the extent of improvement or worsening of a disorder and ensures compliance by requiring that the patient write something on the chart. If the condition is relatively stable, the patient may monitor the grid either weekly or monthly, using a different

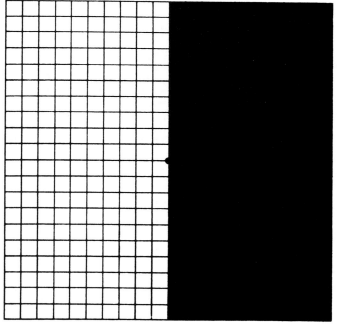

A

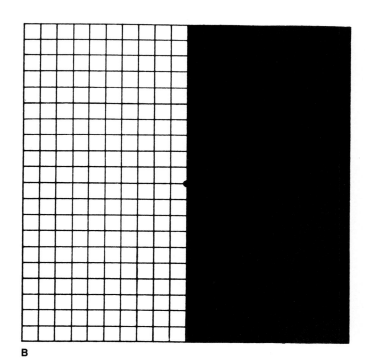

B

FIGURE 48–12. (*A*) Amsler grid testing in the right eye of a patient who suffered severe head trauma in a suicide attempt reveals a right hemianopsia; (*B*) Amsler grid testing in the left eye of the same patient reveals a homonymous defect.

colored pencil each time. The date for each color is written at the bottom of the sheet. The patient should bring marked-up grids to follow-up examinations, regardless of whether any sudden changes in the grid or vision have been noticed. This allows the clinician to observe and evaluate sequential changes and to verify that the patient has been compliant.

In many instances of neovascular maculopathy, the critical combination of patient compliance, meticulous biomicroscopic evaluation on the part of the clinician, and appropriate referral to a retinal specialist for fluorescein angiography and possible laser photocoagulation may prevent significant macular damage and the disabling vision loss that so often accompanies it.

Clinical Interpretation

Diseases that disrupt the retinal architecture may be seen on the standard grid as areas of distortion, or metamorphopsia. As noted before, however, the absence of a defect does not rule out the existence of a lesion, but may, instead, indicate the need for a more sensitive form of testing, such as the threshold method. Nevertheless, numerous macular disorders of minimal to moderate severity may cause the lines of the grid to appear bent or wavy. These include solar retinopathy,[18] coalesced drusen (Fig. 48–4), preretinal gliosis, macular cyst formation, diabetic macular edema, cystoid macular edema, idiopathic detachment of the neurosensory retina (Fig. 48–5) or retinal pigment epithelium, and choroidal neovascular membrane formation.[13–16,19] Severe retinal damage may actually create relative or absolute scotomas on the grid. This may be evident with full-thickness macular hole formation (Fig. 48–6), toxic maculopathy (Fig. 48–7),[20–22] acute macular neuroretinopathy,[23,24] acute posterior uveitis, tapetoretinal degeneration (Fig. 48–8), and the atrophic or fibrovascular scarring seen with diseases such as toxoplasmic retinochoroiditis, serpiginous choroiditis (Fig. 48–9), histoplasmic chorioretinitis, and age-related macular degeneration.

The discovery of holes in the grid in the absence of retinal disease warrants investigation of the optic nerve head or beyond. Optic nerve disorders to consider include glaucoma (Fig. 48–10), ischemic optic neuropathy (Fig. 48–11), optic neuritis, disc drusen, and nutritional optic atrophy. The presence of a unilateral central scotoma without ophthalmoscopic or biomicroscopic evidence of fundus disease may indicate a mass lesion of the anterior visual system. Quadrantic or hemianopic defects will be present most often as a result of mass lesions, vascular accidents, or head trauma (Fig. 48–12).

REFERENCES

1. Amsler M. Quantitative and qualitative vision. Trans Ophthalmol Soc UK 1994;69:397–410.
2. Amsler M. L'examen qualitatif de la fonction maculaire. Ophthalmologica 1974;114:248–261.
3. Slavin ML. The use of the red Amsler grid and red–green lenses in detecting spurious paracentral visual field defects. Am J Ophthalmol 1987;103:338–339.
4. Yannuzzi LA. A modified Amsler grid. A self-assessment test for patients with macular disease. Ophthalmology 1982;89:157–159.
5. Potter JW, Wild BW. A new self-assessment test for age-related macular degeneration patients. South J Optom 1986;4:15–19.
6. Miller D, Lamberts DW, Perry HD. An illuminated grid for macular testing. Arch Ophthalmol 1978;96:901–902.
7. Bernth–Petersen P. Evaluation of the transilluminated Amsler grid for macula testing in cataract patients. Acta Ophthalmol 1981;59:57–63.
8. Wall M, Sadun AA. Threshold Amsler grid testing. Cross-polarizing lenses enhance yield. Arch Ophthalmol 1986;104:520–523.
9. Wall M, May DR. Threshold Amsler grid testing in maculopathies. Ophthalmology 1987;94:1126–1133.
10. Chen KFS, Frenkel M. Dynamic visual field testing using the Amsler grid patterns. Trans Am Acad Ophthalmol 1975;79:761–771.
11. Lang J. Binocular Amsler's charts. Br J Ophthalmol 1971;55:284–285.
12. Lederman ME. Demonstration of scotoma on an Amsler grid examination. Am J Ophthalmol 1985;100:740.
13. Folk JC. Aging macular degeneration. Clinical features of treatable disease. Ophthalmology 1985;92:594–602.
14. Fine AM, Elman MJ, Ebert JE, et al. Earliest symptoms caused by neovascular membranes in the macula. Arch Ophthalmol 1986;104:513–514.
15. Fine SL. The Macular Photocoagulation Study Group. Early detection of extrafoveal neovascular membranes by daily central field evaluation. Ophthalmology 1985;92:603–609.
16. Singerman LJ. Important points in management of patients with choroidal neovascularization. Ophthalmology 1985;92:610–614.
17. Chang MA, Morgan CM, Schatz H. Letter to the editor. Retina 1987;7:279.
18. Wergeland FL, Brenner EH. Solar retinopathy and foveomacular retinitis. Ann Ophthalmol 1975;7:495–503.
19. Grand MG, Burgess DB, Singerman LJ. Choroidal osteoma. Treatment of associated subretinal neovascular membranes. Retina 1984;4:84–89.
20. Maltzman B, Sutula F, Cinotti AA. Toxic maculopathy. Part I. A result of quinine usage. Ann Ophthalmol 1975;7:1321–1326.
21. Easterbrook M. The use of Amsler grids in early chloroquine retinopathy. Ophthalmology 1984;91:1368–1372.
22. Easterbrook M. The sensitivity of Amsler grid testing in early chloroquine retinopathy. Trans Ophthalmol Soc UK 1985;104:204–207.
23. Rush JA. Acute macular neuroretinopathy. Am J Ophthalmol 1977;83:490–494.
24. Miller MH, Spalton DJ, Fitzke FW, et al. Acute macular neuroretinopathy. Ophthalmology 1989;96:265–269.

Quantitative Perimetry

T. David Williams

INTRODUCTION

Definition

Since Goldmann's pioneering work started in the 1940s, the results of perimetric investigation have become increasingly quantitative, hence the term. Instruments that permit a wide variation in stimulus size, color, and intensity are now in routine clinical use. These instruments also permit direct mechanical recording of findings. This simplifies the task of the examiner, but in no way assures that the procedure will be fruitful. An oft-quoted line from Traquair is apposite: "Perimetry is not done by the perimeter but by the perimetrist, and simple tools properly used are much less productive of wrong conclusions than undue reliance on the dicta of an elaborate instrument."[1]

History

Förster, in 1857, reported the use of an arc perimeter. The hemispheric perimeter was described in 1872. Walker, in 1917, described use of an umbrella the black surface of which (1000-mm radius) was used to test a field of 45°. The projection perimeter we know today owes its origin to the work of Goldmann, who described his design in 1945.[2]

Clinical Use

Quantitative perimetry is employed when peripheral function is to be assessed or when the results of confrontation or tangent screen testing are inconclusive or nonproductive. It is especially helpful to confirm and to evaluate the extent of visual field defects detected by other methods. In recent years, quantitative field tests have become automated and now represent a common method for performing visual field assessments in office practice.

INSTRUMENTATION

To test the field up to 90° from fixation, perimeters are built in the shape of a bowl, frequently of a 33-cm radius. The patient's eye is placed as nearly as possible at the center of curvature of the bowl, and the head is comfortably positioned by means of a chin rest. A fixation device is placed directly ahead of the patient's eye.

Both manual and automated perimeters are presently in use. Manual ones (e.g., the Goldmann perimeter) allow either kinetic or static perimetry to be done under control of the examiner. Automated ones (e.g., the Humphrey Visual Field Analyzer) allow static perimetry to be done under computer control, and some instruments perform kinetic tests.

Theory

Manual Perimetry

For manual perimeters, test targets are presented either by projection onto the inner surface of an opaque bowl or by means of light sources that are seen through a transparent bowl material. The recording of test results for opaque bowls is by a pantograph arrangement that permits marking on a chart or, with transparent bowls, by making marks directly on the bowl's outer surface and then transferring the results to a recording sheet.

Goldmann Test Targets

In the notation for the Goldmann perimeter (Fig. 49–1), the stimulus is written with the size (in Roman numerals) first, the intensity

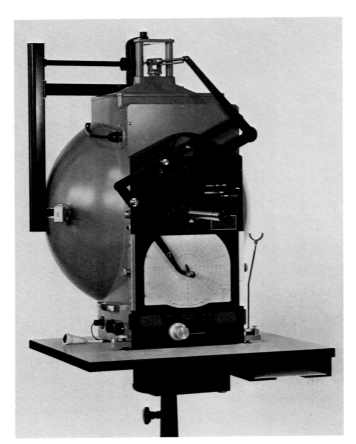

FIGURE 49–1. Haag–Streit Goldmann perimeter 940 (examiner's side).

(in Arabic numerals) second, followed by an optional lower-case letter to indicate the use of auxiliary filters. If the last item is omitted, it is understood that the filter is *e*; thus, I-2-e and I-2 are used to describe the same stimulus. Tables 49–1 and 49–2 give details.

In designing the perimeter that bears his name, Goldmann took into account several well-known attributes of the visual system. Among these was Ricco's law, which states that, for threshold detection of small stimuli, the product of stimulus area and stimulus intensity is a constant. Another major consideration was the

Table 49–3
Effects of Filters a–e

Intensity	1-e	2-a	2-b	2-c	2-d	2-e
Apostilbs	31.5	40	50	63	80	100
Log intensity	1.5	1.6	1.7	1.8	1.9	2.0

Table 49–4
Lowering Intensity by 2-log Units

Intensity	$\overline{1}$-e	$\overline{2}$-a	$\overline{2}$-b	$\overline{2}$-c	$\overline{2}$-d	$\overline{2}$-e
Apostilbs	0.315	0.40	0.50	0.63	0.80	1.00
Log intensity	−0.5	−0.4	−0.3	−0.2	−0.1	0

Weber–Fechner fraction; that is, the observation that, to be perceived, changes in stimuli must be proportional to the strength of the stimulus.

Goldmann made the experimental observation that an increase of 0.5-log intensity unit produced the same increase in field size as an increase of 0.6-log area unit. This is the reason for the size of the stimulus intervals used. In clinical terms, this is the basis for referring to the stimulus value for a given target: this is obtained by adding together the Roman numeral for the target size and the Arabic numeral for the target intensity: thus an I-4 stimulus has a stimulus value of 5, which is equivalent (in terms of its effect

Table 49–1
Goldmann Target Sizes

Target No.	0	I	II	III	IV	V
Area (mm²)	1/16	1/4	1	4	16	64
Log area	−1.2	−0.6	0	0.6	1.2	1.8
Angular size (min)	2.9	5.8	11.6	23.3	46.6	93

Table 49–2
Goldmann Target Intensities

Intensity	1-e	2-e	3-e	4-e
Apostilbs	31.5	100	315	1000
Log intensity	1.5	2.0	2.5	3.0

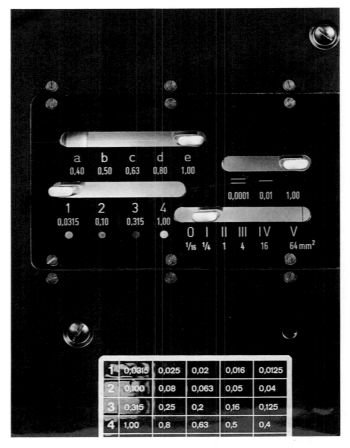

FIGURE 49–2. Stimulus controls for the Goldmann perimeter.

Table 49–5
Lowering Intensity by 4-log Units

Intensity	$\overline{\overline{1}}$-e	$\overline{\overline{2}}$-a	$\overline{\overline{2}}$-b	$\overline{\overline{2}}$-c	$\overline{\overline{2}}$-d	$\overline{\overline{2}}$-e
Apostilbs	0.00315	0.0040	0.0050	0.0063	0.0080	0.01
Log intensity	−2.5	−2.4	−2.3	−2.2	−2.1	−2.0

on the visual field) to a II-3 stimulus or a III-2 stimulus, both of which also have stimulus values of 5.

The main stimulus controls on the Goldmann perimeter are shown in Fig. 49–2. The lower two slides are used for controlling stimulus parameters during kinetic perimetry. For the usual kinetic perimetry, the upper two slides are kept in their right-most positions (i.e., position *e* and 1.00).

The upper two slides are used to provide an extension of the intensity range for static perimetry. The slide lettered *a, b, c, d, e* provides 0.1-log intensity steps that may be used between the Arabic-numbered intensities. Table 49–3 shows how these are used.

The slide marked 0.0001, 0.01, and 1.00 controls a further set of filters that can lower the stimulus intensity by 4-, 2-, and 0-log units, respectively. When these filters are in use, a double-bar, single-bar, or no bar are written above the Arabic numeral of the stimulus. Their use and notation are shown in Tables 49–4 and 49–5.

Use of the three intensity controls thus permits use of an intensity range of nearly 6-log units, from intensity $\overline{\overline{1}}$-a to 4-e, which corresponds to a range extending from 0.00125 apostilb (an *apostilb* is a unit of brightness equal to 1 millilambert) to 1000 apostilb (−2.9-log apostilb to 3-log apostilb). This range of intensities is somewhat less than the 10-log unit range of intensities to which the eye is responsive, but is more than adequate for clinical measures of visual threshold in static perimetry.

Automated perimetry

Most of these instruments are based on a 1/3-m radius bowl, as is the Goldmann perimeter, and they similarly present test targets on the inside surface of the bowl. In some instruments, the test targets are projected onto the inner surface of the bowl; in others, the targets are in the form of light-emitting diodes placed behind the inner surface of the bowl. For automated perimeters, test targets are presented at predetermined locations within the bowl. Records of test results are in the form of computer printouts, in which various levels of analysis are presented. For some instruments, the target sizes and intensities are frequently described in the terms used for Goldmann perimetry.

The field-testing strategy employed by most automated instruments is that of static field testing. The test target is placed at a preselected field position, and its intensity is gradually raised until the patient detects it. The output resulting from this testing is in the form of gray-scale charts, with the darkness of shading corresponding to the decreased sensitivity in the field. Because these charts are concerned with sensitivity, the stimulus is described not in terms of its intensity, but in terms of how much its intensity is reduced, relative to maximum intensity. This reduction is referred to as *attenuation* and is usually given in decibels (dB). The greater the attenuation at which the stimulus is detected, the greater the retinal sensitivity at that point. Table 49–6 gives one system of equivalent values for attenuation and Goldmann stimulus intensity.

COMMERCIALLY AVAILABLE INSTRUMENTS

Manual Perimeters

The Goldmann perimeter 940, made by Haag–Streit AG (Switzerland), is shown in Figures 49–1 and 49–2 (from the examiner's side) and Figure 49–3 (from the patient's side). The salient features shown in Figure 49–1, moving from left to right include the large vertical black projector arm, which swings about the vertical central axis of the instrument; the small white light meter for calibrating the instrument, immediately below which (on the table) one sees the hand-operated button that the patient presses to

Table 49–6
Decibels and Goldmann Intensities

Stimulus Intensity (apostilbs)	Goldmann Description	Attenuation log I	Attenuation (dB)
1000	4-e	0.0	0
316	3-e	0.5	5
100	2-e	1.0	10
32	1-e	1.5	15

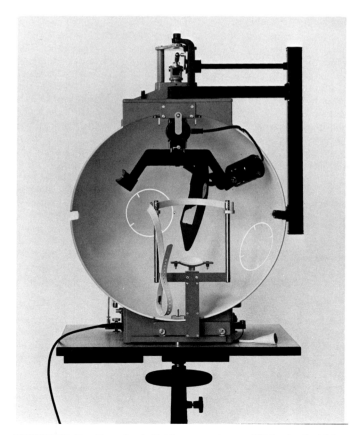

FIGURE 49–3. Haag–Streit Goldmann perimeter 940 (patient's side).

record seeing (or not seeing) the target. Immediately to the right of the switch are two black knobs: the one farther from the examiner is used to adjust background and target intensity, whereas the one nearer the examiner is used to adjust intensity of the recording chart, which is shown in position. At the center of the recording chart is the index of the instrument: the examiner uses a pencil (preferably) to record points on the chart at the tip of the index. Immediately above the index is an observation tube projecting toward the examiner through which the patient's eye may be observed: if the patient has been properly instructed, his or her fixation probably will not wander much, but should still be monitored. Immediately below the index is a pair of silver concentric knobs that are used to adjust the patients' horizontal and vertical position. Above and to the right of the observation tube is the set of four levers that are shown in more detail in Figure 49–2. To the right of the instrument is the trial case lens holder in its storage position.

The index of the instrument is freely moveable over the surface of the chart. Although mechanical limitations of the instrument allow only one hemifield to be tested at a time, a change from the right peripheral field to the left peripheral field can be accomplished by the examiner moving the index across the midline following around the outermost ring of the chart. The examiner is reminded of this by instructions printed on the chart itself. The instrument, as shown, is setup for conventional kinetic perimetry: static perimetry is performed by removing the index and connecting it to a ratchet system that holds the stimulus at a preplaced location in the field and permits its movement in 1° steps across a predetermined meridian of the field, for measurement of retinal sensitivity at each position along the meridian.

In Figure 49–3, one sees the perimeter set up for a relatively uncommon situation: the black structures visible within the bowl are accessories used in testing the visual field of a patient with a left central scotoma and a normal right central field. At the 2-o'clock position by the edge of the bowl is an auxiliary projector that is producing two additional images within the bowl: the right-hand one is viewed by the patient's right eye through a mirror. The patient is instructed to look at the center of the five-dot pattern in the center of the circle. Provided the patient has normal sensory fusion, he or she would see a single large circle binocularly. Because of the septum within the bowl, the space within the circle is seen by the left eye alone and may be tested. For routine testing, the black accessories are removed, and the patient is instructed to look into the hole in the center of the bowl. Because of the ingenious arrangement of the projection system, the stimulus moves in the patient's field exactly as it moves on the recording chart: moving the index to the examiner's left causes movement of the projected stimulus to the patient's left. The test target may be presented anywhere in the field, up to 90° from fixation. The projector of the stimulus may be seen at the end of the vertical black arm, nestled into the horizontal cutout on the right side of the bowl. This vertical black arm moves at times behind the patient's head, hence, it is advisable to instruct the patient to keep his or her chin in the chin rest while the test is performed. Otherwise, it is possible to have the black arm collide with the side of the patient's head.

The Topcon projection perimeter SBP-20 (Fig. 49–4) is based on the Goldmann design and is similar in all major respects. This instrument has an attachment that will make marks on the recording chart whenever the patient pushes the response button. As long as the patient is not too quick with responses, this feature is quite useful.

The Good-lite Universal Perimeter (Fig. 49–5) is a nonprojection system in which the examiner moves the target on the outside of a translucent or transparent hemisphere. The bowl has a radius of 25 cm. Stimulus intensities and sizes equal to those ranging

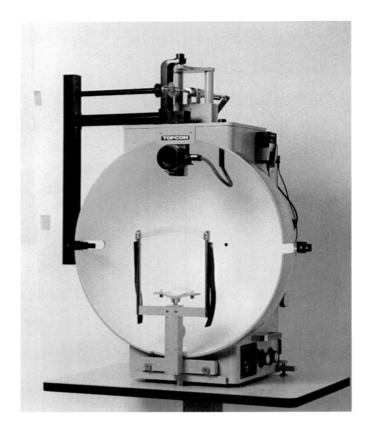

FIGURE 49–4. Topcon perimeter SBP-20.

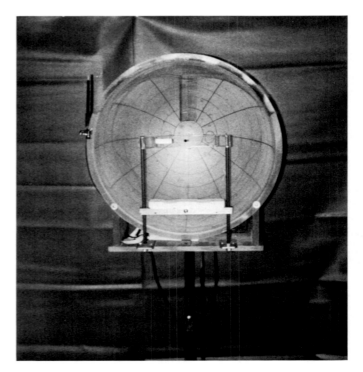

FIGURE 49–5. Good-lite Universal Perimeter.

from the Goldmann I-1 to V-4 may be produced using a fiber-optic system. Responses are marked on the outside of the bowl with a china pencil for later transfer to recording charts.

Automated Perimeters

The Humphrey Field Analyzer Model 640 (Allergan Humphrey), a projection perimeter, is shown in Figure 49–6. This is one of six models offered by Humphrey. The hemispheric bowl is contained within the box of the instrument, and a computer-driven projection system is used to produce test spots of Goldmann sizes I to V on the inner surface of the bowl. A total of 246 predetermined positions in the field may be tested, out to a maximum radius of 60° from fixation. The controls for the instrument are in the black area on the right of the instrument: on the bottom left of the black area hangs the patient's response button (on a cord). Immediately above this are two knobs that are used to produce horizontal and vertical adjustments of the patient's eye, which is observed in a videocamera view in the upper left portion of the computer monitor. The entire test procedure, from recording patient identification to printing out the results, is under control of a clearly understandable, menu-driven computer program. The examiner makes selections from the menu by using the light pen which is hanging in the upper right side of the picture. The paper output from the computer emerges from the slot below the monitor screen. Above the monitor screen are shown two of the data storage devices of the instrument: the upper slot is a floppy disk drive, whereas the

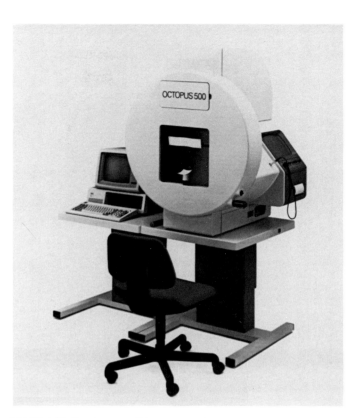

FIGURE 49–7. Octopus 500E Automated perimeter.

lower cartridge is inserted in a streaming tape device, which is used to produce copies of data from the instrument's hard disk drive (not visible in this photograph). As mentioned previously, this device gives the examiner the ability to store the results of a series of field tests. By using the optional STATPAC program, it is possible to analyze groups of test results to detect changes over time. The examiner may select from numerous field test strategies, depending upon the suspected problem. Each of these strategies involves selecting a particular group of test positions from the 246 possible. The examiner may also design his or her own customized test procedures. This instrument is self-calibrating and uses the same background illumination of the bowl as the Goldmann instrument (31.5 apostilbs).

The Octopus 500E Automated perimeter (Interzeag, Switzerland), a projection perimeter, is shown in Figure 49–7. This instrument also permits use of a wide variety of testing routines, and is coupled with an IBM personal computer. The latter feature permits use of a wide range of programs available from the manufacturer (under the name OCTOSOFT), as well as commercially available programs such as Lotus-123 or dBASE. Furthermore, it is possible through the computer's RS232C interface to exchange field data with other centers. Field data may be stored as standard ASCII files. This instrument makes use of two stimulus sizes (Goldmann III and V) and two background illuminances (4 and 31.5 apostilbs), and presents the stimuli in 132 predetermined locations within a radius of 60° from fixation. The examiner may also design his or her own individual testing strategies, within these limitations. Selection of test parameters is carried out by means of computer menus, and the test results may be presented in various formats. Analysis of a series of field tests may also be performed to detect possible trends.

The Topcon computerized perimeter SBP-1000, a 257-point

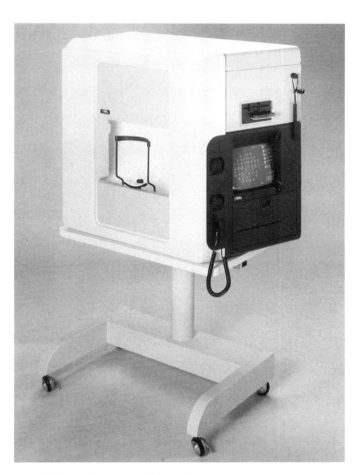

FIGURE 49–6. Humphrey Field Analyzer.

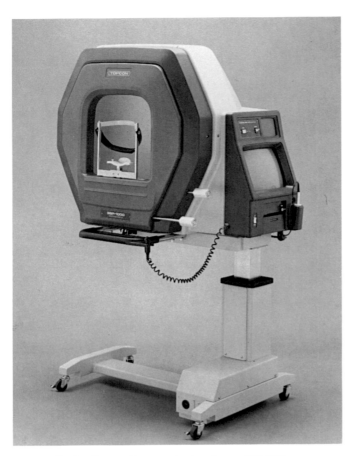

FIGURE 49–8. Topcon Computerized perimeter SBP-1000.

light-emitting diode (LED) instrument, is shown in Figure 49–8. Each LED is 21 minutes in angular size, equivalent to the Goldmann size III target. The LEDs are viewed through holes in the bowl of the perimeter. The background illuminance is 31.5 apostilbs. The examiner may choose from 13 different test programs, which display test targets within a 60° radius from fixation. Stimulus intensity is varied over a range of 2.5-log units (25 dB). Visible to the right of the instrument is the computer monitor, which is

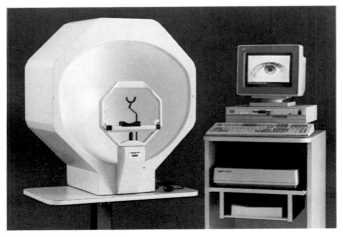

FIGURE 49–9. Digilab 1500 perimeter.

controlled with a light pen to select test parameters. At the upper right of the control panel is a small video screen that is used to monitor patient fixation. The instrument is equipped with a RS232C interface, which permits communication with external computers. Test results are output by a thermal printer just below the main computer monitor.

The Digilab 1500 perimeter, a 310-point light-emitting diode instrument, is shown in Figure 49–9. The patient observes the green LEDs through the translucent bowl of the instrument. Target size is 2 mm (Goldmann size III target), and background intensity may be set to 0.4, 4.0, and 31.5 apostilbs. As seen in Figure 49–9, the instrument is coupled with an IBM Series 30 personal computer and a conventional dot-matrix printer. Results are stored on 3.5-in. diskettes or on the computer's 20-megabyte hard disk, which the manufacturer states can store up to 30,000 fields. Custom field tests may be designed by the examiner. Test targets are presented within a 75° radius from fixation. Four different testing programs are provided.

CLINICAL PROCEDURE

Goldmann Kinetic Perimetry

Preparing the Instrument

Preparing the Goldmann perimeter requires only a few minutes. These calibration steps should be followed regularly, as it is very easy for someone to have pushed a lever or otherwise put the instrument out of calibration. One of the most common errors is using the wrong background illumination. The following steps are recommended:

1. Place a recording chart in the chart holder, with the tallest line on the bottom middle of the chart in the bottom notch of the chart holder.
2. Turn the two knobs at either side of the chart to release the springs that hold the chart in place.
3. Move the index of the perimeter (the pointer that indicates on the chart where the perimeter target is projected on the bowl of the perimeter) to the dot that is located within the right-hand U-shaped area on the chart (which corresponds to the cutout on the examiner's right of the bowl). This places the instrument's projector in the aforementioned cutout, with the projected spot landing on the instrument's light meter. Push in the locking button that is on the pantograph arm up and to the examiner's left.
4. Raise the white opal diffuser out of the light path so that the projected light falls on the sensor of the meter.
5. Place all stimulus control slides to the right-hand side: this permits maximum target intensity and size to fall on the meter.
6. With the rheostat at the base of the instrument on the examiner's left side, adjust the target intensity to 1000 apostilbs (1430 lux).
7. Pull down the white opal diffuser into the path of light from the projector.
8. Move the intensity slide marked with the letters *a* through *e* to the *a* position: this places a 0.0315-density filter in the light path. The light intensity now falling on the diffuser is 1000 × 0.0315 = 31.5 apostilbs.
9. Move to a position where your line of sight follows the path of light from the projector to the diffuser.
10. While holding on to the black shade on the lamp housing, look along the above-described direction and adjust the shade up and down to produce a subjective brightness match between the patch of light falling on the diffuser and the background intensity of the bowl.

11. Release the locking button, and the instrument is now ready for use.

Preparing the Patient

If the patient does not understand the nature of the test, it is unlikely that either valid or reliable visual field test results will be obtained. Consider the position of the patient for a moment: he or she has probably come to the office for a routine eye examination, with no awareness of any problem (aside from the fact that his or her reading glasses are not strong enough, for example). This person is now told or believes that the practitioner suspects a more serious problem (e.g., a brain tumor). At this point, the patient will probably be considerably uneasy, but, nonetheless, strongly interested in helping the clinician determine whether a serious problem exists. Many patients, furthermore, want to give the "right" answer, and this may lead to extremely conservative response criteria. Figure 49–10 shows the right visual field of a 13-year-old girl with an abnormally high intraocular pressure (25 mmHg). Subsequent testing at the perimeter had also indicated a constricted I-2 isopter (inner isopter). On retesting, it was found that the patient's apprehension had caused both the high intraocular pressure and the constricted field. After the patient was persuaded to relax, the intraocular pressure returned to 13 mmHg, and a normal outer I-2 isopter was recorded.

The Goldmann perimeter has attachments that may be used to provide the same effect as that shown in Figure 28–2 for the tangent screen. It is useful to spend several minutes telling the patient about the nature of the test. These few minutes usually yield dividends at the end of the test, in terms of repeatable, valid test results. Counseling for the patient before kinetic field testing may proceed somewhat as follows:

Mrs. Jones, we are going to do some tests of your side vision. We will be doing this one eye at a time, so the eye that is not being tested will be covered with a patch. Your job, while we are doing this testing, will be to look at the middle of the black hole at the center of the bowl. While you are looking at the center, I am going to move a small spot in from various

o'clock positions, starting from where you can't see it and moving in to where you can see it. There are two rather tricky parts to this test. The first one is that you will have a strong urge to peek around to see if you can see my spot: I don't want you do to this, because then we will not be testing your side vision. So please try to keep looking at the center. If I see you starting to wander away from the center, I'll let you know. The second tricky part to this test is that it is what we call a "threshold" test. Now, you know what a threshold is (indicating the bottom of the doorway into the field testing room): when you are standing on a threshold you are sort of nowhere—neither in the room nor out of it. Well, there is a similar kind of threshold in this test: to start with, when I have my little spot way off to the side, you are sure you can't see it; later on, after I've moved it in quite a bit, you will be sure that you do see it; but there will be some in-between place where you will probably say to yourself, "I'm not sure, but I think maybe I see it." **That** is when I want you to push the button. Don't wait until you are certain, but please let me know when you **think maybe you see the spot.** Don't worry about whether you are giving the right answers or not—I'll let you know if your answers aren't making sense. Sometimes you will notice different things: sometimes you may become aware of something moving; other times, you may see something round or something white. I don't mind which of these things you are noticing, just let me know when you think something is happening out there. I am going to move the spot in from various o'clock positions, and I will always tell you which o'clock position it is coming from, so you won't have to be worrying about that. [Author's note: some clinicians prefer not to do this; however, the results presented here were obtained when the patient knew in advance where the spot was coming from. A study by Gandolfo et al.[3] showed improved reliability and savings in time when the patient knew in advance which meridian was being tested.] You may wind up feeling that the whole exercise is rather strange, even to the point of seeing things while it is going on. Don't worry about that: it is just your brain trying to fill in the empty space. You may see spots all over the place after a while. Sometimes you may see the spot through the lens, and sometimes you may see it outside the lens—that doesn't matter: just tell me when you think you see it.

With this sort of introduction, the patient is willing to accept a considerable degree of uncertainty (at least for a short time). After all, if the patient is detecting the target at threshold, he or she should be seeing it only 50% of the time.

Field Testing Strategies

In much the same sense that no patient ever has all possible blood tests performed, no patient ever has all portions of the visual field tested. Rather, the clinician will concentrate his or her search on the portions of the field that are most likely to yield diagnostic information. Visual field testing, like any other clinical procedure, will yield the best results when the examiner is actively looking *for* something, trying to *exclude* something, or trying to *prove* something, rather than simply "doing a test." Of course, there are certain minimum tests that should be done on all patients, regardless of the reason for perimetry:

1. Field testing should be performed on both eyes, regardless of any apparent laterality to the patient's problem.
2. The central field should be assessed, using an I-2 target: this assessment should establish the isopter and rule out any common central or paracentral scotomas.
3. Paracentral scotomas may often be detected by presenting the target at roughly clock intervals around the 15° radius

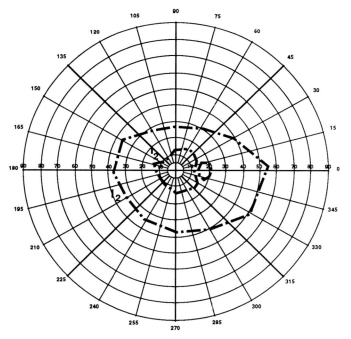

FIGURE 49–10. Visual field constriction caused by apprehension.

from fixation. This is a likely area in which to find arcuate-type scotomas. The target is extinguished, moved to the next point to be tested, then exposed to the patient.

4. The blind spot should be tested with the I-2 target for patients under 40 years of age, and the I-4 target for patients over 40 years of age.

Once these baseline data are recorded, further investigation may proceed, such as establishing the shape of a very peripheral isopter (in case of suspected retinal detachment), or investigation of a particular location in the field (as would occur, for example, in patients for whom a pigment disturbance is to be investigated).

Technique at the Goldmann Perimeter

1. The patient should be seated comfortably.
2. The patient should be appropriately corrected for the viewing distance. Use a full-aperture trial case lens, and be aware of where the rim of the lens is going to obscure the field. It is very easy to plot out the scotoma caused by the lens rim and think it is due to a problem in the visual system. With many lenses, this scotoma will be close to the 30° to 40° radii from fixation. When more peripheral field is being tested, this correcting lens will still enable the patient to maintain accurate fixation.
3. The examiner should be seated comfortably.
4. The nontested eye must be patched.
5. Ask the patient to look at the black hole at the center of the bowl.
6. For baseline testing, working at clock (30°) intervals is adequate. Avoid testing along the vertical or horizontal meridians, but test a few degrees on either side of them. For the vertical meridians, this is useful in detecting hemianopias; for the horizontal meridians, this is useful in detecting nasal steps.
7. Always show the patient the spot in the seeing part of the central field at the outset, so the patient will know what to look for. If this is not done, the patient, not knowing what to expect, may start responding to spurious stimuli or perceptions.
8. Always tell the patient where the test target is coming from, in terms of clock position.[4]
9. Always make encouraging responses to the patient: as the patient responds to the test stimuli, the examiner should say something, such as "OK," "fine," "good," or some such response. The patient may feel rather disoriented during the test, and may even wonder if there is anybody else present in the test room, so it is beneficial to maintain auditory contact with the patient.
10. In retesting situations, it is often helpful to test first the eye that was previously tested second: this serves as a useful check on the validity of the findings.
11. Rate of target movement is important: a useful rate of movement is approximately 5°/sec.[5] Moving it faster than this will usually produce a false constriction of the field (particularly if the patient's reaction time is prolonged), whereas moving more slowly will prolong the test time unduly, resulting in patient fatigue and probably invalid test results.

Goldmann Static Perimetry

There is a fairly close analogy between the two types of Goldmann perimetry and two methods of fundus examination. When assessing the fundus, the practitioner would like to have an initial impression from a technique such as direct or indirect ophthalmoscopy; once an abnormality has been found, it may then be desireable to evaluate it in more detail, for instance using a three-mirror contact lens at the slit lamp, with high magnification and stereopsis.

Similarly in field assessment, it is desirable to have an initial impression by means of some preliminary technique, such as kinetic testing. Once an abnormality is found or suspected, the clinician will then want to concentrate (in some cases) on the abnormal area using a more sensitive method such as static perimetry.

Thus, the practitioner using the Goldmann instrument will locate (by kinetic perimetry) a scotoma or area of depressed sensitivity, determine in which meridian it lies, and then proceed to measure (by static perimetry) retinal sensitivities along that meridian.

A number of attachments are required for this technique. They are necessary for two main reasons: (1) There is a hole in the perimeter bowl at the usual fixation point: measurement of sensitivity in the foveal center cannot be done here. (2) The index of the perimeter must be held stationary at preset degree intervals while the stimulus intensity is adjusted.

These requirements are met by the following:

1. An auxiliary fixation device that projects either a single dot for fixation or a small diamond pattern of dots within which test spots for the very central fovea are projected.
2. An attachment for the recording surface with a series of detents at 1° intervals. This attachment may be rotated through 180°, so that any meridian may be tested. It also carries a ruler with the stimulus intensities marked on it, to be used for recording the retinal sensitivity at each point tested. This attachment may be displaced to one side when the central sensitivities are being measured (to match the amount by which the test spot must be displaced from the central hole in the bowl), and is then returned to the normal position for more remote test locations (the patient is now using the usual fixation target in the center of the bowl).

Instructions to the Patient

The test is somewhat different from kinetic perimetry, as the motion cue is no longer present. It is sometimes advisable to show the patient a suprathreshold test spot so he or she knows where it will appear. The test spot intensity is then dropped below threshold and raised in 0.1-log intensity steps until the patient reports seeing it. The target is extinguished between presentations. If the intensity is lowered by 0.1-log unit after the patient reports seeing it, it will often be detectable at the lower level also.

Automated Perimetry

The clinical procedure with automated perimeters varies greatly according to the instrument in use; however, the same fundamental principles as those described in the foregoing under Goldmann perimetry apply.

With automated perimeters, the patient has no foreknowledge of the meridian or position in which the test target will appear, so he or she should be warned that targets may appear anywhere. One consequence of this is that patients with ptotic lids or overhanging brows may miss large numbers of superior targets during automated perimetry, whereas the same patient, forewarned of the area under test during Goldmann perimetry, will attempt to keep the offending lid out of the way.

The practitioner will have many different options for testing. Most automated perimeters offer different routines to be used in different situations: tests can be confined to the central 30° radius, to the field with a radius greater than 30°, to the central 5° radius, or to other areas at which defects are suspected (e.g., nasal step areas). The practitioner must be careful to select the proper test.

Computer-assisted perimetry offers a long-awaited opportunity for the clinician: the ability to store information, to retrieve it easily at a later date and, more importantly, the ability to do more extensive analysis of data from a single visit and to do longitudinal analyses to see whether a given field parameter is changing over time. The Humphrey system, for example, offers a supplementary program package called STATPAC. With this analytic package, the clinician can examine visual fields from up to 10 visits and assess

whether the patient is recovering or losing field. This is a great boon to the clinician.

Analysis of data from some automated instruments can yield information such as a grand mean that expresses by how much the whole data set (all the individual retinal sensitivities combined) departs from normal. Computer analysis of data produced in isopter form by the Goldmann system provides information concerning shape of the isopter; trends in isopter area may also be assessed from visit to visit.

Like different methods of fundus examination, the two methods of visual field assessment (Goldmann perimetry and auto-

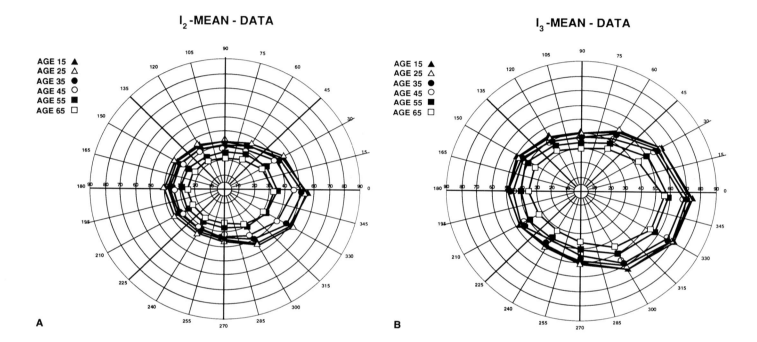

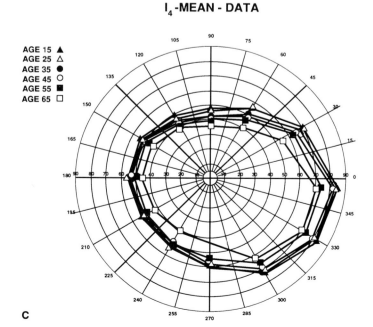

FIGURE 49–11. Age-related Goldmann norms. (A) I-2 isopter; (B) I-3 isopter; (C) I-4 isopter.

mated perimetry) should be regarded as complementary, not mutually exclusive.

CLINICAL IMPLICATIONS

Clinical Significance

Figure 49–11 shows the effect of age on the Goldmann I-2, I-3, and I-4 isopters.[6,7] If the field size is expressed as area on the Goldmann chart, then the I-2 visual field area decreases at the rate of 10% per decade. The I-3 isopter decreases by 8% per decade, and the I-4 isopter decreases by 6% per decade. The I-2 stimulus is equivalent to the 1-mm target commonly used on the 1-m tangent screen, so the I-2 norms may be used to compare with tangent screen results as well.

Clinical Interpretation

Types of Visual Field Disturbance

Broadly speaking, there are four ways in which a given field test results may depart from normal:

1. Abnormality of the blindspot
2. Loss of sensitivity within the limits of the field
3. Overall constriction of the field
4. Abnormality in the shape of isopter(s)

SCOTOMAS. Is the blind spot the only location in which objects are not seen? This question cannot be answered without exhaustive testing. As Portney and Krohn[8] have pointed out, if the visual field is to be tested at degree intervals to a distance of 30° from the fixation point, it would be necessary to present just fewer than 3000 stimuli to the patient. If a wider field were to be tested, for example, to a radius of 90° from the fixation point, then more than 25,000 stimuli would need to be presented. In clinical practice, such exhaustive testing is never done, because the examiner will usually have a strong clue to the most likely location for any field abnormality before field testing. Such clues will arise from the patient's case history or from physical examination of the eye.

Losses of sensitivity within the field are referred to as scotomas, which may be relative or absolute. A *relative scotoma* is one the size (or even existence) of which is influenced by the intensity or size of the test target used. An *absolute scotoma,* on the other hand, has a size that is not dependent upon target size or intensity. In general, new scotomas tend to be relative, whereas older scotomas tend to become absolute. Also, a relative scotoma frequently signals an ongoing disease process, whereas an absolute one is associated with an old, inactive disease process. As scotomas become less sensitive to stimulus changes, they are sometimes described as becoming more dense. A further distinction may be made about scotomas, based on whether the patient is aware of them or not: recent scotomas tend to be positive (i.e., the patient notices them as a dark area in the field), whereas older scotomas tend to be negative (i.e., not noticed by the patient).

The relative scotoma may go undetected if the examiner inadvertently uses a stimulus that is too intense or too large. Equally worrisome is the transient field loss.

OVERALL CONSTRICTION. Determining an overall constriction of the field may be confounded by the fact that the field tends to decrease in size as a function of age. The use of age-related isopter norms (see Fig. 49–11) will make the clinician more confident in interpreting the field of a particular patient.

ABNORMAL ISOPTER SHAPE. Loss of sensitivity within the field may cause a drastic change in the shape of the isopter itself: this will usually be readily noted by the clinician. There is a caveat here, however: when their fields are tested with relatively difficult-to-detect (e.g., Goldmann I-1) targets, some individuals will show considerable abnormality in the shape of the isopter, simply because of the irregularities in the axial length of the eye. In such patients, the use of the next stronger stimulus (e.g., an increase of

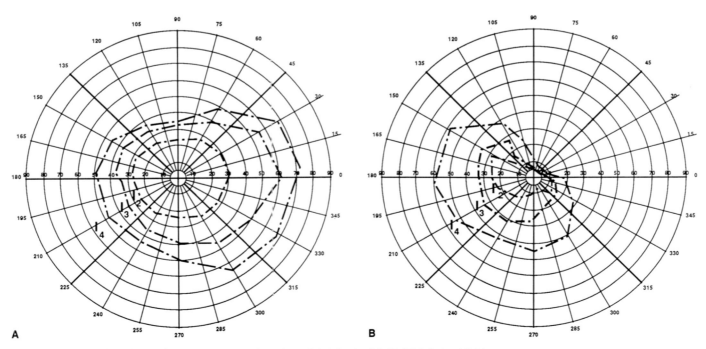

FIGURE 49–12. Glaucomatous loss in superior nasal quadrant: (A) right visual field; (B) left visual field.

0.5-log units in intensity or 0.6-log units in target area) will cause the field anomaly to decrease or vanish; in general, field losses that are significant will persist. Use of the age-related norms shown in Figure 49–11 also facilitates detection of field losses at, for example, the quadrantal level. The I-2, I-3, and I-4 isopters shown in Figure 49–12 are for a patient with chronic open-angle glaucoma. Although the I-2 and I-3 isopters for the right eye agree reasonably well with the norms, the I-4 isopter shows a decreased sensitivity in the superior nasal quadrant. It appears that the superior nasal quadrant is particularly prone to glaucomatous damage, hence, the

long-recognized nasal step. The left visual field shows a near-total loss of the superior nasal field to all targets.

Figure 49–13 shows two visual fields for the left eye of a 75-year-old patient with a notched disk: the cupping reaches the disc margin at the 1- to 2-o'clock position. Goldmann field testing shows a normal I-4 isopter and an I-2 isopter that is indented in the inferior nasal quadrant. Testing of the blindspot itself with the I-4 target is unremarkable, whereas the inferior nasal scotoma is obvious with the I-4 target. The patient's field was retested 4 months later at the Octopus 500 automated perimeter, and this testing

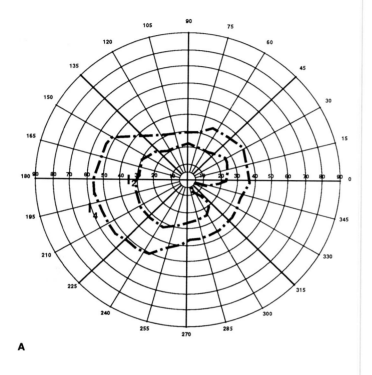

A

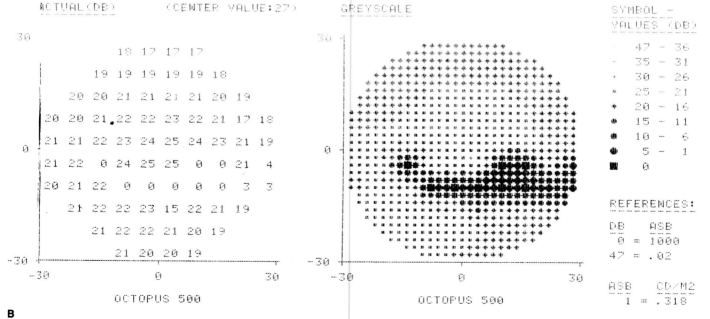

B

FIGURE 49–13. Arcuate scotoma: (*A*) results of Goldmann perimetry; (*B*) results of automated perimetry.

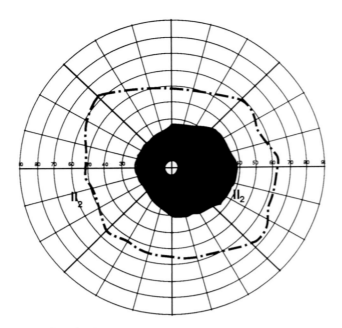

FIGURE 49-14. Ring scotoma.

revealed an arcuate scotoma extending from the blindspot to the inferior nasal scotoma. The practitioner should thus return to the field lying between any new-found scotoma and the blindspot with dimmer targets to see if there are any connecting areas of decreased sensitivity.

Figure 49-14 shows the right visual field of a 32-year-old woman with retinitis pigmentosa. This patient shows a broad ring scotoma when tested with the II-2 target. The diameter of the central field with this stimulus is 10°. If this patient were tested at the tangent screen, the clinician would be impressed by the pa-

tient's severe field constriction. The presence of useful field outside the ring scotoma might be overlooked. The clinician should be alerted to the presence of this outer, viable field by the observation that the patient's mobility is reasonably normal.

Figure 49-15 shows the Goldmann visual fields of a 20-year-old woman who was being treated with isoniazid for tuberculosis. Her dosage was 300 mg daily, and she had been taking it for 9 months at the time of her field testing. Possible adverse effects of isoniazid include paresthesias, optic neuritis, and optic atrophy. Tangent screen testing 3 years before isoniazid treatment was reasonably normal. The Goldmann I-2 isopters measured after she had been receiving treatment for 9 months showed considerable overall constriction. When her internist was advised of this, he discontinued the medication.

Figure 49-16 shows automated perimetry results using the Humphrey instrument. The patient is a 28-year-old man with an arteriovenous malformation affecting the left visual cortex. There is a congruent loss of sensitivity in the superior right field.

It is difficult, and probably inappropriate, to try to convert, for example, Humphrey field test results into equivalent Goldmann isopters, because static perimetry and kinetic perimetry assess somewhat different functions of the visual system: the former is based on retinal light sensitivity, whereas the latter is based on motion detection as well as light sensitivity. The lack of human feedback and the inherent boredom of static field testing can lead to invalid and unreliable test results. Moreover, the patient may very well notice something or make some comments during testing of which the practitioner, not being present, will not be aware. Such missed information may seriously impede the diagnostic process.

A further source of difficulty with automated field testing equipment is related to norms. Published norms for this test are lacking, especially on the effects of aging. The data seem to be regarded as proprietary information by the manufacturers and, as such, are available only as the (implicit) background for the field analyses produced. Most manufacturers seem to have adopted the strategy of using the patient as his or her own control, defining

(Text continues on page 461)

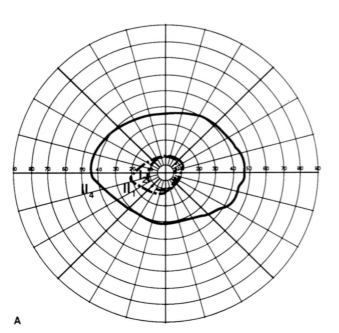

A

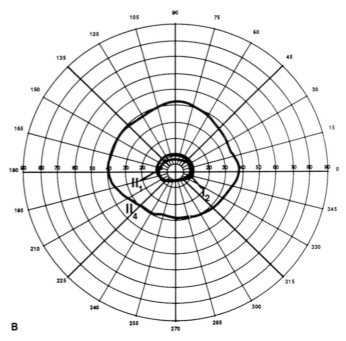

B

FIGURE 49-15. Overall contraction due to isoniazid toxicity: (*A*) right visual field; (*B*) left visual field.

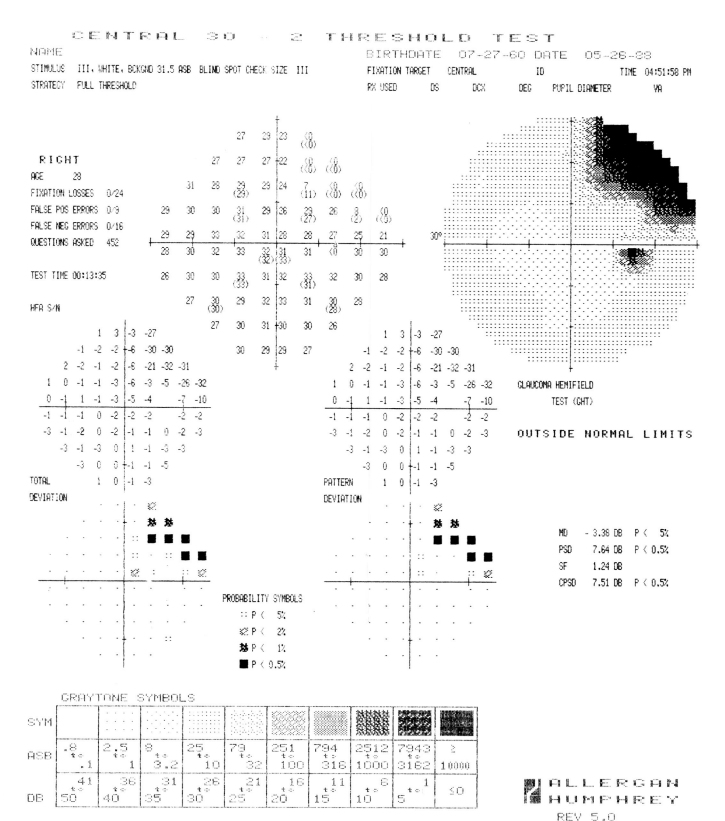

FIGURE 49–16. Humphrey visual field results in a patient with arteriovenous malformation: (*A*) right visual field; (*B*) left visual field.

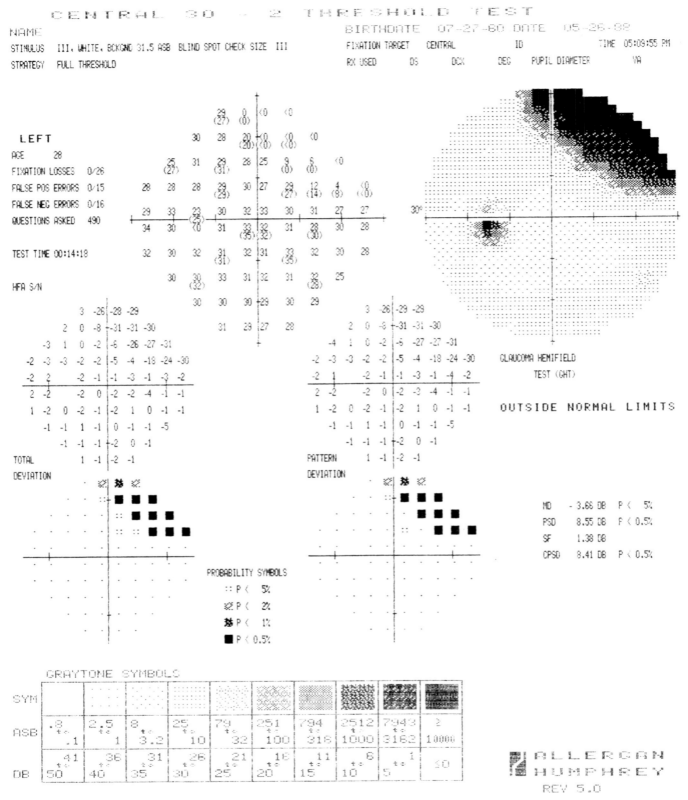

B

FIGURE 49-16, *continued*

scotomas, for example, as a decrease in sensitivity of 15-dB below the sensitivity of adjacent retina.[9] There is some concern about this approach, as normal eyes may show variance of greater than 4 dB from one day to the next.[10–12]

REFERENCES

1. Traquair HM. An introduction to clinical perimetry, 3rd ed. St Louis: CV Mosby Co, 1940:32.
2. Duke–Elder S. System of ophthalmology, vol 7. The foundations of ophthalmology, heredity, pathology, diagnosis, and therapeutics. St Louis: CV Mosby Co, 1962:399.
3. Gandolfo E, Capris P, Corallo G, Zingirian M. Effects of random presentation on kinetic threshold. In: Heijl A, Greve EL, eds. Proceedings of the 6th international visual field symposium. The Netherlands: W. Junk, Dordrecht, 1985:539–543.
4. Gandolfo E, Capris P, Corallo G, Zingirian M. Effects of random presentation on kinetic threshold. In: Heijl A, Greve EL, eds. Proceedings of the 6th international visual field symposium. Dordrecht, Netherlands: W Junk, 1985:539–543.
5. Goldmann H. Grundlagen exakter Perimetrie. Ophthalmologica 1945;109:57–70.
6. Williams TD. Age-related norms for peripheral visual field. Can J Optom 1985;47:140–141.
7. Williams TD. Computer-based analysis of visual fields: age-related norms for the central visual field, Can J Optom 1983;45:166–170.
8. Portney GL, Krohn MA. The limitations of kinetic perimetry in early scotoma detection. Ophthalmology 1978;85:287–293.
9. Mills RP, Hopp RH, Drance SM. Comparison of quantitative testing with the Octopus, Humphrey, and Tuebingen perimeters. Am J Ophthalmol 1986;102:496–504.
10. Wilensky JT, Joondeph BC: Variation in visual field measurements with an automated perimeter. Am J Ophthalmol 1984;97:328–331.
11. Keltner JL, Johnson CA, Lewis RA. Quantitative office perimetry. Ophthalmology 1985;92:862–872.
12. Parrish RK II, Schiffman J, Anderson DR. Static and kinetic visual field testing. Reproducibility in normal volunteers. Arch Ophthalmol 1984;102:1497–1502.

Scleral Indentation

Anthony A. Cavallerano

INTRODUCTION

Definition

Scleral indentation is a supplemental clinical procedure used in concert with stereoscopic indirect ophthalmoscopy to evaluate the most anterior portion of the peripheral ocular fundus. This is accomplished by applying minimal pressure to the sclera for palpation of the underlying retina or for observation of an area of the fundus that may not otherwise be visualized.

History

Many devices have been developed throughout the years to indent or depress the globe. The technique of scleral indentation was first suggested by Trantas in 1900, when he demonstrated that more of the peripheral ocular fundus could be observed by applying pressure to the sclera with the thumbnail.[1] During the era of direct ophthalmoscopy, numerous devices were employed in the art of indenting the sclera, including a coin and a cotton tipped applicator.

Coston and Wilder developed simple instruments to facilitate examination of the fundus periphery by indentation, but it was Charles Schepens who popularized the technique in the early 1950s, when he developed the thimble-type indentor. As indirect ophthalmoscopy became more prevalent and an accepted clinical procedure, attendant interest was kindled, and the importance of scleral indentation became recognized. Scleral indentation has since become a universally accepted and important clinical procedure.[2]

The devices have undergone several evolutionary changes, and in 1968, Schepens introduced the articulated depressor.[3] Mainster refined the design further when he developed a light-weight pencil-like device with an S-shaped shaft that facilitates indentation when using condensing lenses of short focal length.[4] Numerous designs are currently available that have been refined to permit an enhanced view of the structures of the peripheral retina.

Clinical Use

Scleral indentation, when used as an adjunct to stereoscopic indirect ophthalmoscopy, has many important clinical applications in the diagnosis of vitreoretinal disease. It is indicated when the examiner would like to gain an additional perspective of an area of the fundus. Retinal holes and breaks may go undetected if a thorough examination of the periphery is not carried out with this technique. Scleral indentation has a number of important clinical uses (Table 50–1).

1. Application of the indentor permits careful examination and evaluation of the peripheral ocular fundus when it otherwise might not be seen. This is often due to anatomical limitations, and scleral indentation extends the extreme limit of visibility of the retina. These anatomical limitations include the diameter of the dilated pupil, the anterior limit of the extreme peripheral retina, the ora serrata and pars plana, the depth of the anterior chamber angle and the posterior insertion of the root of the iris, and the refractive state of the eye.
2. Application of the indentor to the sclera produces an elevated, rolled section of retinal surface, thus permitting a view of the retina in profile. This maneuver provides a different view and another perspective of the appearance of retinal lesions. Depressing the sclera and manipulating the retina will enable the examiner to better differentiate between raised and excavated lesions in the retina.

Table 50–1
Clinical Uses of Scleral Indentation

1. Extends the extreme limit of visibility of the structures located in the retinal periphery.
2. Rolling the retinal surface gains another perspective and view of retinal lesions.
3. Palpation of the globe provides a critical view of the vitreoretinal interface.
4. To differentiate a retinal break from a retinal hemorrhage or other peripheral retinal lesions.

3. Application of the indentor enables the examiner to palpate the globe and gain a critical perspective of the tissue interaction at the vitreoretinal interface. This is vital when evaluating peripheral retinal disease, since the vitreous plays an intimate role in the pathogenesis of most disorders occurring in this segment of the fundus. The phenomenon of white-with-pressure, for example, can be observed only with the aid of scleral indentation.
4. Application of the indentor abets the detection of retinal breaks, either silent breaks or those occurring in patients with entoptic symptoms.
5. Application of the indentor enables the examiner to make a better distinction between a retinal break and a retinal hemorrhage.

INSTRUMENTATION

Theory

The principle involved in scleral indentation is the relationship between the appearance of the indented area and the surrounding area of the retina. Retinal transparency decreases in the indented area and, therefore, this elevated area appears darker than the surrounding retina. There is an apparent change in tissue density, and anatomical and pathologic structures take on a slightly different shape and appearance.[5]

Use

Scleral indentation allows comparison of the appearance of the same area of retina with and without application of the indentor. Retinal lesions are viewed from different angles, and the perspective provides a profile view or a view "from behind" the lesion. This relationship and comparison provides the examiner with additional information about the peripheral retina and any lesions or abnormalities that may be present.[5–7]

COMMERCIALLY AVAILABLE INSTRUMENTS

Numerous devices are currently available for scleral indentation and, although the clinician can resort to crude implements, such as a cotton-tipped applicator, a coin, or a paper clip, they are not recommended because patient comfort is at stake and the examiner may compromise maneuverability. Commercially available devices are more refined and permit a more exacting view of the structures of the peripheral retina.

One of the more popular types of scleral indentors is the thimble depressor of Schepens, which consists of a slightly fixed curved shaft with a flat, knoblike probe attached to a thimble (Fig. 50–1).[8]

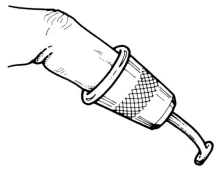

FIGURE 50–1. Thimble-type indentor with typical placement on the index finger. (From Potter J, Semes L, Cavallerano A, Garston M. Binocular indirect ophthalmoscopy. Boston: Butterworth Publishers, 1988, with permission)

This type of indentor is versatile because it can be placed on one finger or simply held between the thumb and the index finger. When placed on the index finger, this frees the other fingers for lid manipulation and, hence, increases the dexterity and maneuverability (Fig. 50–2).

A variation on this theme is a similar, open-ended, thimblelike device with a broader shaft, which is also fixed, but which has a thicker knobbed probe. The design is similar to that of the thimble type, except in some versions, the shaft is longer, which may be an advantage in some indentation situations. There is more flexibility in the holder because it is open-ended and permits placement on the finger in a much lower position (Fig. 50–3).

The third type of scleral depressor is the Mainster S-type, which consists of a stylus-type holder connected to a rather long, curved, fixed probe (Fig. 50–4). The device allows plenty of room for holding and manipulation, especially when used in the close quarters of the orbital area, and, because of this, it permits more efficient examination in patients with prominent orbital or nasal structures or recessed orbital cavities.[9,10] Such examination can be readily accomplished by using the indentor in conjunction with the 30-diopter (D) condensing lens, which has a smaller diameter and is easier to insert into smaller spaces. The device was developed because of a perceived problem with using the indentor with condensing lenses of shorter focal length.[4]

The device comes equipped with a pocket clasp, so it can easily be stored in the coat pocket when not in use. The probe is longer than most scleral depressors, and the end is finer; therefore, it is sometimes easier to apply on tight or anatomically small lids.[4,9,10]

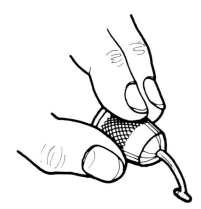

FIGURE 50–2. Thimble-type indentor shown grasped by the thumb and index finger. (From Potter J, Semes L, Cavallerano A, Garston M. Binocular indirect ophthalmoscopy. Boston: Butterworth Publishers, 1988, with permission)

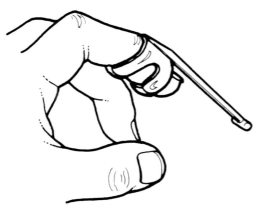

FIGURE 50–3. Open-ended thimble-type indentor. (From Potter J, Semes L, Cavallerano A, Garston M. Binocular indirect ophthalmoscopy. Boston: Butterworth Publishers, 1988, with permission)

Finally, another variation consists of an articulated depressor with a tip similar to the Mainster design, but which is equipped with a movable shaft (Fig. 50–5). The shaft is mounted on a loose spring and allows the examiner to apply only minimal pressure to the globe when performing the procedure.[3] The relatively small holder sometimes makes this device difficult to grasp, but, because there is very little bulk to it, it is sometimes easier to insert into the orbital area when one is attempting to indent the sclera and hold a relatively large condensing lens (e.g., 20-D lens) at the same time.

CLINICAL PROCEDURE

Patient Preparation

As with other indirect ophthalmoscopic procedures, the patient's pupils should be maximally dilated, and the patient should be in the supine position. Preferably, the examiner should have the ability to move freely around the head of the patient so that all areas of the periphery can be examined with minimal encumbrance (Table 50–2).

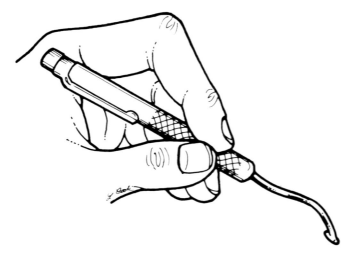

FIGURE 50–4. Mainster S-type indentor. (From Potter J, Semes L, Cavallerano A, Garston M. Binocular indirect ophthalmoscopy. Boston: Butterworth Publishers, 1988, with permission)

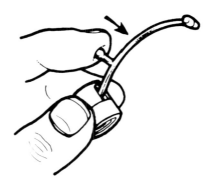

FIGURE 50–5. Schepens articulated indentor. (From Potter J, Semes L, Cavallerano A, Garston M. Binocular indirect ophthalmoscopy. Boston: Butterworth Publishers, 1988, with permission)

Examiner Preparation

1. The indentor should be grasped firmly by the examiner so that it is comfortable, but the fingers should still be able to move freely.
2. The indentor should be held in such a way that it can be manipulated easily about the orbital area. When using the thimble depressor, try to maintain as much freedom of movement as possible with the index finger inserted into the device. This will enable the examiner to use the other fingers to hold the patient's lid without feeling that they are "bound down" (see Fig. 50–1).

   Another option is to hold the depressor in the same manner that a pencil is grasped, remembering once again to maintain as much freedom of movement as possible with the other fingers (see Fig. 50–2). This can be accomplished by either holding the indentor between the thumb and the index finger or between the thumb and the middle finger. Excessive pressure need not be applied to the globe to perform the procedure correctly.
3. The practitioner should learn to hold the indentor in either hand. During the examination it is a constant requirement to exchange hands with the condensing lens and the depressor, depending on the quadrant of the retina being viewed and on the examiner's approach to the patient.

Table 50–2
Clinical Procedure for Scleral Indentation

---

1. Patient preparation
   a. Pupils maximally dilated
   b. Patient reclining
2. Examiner preparation
   a. Indentor grasped firmly
   b. Maintain freedom of movement of fingers
   c. Learn to hold the indentor in either hand
   d. Maintain freedom of movement about the patient
   e. Stand 180° from retina being observed
3. Patient examination
   a. Indent the globe gently through the eyelids
   b. Maintain common axis
   c. Indent 7- to 14-mm posterior to limbus
   d. Observe the indented area of the retina

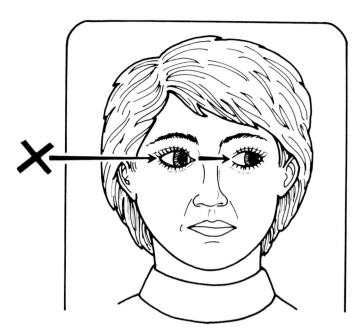

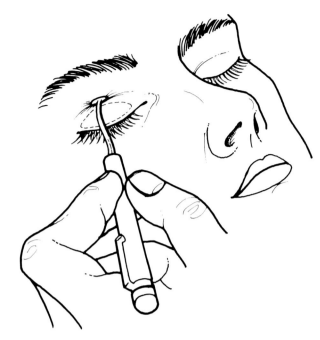

FIGURE 50–6. *X* defines the proper position for scleral indentation, 180° from the area of the retina being examined. (From Potter J, Semes L, Cavallerno A, Garston M. Binocular indirect ophthalmoscopy. Boston: Butterworth Publishers, 1988, with permission)

FIGURE 50–7. Proper placement and position for indenting the superior quadrant of the patient's right eye. (From Potter J, Semes L, Cavallerano A, Garston M. Binocular indirect ophthalmoscopy. Boston: Butterworth Publishers, 1988, with permission)

Patient Examination

It is easiest to indent superiorly, and the proper point of insertion of the device is crucial to the success of the procedure. Most indentation procedures begin superiorly at the 12-o'clock position To examine the superior quadrant of the right eye with the patient in the supine position, the following steps should be taken:

1. As with any indirect ophthalmoscopic technique, a basic tenet calls for the examiner standing 180° away from the area of the fundus to be examined.[9–11] From this point of observation, the pupil appears oval when the patient looks away from the examiner into one of the extreme positions of gaze (Fig. 50–6).
2. With the patient in the supine position, the examiner should stand by the patient's right arm. From this vantage point, to examine the superior quadrant of the right eye, the depressor should be held in the left hand and the condensing lens should be held in the right hand. The patient's gaze should first be directed downward, and the examiner should locate the superior-most lid fold, a point corresponding to the superior border of the tarsal plate (Fig. 50–7).
3. The examiner should then insert the indentor gently into this fold, and the patient is instructed to look up, toward his or her forehead.
4. As the lid retracts, the examiner slides the indentor posteriorly toward the orbit. The shaft of the depressor must remain parallel to the surface of the globe; that is, the tip and the shaft are placed tangentially along the plane of the globe, and the tip must remain at the superior tarsal margin (Fig. 50–8). This maneuver will assure that (1) the indentor is applied at the correct point on the globe, namely 7 to 14 mm from the limbus; and (2) the upper lid is raised up and moved away from the pupillary area, thereby permitting full illumination of the retina[12–14] (Fig. 50–9).

5. The next step requires that the examiner introduce the light from the binocular indirect ophthalmoscope into the pupillary area and look for the red reflex. An important clue to proper placement of the indentor is a darkening of the red reflex along the visual axis while observing it through the oculars of the ophthalmoscope. All of this takes place before the condensing lens is introduced; the examiner should attempt to keep the fingers away from the ocular area to allow enough room for the condensing lens.
6. The condensing lens is then introduced into the light path, remembering to maintain the common axis with the oculars of the ophthalmoscope and the area of the retina being observed.[13] Application of the indentor introduces the fourth point along the common visual axis; namely, the eyepieces of the ophthalmoscope, the light source, the condensing lens, and the indented area of the retina (Fig. 50–10).

At this point, the examiner should observe an elevated greyish area in the inferior part of the lens (that portion of the lens closest to the examiner) (Fig. 50–11). This is sometimes referred to as the "mouse under the blanket"; rolling the depressor will produce this effect. The indentor can now be moved from side to side and front to back (Fig. 50–12). If the greyish mound is not observed, then either the light source is not directed to the proper location on the retina or the indentor should be removed and placed along the common axis with the light source and the oculars. If the indentor is not seen, additional pressure should not be applied. Rather, move very slightly from one side to the other, looking for the indented retina.

The condensing lens should now be filled with the image of the retina. Fine adjustments of the lens or the ophthalmoscope are sometimes necessary to eliminate reflections and improve the quality of the image. The indentor can then be moved anteriorly to examine the far periphery and the ora serrata. The patient should

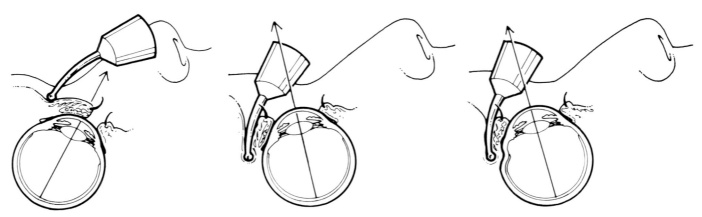

FIGURE 50–8. Movement of the indentor as the lid retracts and the patient looks away from the examiner. (From Potter J, Semes L, Cavallerano A, Garston M. Binocular indirect ophthalmoscopy. Boston: Butterworth Publishers, 1988, with permission)

be instructed to look away from the examiner when one is trying to observe the more peripheral areas; he or she should look more in the direction of the examiner or the ophthalmoscope for examination of the equatorial areas.

Concerning the condensing lens, remember that the larger lenses generally have more magnification and a smaller field of view. In addition, they are sometimes more difficult to manipulate because of their size. Therefore, consider using higher-powered lenses, which are smaller in diameter, but provide a greater field of view, and thus permit more visualization of the peripheral retina. They will also fit more easily into tight quarters and permit the examiner to insert the indentor into the orbital area with one hand and hold the condensing lens in the other hand.

This principle should also be adhered to when examining patients with smaller pupils; namely, the smaller the pupil, the more deeply one must insert the indentor to successfully perform the procedure. The indentor can then be moved laterally to scan the remaining portion of the superior fundus.

Scleral indentation is a dynamic technique requiring continual movement of the indentor and concomitant movement on the part of the examiner, always remembering to maintain the common axis along the four points (see Fig. 50–10). The amount of pressure necessary to view the fundus is less than one would

anticipate and is approximately equivalent to the force one applies to the globe when performing tactile tensions. The patient should experience no discomfort if the procedure is carried out properly. The examiner can ensure continued patient comfort by (1) remembering not to indent the tarsal plate, (2) not indenting too close to the limbus (pressure is then exerted on the ciliary body), (3) not pinching the lid against the orbital rim, since this can cause the patient to attempt to squeeze the eyelids shut.

Scleral indentation is routinely performed through the eyelids. The technique for examining the inferior retina is identical to that described in the foregoing, and the nasal and temporal areas can be examined by "dragging or hooking" the upper lid and aligning it with the area to be examined (Fig. 50–13).

If this procedure is not possible, then a topical anesthetic can be instilled and the indentor can be applied directly to the bulbar conjunctiva overlying the sclera (Fig. 50–14). If this technique is required, one should remember to take proper precautions to sterilize the tip of the indentor and avoid coming close to the cornea. This method is sometimes necessary when examining a patient with tight lids or a patient who is a "squeezer." It should be noted that the application of a topical anesthetic may cloud the cornea and obscure view of the peripheral retina; therefore, topical anesthetics should be used only when necessary.

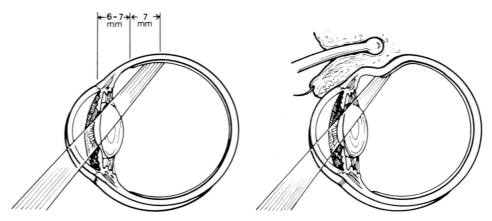

FIGURE 50–9. Scleral indentation is performed on the area of the retina corresponding to 7 to 14 mm behind the limbus. (From Potter J, Semes L, Cavallerano A, Garston M. Binocular indirect ophthalmoscopy. Boston: Butterworth Publishers, 1988, with permission)

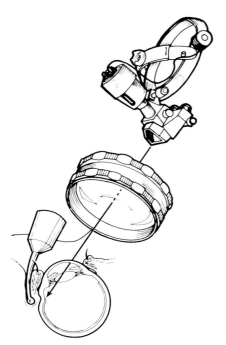

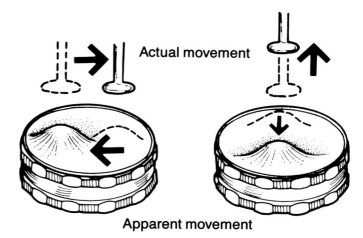

FIGURE 50–12. "Rolling" the retina by moving the indentor laterally and from front to back. (From Potter J, Semes L, Cavallerano A, Garston M. Binocular indirect ophthalmoscopy. Boston: Butterworth Publishers, 1988, with permission)

FIGURE 50–10. Common axis between the indented retina, the patient's pupil, the condensing lens, and the examiner's eyepiece. (From Potter J, Semes L, Cavallerano A, Garston M. Binocular indirect ophthalmoscopy. Boston: Butterworth Publishers, 1988, with permission)

CLINICAL IMPLICATIONS

Clinical Significance

Scleral indentation has become a fundamental procedure in primary eye care. This important technique should be mastered by the clinician to enhance diagnostic capabilities and reinforce clinical judgments.

Since scleral indentation is a dynamic technique, important information can be gathered by moving the indentor across and along the globe. This permits the examiner to obtain different views of lesions and gain a different perspective on the significance of findings.

Clinical Interpretation

Scleral indentation in conjunction with the stereoscopic view obtained with the binocular indirect ophthalmoscope enables a more refined differentiation between raised and excavated lesions. The technique also helps to differentiate between a retinal break (the margins of which blanche with indentation) and a retinal hemorrhage (which remains constant in color and appearance with indentation).[7-10]

The presence and amount of vitreoretinal adhesion or traction can also be evaluated more precisely. The phenomenon of white-with-pressure can be visualized only with the aid of scleral indentation, and a retinal break, lying anterior to an area of vitreous adhesion or traction, may not be seen unless the technique is employed. Passing the depressor beneath the lesion will allow the examiner to view it "on end" or "from behind." This is evident, for example, when viewing an area of lattice retinal degeneration in which the anterior border is torn secondary to vitreoretinal traction: it can be seen to "fishmouth" or open up upon indentation.[7,8,12,14]

Scleral indentation is indicated when the clinician would like to get a different perspective of an area of the equatorial or peripheral fundus. Retinal holes or breaks may go undetected if a thorough examination of the periphery is not carried out with the technique. In addition to viewing the retina in profile, this procedure enables the examiner to evaluate the vitreous cortex and make clinical determinations about the important role the vitreous

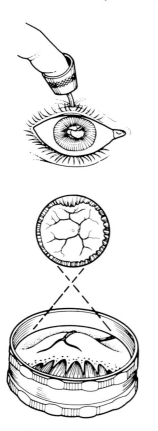

FIGURE 50–11. Elevated portion of the indented retina. (From Potter J, Semes L, Cavallerano A, Garston M. Binocular indirect ophthalmoscopy. Boston: Butterworth Publishers, 1988, with permission)

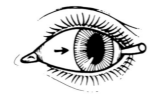

FIGURE 50–13. Dragging the lids to indent the nasal and temporal aspects of the retina. (From Potter J, Semes L, Cavallerano A, Garston M. Binocular indirect ophthalmoscopy. Boston: Butterworth Publishers, 1988, with permission)

plays in peripheral retinal changes. Adhesion of the vitreous to the retina may give the examiner the illusion of an intact retina, when, in fact, there may be an insidious break and subsequent separation of the retina (Table 50–3).

Scleral indentation also permits evaluation of areas in the most anterior periphery and in the pars plana, which would otherwise not be seen because of limitations of pupil size and viewing angle. Without indentation, anatomic variations (e.g., prominent orbital bones or deeply recessed globes) sometimes make it difficult or impossible to observe the fundus out to the ora serrata.

When properly performed, scleral indentation is an extremely safe and effective procedure, causing a minimal amount of patient discomfort. The procedure will not initiate or worsen retinal breaks or detachments. In fact, when attempting to discover small breaks, especially those lesions anterior to the equator, or to view retinal breaks directly (e.g., to determine if a break is partial or full thickness) it is an invaluable technique.[7–10]

Scleral indentation does increase the intraocular pressure and, therefore, can be painful when performed on patients with elevated pressure. These patients should be examined gently and

Table 50–3
Indications for Scleral Indentation

To enhance recognition of a retinal break

To enhance determination of the thickness of a retinal break

To evaluate areas of degeneration of the peripheral retina

To rule out retinal breaks and detachment in patients presenting with entoptic symptoms

To evaluate the presence and amount of fluid surrounding a retinal break

To evaluate the presence and amount of vitreous traction surrounding a retinal break or degenerative lesion

carefully; giving them frequent respites from the procedure is strongly recommended.[5,14]

The prudent clinician should avoid scleral indentation when increasing intraocular pressure might harm the eye. Some examples include patients having or suspected of having penetrating ocular or orbital injuries. Similarly, it should be deferred until approximately 8 weeks after intraocular surgery for fear of precipitating wound leak.[9,10,15]

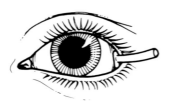

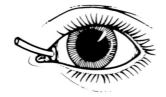

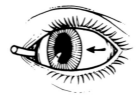

FIGURE 50–14. Indenting directly on the bulbar conjunctiva after instillation of a topical anesthetic. (From Potter J, Semes L, Cavallerano A, Garston M. Binocular indirect ophthalmoscopy. Boston: Butterworth Publishers, 1988, with permission)

REFERENCES

1. Trantas A. Moyens d'explorer par l'ophthalmoscopie—et par translucidite-la partie anterieure du fond oculaire, le cercle ciliaire y compris. Arch d'Ophthalmol 1900;20:314–326.
2. Schepens CL, Bahn GC. Examination of the ora serrata: its importance in retinal detachment. Arch Ophthalmol 1950;44:677.
3. Hovland KR, Tanenbaum HL, Schepens CL. New scleral depressor. Am J Ophthalmol 1968;66:117.
4. Mainster MA, Tolentino FI. Scleral depressor for short focal length lenses. Ann Ophthalmol 1982;14:46.
5. Walters GB. The technique of scleral indentation. Am J Optom Physiol Opt 1982;7:569–573.
6. Eisner G. Biomicroscopy of the peripheral fundus: an atlas and textbook. Berlin: Springer-Verlag, 1973:3–11.
7. Benson WE. Retinal detachment: diagnosis and management. Hagerstown: Harper & Row, 1987:82–94.
8. Schepens CL. Progress in detachment surgery. Trans Am Acad Ophthalmol 1951;55:607–615.
9. Cavallerano AA, Semes LP. How to perform scleral indentation. Rev Optom 1987;126(11):51–59.
10. Potter J, Semes L. Cavallerano A, Garston M. Binocular indirect ophthalmoscopy. Boston: Butterworth Publishers, 1988:54–67.

11. Eisner G. The principles of indentation. In: Biomicroscopy of the peripheral fundus: an atlas and textbook. Berlin: Springer-Verlag, 1973: 3–11.
12. Schepens CL. Techniques of examination of the fundus periphery. In: Symposium on retina and retinal surgery. Transactions of the New Orleans Academy of Ophthalmology. St Louis: CV Mosby Co, 1969: 39–51.

13. Rosenthal MR, Fradin S. The technique of binocular indirect ophthalmoscopy. Highlights Ophthalmol 1967;9:179–257.
14. Havener WH, Gloeckner S. Atlas of diagnostic techniques and treatment of retinal detachments. St Louis: CV Mosby Co, 1967:22–34.
15. Draeger J, Guthoff R, Moeller J. Correlations between intraocular pressure and resulting scleral indentation after retinal detachment surgery. Ophthal Res 1982;14:466–472.

Potential Acuity Assessment

Anthony A. Cavallerano

INTRODUCTION

Patients with cataracts often suffer from visual loss as a result of concurrent or related macular disease. Removing the opacity may not restore the vision to an acceptable and comfortable level. Surgical decisions can often be facilitated if accurate presurgical assessment of retinal and optic nerve function can be accomplished.

Until recently there has been no quantitative method of predicting postoperative visual acuity in patients with cataracts. A variety of crude methods have been employed, but some of these are subjective and, to a large degree, rely on examiner observation or patient response. These methods include the pinhole test, the swinging flashlight test, and the "blue field" entoptic test. Appreciation of the Purkinje vessel shadows and elicitation of the Haidinger brush phenomenon have also been used, as well as two-point discrimination, color vision, and central light fixation. Electrophysiologic tests are cumbersome and yield inconclusive results, providing information that may serve to only perplex the already shrouded issue of postoperative visual outcome.

Visual discrimination and entoptic imagery have given rise to more direct and quantitative methods of measuring visual acuity behind a media opacity. This most popular devices for this purpose include the Potential Acuity Meter and the clinical interferometer. Each of these systems has been developed and implemented into clinical practice within the last decade. When properly used, each can provide a reasonably accurate assessment of macular and optic nerve function through lenticular opacities. This chapter will address the clinical application and interpretation of findings using the Potential Acuity Meter (PAM) and two types of clinical interferometers, the Randwal IRAS Interferometer and the Haag–Streit Lotmar Visometer.

POTENTIAL ACUITY TESTING

Definition

Potential acuity testing is used to measure or predict the retinal visual acuity behind cataracts or other opacities in the media. The technique can also be used as an index for predicting visual outcomes or results whenever a view of the macula is obscured or if visual acuity measurement is desired without refraction.

Clinical Use

Potential acuity testing has many possible clinical applications when used as an adjunct test for subjectively predicting retinal visual acuity. Predicting visual outcomes often depends on the integrity of the macula, which is not visualized when corneal or media opacities are present. Potential acuity testing provides the clinician with information that serves as an index of potential visual function when the macula may not be visualized. This information can then be used to determine whether or not cataract surgery will significantly improve the visual acuity. The results can also provide important prognostic information on the outcome of certain disorders or conditions, such as trauma. The primary clinical uses are listed in Table 51–1.

Diffraction Theory and Maxwellian View

Devices used for potential acuity testing operate on the optical principle of Maxwellian view. Diffraction limits the clinically useful

Table 51–1
Clinical Uses of Potential Acuity Information

Predicting visual outcomes following:
  Cataract surgery
  Nd:YAG capsulotomy
  Penetrating keratoplasty
Estimation of visual function in amblyopes
Determination of retinal acuity in glaucoma
Rapid retinal visual acuity screening in large or irregular refractive states
Vision screening without refraction for vitreoretinal, retinal vascular, or
    neuroophthalmic patients

conventional pinhole to a diameter of 1.0 mm. An aperture smaller than this would produce significant diffraction, as well as diminished illumination, thus preventing 20/20 information from passing to the retina. The transilluminated aerial aperture is not a physical entity and, therefore, has no edges to diffract the light. There is some diffraction originating from the edges of the letters in the PAM. This effect was analyzed by Westheimer in such "Maxwellian view" optical systems.[1]

With the PAM, patients can read the 20/20 optotype letters due to diffraction from the edges of the letters on the projected Snellen chart. This diffracted light diverges to pass through the optics of the eye and produces legible 20/20 letters for the patient. The diffracted light carries high spatial frequency information, and there is a depth of focus of only 0.75 D to 1.00 D on either side of the best focus when working with a 6-mm pupil.

With the interferometer, light waves are produced from two sources behind the lenticular opacity. Moire fringes or grate patterns are created when light waves overlap. Where the crest of one wave overlaps the trough of another, a black band is created. When the crests are coincident, the additive effect produces a bright band.

Instrumentation: The Potential Acuity Meter

History

The PAM was conceived and designed by David Guyton and John Minkowski in early 1980.[2] Before that time, a prototype device, using Landolt broken rings, was reported by Cavonius and Hilz.[3] This early device was tested on a small sample of normal individuals with simulated media opacities, but the development was not carried any further. Other attempts have been made to estimate or predict the final visual acuity after cataract surgery using various primitive devices.[4]

Theory

The PAM mounts on a slit lamp biomicroscope and projects an image of a Snellen visual acuity chart through a 0.1-mm aerial aperture onto the retina (Fig. 51–1). The light beam narrows to pass through the aerial aperture at the focal plane of the slit lamp binoculars and takes advantage of the fact that not all lenticular or media opacities are homogeneous. Restricting the light to a narrow beam reduces the scatter produced by the cataract. The beam is then directed through a clear "window" of the immature cataract and focused on the retina. The result is a pinhole vision test produced without significant diffraction and without a decrease in illumination.[2,5,6]

The PAM visual acuity chart has black optotypes on a white background. The illumination of the chart is brighter than a conventional Snellen chart, and optotypes are available in number or letter format.

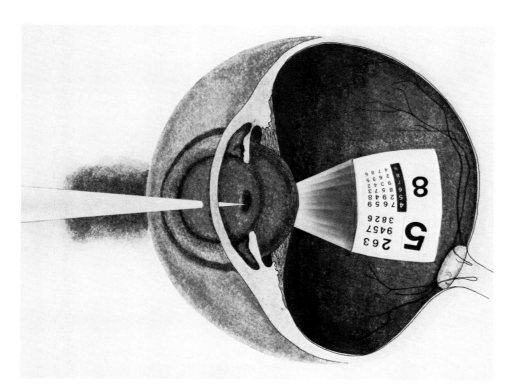

FIGURE 51–1. Concept of the PAM with a cataractous lens depicting the projected acuity chart on the retina. (Courtesy of Mentor)

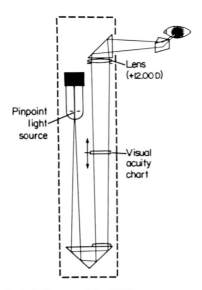

FIGURE 51–2. Optical diagram of the PAM.

There are five fundamental components to the PAM (Fig. 51–2). These include:

1. The pinpoint light source that defines the aperture.
2. A transilluminated Snellen visual acuity chart, providing visual acuity levels from 20/400 to 20/20.
3. A +12.00-diopter achromatic condensing lens that forms an image of the light source in the patient's pupil. This lens serves as an optometer lens so that when the transilluminated light beam is imaged into the plane of the patient's cataract, the optometer arrangement provides refractive correction referenced to the spectacle plane.[2]
4. Three reflecting prisms to appropriately direct the optical path of the light.
5. An additional +3.00-diopter lens to assist in imaging the light source at the patient's pupil.

THE IMAGING PRINCIPLE. The acuity chart may be moved along the optical axis within the instrument to compensate for refractive correction. The examiner or the patient can alter this distance along the axis by adjusting the external knob provided as the sphere power control. The dioptric scale ranges from −10.00 to +13.00, and the arrangement simulates a spherical spectacle lens. The end result is an acuity chart imaged on the retina, and the magnification of the characters varies to the same extent as with corrective lenses placed in the spectacle plane.[7] This principle is illustrated in Figure 51–3.

The PAM is more effective than a conventional pinhole aperture because most windows through immature cataracts are large enough to pass sufficient information to achieve at least 20/30 resolution. However, a pinhole 1.2 mm in diameter reduces the illumination through a normal-sized pupil by approximately 91%,[2] whereas with the PAM there is no decrease in illumination. It appears that it is the level of illumination, as much as the small size of the projected aerial image, that is responsible for the effectiveness of the PAM.[2]

Commercially Available Instruments

The Mentor Guyton–Minkowski Potential Acuity Meter (Fig. 51–4) is the only one of its kind commercially available and is designed to fit onto the central column of most slit lamp biomicroscopes.

The device consists of the following features:

1. A power on/off switch
2. A patient viewing window, which is a small aperture through which the patient observes the Snellen acuity chart.
3. Background illumination light that provides red background illumination to the patient's eye.
4. Background illumination control that changes the intensity of the illumination being directed to the external surface of the patient's eye.
5. A two-target knob to adjust between Snellen and numbered optotypes.
6. Sphere power control and scale, which provide a reading of simulated spherical power in the instrument.
7. Mounting pin, locking knob, and alignment notch, which holds the PAM on the slit lamp biomicroscope.

Two visual acuity charts are available with the PAM, one with numbers, the other with letters (Fig. 51–5). The key for the various letter and number charts is printed in the instruction manual and becomes familiar to the examiner with repeated useage. Selection of the Snellen letters corresponds to the American Optical projected Snellen acuity chart. With the proper adaptor, the PAM can be mounted to virtually any type of slit lamp biomicroscope.

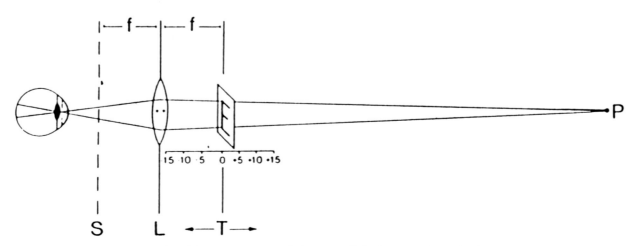

FIGURE 51–3. Optical principles of the PAM. *P*, pinpoint light source; *T*, Snellen target; *L*, condensing lens, with focal length *f*, and spectacle plane *S*. Refractive changes are made by displacing *T* relative to *L*, thereby changing magnification as if the lens were in the spectacle plane.

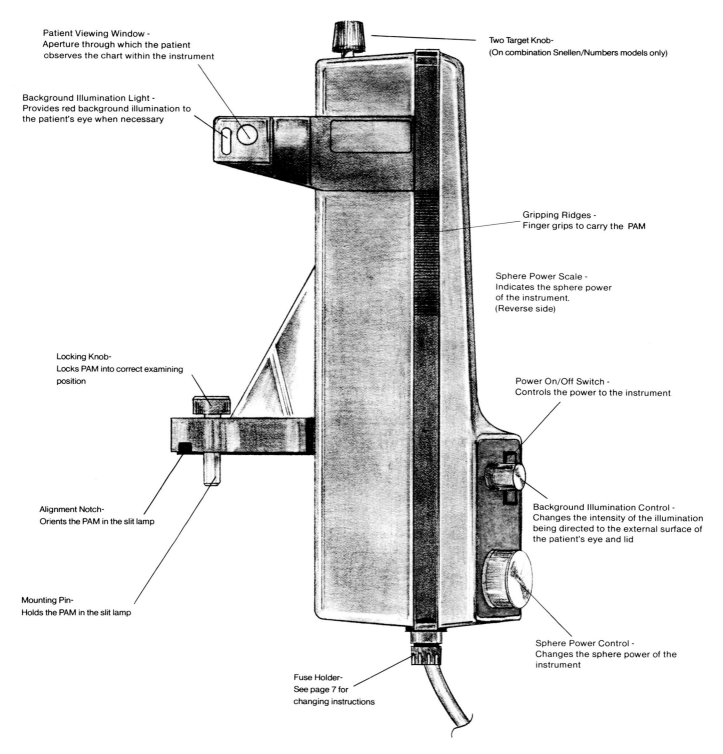

FIGURE 51–4. The Guyton–Minkowski Potential Acuity Meter (PAM). (Courtesy of Mentor)

Clinical Procedure

The recommended clinical procedure in using the Guyton–Minkowski Potential Acuity Meter is the following (Table 51–2):

1. *The examination room should be dimly lighted.* Ensure that there are no distractions, such as open doors, points of

light, or projected Snellen charts on the wall. Minimal background ambient illumination can be provided by a small light source directed to a rear wall.

2. *Position and prepare the patient.* The patient should be seated comfortably at the slit lamp biomicroscope. Advise the patient to remain still and to communicate by talking through his or her teeth without moving the chin. If neces-

Visual Acuity Chart (Letters)

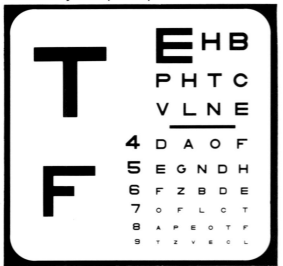

Visual Acuity Key (Letters)	
T	20/400
F	20/300
E	20/200
H B	20/100
P H T C	20/80
V L N E	20/70
4 D A O F	20/60
5 E G N D H	20/50
6 F Z B D E	20/40
7 O F L C T	20/30
8 A P E O T F	20/25
9 T Z V E C L	20/20

Visual Acuity Key (Numbers)	
5	20/400
8	20/300
2	20/200
6 3	20/100
9 4 5 7	20/80
3 8 2 6	20/70
4 7 6 5 9	20/60
5 2 9 4 8	20/50
6 8 5 7 3	20/40
7 9 3 4 2	20/30
8 2 6 3 5	20/25
9 4 7 8 6	20/20

Visual Acuity Chart (Numbers)

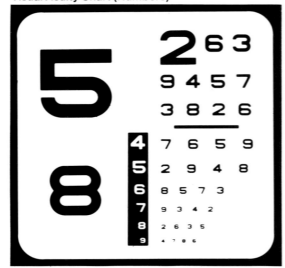

FIGURE 51–5. Sample visual acuity charts available with the two-target PAM.

Table 51–2
Clinical Procedure for Potential Acuity Testing

1. Dimly lighted examination room
2. Maximum pupillary dilatation
3. Position and prepare the patient
4. Focus and adjust the instrument
5. Instruct the patient
6. Look for clear windows
7. Make the measurement
8. Record the measurement

sary, the chin rest can be lowered once the patient is aligned so that he or she may talk more easily while maintaining the chart in view.

The pupils should be maximally dilated to expose the largest number of lucent or semilucent windows, but the procedure can be performed through miotic pupils, if necessary. With children, amblyopes, or uncooperative adults, it may be necessary to patch the better eye and, as with any visual acuity measurement, refrain from exposing the eye to bright lights immediately before the examination.

3. *Focus and adjust the instrument.* First, use the lowest viewing magnification on the slit lamp biomicroscope or look around the slit lamp to locate the dot of light. The slit lamp illumination should be turned off to avoid unnecessary glare. Observe the red background light and the small white dot as it traverses the media. Move the slit lamp and use the iris as a background to find the white dot if it is not readily visible. Look through the slit lamp under low magnification and direct the beam into the pupillary area (Fig. 51–6). The beam is visible to the examiner as it passes through the crystalline lens. While the patient holds the eye steady, the examiner looks for clear windows. If the beam strikes an opacity, the scattering will be obvious to the examiner.

The spherical power control should be set to 0 diopters initially or, if known, to the approximate spherical equivalent of the patient's refractive error before the onset of cataracts. Alternately, the patient may be tested through glasses or contact lenses. For uncorrected aphakes, set the power control initially to +12.00 diopters (D).

4. *Instruct the patient.* The patient should be instructed to look at the light by directing the gaze down approximately 14° from horizontal. The patient is then instructed to read the smallest line of numbers or letters that can be seen clearly. Once the patient successfully identifies three characters on the line, he or she is encouraged to move to the next line. The examiner should move quickly to avoid line fatigue.

5. *Look for clear windows.* This is accomplished by moving the slit lamp in all directions, vertically, laterally, and front to back to find neighboring windows. A brief slit lamp examination before using the PAM will help to locate the potential clear windows. If the patient reports that the letters were instantaneously clear, but that there was no time to read them, the area should be rescanned.

6. *Attempt to focus the chart better.* Move the diopter control setting in combination with making the foregoing slit lamp adjustments. Begin by moving in 3-D increments. A good setting for one window is often appropriate for others. Fine adjustments of the dioptric setting are made by moving in a plus or minus direction until the patient reports

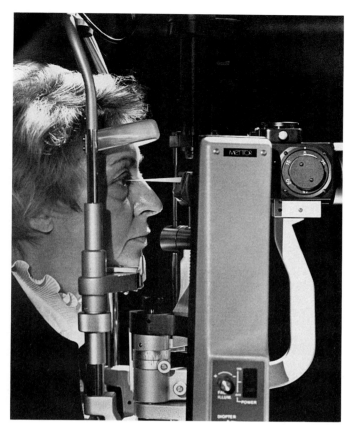

FIGURE 51–6. Patient aligned at the slit lamp for a PAM procedure. (Courtesy of Mentor)

optimal clarity. Once set, avoid dioptric changes greater than plus or minus 2.00 D.

Certain patients can control the dipoter setting and move their heads to obtain the most precise view. Once the optimal dioptric setting is obtained, these small self-scanning movements become the most important adjustment.

7. *Record the measurement.* The end point is reached if the patient correctly identifies three characters on a line and the examiner cannot encourage extra lines. If the patient cannot read additional lines by self-scanning, then the end

point has been reached. The examination should take only 1 to 5 minutes per eye and increasing the test time may produce fatigue, especially among elderly patients.

If the light is not seen, be sure the patient is looking toward the beam of light. If, after making adjustments the light is still not seen, then a "no light seen" reading is recorded.

CLINICAL INTERFEROMETRY

Definition

Another device that provides a useful estimation of the retinal acuity behind lenticular opacities is the clinical interferometer. The interferometer uses two coherent beams of light to create a three-dimensional fringe or striped pattern on the retina. The pinpoint beams of light are directed through opacities in the optical system of the eye in Maxwellian view.

Instrumentation

History

In 1935 Le Grand was the first to describe a method for obtaining a quantitative measurement of retinal visual acuity using interference fringes in Maxwellian view.[8] The theory was further evaluated independently by Green and Cohen[9] and Goldmann and Lotmar.[10] In the early 1970s monochromatic light from a laser source was used to generate fringe patterns.[10,11] Lotmar later developed an apparatus that generated moire fringes with variable pitch using a normal low-voltage incandescent lamp.[11] This achromatic interferometer, the Lotmar Visometer, and other similar devices, are now in widespread clinical use.

Theory

Clinical interferometers are devices that are hand-held or mounted on a slit lamp biomicroscope that produce two coherent pinpoint sources of light, each less than 0.1 mm in diameter. These point sources are generated in the vicinity of the pupillary plane, and interference fringes are produced on the retina at the point the two beams overlap (Fig. 51–7). The examiner adjusts the spacing between the fringes until the patient can no longer detect their orientation (Fig. 51–8). Refractive correction is not required, but a Scheiner's disk may be seen by the patient with a large uncorrected refractive error.[12]

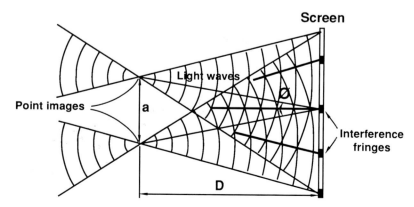

FIGURE 51–7. Interaction of wavefronts from two coherent light sources, producing interference fringes.

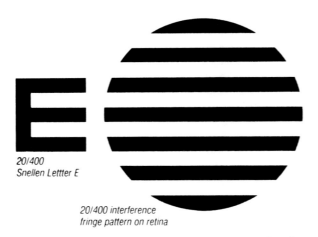

20/400
Snellen Lettter E

20/400 interference
fringe pattern on retina

FIGURE 51–8. Correlation between interference acuity and Snellen acuity at 20/400.

Clinical interferometers use either a neon–helium laser or a white incandescent bulb as a source of the coherent light. Production of the interference fringes is independent of the intensity of the source and, therefore, the procedure does not rely on high transmissability of light. In Maxwellian view, the formation of a retinal image is also independent of refractive error.[1,12]

Maxima refers to the points on the retina at which both beams are in phase and are seen as bright white or red bars. Black bars are observed at minima, the point at which the beams are out of phase. Varying the lateral separation between the two light sources will change the frequency of the interference pattern. The laser light source produces interference fringes by producing light waves that occupy different positions in space. This system does not rely on frequency to generate the two periodic waves.[13]

The field size of the interference fringe ranges from 1.5° to 8° and varies with different instruments. The orientation of the fringe pattern provides an indication of the patient's resolving capability.

Thirty-three maxima per degree of visual angle corresponds to a Snellen equivalent of 20/20.[14]

Commercially Available Instruments

Randwal IRAS Interferometer

The Randwal IRAS Interferometer (Fig. 51–9) can be hand held or adapted for use with the slit lamp biomicroscope. Clinical application of the instrument is identical regardless of the method of use. The device consists of the following features (Fig. 51–10):

1. A power on/off switch. A barrel switch located at the bottom of the instrument has three settings: HI, LO, and OFF. An illuminated red light at the base of the instrument indicates that the instrument is turned *on.*
2. A retinal acuity sleeve used to increase and decrease the spacing of the targets. The Snellen acuity equivalent is visible through the sleeve window.
3. Pattern orientation varies the direction of the pattern lines by rotating the body of the instrument while holding the head steady.
4. The iris diaphragm lever continuously regulates the field size between 3° and 8°. A field size of 5.5° occurs with the lever in the middle position.
5. The power module can be plugged into a wall outlet and comes equipped with a flexible retractible cord.
6. A toggle switch activates an optional glare-testing function. Glare sources are not controlled by the barrel switch. (Glare testing is discussed in Chap. 53).

Haag–Streit Lotmar Visometer

The Lotmar Visometer (Fig. 51–11) is mounted on a slit lamp biomicroscope and produces moire fringes generated by two gratings. The fringe pitch is controlled by the angle between the gratings, and a striped pattern of variable pitch provides an assessment of visual acuity. As the beam separation is increased, the fringe pattern becomes finer (Fig. 51–12). The instrument consists of the features shown in Figure 51–13.

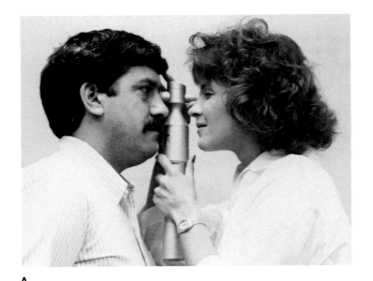

A

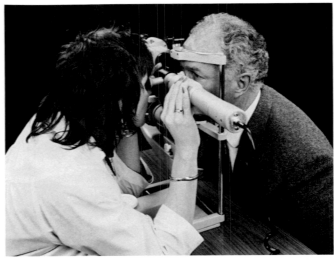

B

FIGURE 51–9. Randwal IRAS hand-held (*A*) and slit lamp-mounted (*B*) interferometer. (Courtesy of Randwal)

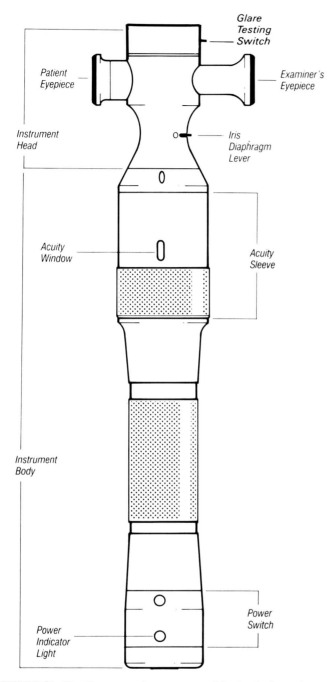

FIGURE 51–10. Features and components of the Randwal Interferometer. (Courtesy of Randwal)

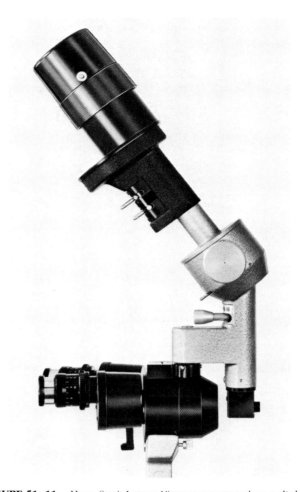

FIGURE 51–11. Haag–Streit Lotmar Visometer mounted on a slit lamp biomicroscope. (Courtesy of Haag–Streit)

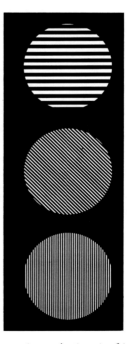

FIGURE 51–12. Progressive reduction in fringe pattern requiring greater resolving capability.

Clinical Procedure

The recommended clinical procedure for using any interferometer is as follows:

Patient Preparation

1. The examination room should be dimly lighted. Minimal background illumination is helpful for observing the patient's pupillary area while aligning the instrument.

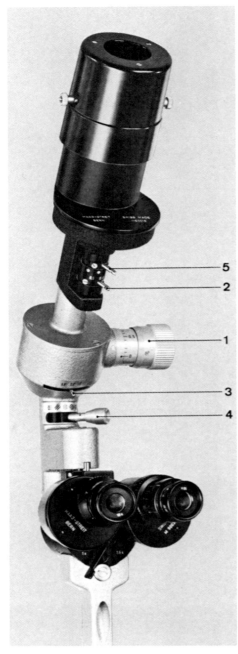

FIGURE 51–13. Features and components of the Haag–Streit Lotmar Visometer: (*1*) knurled knob with graduated drum for setting the fringe pitch and reading the visual acuity; (*2*) lever for forming an entrance pupil of 0.5-mm or 0.15-mm diameter; (*3*) lever for selecting visual fields of 1.5°, 2.5°, or 3.5°; (*4*) handle for changing fringe direction, with push button for obscuring the visual field; (*5*) lever for interposing filter; stop positions: right = green, middle = empty, left = grey. (Courtesy of Haag–Streit)

2. The patient's pupils should be maximally dilated; do not shine bright lights into the eye before testing.
3. No patient refractive correction is necessary unless there is a high refractive error. The examiner should be corrected for distance vision to clearly see the slit sources.
4. The patient should be comfortably seated with the head against the headrest. He or she should refrain from talking

except to indicate the fringe orientation. If the slit lamp is used the patient should be properly positioned.
5. Familiarize the patient with the test target by demonstrating the test pattern. Explain that partial patterns may be seen and that the patient should ignore wavy or distorted lines.
6. The patient should be told to indicate only the direction of the lines seen.

Randwal Interferometer Instructions

The recommended procedure in using the Randwal IRAS Interferometer is the following:

1. Set the power switch to HI intensity, the acuity sleeve to 20/80, and the field size to 8°.
2. Set the pattern orientation to horizontal.
3. Position the interferometer approximately 1.5 in. (4 cm) from the patient's cornea.
4. Direct the light source into the pupillary plane along the optical axis looking for less dense areas of cataract.
5. Proper operation occurs when the patient's iris and the operator's slit sources are in focus.
6. Begin testing the better eye with an 8° field size and an acuity setting two lines worse than the patient's best corrected visual acuity.
7. If the patient can see and correctly identify the orientation

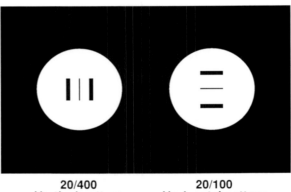

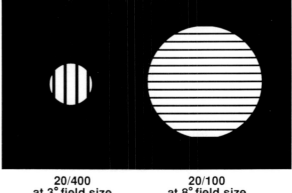

FIGURE 51–14. Patient acuity target and operator slit view with the Randwal Interferometer.

of the coarse line pattern, quickly move to the next finer line spacing.

8. Monitor the patient's fixation during the test.
9. The orientation of the examiner's slit indicates the orientation of the lines seen by the patient (Fig. 51–14).

MEASUREMENT

1. Obtain a direct measurement by observing the sleeve window. The Snellen equivalent is visible in the window, with 80 corresponding to 20/80, 40 to 20/40, etc.
2. Determine the finest grating the patient can observe 50% of the time. Once a threshold acuity is determined at 8°, repeat the procedure with 3° target size.
3. A variation of two or more lines between the 8° and 3° acuity thresholds may require further evaluation for macular or optic nerve abnormalities.

Lotmar Visometer Instructions

The recommended clinical procedure in using the Lotmar Visometer is the following:

1. Demonstrate the target to the patient (Fig. 51–15). It is useful to explain to the patient and illustrate by this example that the stripes may not be uniform or complete.
2. Set the filter lever (5) to the middle position (empty).
3. Set the entrance pupil lever (2) to 0.5 mm.
4. Set the knurled knob designating the fringe pattern (1) to 0.05.
5. Set lever (3) to a visual field of 3.5°.
6. Adjust the prism to orientate the fringe pattern (4) to the vertical direction. When changing the direction during the test, depress the handle to obscure the field during manipulation.
7. Adjust the voltage switch to 5 V.
8. Find the region of highest transparency in the crystalline lens and switch to stop 0.15 mm.

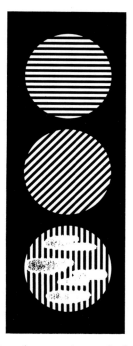

FIGURE 51–15. Patient demonstration card of the Lotmar Visometer target with incomplete stripe pattern demonstrated on the lower target example. (Courtesy of Haag–Streit)

Table 51–3
Lotmar Visometer Reference Card

| | Snellen | |
Decimal System	6-m Table	20-ft Table
1.0	6/6	20/20
0.8	5/6	20/25
0.7	6/9	20/30
0.6	5/9	15/25
0.5	6/12	20/40
0.4	5/12	20/50
0.3	6/18	20/70
0.1	6/60	20/200

MEASUREMENT

1. Maintain a constant distance from the corneal surface.
2. Direct the light source into the pupillary plane along the optical axis looking for less dense areas of cataract.
3. After the patient recognizes the fringe pattern, switch the entrance pupil (lever 2) to 0.15 mm and introduce the green filter.
4. Increase the fringe pitch in steps of 0.1, asking the patient to designate the azimuthal direction of the fringes.
5. Vary the direction of the fringes at random and, as the end point is reached, four correct responses are required for a final visual acuity reading.
6. Obtain the reading of the fringe pitch directly from the instrument and convert to the Snellen equivalent using Table 51–3.

CLINICAL IMPLICATIONS

Clinical Significance

Potential acuity testing can be important for predicting the level of visual function after surgery. It is an important index of retinal acuity when advising a patient about surgery if the posterior segment cannot be observed directly with an ophthalmoscope or by fundus biomicroscopy. The information derived from the measurement of vision can be of diagnostic importance when deciding if cataract surgery or keratoplasty will improve the level of visual function.

The patient and the examiner recognize the importance of this mode of testing, and the patient is often reassured that visual function can be restored if surgery is performed.[7] The measurement of foveal function is useful information, and with potential acuity testing, only one small window is required for the measurement to be made.

Interferometers tend to penetrate dense cataracts better than the PAM and, therefore, give more falsely good predictive results because of the nature of the light stimulus.

Clinical Interpretation

Potential Acuity Meter

The ability of the PAM to penetrate an opacified lens decreases as the density of the cataract increases, and the accuracy of the PAM reading may diminish slightly with denser cataracts. Cataracts denser than 20/300 may cause a clinically significant disparity between the PAM findings and true retinal visual acuity.[2,6,7,15] In general, the PAM gives more falsely poor results (postoperative acuity better than predicted) because of its poor ability to penetrate dense opacities.

An advantage of the PAM is that it relies on Snellen letters or numbers. An additional advantage is the ability of a single beam of light to penetrate the cataract. The results obtained with the PAM are more accurate if no preexisting retinal disease is present or if the macula can be directly observed with the ophthalmoscope and no abnormalities detected. Under most circumstances, the results compare favorably with the true retinal acuity, as determined by conventional Snellen measurement after cataract extraction or resolution of media opacities.[16,17] It has been demonstrated that if the macula cannot be directly observed, the PAM seems to be more reliable when maculopathy is present.[2]

Clinical judgment is always required in the interpretive process, but true retinal acuity is usually equal to, or better than, the PAM acuity. The PAM acuity represents the worst level of acuity attainable postoperatively (unless macular edema or an irregular cornea is present) and, therefore, significant improvement is a good recommendation for surgery.[18–20] If the PAM acuity is 20/40 or better, or three-lines better than the best-correctable visual acuity, then there is sufficient reason to believe that beneficial surgical results are strongly suggested. If the PAM acuity is not 20/40 or better, or if it is not three-lines better than the best-corrected acuity, then postoperative improvement may not occur.

If any posterior pole disease is visible ophthalmoscopically or by fundus biomicroscopy, then the media are most likely not responsible for poor PAM acuity.[18]

Interferometers

Interferometers penetrate denser cataracts because they do not depend on clear zones in the crystalline lens.[19,20] Other advantages include independence from refractive error and the use of a single variable target. If the opacity is dense enough to prevent penetration, then the test will yield false-negative results. Penetration of the light beam can be monitored by the examiner by observing the passage of the light with the slit lamp biomicroscope. Problems also occur with vitreous hemorrhage and advanced glaucoma; both will result in falsely poor predicted vision. Interferometers tend to overestimate retinal acuity in amblyopia.[14,18,19]

False-Positive and False-Negative Results

Potential acuity testing is more reliable when dealing with immature cataracts or with discrete opacities in the crystalline lens. As with any clinical procedure, there are some limitations (Table 51–4). Diffuse posterior subcapsular cataract or dense cortical opacities may be disruptive, especially to the light rays of the PAM and, therefore, produce false-negative results, that is, better vision postoperatively than expected. Other causes of false-negative results or pessimistic acuity (resulting from insufficient light reaching the retina) include vitreous hemorrhage or testing without adequate pupillary dilatation.[16,18]

Falsely optimistic or positive results can occur if there are residual capsular opacities after extracapsular cataract extraction or if irregular astigmatism resulting from the surgery produces a distorted cornea. Falsely optimistic results are also obtained in the presence of cystoid macular edema. Scattering of light from the inner retinal layers blurs the image of the photoreceptor layer when the entire pupil is used for viewing. Restriction of the light to a small part of the pupil causes less scattering and a better image on the photoreceptor layer. If the photoreceptor layer is healthy, good vision will be predicted, representing a falsely optimistic result. However, false-positive results will not be obtained if the photoreceptor layer is not healthy. Macular edema will produce falsely good results and this has been attributed to better stimulation of photoreceptors by the fringe patterns.[21] It has also been reported that wet macular degeneration tends to produce false-positive results more frequently than the dry type.[19]

Causes of false-positive results from macular edema include:

Serous detachment of the macula

Macular edema from any cause

Early postoperative retinal detachment

If the posterior pole can be visualized and it is determined that macular edema is not present and there is no corneal irregularity, then suspect amblyopia, a macular scotoma from a foveal lesion, glaucoma, optic neuropathy, or a field defect of neurologic origin.

Other causes of falsely good results following surgery are listed in Table 51–5.

False-positive findings are disquieting to the patient and examiner alike. Therefore, any findings with potential acuity testing method requires caution in the presence of macular edema or corneal irregularity.

Table 51–4

Limitations That May Affect the Results with Potential Acuity Testing

Poor pupillary dilation
Dense, diffuse media
Poor patient posture at the slit lamp
Poor patient fixation and cooperation
Nystagmus
Senility
Fatigue
Language barrier

Table 51–5

Falsely Good Results with Potential Acuity Testing

Cystoid macular edema
Serous detachment of the macular RPE
Geographic atrophy of the RPE
Visual field cut through fixation
Recent reattached retina
Macular hole
Amblyopia
Corneal irregularities

REFERENCES

1. Westheimer G. Retinal light distribution for circular apertures in Maxwellian view. J Opt Soc Am 1959;49:41–44.
2. Minkowski JS, Palese M, Guyton DL. Potential acuity meter using a minute aerial pinhole aperture. Ophthalmology 1983;90:1360–1368.
3. Cavonius CR, Hilz R. A technique for testing visual function in the presence of opacities. Invest Ophthalmol 1973;12:933–936.
4. Worst J. Prediction of the aphakic vision. Ophthalmologica 1966; 151:659–661.
5. Boyd BF. Tri-weekly letter. Highlights Ophthalmol 1983;4:1–8.
6. Guyton DL. Instruments for measuring retinal visual acuity behind cataracts. Ophthalmology 1982;89(suppl 8):34–39.
7. Minkowski JS. Preoperative evaluation of macular function. *In:* Cataract surgery. Baltimore: Grune & Stratton, 1983:327–341.
8. Bernth-Petersen P, Naeser K. Clinical evaluation of the Lotmar Visometer for macular testing in cataract patients. Acta Ophthalmol 1982; 60:525–532.

9. Green DG, Cohen MM. Laser interferometry in the evaluation of potential macular function in the presence of opacities in the ocular media. Trans Am Acad Ophthalmol Otolaryngol 1971;75:629–636.
10. Lotmar W. Use of moire fringes for testing visual acuity of the retina. Appl Opt 1972;11:1266–1268.
11. Lotmar W. Apparatus for measurement of retinal visual acuity by moire fringes. Invest Ophthalmol Vis Sci 1980;19:393–401.
12. Enoch JM, Bedell HE, Kaufman HE. Interferometric visual acuity testing in anterior segment disease. Arch Ophthalmol 1979;79:1916.
13. Green DG. Laser devices in measuring visual acuity. In: Duane TD, ed. Clinical ophthalmology, vol 1. Philadelphia: Harper & Row, 1988: chap 66, 1–7.
14. Minkowsi JS, Guyton DL. New methods for predicting visual acuity after cataract surgery. Ann Ophthalmol 1984;16:511–516.
15. Carpel EF, Henderson V. The influence of cataract types on potential acuity meter results. J Cataract Refract Surg 1986;12:276–277.
16. Miller ST, Graney MJ, Elam JT, et al. Predictions of outcomes from cataract surgery in elderly persons. Ophthalmology 1988;95:1125–1129.
17. Graney MJ, Applegate WB, Miller ST, et al. A clinical index for predicting visual acuity after cataract surgery. Am J Ophthalmol 1988;105:460–465.
18. Faulkner W. Macular function testing through opacities. In: Focal points 1986: clinical modules for ophthalmologists, vol 4, module 2. American Academy of Ophthalmology, 1986.
19. Guyton DL. Preoperative visual acuity evaluation. Int Ophthalmol Clin 1987;27(3):140–148.
20. Guyton DL. Prediction of postoperative vision in cataract patients. Ophthalmol Clin North Am 1989;2:431–442.
21. Faulkner W. Laser interferometric prediction of postoperative visual acuity in patients with cataracts. Am J Ophthalmol 1983;95:626.

Photostress Recovery Testing

Charles J. Patorgis

INTRODUCTION

Definition

Photostress recovery time,[1] also referred to as dazzling time[2,3] and readaptation time,[4] is the period required for the macula to return to a normal level of function after being exposed to an intense light source.

History

Bailliart[5] first reported on the concept and technique of photostress recovery testing in 1954. Not until 1960, however, did its clinical applicability appear in the American literature.[6] Between the years of 1962 and 1968, 11 additional papers were published by several investigators on various clinical techniques, assorted instrumentation, and the results of clinical research.[1–3,7–14] As a consequence of this flurry of publications, the procedure became widely accepted as a simple, rapid, and inexpensive means of evaluating patients suspected of having macular edema or photoreceptor dysfunction. Glaser et al.[15] updated the literature in 1977 and provided procedural and diagnostic guidelines that continue to be used by many clinicians. Three papers published in the 1980s reaffirmed the practicality of this procedure.[16–18]

Clinical Use

The photostress test is a simple, easy to administer, and inexpensive test of macular function. It is based on the ability of the macular photoreceptors to recover from exposure to intense light. More specifically, bleaching the macular photoreceptors with intense light results in the formation of a positive afterimage, which cre-

ates a dense central scotoma and reduces visual acuity.[19] As photopigments are regenerated, visual acuity slowly improves, with disappearance of the scotoma. A delay in resynthesis, which may occur with various disorders of the photoreceptors, retinal pigment epithelium (RPE), or choriocapillaris, results in a prolonged recovery time.

The basis of this readaptive response lies in the mechanisms governing photopigment regeneration. For photochemical synthesis to occur, vitamin A must be converted to the aldehyde retinene by either of the cofactors diphosphopyridine (DPN) or triphosphopyridine nucleotide (TPN). Retinene, in turn, combines with photopsin to form rhodopsin, a photopigment (Fig. 52–1).[14] This sequence of events occurs normally when retinal metabolic processes or connections between the RPE and photoreceptors are intact.[1]

INSTRUMENTATION

Theory

Several illumination sources have been used for photostress testing (Table 52–1). The disposable penlight is the simplest and least expensive of these. The primary drawback to this light source is its fluctuation in intensity, which may create problems with reliability and reproducibility of data. This may be minimized either by refrigerating the penlight[17] or by replacing it every 1 or 2 weeks. Glaser et al.,[15] in calibrating their penlights daily, found a variance in intensity of up to 24%. A disposable penlight, therefore, is not the most reliable device if constant luminance of the light source is desired.[10]

Consequently, the light from a direct ophthalmoscope or transilluminator is most often employed to clinically assess photostress recovery time (Fig. 52–2). Bailliart[5] was the first to docu-

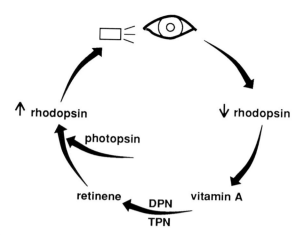

FIGURE 52–1. Biochemical process of photopigment regeneration after photostress. The introduction of a light source diminishes the supply of rhodopsin in the photoreceptors and sets the metabolic cycle of photopigment regeneration into motion. An interruption of this process, either by macular edema or photoreceptor breakdown, may result in a prolonged photostress recovery time.

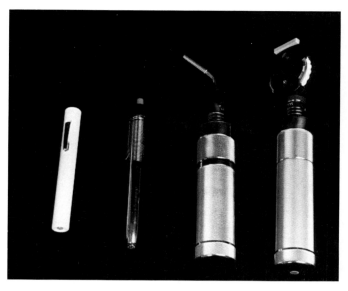

FIGURE 52–2. Instrumentation used for clinical assessment of photostress recovery. From left to right: disposable penlight, battery-powered penlight, transilluminator, and direct ophthalmoscope.

ment the use of the direct ophthalmoscope as a dazzling source. Subsequent reports[2,3,6,7,9,10,16] confirmed the clinical practicality and effectiveness of this instrument. Although white light is characteristically employed to induce photostress, two reports[8,9] concluded that red and green filters were quite reliable in eliciting delayed recovery times in patients with macular disease who had otherwise normal recovery times with white light. Schlaegel and Weber,[18] in evaluating 60 cases of active toxoplasmic retinochoroiditis for the presence of macular edema, advocated the use of a transilluminator as a dazzling source.

The Scotometer, a device developed in the late 1960s by Henkind and Siegel,[11] was a T-shaped instrument comprising a vertical cylindric hand grip that contained batteries and supported a short horizontal boxlike rectangular body. As the subject attained best visual acuity on a chart focused at optical infinity inside the instrument, the examiner activated a 10-second dazzling source located directly in the line of sight. The time required for the subject to achieve prestress visual acuity was then recorded.

Sloan[13] positioned an electronic flash unit 15 cm from the eye and instructed the subject to fixate on the center of the flash tube. The flash, which emitted an energy of 24 mJ for 1/1500 second, was then activated. The subject was quickly positioned behind a phoropter containing the best correction and was asked to read the red letters of a bichrome visual acuity chart without hesitation. Recovery times for reading the second letter of both the 20/25 and 20/20 lines were then measured from the time of the flash.

The most comprehensive studies of measuring recovery times for both prestress contrast discrimination and visual acuity were conducted by Severin et al.[1,8,12,14] Elaborate instrumentation to illuminate the retina was utilized. Initial flash sources consisted of a Meyer–Schwickerath Zeiss xenon arc photocoagulator and a 500-W projection bulb used alternately.[1,8] Eventually, a modified nuclear-flash unit was employed.[12,14] Other components of the system included a Goldmann–Weekers adaptometer and timing clocks. After each subject had been dazzled by an intense flash from the light source positioned 50 cm away, recovery times for observing a small patch of light blinking at 1-second intervals (contrast discrimination), and identifying prestress letter symbols (visual acuity) in the adaptometer were recorded sequentially by two remote-control timing clocks.

COMMERCIALLY AVAILABLE INSTRUMENTS

The complicated instrumentation designed specifically for photostress recovery testing has never been marketed for clinical practice. This is probably the result of the availability and low cost of such commonplace illuminating sources as the penlight, transilluminator, and direct ophthalmoscope.

CLINICAL PROCEDURE

The values obtained by the photostress recovery test will depend upon a variety of factors. These include (1) the type, duration, intensity, and distance of the light source; (2) the type and luminance of the visual acuity chart; (3) the line of the visual acuity chart used as an end point; (4) the prestress level of dark adaptation; (5) the clarity of the ocular media; and (6) the fixation ability and perceptiveness of the patient. In clinically oriented studies, the light source has been positioned 2 cm,[15,17] 15 cm,[18] and 30 cm[2,3] from the eye; the duration of exposure has been recorded as 10 seconds,[11,15,17] 15 seconds,[2,3,6,16] 20 seconds,[18] and 30 seconds.[7,9,10] The means and methods of testing, however, are not as significant as the consistency with which the test is administered. The basic clinical procedure, adapted from Glaser et al.[15] and summarized in Table 52–2, is as follows:

Table 52–1
Illumination Sources Utilized for Photostress Recovery Testing

Penlight[15,17]
Transilluminator[18]
Direct ophthalmoscope[2,3,5–7,9,10,16]
Scotometer[11]
Electronic-flash unit[13]
500-W projection bulb[1,8]
Xenon arc photocoagulator[1,8]
Modified nuclear-flash unit[12,14]

---

1. Obtain and use the most current optical correction to determine distance visual acuity for each eye through an undilated pupil. Recovery time should not be influenced by pupillary dilation.[2]
2. Test the uninvolved eye while the involved eye is occluded. If both eyes are involved, begin with the right eye. Dim the

Table 52–2
Clinical Procedure for Photostress Recovery Testing

1. Determine the best-corrected distance visual acuity for each eye
2. Allow the right eye to dark-adapt for 1 minute while the left eye is occluded
3. Position the light source 1 in. (2.5 cm) from the right eye and instruct the patient to view it directly for 10 seconds
4. Remove the light source and immediately show the patient the line above best visual acuity
5. Measure and record the time required for the patient to read at least one-half of the line
6. Repeat the procedure for the left eye and compare the results

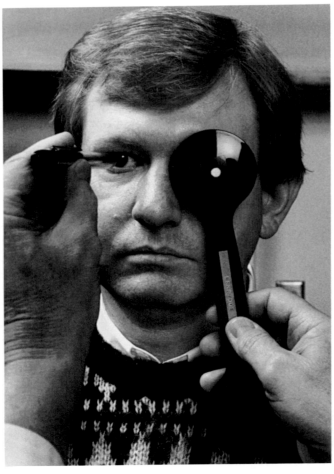

FIGURE 52–3. Right eye undergoing photostress while left eye is occluded. Note that the light source is about 1 in. (2.5 cm) from the eye as the patient looks directly at it for approximately 10 to 15 seconds. The time required for the patient to read at least half of the line above best acuity is then recorded in seconds. The procedure may then be performed in the same manner for the left eye.

room lights and allow the patient to dark-adapt for about 1 minute.
3. Instruct the patient to fixate on the center of the light source while it is positioned approximately 1 in. (2.5 cm) from the eye. If the source is a direct ophthalmoscope, the visuoscopic target may be used to ensure fixation. The duration of viewing is typically 10 to 15 seconds, but may be any value if tested using this time consistently (Fig. 52–3).
4. Remove the light source and immediately show the patient the line above best visual acuity.[2,15] If the prestress visual acuity is 20/30, isolate the 20/40 line. If the prestress visual acuity is 20/80 to 20/100 or less, photostress recovery testing becomes diagnostically meaningless, since a macular lesion causing such visual acuity loss is often obvious to the clinician. The patient with this level of visual acuity may also be utilizing an extramacular area to see the chart, which limits the validity of test results.[18]
5. Measure and record the time required (in seconds) for the patient to read at least one-half of the line. If the line has five letters, the patient should read a minimum of three letters. An average value of 30 seconds or less is expected in normal eyes,[15,16] with 50 to 60 seconds being the upper limit of normalcy.[1,6,7] As mentioned before, however, a number of factors may contribute to the variability of these values. Patients who are 40 years of age or older typically have a slower recovery time than younger patients.[3,14–16]
6. Repeat the procedure for the fellow eye and compare results. The difference between normal eyes averages 5 to 6 seconds, although as much as a 20-second difference may exist.[15] If testing conditions are consistent and the patient is observant, no remarkable difference in recovery times should occur between the right and left eyes in subsequent testing sessions.[1]

CLINICAL IMPLICATIONS

Clinical Significance

Photostress recovery testing may be applied to several clinical situations (Table 52–3). A prolonged recovery time implies either that (1) the adherence between sensory retina and RPE has been

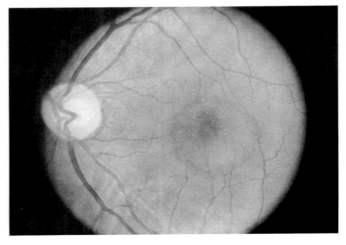

FIGURE 52–4. Left eye of patient with central serous chorioretinopathy. Note well-defined circular dome-shaped lesion in macular area. Photostress recovery time is longer than 3 minutes, yet visual acuity is 20/20–. The fellow eye is uninvolved and has recovery time of 44 seconds.

Table 52–3
Clinical Applications of Photostress Recovery Testing

To detect subtle unilateral or bilateral macular disease
To monitor advancement or resolution of macular disease
To distinguish macular disease from optic nerve disease

Table 52–4
Documented Macular Disorders with Prolonged Recovery Times

Edematous Disorders
 Central serous chorioretinopathy[1,2,6,7,10,11,13,15]
 Macular edema secondary to toxoplasmic retinochoroiditis[3,18]
 Cystoid macular edema[15,17]
 Diabetic macular edema[15]
 Serous detachment of the retinal pigment epithelium[15]
 Neovascular age-related macular degeneration[3]
 Macular cyst[1]

Nonedematous Disorders
 Atrophic age-related macular degeneration[1,7,13,15]
 Chloroquine maculopathy[1,10,13]
 Active/inactive macular chorioretinitis[1,6,13,15]
 Juvenile macular degeneration[1]
 Macular involvement in high myopia[13]
 Macular involvement in retinal detachment[7]
 Macular involvement in tapetoretinal degeneration[1,3]

Table 52–5
Clinical Indicators of Early Macular Disease

Normal to mildly reduced visual acuity
Defective Amsler grid
Prolonged photostress recovery time
Ophthalmoscopic or biomicroscopic evidence

Clinical Interpretation

Once photostress recovery times are obtained, the clinician must then combine past experience with present history and examination findings to arrive at a diagnostic decision. This may not always be simple or straightforward. For example, consider the patient with coalesced macular drusen and 20/25− acuity in each eye with Amsler grid distortions. What if recovery time is prolonged in both eyes but more so in the right eye? Does this mean that the right macula has greater damage to the photoreceptors or that it has been affected by edema secondary to a shallow RPE detachment or, more seriously, a leaking choroidal neovascular membrane? If the clinician is unable to answer these questions on the basis of history or additional examination findings, referral for fluorescein angiography may then be warranted to exclude edema or choroidal neovascularization as a reason for delayed recovery.

Photostress recovery testing may be useful for monitoring the progression or regression of an active disease process. An increase in recovery time will occur with progression of the disorder, a decrease with regression. In central serous chorioretinopathy, complete recovery from photostress may take anywhere from 20 minutes[7] to more than 1 hour[6] once vision has been affected (Table 52–4).[2] As the disorder resolves over a period of weeks or months, however, recovery time gradually returns to a normal level.

The results of photostress testing may also assist the clinician in differentiating between macular disease and optic nerve disease. As optic nerve diseases that create a conduction defect, such as glaucoma, optic neuritis, and ischemic optic neuropathy, are independent of photochemical processes, recovery time should remain unimpaired.[15]

Another dilemma may arise when photostress recovery time is prolonged without evidence of disease. Henkind and Siegel[11] found this to be true in patients taking chloroquine who had otherwise normal visual acuities and eye findings. Forsius et al.[3] reported delayed recovery times in four unaffected members of a family with tapetoretinal degeneration. A positive finding, therefore, may be somewhat misleading, but generally deserves further investigation to rule out early macular involvement.

In summary, macular disorders characterized by edema or photoreceptor breakdown may not always be apparent to the clinician in the early stages. This is particularly true when clinical indicators of macular disease are absent, such as reduced visual acuity, Amsler grid defects, or ophthalmoscopic or biomicroscopic evidence (Table 52–5). Photostress recovery testing, therefore, may be a means of detecting a subtle macular disturbance that is otherwise difficult to confirm with standard clinical tests or ocular health assessment procedures.

compromised, as in central serous chorioretinopathy (Fig. 52–4), or (2) the photoreceptors are not functioning optimally, as in atrophic age-related macular degeneration. Delayed recovery times have been documented in various disorders involving the macula directly or secondarily and may be classified as either edematous or nonedematous (Table 52–4 and Fig. 52–5). No distinction can be made between the two types, however, on the basis of values obtained. An abnormal recovery time in one or both eyes simply alerts the clinician to the possibility that macular compromise is present. A value of 120 seconds or greater in either eye is strongly suggestive of an active disease process.[18]

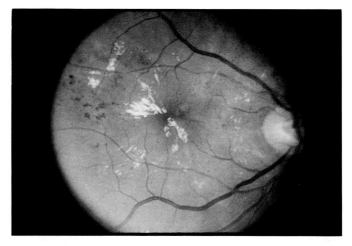

FIGURE 52–5. Right eye of patient with diabetic macular edema. Note hard exudate formation in macula, implying chronic vascular leakage. Photostress recovery time is 105 seconds with visual acuity of 20/50−. The fellow eye has 20/20− visual acuity, with no clinical evidence of macular edema and a recovery time of 25 seconds.

REFERENCES

1. Severin SL, Harper JY, Culver JF. Photostress test for the evaluation of macular function. Arch Ophthalmol 1963;70:593–597.
2. Forsius H, Krause U, Eriksson A. Dazzling test in central serous retinopathy. Acta Ophthalmol 1963;41:25–32.
3. Forsius H, Eriksson AW, Krause U. The dazzling test in diseases of the retina. Acta Ophthalmol 1963;41:55–63.
4. Tengroth B, Hogman B, Linde CJ, et al. Readaptation time after photo-

stress. Readaptation time as a function of oxygen concentration. Acta Ophthalmol 1976;54:507–516.

5. Bailliart JP. Examen fonctionnel de la macula. Bull Soc Ophthalmol Fr 1954;4:71–81.

6. Magder H. Test for central serous retinopathy based on clinical observations and trial. Am J Ophthalmol 1960;49:147–150.

7. Chilaris GA. Recovery time after macular illumination as a diagnostic and prognostic test. Am J Ophthalmol 1962;53:311–314.

8. Severin SL, Newton NL, Culver JF. A new approach to the study of flash blindness. Use of the Zeiss light coagulator. Arch Ophthalmol 1962;67:578–582.

9. Paul SD, Batra DV. Macular illumination tests. Variations in recovery time. Am J Ophthalmol 1966;61:99–103.

10. Batra DV, Paul SD. Macular illumination test in central serous retinopathy. Am J Ophthalmol 1967;63:146–149.

11. Henkind P, Siegel IM. The Scotometer. A device for measuring macular recovery time. Am J Ophthalmol 1967;64:314–315.

12. Severin SL, Tour RL, Kershaw RH. Macular function and the photostress test 2. Arch Ophthalmol 1967;77:163–167.

13. Sloan PG. Clinical application of the photostress test. Am J Optom 1968;45:617–623.

14. Severin SL, Tour RL, Kershaw RH. Macular function and the photostress test 1. Arch Ophthalmol 1967;77:2–7.

15. Glaser JS, Savino PJ, Sumers KD, et al. The photostress recovery test in the clinical assessment of visual function. Am J Ophthalmol 1977;83:255–260.

16. Severin SL. Qualitative photostress testing for the diagnosis of cystoid macular edema. Am Intraocul Implant Soc J 1980;6:25–27.

17. Lovasik JV. An electrophysiological investigation of the macular photostress test. Invest Ophthalmol Vis Sci 1983;24:437–441.

18. Schlaegel TF Jr, Weber JC. The macula in ocular toxoplasmosis. Arch Ophthalmol 1984;102:697–698.

19. Brindley GS. The discrimination of afterimages. J Physiol 1959;147:194–199.

Glare Testing

Charles J. Patorgis

INTRODUCTION

Definition

Glare is a visual perception created when external light becomes scattered within the eye to cast a hazy veil over the retinal surface, thus reducing the quality of the image. It may occur in the presence of an extremely bright axial or peripheral light source and may be compounded by opacifications or irregularities of the ocular media.[1-3]

Glare discomfort relates to the bothersome aspect of light scatter that has a negligible impact on visual performance.[4] *Glare disability* is the reduction in visual performance that occurs when the person with clinically significant media opacities is exposed to bright sunlight, oncoming headlights at night, or reflections off glossy surfaces.[2,3]

Glare testing is an objective means of quantifying the deleterious effects of light scatter on visual performance.

History

The adverse effect of glare on overall visual function has been recognized for many years.[5-9] The realization that Snellen visual acuity testing is highly misleading in assessing functional vision impairment has led a number of researchers to develop instrumentation that provides the clinician with a clearer understanding of glare disability.[4,10-16]

Prior to 1983, methods for determining the extent of glare disability in the office or clinical setting were limited. Nevertheless, these methods were simple, quick, and inexpensive, and continue to be used. The contralight test, in which visual acuity is measured from a cardboard wall chart placed against a sunlit window, provides the clinician with some idea of how the patient may function on a bright or hazy day.[17] The penlight test, in which visual acuity is measured in darkness while a penlight is directed into the eye at a 15° to 30° angle from a distance of 12 to 18 in. (30 to 46 cm), gives the clinician some insight on how the patient may function at night.[18] Another means of evaluating glare disability involves measuring visual acuity from a projector chart while the examining room lights are on.

In 1972, Miller et al.[11] first reported the results of a prototypical clinical glare tester. The instrument underwent several design modifications and was eventually released commercially in 1983 as the Miller–Nadler GlareTester.[12] Since its introduction, several other glare testers have been developed and marketed for clinical use (see under "Commercially Available Instruments"). All of them are tabletop models, with the exception of the Brightness Acuity Tester (BAT), which is hand-held.

The majority of recent studies on glare testing have used either a single instrument for obtaining data on a particular study population[4,10-16,19-22] or have made comparisons between instruments.[23-25] The Miller–Nadler GlareTester, considered the standard device in the field, has been utilized in seven of the single-instrument studies[11-13,19-22] and all of the comparison studies.

Clinical Use

Glare testing is rapidly becoming recognized as an essential and necessary adjunct to preoperative evaluation of patients with corneal or lenticular opacities and to postoperative evaluation of patients who have undergone corneal transplantation, keratorefractive surgery, or extracapsular cataract removal, with or without intraocular lens implantation (Table 53–1).

Table 53–1
Pre- and Postoperative Indications for Glare Testing

Preoperative	Postoperative
Cornea	Cornea
Infectious scarring	Penetrating keratoplasty
Traumatic scarring	Radial keratotomy
Degenerative scarring	Epikeratophakia
Dystrophic scarring	Keratomileusis
Lens	Repaired laceration
Age-related cataract	Lens
Traumatic cataract	Posterior capsular opacification
Drug-induced cataract	following extracapsular
Disease-induced cataract	cataract removal/intraocular
	lens implantation

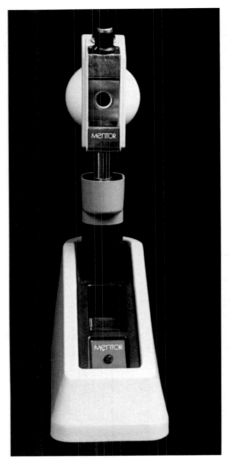

FIGURE 53–1. Brightness Acuity Tester (BAT).

INSTRUMENTATION

Theory and Use

A glare source of either axial or peripheral origin should not impair visual performance in an eye lacking opacification of the cornea or lens. Introduction of a glare source to an eye with media opacification, however, may result in some degree of visual disability, much the same as when a projected image is viewed with the room lights on or when road signs are observed as sunlight strikes a dirty windshield. Current glare testing devices give the clinician some idea of the extent of this disability in the form of diminished visual acuity or contrast sensitivity.

COMMERCIALLY AVAILABLE INSTRUMENTS

Brightness Acuity Tester

The Mentor* Brightness Acuity Tester (BAT) (Fig. 53–1) is a hand-held instrument that consists of a white, ice cream scoop-shaped, 6-cm diameter hemisphere situated atop a 16-cm handle. A 12-mm circular aperture in the center of the hemisphere allows the patient to view a standard projector chart while holding the instrument against the spectacle correction or eyebrow. The hemisphere is then illuminated by a surrounding uniform glare source of low (bright overhead commercial lighting), medium (partly cloudy day), or high (direct overhead sunlight) intensity. Visual acuity obtained under these simulated environmental conditions is then recorded.

Optec 1500 Glare Tester

The Stereo Optical† Optec 1500 Glare Tester (Fig. 53–2) is an automated tabletop instrument with a central rectangular glare source that simulates the halogen headlight of an automobile 60 ft (18.3 m) away. Slides consisting of variably sized Snellen letters distributed in a circle around the glare source are presented with and without glare. Visual acuity is measured in both situations and a comparison made between the two values to determine the extent of functional vision impairment. The slides are illuminated uniformly against a dark background by an electroluminescent lamp to ensure repeatability. A separate control panel is employed by the examiner for convenience.

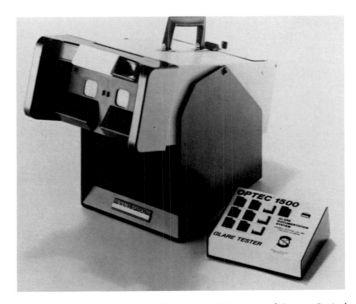

FIGURE 53–2. Optec 1500 Glare Tester. (Courtesy of Stereo Optical Company)

* Mentor O&O, Inc., 3000 Longwater Drive, Norwell MA 02061
† Stereo Optical Company, 3539 N. Kenton, Chicago IL 60641

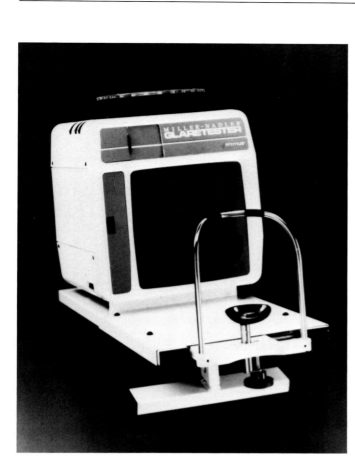

FIGURE 53–3. Miller–Nadler GlareTester. (Courtesy of Titmus Optical, Inc)

Miller–Nadler Glare Tester

The Titmus* Miller–Nadler GlareTester (Fig. 53–3) utilizes a series of 19 35-mm slides containing 20/400 black Landolt Cs set against a 4-cm diameter circular gray background. The slides are surrounded by a rectangular, uniformly bright glare source emanating from a modified tabletop carousel projector. They are presented sequentially in one of four orientations from highest (80%) to lowest (2.5%) contrast between the Landolt C and the gray background until the opening of the letter cannot be visualized. The results are expressed in percentage glare disability, which may then be converted to expected outdoor Snellen acuity with the use of an accompanying graph (Fig. 53–4).[13]

MCT 8000

The Vistech† MCT 8000 Multivision Contrast Tester (Fig. 53–5) is an automated tabletop instrument that primarily uses sine wave gratings as targets. Contrast sensitivity may initially be measured without glare and equivalent Snellen visual acuity derived from an accompanying chart. One of three glare sources may then be presented while the patient attempts to determine grating orientation. The glare source may be a point of light in the center of the target (central glare), a horizontally oval ring of 12 points of light that surrounds the target (peripheral glare), or any one of the 12 points

of light individually (radial glare). A separate control panel facilitates examination.

Terry Vision Analyzer (TVA)

The InnoMed* Terry Vision Analyzer (TVA) (Fig. 53–6) is an automated tabletop instrument that uses computer-assisted letter optotypes and square wave gratings ranging in contrast value from 0.7% to 83.0% over nine levels. Data for determining contrast sensitivity function are initially obtained with optotypes of various contrast levels and sizes. A spot glare source of constant luminance, which is located 19 cm (7.5 in.) below the viewing screen and within 10° of the line of sight, is then turned on to assess glare disability.

CLINICAL PROCEDURE

Both the BAT and the Miller–Nadler GlareTester are commonly used in clinical practice. They are the only two commercially available glare testers that were developed in accordance with the results of actual outdoor visual acuity testing of patients with cataracts. The basic clinical procedure for each instrument is as follows:

Brightness Acuity Tester

1. The patient should be comfortably seated in a darkened examination room. Best-corrected distance visual acuity should be obtained in the test eye with a regular projector chart through an undilated pupil. The fellow eye should be occluded.
2. The patient should be given the BAT and asked to hold it vertically in front of the test eye. The chart should then be located by the patient through the 12-mm central aperture (Fig. 53–7).
3. The BAT should be turned to MED and best visual acuity measured after the patient has had 20 to 30 seconds to adapt to the glare source. (Note: The LO and HI settings may result in underestimates or overestimates of glare disability, respectively, and, therefore, are not suggested for routine evaluation.)
4. The procedure should then be repeated for the fellow eye if indicated.

Miller–Nadler GlareTester

1. The patient should be centered directly in front of the viewing screen at a distance of 36 cm by means of chin and forehead rests (Fig. 53–8). The best correction should be in place and the fellow eye occluded.
2. Slides of highest contrast should be presented initially and the patient asked to identify the orientation of the Landolt C in the presence of a background glare source.
3. Slides of progressively lower contrast between the C and the circular gray surround should then be presented in sequence until the patient is no longer able to distinguish orientation. The final slide identified correctly is considered the contrast threshold.
4. The procedure should then be repeated for the fellow eye if indicated.

* Titmus Optical, Inc., PO Box 191, Petersburg VA 23804

† Vistech Consultants, Inc., 4162 Little York Road, Dayton OH 45432

* InnoMed Corporation, 620 Lunar Avenue, Brea CA 92621

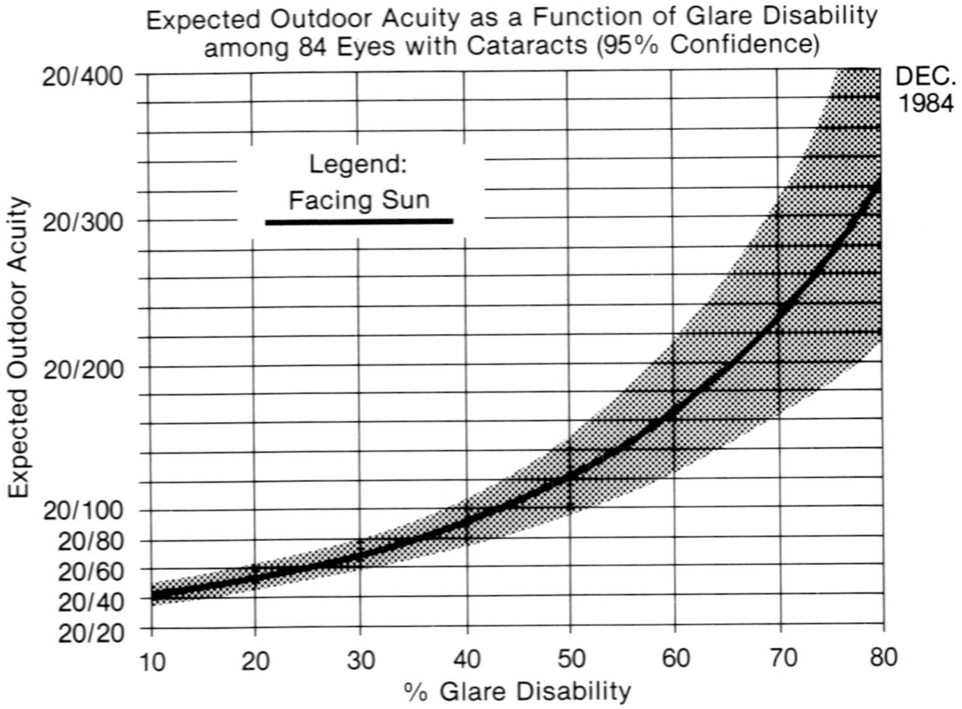

Expected Outdoor Acuity as a Function of Glare Disability
among 84 Eyes with Cataracts (95% Confidence)

FIGURE 53–4. Equivalence chart that accompanies Miller–Nadler GlareTester and relates expected outdoor visual acuity to glare scores. To interpret, find the percent glare disability score of the patient at the bottom of the graph and sight vertically to the line in the shaded area. From its intersection at this point, follow the horizontal grid line to the Snellen value at the left. This is the mean outdoor visual acuity of the patient. (Courtesy of Titmus Optical, Inc)

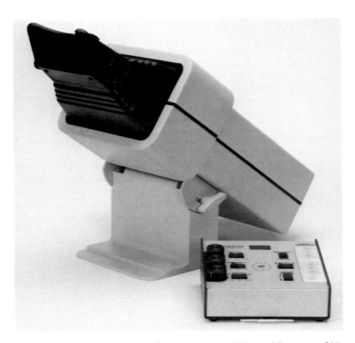

FIGURE 53–5. MCT 8000 Multivision Contrast Tester. (Courtesy of Vistech Consultants, Inc)

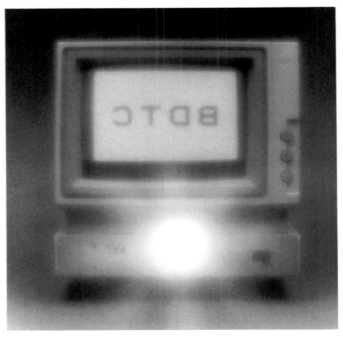

FIGURE 53–6. Terry Vision Analyzer (TVA) as it appears for use in a mirrored examining room with the glare source activated. (Courtesy of InnoMed Corporation)

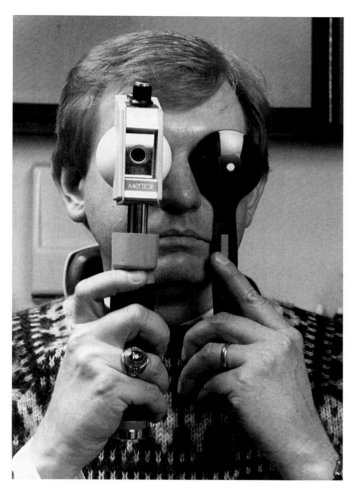

FIGURE 53–7. Proper positioning of BAT before test eye.

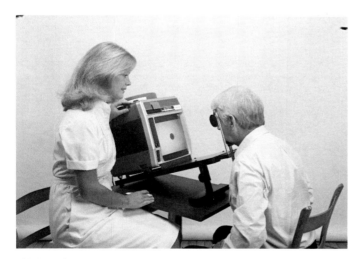

FIGURE 53–8. Proper positioning of patient before Miller–Nadler GlareTester. (Courtesy of Titmus Optical, Inc)

CLINICAL IMPLICATIONS

Clinical Significance

The clinician cannot rely on Snellen visual acuity alone for determining whether patients with cataracts are in need of surgery. Standard Snellen testing in a darkened examining room is an inaccurate and unrealistic indicator of visual performance, mainly because it is performed at 90% to 100% contrast. The normal visual environment consists of many objects and situations of low and medium, but rarely high, contrast. With Snellen testing, many patients with cataracts may have good visual acuity in the office, but will emphatically complain of not being able to see people, road signs, or airborne golf balls during the day, or of ceasing to drive at night because of the glare from streetlights or oncoming headlights.

Aphakic and pseudophakic patients will often display more glare sensitivity than noncataractous phakic patients.[12] This may not necessarily be due simply to absence of the crystalline lens. Patients with extracapsular cataract removal may experience glare disability because of moderate central or peripheral posterior capsular clouding,[23] Elschnig's pearls, or capsular fibrosis that develops within the first 10 months of surgery.[19] The degree of capsular clouding may, in fact, be more of a limiting factor than dense capsular fibrosis. This can be especially true in the presence of a peripheral iridectomy or a pupil of more than 2 mm in diameter.

Consequently, glare testing after extracapsular cataract removal may provide the clinician with some basis for the vague visual complaints that patients with capsular opacification often experience in the absence of vision loss per se. Confirmation of glare disability may also justify consultation with a cataract surgeon for YAG laser capsulotomy, especially when combined with reduced visual acuity attributed to a cloudy capsule.[20,22]

The results of glare testing may ultimately yield information on how the patient functions in a world filled with gray tones, subtle hues, and generally innocuous light sources. It may lend credence to patient symptoms that otherwise seem unjustified on the basis of Snellen testing. In addition, increasing intervention of peer review organizations (PROs) and the reshaping of Medicare reimbursement policies by the Health Care Financing Administration (HCFA) necessitate the utilization of objective tests and criteria for evaluating the pre- and postoperative level of functional visual impairment in cataract patients.

The clinician must use a combination of clinical findings in assessing the need for cataract surgery and recommending such to the patient. These would include the general health of the patient, symptomatic complaints, best-corrected distance and near visual acuities, glare scores, potential acuity measurement, and existing ocular disease. Regardless of clinical data, however, the decision to proceed with surgery lies with the patient in most instances. The clinician must understand the fears and desires of each patient as well as the risks and benefits of cataract surgery to intelligently present it as an alternative. The degree to which occupational or avocational performance is impaired by cataracts is the most critical factor in determining the need for surgery.

Clinical Interpretation

Glare testing may be useful in quantifying the decline in visual function experienced by patients with cataracts. All too often, indoor Snellen testing is an invalid predictor of visual performance outdoors. Neumann et al.[26] demonstrated that patients with cataracts have lower visual acuity outdoors while facing the sun by a median difference of three Snellen lines when compared with indoor visual acuity. In 106 eyes of 78 subjects, those with pure nuclear sclerosis generally experienced less visual decline outdoors than eyes with mixed cataracts or a combination of nuclear sclerosis and posterior subcapsular cataract. In fact, three eyes with nuclear sclerosis had better visual acuity outdoors than indoors. Another report of the same study population[21] revealed that Miller–Nadler glare testing predicted actual outdoor visual acuity within one Snellen line for nearly half of all eyes (46.7%) and was more accurate than indoor Snellen testing in 59 eyes (64.1%).

Hirsch and coworkers[13] compared 81 noncataractous eyes of 48 subjects with 84 cataractous eyes of 52 subjects. They found that Miller–Nadler glare scores and actual outdoor visual acuity in noncataractous eyes were closely correlated over a narrow range. In cataractous eyes, however, glare scores were almost twice as reliable as indoor visual acuity in predicting actual outdoor visual acuity for subjects facing the sun. Subjects turned away from the sun had glare scores that were very similar to indoor visual acuity.

Nadler et al.[19] claimed that pseudophakic patients with posterior chamber intraocular lenses may encounter glare disability when light is reflected off the edges or the positioning holes of the implant in the presence of a dilated or surgically distorted pupil. Koch and coworkers,[23] however, indicated that exposure of the implant edge is not as significant as proximity of the edge to the visual axis. They also determined that patient age, eye color, and implant optic design did not contribute to poor glare scores. Although ultraviolet-absorbing implants have considerably reduced the potential for glare disability in many pseudophakic patients, an implant edge decentered onto the visual axis can easily negate this benefit and may warrant a surgical exchange of intraocular lenses.

Unfortunately, present methods of glare testing are flawed. No two glare testers are alike in the type or consistency of information they provide, nor should one instrument be considered valid for all situations.[24,25] For example, some instruments test with a point glare source to create directional glare, others test with a surrounding glare source to create veiling glare. Advocates of point glare sources argue that they give a truer picture of intraocular light scatter,[16] whereas detractors state that point sources prove more fatiguing, may create negative afterimages, and may be more distracting in terms of maintaining fixation.[4,13] Some instruments test visual acuity, others test contrast sensitivity function, still others test both. Although the standard Snellen chart has its drawbacks in terms of optotypes used, spacing of optotypes, acuity increments, and chart contrast, the introduction of sine wave gratings has, in some respects, added to the confusion of interpreting patient responses.

Such an absence of uniform standards for glare testing precludes its exclusive use for determining functional impairment from cataracts or any other type of media opacity. Its value may eventually be realized in industries in which glare disability has a potential impact on employee performance, such as transportation or factory settings, but too much room for interpretation currently exists.

REFERENCES

1. Knott RL, Amick CL, Bachler JM, et al. Proposed American national standard practice for industrial lighting. Light Design Appl 1983; 13:29–68.

2. Jaffe NS. Glare and contrast: indications for cataract surgery. J Cataract Refract Surg 1986;12:372–375.

3. Koch DD. Glare and contrast sensitivity testing in cataract patients. J Cataract Refract Surg 1989;15:158–164.

4. Abrahamsson M, Sjostrand J. Impairment of contrast sensitivity function (CSF) as a measure of disability glare. Invest Ophthalmol Vis Sci 1986;27:1131–1136.

5. Cobb PW, Moss FK. Glare and the four fundamental factors in vision. Trans Illuminat Eng Soc 1923;23:1104–1120.

6. Holladay LL. The fundamentals of glare and visibility. J Ophthalmol Soc Am 1926;12:492–531.

7. Fry GA, Alpern M. The effect of a peripheral glare source upon the apparent brightness of an object. J Opt Soc Am 1953;43:189–195.

8. Wolfe E. Glare and age. Arch Ophthalmol 1960;64:502–514.

9. Hess R, Woo G. Vision through cataracts. Invest Ophthalmol Vis Sci 1978;17:428–435.

10. Paulsson L-E, Sjostrand J. Contrast sensitivity in the presence of a glare light. Theoretical concepts and preliminary clinical studies. Invest Ophthalmol Vis Sci 1980;19:401–406.

11. Miller D, Jernigan ME, Molner S, et al. Laboratory evaluation of a clinical glare tester. Arch Ophthalmol 1972;87:324–332.

12. LeClaire J, Nadler MP, Weiss S, et al. A new glare test for clinical testing. Results comparing normal subjects and variously corrected aphakic patients. Arch Ophthalmol 1982;100:153–158.

13. Hirsch RP, Nadler MP, Miller D. Glare measurement as a predictor of outdoor vision among cataract patients. Ann Ophthalmol 1984;16:965–968.

14. Smith J, Downing J. Visual function tester. A new test for glare. J Ocular Ther Surg 1984;3:226–228.

15. Holladay JT, Trujillo J, Prager TC, et al. Brightness acuity test and outdoor visual acuity in cataract patients. J Cataract Refract Surg 1987; 13:67–69.

16. Terry CM, Brown PK. Clinical measurement of glare effect in cataract patients. Ann Ophthalmol 1989;21:183–187.

17. Junker C. Vision against the light as an aid to indication for cataract operation. Klin Monatsbl Augenheilkd 1976;169:348–351.

18. Maltzman B, Horan C, Rengel A. Penlight test for glare disability of cataracts. Ophthal Surg 1988;19:356–358.

19. Nadler DJ, Jaffe NS, Clayman HM, et al. Glare disability in eyes with intraocular lenses. Am J Ophthalmol 1984;97:43–47.

20. Knighton RW, Slomovic AR, Parrish RK II. Glare measurements before and after neodymium-YAG laser posterior capsulotomy. Am J Ophthalmol 1985;100:708–713.

21. Neumann AC, McCarty GR, Steedle TO, et al. The relationship between cataract type and glare disability as measured by the Miller–Nadler glare tester. J Cataract Refract Surg 1988;14:40–45.

22. Masket S. Reversal of glare disability after cataract surgery. J Cataract Refract Surg 1989;15:165–168.

23. Koch DD, Jardeleza TL, Emery JM, et al. Glare following posterior chamber intraocular lens implantation. J Cataract Refract Surg 1986; 12:480–484.

24. Neumann AC, McCarty GR, Locke J, et al. Glare disability devices for cataractous eyes: a consumer's guide. J Cataract Refract Surg 1988; 14:212–216.

25. Prager TC, Urso RG, Holladay JT, et al. Glare testing in cataract patients: instrument evaluation and identification of sources of methodological error. J Cataract Refract Surg 1989;15:149–157.

26. Neumann AC, McCarty GR, Steedle TO, et al. The relationship between indoor and outdoor Snellen visual acuity in cataract patients. J Cataract Refract Surg 1988;14:35–39.

Brightness and Color Comparison

John C. Townsend

INTRODUCTION

Definition

Brightness and color comparison testing are clinical procedures that can be used to subjectively assess the difference in the integrity of the visual pathway between the two eyes.

History

Several clinicians have reported that diseases affecting the visual pathway may result in reduced light and color perception. R. Marcus Gunn is attributed with the alternate-cover or illumination testing of the afferent pupillary reflex arc that subjectively and objectively tested for brightness comparison.[1]

Traquair advocated the use of colored test targets, especially red, in certain types of visual field defects (e.g., nutritional optic neuropathy) but felt that the usefulness of color perimetry was limited.[2] It was Bender and Kanzer who believed that defects for colored objects appeared before those obtained with black-and-white stimuli.[3] In general, if the visual field is defective for colors, it will be altered for a white stimulus; however, it may be easier to elicit with a colored target.[4]

Clinical Use

This testing is useful in detecting retinal, optic nerve, chiasmal, or postchiasmal disorders. It requires an alert, coherent, and cognizant patient.

INSTRUMENTATION

Theory

Disease conditions can asymmetrically affect the eyes. With unilateral structural damage to the retina or optic nerve, there may be diminished perception of light or color when compared with the normal eye.[1,5] Approximately 70% of the optic nerve is composed of macular fibers, which are primarily responsible for daytime and color vision.[1,5,6] Since the visual pathway decussates at the chiasm, a hemifield loss may be present, and may be uncovered by using a red stimulus, thereby preferentially stimulating cone or macular function.[5,7–10]

Use

The light brightness test may be performed with a penlight, transilluminator, or binocular indirect ophthalmoscope. It is important for the source of light to be as bright as possible so that media opacities (i.e., cataracts) are not a factor. Neutral-density filters may be utilized to quantify the perceived difference in brightness.[1,5,7]

Color comparison testing using a red object is helpful in uncovering subtle disorders as the target becomes desaturated. Media opacities may affect the results of testing.[1,4,5,7,9]

COMMERCIALLY AVAILABLE INSTRUMENTS

For brightness comparison testing, most optometric diagnostic kits have a transilluminator attachment available. Binocular indirect ophthalmoscopes may be purchased from vendors of ophthalmic equipment. Penlights may be found at local drugstores. Neutral-density filters may be obtained from Kodak (e.g., Kodak No. 96, ND 2.00) for quantification.

Color comparison testing for this chapter will only utilize the colored caps on the top of bottles of ocular pharmaceutics. Parasympatholytic ophthalmic pharmaceutic agents such as tropicamide, cyclopentolate, homatropine, and others have red caps that are ideal for color comparison testing.

CLINICAL PROCEDURE

Brightness Comparison Testing

1. Instruct the patient to fixate an object 4 to 6 m away. The patient should be wearing the best refractive correction. The patient's pupils may be dilated or undilated. The room should be normally illuminated.
2. Hold the penlight, transilluminator, or binocular indirect ophthalmoscope approximately 3 cm from the eye being illuminated, and direct the light toward the macular area (Fig. 54–1).

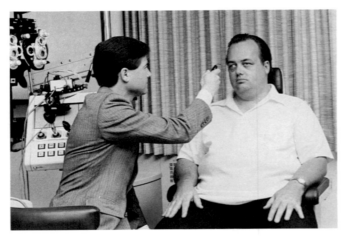

FIGURE 54–1. Stimulation of the right eye with the transilluminator in brightness comparison testing.

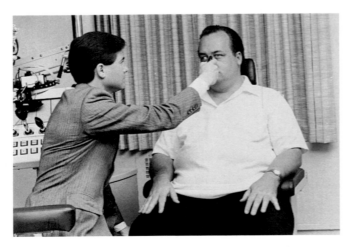

FIGURE 54–2. Stimulation of the left eye with the transilluminator in brightness comparison testing.

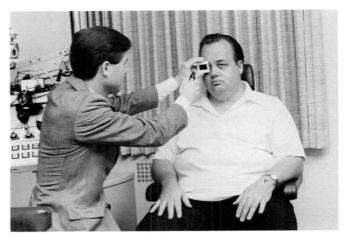

FIGURE 54–3. Use of a neutral-density filter placed before the right eye to equalize the perception of light brightness between the two eyes.

3. Present the light source for no more than 5 seconds to one eye and then quickly present the light source to the other eye (Fig. 54–2). Be careful not to stimulate one eye longer than the other.
4. While illuminating each eye separately, the following questions are asked (assuming the right eye to be normal):

   "In which eye is the light the brightest?"
   "If the brightness of the light in your right eye equals $1.00, how many cents does it equal in the left eye?"[1,5]

   If the patient responds 90 cents to $1.00, that is a normal, negative, and unequivocal test result. A positive response is that one eye perceives the light at a value less than 90 cents.
5. Another technique for assessing the difference in the perception of the brightness between the two eyes is to quantify the asymmetry by the use of neutral-density filters. Instead of asking for the difference in brightness in terms of dollars or cents, neutral-density filters are placed before the eye in which the light is perceived as the brightest in increasing strengths until there is no apparent difference (Fig. 54–3). The amount may be recorded as a percentage or logarithmic difference for the contralateral eye.[1,5,7]

Color Comparison Testing

1. The patient should be sitting in the examination chair. The room should be fully illuminated.
2. While holding a mydriatic bottle at approximately 40 cm from the patient, ask the patient to look directly at the red cap.
3. Occlude the left eye and ask the patient to look at the red cap, then occlude the right eye and ask the patient to look at the red cap (Figs. 54–4 and 54–5).
4. The following directions are given as each eye is alternately occluded:

   "If the cap is worth $1.00 in brightness or color with the right eye, how much is it worth when viewed with the left eye?"[1,5,7,8]

   A normal or negative response is 90 cents to $1.00. A positive response is that one eye perceives the red cap at a value less than 90 cents.

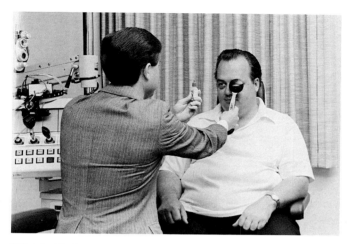

FIGURE 54–4. Occlusion of the left eye with the right eye viewing the red cap of a tropicamide bottle in color comparison testing.

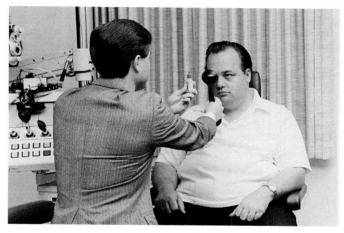

FIGURE 54–5. Occlusion of the right eye with the left eye viewing the red cap of a tropicamide bottle in color comparison testing.

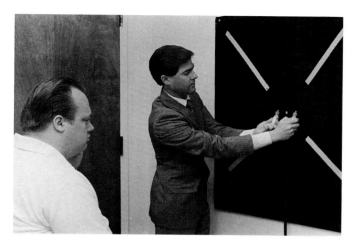

FIGURE 54–6. Monocular presentation of two red caps using the tangent screen in search of a hemianopic desaturation to red.

Modified Color Comparison Testing

If a chiasmal or postchiasmal lesion is suspected, these additional procedures should be performed using a black felt tangent screen:

1. Seat the patient 1 m away from the center of the tangent screen with one eye occluded. The room should be fully illuminated.
2. Instruct the patient to look at the central button of the black felt screen.
3. Present two red tropicamide caps simultaneously within the central 5°, equidistant from the central button on either side of the vertical midline (Fig. 54–6).
4. The following directions are given:

   "While looking at the central button on the black felt screen, you will see a red cap on either side."

   "Tell me if you notice any difference in color or brightness between the two caps."

   "If the cap on the left side is worth $1.00 in redness, how much is the cap on the right side worth?"[1,5,7,10]

A normal or negative response is 90 cents to $1.00. A positive response is that one cap is perceived at a value less than 90 cents.

CLINICAL IMPLICATIONS

Clinical Significance

A positive response to brightness or color comparison testing may be due to an anomaly or disease in the retina, optic nerve, optic chiasm, or postchiasmal region. This testing may also reveal asymmetric chiasmal or tract lesions. Table 54–1 includes a list of some of the diseases that produce unilateral brightness and color losses.[10] Such patients need additional testing and evaluation so that the anomaly or disease can be identified and proper health care delivered.

Clinical Interpretation

When doing the brightness comparison testing, if the patient reports that the right eye was worth $1.00 in brightness and the left eye was worth 70 cents, this would be a positive subjective afferent defect of the left eye. If the media were clear and there were no observable lesions in the papillomacular area or retina, one would suspect optic nerve disease.[1,5,7,8]

In chiasmal disorders, the patient may perceive no difference in brightness between the two eyes, whereas in unilateral optic nerve or tract disease an asymmetry in brightness is commonly reported.[10] For tract lesions, this occurs because between 53% to 60% of the optic nerve fibers, which are composed primarily of macular fibers, decussate at the chiasm.[6,10,11] This results in a reduced perception of brightness in the eye opposite the side of the lesion. In retrobulbar neuritis, the light brightness test would be positive long before the observation of optic atrophy, which may become apparent within 2 to 4 months.[10]

With an alert and cognizant patient, subjective quantification of brightness loss correlates well with the observation of an afferent pupillary defect.[1,5,10] Additionally, it is comparable with a correspondingly reduced amplitude found with visual-evoked cortical potential (VER or VECP).[10]

If there is unilateral macular or optic nerve disease, a reduced perception of red may be apparent in the affected eye. For exam-

Table 54–1
Diseases That Produce Unilateral Brightness and Color Losses

Unilateral Macular or Retinal Lesions
Toxoplasmosis: common; congenital or acquired
Macular coloboma: rare; congenital
Traumatic retinopathy: macular or retinal detachment
Central serous chorioretinopathy: common; males > females; age 30–50s
Histoplasmosis maculopathy: common; males > females; age 30–50s
Age-related maculopathy: common, if asymmetric; age 50+
Vascular occlusive disease: CRA and CRV, total and branch; age 40+
Diabetic maculopathy: if asymmetric, any age

Unilateral Optic Nerve Disorders
Extreme hypoplasia: rare; congenital
Segmental hypoplasia: common; congenital
Relative hypoplasia: common; congenital
Coloboma: uncommon; congenital (inclusive of pits)
Traumatic optic neuropathy: acquired; any age
Optic neuritis and demyelinating disease: acquired; age 20+
Glaucomatous optic neuropathy: if asymmetric, any age
Hyaloid bodies: if asymmetric, hereditary, any age
Ischemic optic neuropathy: anterior or posterior; age 50+
Compressive optic neuropathy: glioma, meningioma, hemangioma, thyroid eye disease; any age

Chiasmal Disorders
Pituitary adenoma (acidophilic, basophilic, chromophobic); age 30–50s
Craniopharyngioma: age 5–20 and 50–60
Aneurysm: congenital or acquired from atherosclerosis, especially of internal carotid artery or circle of Willis; any age
Meningioma: any age
Demyelinating disease: age 20+
Sinusitis: sphenoid bone; any age
Hydrocephalus: congenital affecting third ventricle
Trauma: any age
Sarcoidosis: age 20+

Tract Lesions
Demyelinating disease: age 20+
Cerebrovascular accidents: hemorrhagic or ischemic stroke; any age
AV malformations: congenital or acquired
Hydrocephalus: congenital
Sarcoidosis: age 20+
Meningiomas: any age
Trauma: any age

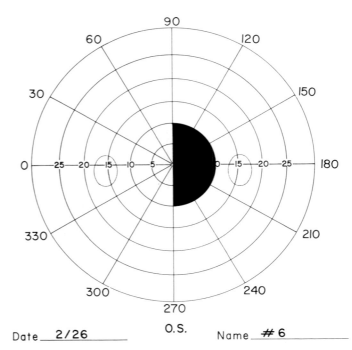

Date 2/26   O.S.   Name # 6

FIGURE 54–7. Visual field of a patient with a chiasmal mass who reported temporal hemianopic desaturation to red of the right eye.

color vision with either the AO Pseudoisochromatic or Ishihara Plates. Monocular testing of the hemifields in the central 5° may reveal bitemporal desaturation to red respecting the vertical midline, which is pathognomonic of a chiasmal mass (Figs. 54–7 and

ple, if the right eye equaled $1.00 in redness and the left eye was worth 50 cents when the stimulus was presented monocularly, this would be a positive response of the left eye. Often a corresponding afferent pupillary defect will be observed.[1,5,10]

The red stimulus is useful in eliciting subtle optic neuropathy or macular disease. This occurs because about 70% of the normal optic nerve is composed of macular fibers, which represent cone function. The light-adapted eye responds maximally to a wavelength of 555 nm. Under scotopic conditions, the most efficient wavelength is 510 nm.[12,13] Physiologically, cones have a peak response to stimulation by the use of a broad-band filter (e.g., Wratten 26, wavelength > 600 nm), which approximates the color red, wavelength 650 nm, in the visible spectrum.[12]

This ability to preferentially stimulate cones with the color red under high room illumination is useful in uncovering subtle chiasmal lesions. A patient may have full fields by confrontations, normal visual acuity, an equal light brightness test, and normal

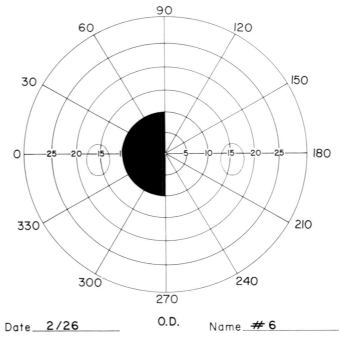

Date 2/26   O.D.   Name # 6

FIGURE 54–8. Visual field of a patient with a chiasmal mass who reported temporal hemianopic desaturation to red of the left eye.

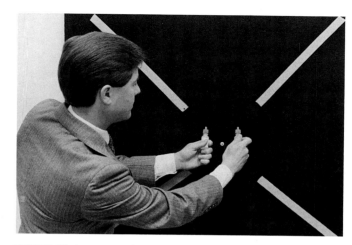

FIGURE 54–9. Monocular testing for superior temporal desaturation to red from a pituitary tumor.

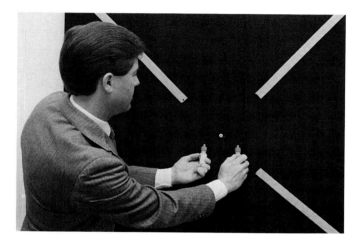

FIGURE 54–10. Monocular testing for inferior temporal desaturation to red from a craniopharyngioma.

54–8).[7,10] The patient may report that both caps are observed; however, the cap in the temporal field may appear colorless.[1,5,7,10] With a positive finding on the monocular testing, the value of each quadrant should then be assessed to determine whether the lesion arises inferior to the chiasm, resulting in superior temporal desaturation to red, as commonly observed with a pituitary adenoma, or arises superiorly, as in a craniopharyngioma, resulting in inferior temporal desaturation[7,9,11] (Figs. 54–9 and 54–10). To affect the chiasmal fibers, a pituitary tumor must be at least 1 cm in size.[10] With the advent of more sophisticated diagnostic imaging techniques such as computed tomography (CT scan) and magnetic resonance imaging (MRI), pathologic corroboration of visual field loss may be revealed. Additionally, neuroendocrine signs and symptoms may be present.[7,10]

REFERENCES

1. Duanes TD. Clinical ophthalmology, vol 2, chap 2. Philadelphia: Harper & Row, 1981:3–6, 10–13, 25.
2. Scott GI, Dott NM. Traquair's clinical perimetry, 7th ed. London: Henry Kimpton, 1957:10–11.
3. Bender MB, Kanzer M. Dynamics of homonymous hemianopias and preservation of central vision. Brain 1939;62:404–421.
4. Harrington DO. The visual fields—a textbook and atlas of clinical perimetry, 4th ed. St Louis: CV Mosby Co, 1976:59–60, 265.
5. Glaser JS. Neuro-ophthalmology. New York: Harper & Row, 1978:12–20.
6. Pavan-Langston D. Manual of ocular diagnosis and therapy. Boston, Mass: Little, Brown & Co, 1980:303–309.
7. Barresi BJ. Ocular assessment the manual of diagnosis for office practice. Woburn, Mass: Butterworth Publishers, 1984:444–446, 490–491, 502–505.
8. Anderson DR. Testing the field of vision. St Louis: CV Mosby Co, 1982:236–239, 256.
9. Frisen L. A versatile color confrontation test for the central visual field: a comparison with automatic perimetry. Arch Ophthalmol 1973;89:3–9.
10. Townsend JC, et al. Visual fields: clinical case presentations. Boston, Mass: Butterworth-Heinemann, 1991.
11. Scheie HG, Albert DM. Textbook of ophthalmology, 9th ed. Philadelphia: WB Saunders Co, 1977:187–194.
12. Moses RA. Adler's physiology of the eye. St Louis: CV Mosby Co, 1975:456, 458–462, 530.
13. Davson H. The physiology of the eye, 3rd ed. New York: Academic Press, 1972:181–183.

Contrast Sensitivity

Charles J. Patorgis

INTRODUCTION

Definition

Contrast is most simply defined as the degree of blackness to whiteness of a target.[1] Given a test stimulus of alternating light (maximum luminance) and dark (minimum luminance) stripes, contrast is the difference between the maximum and minimum luminances divided by their sum. This is represented by the ratio

$$(L_{max} - L_{min})/(L_{max} + L_{min})$$

Multiplying this ratio by 100 gives the percentage contrast of a particular target. As an example, the optotypes of a standard Snellen chart are measured at 90% to 100% contrast, since dark black letters (minimum luminance) are set against a white background (maximum luminance).

One pair of light and dark stripes is known as a cycle. The number of cycles per degree (c/d) of visual angle is the *spatial frequency*. The thinner the stripes, the higher the spatial frequency; the broader the stripes, the lower the spatial frequency.

History

Contrast sensitivity testing was once confined to the research laboratory where gratings were produced on oscilloscopes or television monitors. It was conducted primarily to determine how the visual systems of animals and humans processed information relating to pattern recognition. Accordingly, Schade[2] drew mathematical comparisons of Fourier analysis to contrast sensitivity in 1956, and Campbell and Green[3] plotted the contrast sensitivity function (CSF) of the human visual system in 1965.

In 1972, Bodis-Wollner[4] was the first to apply contrast sensitiv-

ity testing to clinical practice by introducing the concept of a visuogram, which charted the CSF of a patient with ocular disease against that of a normal CSF. In 1978, Arden and Jacobsen[5] reported the results of their work with the first commercially available contrast sensitivity test. Called the Arden gratings, the test consisted of a set of six photographic plates containing a demonstration grating and six sinusoidal gratings of relatively low spatial frequency. These frequencies were selected to increase sensitivity to neural changes and to minimize the effect of optical aberrations. Many studies have used the Arden gratings, with variable and sometimes conflicting results.[6-20] Although the system is still available, production problems have limited its supply and distribution.

In 1984, Ginsburg[21] formally introduced his Vision Contrast Test System after several years of research. The system, which has since undergone several modifications and refinements, consists of a photographic series of computer-generated sinusoidal gratings. The spatial frequencies of the gratings are generally higher than those of the Arden gratings. They were selected on the premise that visual acuity relates poorly to contrast sensitivity for spatial frequencies below 18 c/d.

In addition to the grating systems described, Regan et al.[22] have demonstrated the effectiveness of variable-contrast Snellen charts in assessing the functional ability of patients.

Clinical Use

Discrete alternating black and white bars representing square waves have been used since the 18th century to measure visual acuity, but sine wave gratings, which have softer bar edges, are now used in clinical practice to measure both visual acuity and contrast sensitivity (Fig. 55–1).

Commercially available contrast sensitivity systems that utilize

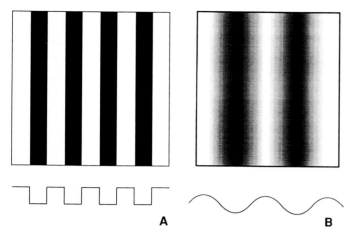

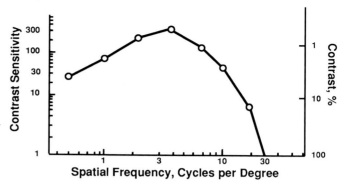

FIGURE 55–1. Diagrammatic illustration of (A) square wave gratings and (B) sine wave gratings. Note the difference in the distinction of borders between the two types.

FIGURE 55–2. Normal contrast sensitivity curve for the human visual system.

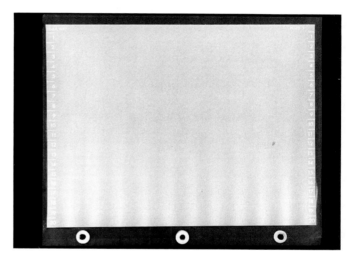

FIGURE 55–3. Arden Contrast Sensitivity Plate.

these gratings have made it possible for the clinician to investigate the functional capabilities of patients having or suspected of having corneal, retinal, optic nerve, anterior visual pathway, or cerebral disorders. These systems are most effective as screening tools and contribute minimally to diagnosis.

INSTRUMENTATION

Theory and Use

To evaluate contrast sensitivity clinically, a sinusoidal grating of given spatial frequency may be presented and its contrast reduced until the pattern is visible to the subject only 50% of the time. This is known as the *contrast threshold* for that spatial frequency, and its reciprocal is defined as *contrast sensitivity*. In other words, the lower the contrast threshold, the higher the contrast sensitivity. Spatial contrast sensitivity is measured with stationary gratings, whereas temporal contrast sensitivity is measured with gratings that reverse contrast at various rates over time.[23]

After contrast sensitivity has been determined for a wide range of spatial frequencies, its logarithmic value is plotted as the ordinate (vertical axis) and spatial frequency as the abscissa (horizontal axis) to obtain the contrast sensitivity curve, or modulation transfer function, of the patient (Fig. 55–2). This curve, which is governed by both optical and neural factors, represents the resolving capability of the human visual system for every contrast level and spatial frequency.

The peak of the curve generally occurs at 3–4 c/d for the patient with normal vision. A shift of the peak from 4 c/d to 2 c/d and reduced sensitivity to intermediate and high spatial frequencies occurs in the normally sighted patient over 60 years of age.[24–26] This reduction is most likely due to decreased retinal illuminance from pupillary miosis and lenticular opacification.[25]

The point at which the curve crosses the abscissa is known as the *cutoff frequency*, and denotes the maximum resolving capacity of the visual system at 100% contrast. Although this value is in cycles per degree, it may be converted into the denominator of Snellen acuity by dividing it into 600. For example, a cutoff frequency of 15 c/d should yield a Snellen acuity of 20/40 (600/15 = 40; therefore, Snellen = 20/40). It then follows that the patient with 20/20 Snellen acuity or better should have a cutoff frequency of 30 c/d or higher. If disease is present, this cutoff frequency, as well as other points along the curve, may be considerably reduced.

Instrumentation for contrast sensitivity testing has been developed as a means of establishing a better overall picture of visual performance. Visual acuity measurement alone is inadequate, since it represents only one point along the contrast sensitivity curve and bears little relationship to the countless contrast levels and environmental details one encounters on a daily basis. In fact, certain patients may prefer an eye with higher peak contrast sensitivity over one with better visual acuity.

COMMERCIALLY AVAILABLE INSTRUMENTS
(sequenced in order of ascending cost)

Arden Contrast Sensitivity System

The Arden Contrast Sensitivity System* (Fig. 55–3) consists of six photographic plates measuring 23 × 30.5 cm (9 × 12 in.), which subtend a visual angle of 28° at 57 cm. The first plate of sinusoidal gratings is for demonstration and the other five have spatial frequencies of 0.2, 0.4, 0.8, 1.6, 3.2, and 6.4 c/d, respectively. The last plate contains the two highest spatial frequencies, each of which occupies half the plate. Contrast of each plate increases from top to bottom over a range of 1.76 log units, and contrast levels are numbered from 1 to 20 on a vertical scale. The testing procedure

* Richmond Products, 1021 S. Rogers Circle, Boca Raton, FL 33487

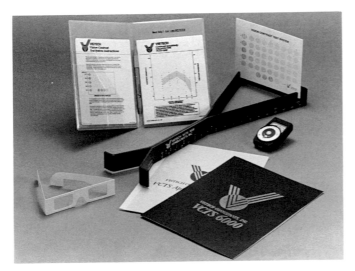

FIGURE 55–4. VCTS 6000 near system. (Courtesy of Vistech Consultants, Inc)

involves removing each plate from its folder at a rate of 1 scale unit/sec until the gratings are visible to the subject. The contrast levels selected for each grating are then totaled and compared with normal values.

VCTS 6000

The Vistech* VCTS 6000 (Fig. 55–4) is a set of three portable near-vision charts measuring 14 × 17.5 cm (5.5 × 7 in.). Each chart contains five horizontal rows of nine circular sinusoidal grating patches oriented vertically or tilted 15° to the left or right. The spatial frequency of each of the five rows from top to bottom is 1.5, 3.0, 6.0, 12.0, and 18.0 c/d, respectively. The contrast level of each of the nine patches decreases progressively (33% to 0%) from left to right in approximately 0.2-log unit steps. Each patch subtends a visual angle of 1.4° at 46 cms (18 in.).

VCTS 700S

The Vistech* VCTS 700S (Fig. 55–5) is a projector slide that utilizes circular sinusoidal grating patches having the same spatial frequencies as the VCTS 6000 and VCTS 6500 (see following). Test results cannot be standardized because of the variability inherent in projection systems. Due to its reduced number of contrast levels (four to six per spatial frequency), the manufacturer suggests using the slide in conjunction with standard Vistech charts to verify and quantify functional vision loss.

VCTS 6500

The Vistech* VCTS 6500 (Fig. 55–6) is the distance analog of the VCTS 6000 and consists of a set of three wall posters each measuring 68 × 94 cm (27 × 37 in.). The spatial frequencies of the five rows from top to bottom and the contrast levels of the nine circular sinusoidal grating patches from left to right are identical with those of the VCTS 6000. Each patch subtends a visual angle of 1.4° at 3.05 m (10 ft).

* Vistech Consultants, Inc., 4162 Little York Road, Dayton, OH 45414

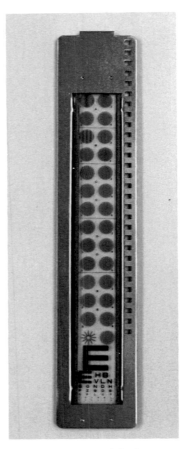

FIGURE 55–5. VCTS 700S projection slide. (Courtesy of Vistech Consultants, Inc)

B-VAT II-SG

The Mentor* B-VAT II-SG Video Acuity Tester (Fig. 55–7) is an automated tabletop instrument with multiple capabilities, including contrast sensitivity testing. Sinusoidal gratings of vertical orien-

* Mentor O&O, Inc., 3000 Longwater Drive, Norwell, MA 02061

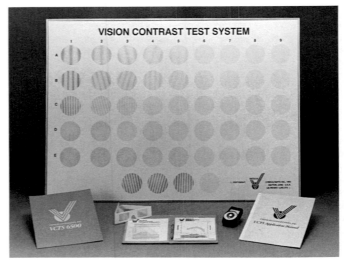

FIGURE 55–6. VCTS 6500 distance system. (Courtesy of Vistech Consultants, Inc)

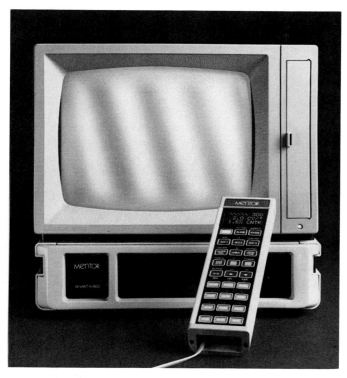

FIGURE 55–7. B-VAT II-SG Video Acuity Tester. (Courtesy of Mentor O&O, Inc)

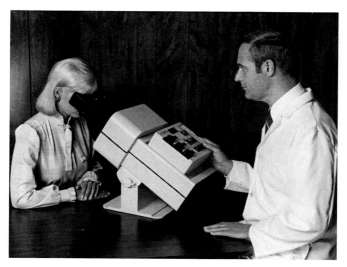

FIGURE 55–8. MCT 8000 Multivision Contrast Tester. (Courtesy of Vistech Consultants, Inc)

tation, or tilted 14° to the left or right, are generated on a television monitor measuring 28 cm diagonally. Sixteen spatial frequencies ranging from 1.5 to 40 c/d may be presented at 20 different contrast levels ranging from 0.10% to 98% in approximately 0.1-log unit steps. Testing may be performed between 3 and 6 m (10 and 20 ft). A hand-held keypad control unit facilitates examination.

MCT 8000

The Vistech* MCT 8000 (Fig. 55–8) Multivision Contrast Tester is an automated tabletop instrument that primarily utilizes sinusoidal gratings as targets. Two separate sets of six slides consist of one visual acuity slide and five contrast sensitivity slides made of the same spatial frequencies described for other Vistech systems. The contrast sensitivity slides comprise seven grating patches arranged in a circle around a central potential glare source. Both distance and near testing may be performed with and without activation of the glare source.

Terry Vision Analyzer

The InnoMed† Terry Vision Analyzer (TVA) (Fig. 55–9) is an automated tabletop instrument that utilizes letter optotypes and square wave gratings, ranging in contrast value from 0.7% to 83.0% over nine levels. The largest letter optotypes (20/400) are initially presented at low contrast levels between letter and surround. Contrast is then slowly and systematically increased until three letters of the display can be correctly named. This is considered the contrast threshold for that letter size. The same procedure is then followed for the next smallest letter size.

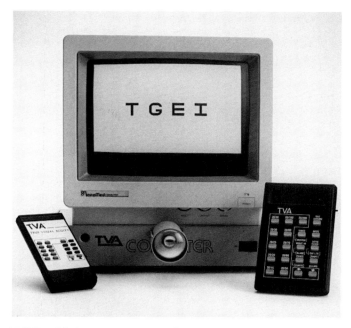

FIGURE 55–9. Terry Vision Analyzer (TVA). (Courtesy of InnoMed Corporation)

CLINICAL PROCEDURE

The Vistech series of contrast sensitivity testers is perhaps the most affordable and accessible to the clinician. Accordingly, the clinical procedure for performing near and distance testing with these systems is outlined in the following:

VCTS 6000/VCTS 6500*

1. Light reflected off the chart (luminance) should be measured with a photometer. This should be adjusted ac-

* Vistech Consultants, Inc., 4162 Little York Road, Dayton, OH 45414
† InnoMed Corporation, 620 Lunar Ave., Brea, CA 92621

* Adapted from the Vistech manual.

cordingly if not within the range of 30 to 70 ft-lamberts. It should be constant and uniform across the entire chart.

2. The patient should be positioned at the proper distance from the chart. Best optical correction should be worn for the test distance, regardless of the level of visual acuity, since contrast sensitivity may decline dramatically for all spatial frequencies if optical blur is present.[3,20]

3. The patient should be instructed to observe the sample circular sinusoidal grating patches at the bottom of the chart. The four possible responses (left, right, up, and blank) should then be reviewed.

4. With the fellow eye occluded, the patient should be instructed to begin with the top row (row A) and identify the orientation of as many patches as possible from left to right. The first incorrect response should serve as the end point for that row. Proceed to the next row (row B) and follow the same steps.

5. The end point for each of the five rows should be documented by marking the associated encircled number on the evaluation form (Fig. 55–10). The vertical rows on the form directly correspond to the horizontal rows on the chart. The numbers marked should be connected to form a contrast sensitivity curve for the patient. Results should then be compared with the shaded normal population range on the evaluation form.

6. The procedure should be repeated for the fellow eye, if indicated.

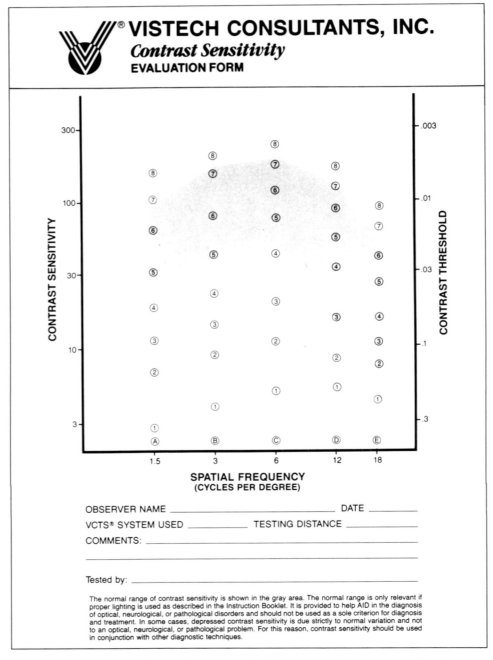

FIGURE 55–10. Evaluation form used to chart results of contrast sensitivity testing using Vistech systems.

CLINICAL IMPLICATIONS

Clinical Significance

Visual acuity and contrast sensitivity are simply two components of vision that occur as a result of a complex interaction of sensory and nonsensory factors. As essential as visual acuity testing is, it may mislead the clinician in assessing the functional vision of patients with ocular disease. Visual acuity provides tangible guidelines for "visual quantity," but reveals little in the way of "visual quality." Every clinician has encountered the patient who reads the bottom line of the chart, yet complains of dim, foggy, or unclear vision. All too often, such complaints may indicate diminished contrast sensitivity, yet are readily dismissed in the presence of favorable Snellen results.

Over the last 25 years, a voluminous amount of research has been conducted in the area of contrast sensitivity function as it relates to amblyopia,[19,28] contact lens wear,[29,30] keratoconus,[31] penetrating keratoplasty,[32] radial keratotomy,[33] intraocular lens implantation,[34] cataracts,[10,35] glaucoma,[5] optic neuritis,[36] papilledema,[37] anterior visual pathway and cerebral lesions,[38] multiple sclerosis,[39] and hemodialysis.[40] Several retinal diseases have also been studied, including retinitis pigmentosa,[11,17,41,42] toxic retinopathy,[17,18] central serous choroidopathy,[41,43,44] age-related macular degeneration,[41,44–46] diabetic maculopathy,[13] vitelliform dystrophy,[17] Stargardt's dystrophy,[17] and cone–rod dystrophy.[11]

In general, the results of these studies indicate that certain diseases demonstrate selective spatial frequency deficits, whereas others show more uniform loss across a wide range of frequencies (Table 55–1). Low and medium spatial frequency losses have been linked to problems with mobility and reduced ability to recognize faces and large objects,[47] whereas high-frequency loss is more closely correlated with decreased visual acuity.

Clinical Interpretation

The many studies associated with contrast sensitivity testing indicate that it is assuming greater importance in the assessment of visual function. However, it has not yet attained the widespread acceptance in the ophthalmic community that its advocates had hoped. Despite exhaustive clinical research, the literature continues to pose the same questions.[48–50] Can the results of contrast sensitivity testing be applied to everyday situations, or are they purely academic? How can our knowledge of diminished contrast sensitivity improve the quality of life for affected patients? Should it be tested routinely along with visual acuity to provide a clearer explanation of one's visual performance? Although the answers may be forthcoming, these and other questions remain unanswered.

The clinician should remember that the results of contrast sensitivity testing are merely one part of a complete visual profile and must be analyzed along with other clinical data. At its current level of evolution, contrast sensitivity testing may provide the clinician with the insight necessary for (1) detecting subtle or insidious disease processes that have not yet affected visual acuity, such as early keratoconus or multiple sclerosis; (2) monitoring the course of diseases that have already compromised visual acuity, such as cataracts or age-related macular degeneration; and (3) understanding how patients with various ocular diseases function when engaged in routine visual activities.[17]

REFERENCES

1. Arden GG. The importance of measuring contrast sensitivity in cases of visual disturbance. Br J Ophthalmol 1978;62:198–209.
2. Schade OH. Optical and photoelectric analog of the eye. J Opt Soc Am 1956;46:721–739.
3. Campbell FW, Green DG. Optical and retinal factors affecting visual resolution. J Physiol 1965;181:576–593.
4. Bodis-Wollner I. Visual acuity and contrast sensitivity in patients with cerebral lesions. Science 1972;178:769–771.
5. Arden GB, Jacobson JJ. A simple grating test for contrast sensitivity: preliminary results indicate value in screening for glaucoma. Invest Ophthalmol Vis Sci 1978;17:23–32.
6. Sokol S, Domar A, Moskowitz A. Utility of Arden grating test in glaucoma screening: high false-positive rate in normals over 50 years of age. Invest Ophthalmol Vis Sci 1980;19:1529–1533.
7. Skalka HW. Effect of age on Arden grating acuity. Br J Ophthalmol 1980;64:21–23.
8. Skalka HW. Comparison of Snellen acuity, VER acuity, and Arden grating scores in macular and optic nerve diseases. Br J Ophthalmol 1980;64:24–29.
9. Weatherhead RG. Use of the Arden grating test for screening. Br J Ophthalmol 1980;64:591–596.
10. Skalka HW. Arden grating test in evaluating "early" posterior subcapsular cataracts. South Med J 1981;74:1368–1370.
11. Marmor MF. Contrast sensitivity and retinal disease. Ann Ophthalmol 1981;13:1069–1071.
12. Brown B. Reading performance in low vision patients: relation to contrast and contrast sensitivity. Am J Optom Physiol Opt 1981;58:218–226.
13. Ghafour IM, Foulds WS, Allan D, et al. Contrast sensitivity in diabetic subjects with and without retinopathy. Br J Ophthalmol 1982;66:492–495.
14. Woo GC, Prentice VDM. An evaluation of the Arden grating test. J Am Optom Assoc 1983;54:985–989.
15. Yap M, Grey C, Collinge A, et al. The Arden gratings in optometric practice. Ophthal Physiol Opt 1985;5:179–183.
16. Corwin TR, Richman JE. Three clinical tests of the spatial contrast sensitivity function: a comparison. Am J Optom Physiol Opt 1986;63:413–418.
17. Marmor MF. Contrast sensitivity versus visual acuity in retinal disease. Br J Ophthalmol 1986;70:553–559.
18. Salmon JF, Carmichael TR, Welsh NH. Use of contrast sensitivity measurement in the detection of subclinical ethambutol toxic optic neuropathy. Br J Ophthalmol 1987;71:192–196.
19. Glover H, Bird S, Yap M. Performance of amblyopic children on printed contrast sensitivity test charts. Am J Optom Physiol Opt 1987;64:361–363.
20. Marmor MF, Gawande A. Effect of visual blur on contrast sensitivity. Clinical implications. Ophthalmology 1988;95:139–143.
21. Ginsburg AP. A new contrast sensitivity vision test chart. Am J Optom Physiol Opt 1984;61:403–407.
22. Regan D, Neima D. Low-contrast letter charts as a test of visual function. Ophthalmology 1983;90:1192–1200.

Table 55–1
Spatial Frequency Deficits in Selected Ocular Disorders

	Low	Middle	High
Anterior Segment			
Keratoconus	−	+	+
Corneal edema	+	−	+
Cataracts	−	+	+
Posterior Segment			
Optic neuritis	+ (Acute)	+	+ (Acute)
Pseudotumor cerebri (± disc edema)	+	+	−
Glaucoma	+	+	−
Age-related macular degeneration	+ (Advanced)	+	+
Central serous choroidopathy	−	+	+
Retinitis pigmentosa	−	−	+
Miscellaneous			
Strabismic amblyopia	−	−	+
Uncorrected refractive error	+	+	+

23. Jindra LF, Zemon V. Contrast sensitivity testing: a more complete assessment of vision. J Cataract Refract Surg 1989;15:141–148.

24. Arundale K. An investigation into the variation of human contrast sensitivity with age and ocular pathology. Br J Ophthalmol 1978;62:213–215.

25. Owsley C, Sekuler R, Siemsen D. Contrast sensitivity throughout adulthood. Vision Res 1983;23:689–699.

26. Ross JE, Clarke DD, Bron AJ. Effect of age on contrast sensitivity function: uniocular and binocular findings. Br J Ophthalmol 1985;69:51–56.

27. Young DA, McKee MC, Coffey B, et al. Comparison of Snellen letter and Vistech grating charts as refraction targets. J Am Optom Assoc 1988;59:364–371.

28. Levi DM, Harwerth RS. Spatiotemporal interactions in anisometropic and strabismic amblyopia. Invest Ophthalmol Vis Sci 1977;16:90–95.

29. Kirkpatrick DL, Roggenkamp JR. Effects of soft contact lenses on contrast sensitivity. Am J Optom Physiol Opt 1985;62:407–412.

30. Grey CP. Changes in contrast sensitivity during the first hour of soft lens wear. Am J Optom Physiol Opt 1986;63:702–707.

31. Zadnik K, Mannis MJ, Johnson CA, et al. Rapid contrast sensitivity assessment in keratoconus. Am J Optom Physiol Opt 1987;64:693–697.

32. Mannis MJ, Zadnik K, Johnson CA. The effect of penetrating keratoplasty on contrast sensitivity in keratoconus. Arch Ophthalmol 1984;102:1513–1516.

33. Trick LR, Hartstein J. Investigation of contrast sensitivity following radial keratotomy. Ann Ophthalmol 1987;19:251–254.

34. Roel L, Zemon V, Jindra LF, et al. Contrast sensitivity and Snellen acuity of patients with intraocular lens implants. ARVO abstracts. Invest Ophthalmol Vis Sci 1988;29(suppl):434.

35. Hess RT, Woo G. Vision through cataracts. Invest Ophthalmol Vis Sci 1978;17:428–435.

36. Fleishman JA, Beck RW, Linares OA, et al. Deficits in visual function after resolution of optic neuritis. Ophthalmology 1987;94:1029–1035.

37. Wall M. Contrast sensitivity testing in pseudotumor cerebri. Ophthalmology 1986;93:4–7.

38. Bodis-Wollner I, Diamond SP. The measurement of spatial contrast sensitivity in cases of blurred vision associated with cerebral lesions. Brain 1976;99:695–710.

39. Regan D, Silver R, Murray TJ. Visual acuity and contrast sensitivity in multiple sclerosis—hidden visual loss. Brain 1977;100:563–579.

40. Woo GC, Mandelman T, Liu TT, et al. Effect of hemodialysis on contrast sensitivity in renal failure. Am J Optom Physiol Opt 1986;63:356–361.

41. Wolkstein M, Atkin A, Bodis-Wollner I. Contrast sensitivity in retinal disease. Ophthalmology 1980;87:1140–1149.

42. Hyvarinen L, Rovamo J, Laurinen P, et al. Contrast sensitivity function in evaluation of visual impairment due to retinitis pigmentosa. Acta Ophthalmol 1981;59:763–773.

43. Kayazawa F, Yamamoto T, Itoi M. Temporal contrast sensitivity in central serous choroidopathy. Ann Ophthalmol 1982;14:272–275.

44. Sjostrand J. Contrast sensitivity in macular disease using a small-field and a large-field TV-system. Acta Ophthalmol 1979;57:832–846.

45. Loshin DS, White J. Contrast sensitivity. The visual rehabilitation of the patient with macular degeneration. Arch Ophthalmol 1984;102:1303–1306.

46. Kleiner RC, Enger C, Alexander MF, et al. Contrast sensitivity in age-related macular degeneration. Arch Ophthalmol 1988;106:55–57.

47. Marron JA, Bailey IL. Visual factors and orientation–mobility performance. Am J Optom Physiol Opt 1982;59:413–426.

48. Legge GE, Rubin GS. Contrast sensitivity function as a screening test: a critique. Am J Optom Physiol Opt 1986;63:265–270.

49. Mannis MJ. Making sense of contrast sensitivity testing. Has its time come? Arch Ophthalmol 1987;105:627–629.

50. Prager TC, Holladay JT, Ruiz RS. The other side of visual acuity testing: Contrast sensitivity. CLAO 1986;12:230–233.

Electroretinography

Vesna G. Sutija
Jerome Sherman

INTRODUCTION

Definition

The *electroretinogram* (ERG) is a field potential recorded from the cornea of the intact eye in response to light. It reflects summed electrical activity of populations of different cell types and structures within the retina. The technique is used in research to study basic visual functions or, in clinical practice, as a diagnostic tool. The potential diagnostic usefulness of the technique depends on the understanding of the mechanism that generates it and on the precise neuronal site of origin of its components.

History

The ERG was first recorded by Holmgren in 1865, and its intraretinal origin suggested by Dewar and McKendrick in 1873.[1,2] The first ERG component analysis was attempted by Granit (1933), who was able to distinguish three major ERG components, PI, PII, and PIII, in order of their disappearance under ether anesthesia.[3] The PI formed the c-wave; the PII, the b-wave; and the PIII was later shown to have a fast and a slow subcomponent. Only the early, fast PIII subcomponent is generated by the neurons, the photoreceptors; the rest are generated by nonneuronal retinal structures, the Muller cells and the retinal pigment epithelium (RPE), in response to changes in the concentration of extracellular potassium. The changes in concentration of extracellular potassium, however, result from neuronal activity; hence, ultimately, the ERG does reflect the integrity of neuronal functioning within the retina.

Clinical ERG was promoted by Karpe (1945) in Europe, who became the first president of the International Society for Clinical Electroretinography, today's ISCEV (International Society of Clinical Electrophysiology of Vision), and Riggs (1941) in the United States, who developed the first ERG electrode embedded in a contact lens.[4,5]

The b-wave has been studied most extensively, because it is the largest, most prominent and easiest to record. It is also the most sensitive (i.e., it needs the least amount of light to appear) and is recordable over the range of 6 log units. The a-wave, for example, needs 100 times more light, so that there is about 2 log units of threshold difference between the two waves. The b-wave's threshold is comparable to psychophysical threshold in humans.

It has been shown that the b-wave is useful in assessment of the functional state of the retina in ocular disease, which created a lively interest in this ERG component. There is little doubt that it originates from retinal structures postsynaptic to the photoreceptors, since it is blocked by virtually any pharmacologic agent that impairs the synaptic transmission between the photoreceptors and the second order neurons. On the other hand, it can be recorded in eyes after optic nerve transsection in patients whose ganglion cells have degenerated. Thus the ganglion cells and the photoreceptors do not contribute directly to its formation. Currently, the most popular hypothesis about the origin of the b-wave is the "Muller cell hypothesis." This assumes that the b-wave is the extracellular expression of radial current flow generated by a potassium ion-mediated depolarization of the Muller cells.[6,7]

Clinical Use

Structural and functional retinal integrity can be assessed and monitored by the following means:

1. Visually, by various forms of ophthalmoscopy, fundus photography, and fluorescein angiography
2. Psychophysically, by tests of visual acuity, visual fields, contrast sensitivity, dark adaptometry, color vision, glare, and macular dazzle

3. Electrophysiologically, by ERG, electro-oculography (EOG), and visual-evoked potentials (VEP)

Among these procedures, the single objective test that best reflects overall retinal function is the standard full-field flash ERG. In some retinal diseases, the structure of the retina may appear uncompromised when visualized ophthalmoscopically, yet the function may be severely impaired when measured by retinography. In other conditions, an ERG abnormality may precede subjective awareness of visual loss and permit a diagnosis years in advance of a psychophysically measurable deficit. To be of clinical importance, the ERG must be able to separate rod and cone function, compare the activity of local retinal areas, and test the function at different retinal depths. The clinical protocols usually indicate whether the responses are obtained under scotopic (dark-adapted) or photopic (light-adapted) conditions, but this description does not necessarily define the receptor system (rod or cone) that has generated the response. Responses to dim white or blue light flashes under dark adaptation can be attributed to rods alone, but scotopic ERGs to intense white light flashes reflect a mixed rod–cone contribution. Photopic ERGs may reflect the activity of either light-adapted or dark-adapted cones. The wavelength and the brightness of the light flash, the state of adaptation, and the flash frequency, all are contributing factors that must be taken into consideration when describing the involvement of either receptor system in abnormal ERG responses. The rod response, for example, is useful in documentation of hereditary night-blinding disorders that involve the retinal periphery. The cone response, on the other hand, is useful to diagnose cone dysfunction associated with hereditary or acquired diseases. A normal ERG (flash and pattern reversal) rules out a retinal involvement and strongly suggests a visual pathway dysfunction, indicating a need for further neurologic testing.

INSTRUMENTATION

Theory

Vision begins in the photoreceptors, where light is absorbed and the first in a long series of neural signals is initiated. The signal, in the form of a membrane hyperpolarization, communicates with the second-order retinal neurons by reducing the rate of neurotransmitter release from the photoreceptor's synaptic terminals. All the steps by which light generates the photoreceptor hyperpolarization are not yet known. In darkness, there is a steady influx of ions into the outer segment, and this "dark current" partially depolarizes the cell, maintaining a high rate of transmitter release from the synaptic terminals. In the light, the permeability decreases, reducing the ion influx: the membrane hyperpolarizes, and the transmitter release is stopped. The photoreceptors communicate directly with horizontal and bipolar cells, the second-order neurons. The continuous release of the photoreceptor neurotransmitters in the dark, depolarizes the horizontal cells and one of the two kinds of bipolar cells, the hyperpolarizing (off) bipolar cell, while it hyperpolarizes the other kind, the depolarizing (on) bipolar cell. The light hyperpolarizes the horizontal cells and the off-center bipolars, effectively stopping the release of the transmitter from their terminals, but depolarizes the on-center bipolars, effectively initiating the release of transmitter from their terminals. The communications of the photoreceptors with the horizontal and bipolar cells within the outer plexiform layer are transmitted into more proximal retinal layers, influencing the function of Muller cells, until, at the end, they leave the retina by the optic nerve axons to send the retinal signal to the brain for further refinement.

The neuronal retinal activity mirrors the changes in membrane permeabilities to different species of ions and resultant currents that flow through cell membranes. Observed from extracellular space on a larger scale, they appear as sinks and sources. If the outward currents dominate, a current source results; if the inward currents dominate, a current sink is created. These sinks and sources are the physical substrates of field potentials, such as the ERG. The field potentials are relatively easy to record, but often difficult to interpret, because they are only an indirect and a somewhat ambiguous reflection of the underlying neuronal activity.

The vertebrate ERG has a complex waveform, composed of several major wave components known as the a-wave, b-wave, c-wave, and d-wave, and other minor components, including the oscillatory potentials. Figure 56–1 shows a typical ERG in response to a single bright white flash after 30 minutes of dark adaptation recorded from the right eye of a healthy visually normal 29-year-old woman and depicts only the a- and b-waves.

Experimental evidence from the intraretinal current–source–density (CSD) analysis and the intracellular recording from Muller cells places the b-wave origin in Muller cells.[8,9] Intracellularly recorded Muller cell responses and ERG b-wave have similar latencies and show similar waveforms. The CSD analysis indicates a large sink for b-wave current in the region of the outer plexiform layer. The Muller cells are known to act as potassium electrodes (i.e., they are sensitive to extracellular potassium concentrations). There are three light-evoked changes in extracellular potassium that can be measured directly with ion selective (potassium sensitive) electrodes: a "distal decrease" and two increases, a smaller "distal increase" and a larger "proximal increase"; distal and proximal referring to the general regions of the outer and inner plexiform layers, respectively. The distal decrease is unrelated to the b-wave, but contributes to other ERG components, the c-wave and the slow PIII. Although the smaller of the two increases, it has recently been established that the distal increase in extracellular potassium is mostly responsible for the generation of the b-wave. It is attributed to the depolarizing bipolar cells.

The ERG b-wave is formed by two current sinks, one in the outer plexiform layer and the other in the inner plexiform layer, and a current source along the inner margin of the retina. The light-evoked increases in potassium in the two plexiform layers cause potassium influxes into the Muller cells and the consequent

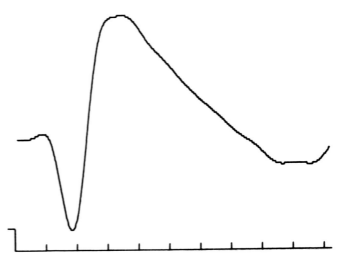

FIGURE 56–1. Human ERG in response to a single "standard" white flash after 30 min of dark adaptation recorded from the right eye of a healthy, visually normal 29-year-old woman. The a-wave implicit time at 17 msec; b-wave implicit time at 48 msec; amplitude of 496 μV.

depolarization of the Muller cell membrane. Almost all of the potassium current exits from the high-conductance endfoot region of the cell. The extracellular current flow thereby established around the Muller cells, particularly by the distal potassium increase, gives rise to the b-wave of the ERG.

The a-wave can be isolated from the b- and c-waves by experimental manipulation. The a-wave and the PIII component have subcomponents, an early fast subcomponent, arising from the photoreceptors, and a slower PIII, originating in the Muller cells. The slow PIII reflects the activity of the rods.

The c-wave cannot be recorded from an isolated retina, which clearly shows that it does not arise from within the retina. The c-wave is generated by the RPE in response to the decrease in potassium concentration in the subretinal space initiated by the photoreceptor's response to light.

In summary, the c-wave, the slow PIII and the b-wave, all result from the changes in potassium fluxes induced by light. Intracellular recording from RPE cells and the c-wave show that these potentials are correlated.[10] Pigment epithelial cells, just as the Muller cells, are very sensitive to the changes in extracellular potassium concentration and behave like potassium electrodes.

The small wavelets superimposed on the raising arm of the b-wave, and called the oscillatory potentials (OPs), are not seen in the intracellular Muller cell recordings, suggesting a different origin from the b-wave. The OPs are most readily observed under mesopic conditions, because their light threshold is higher than that of the b-wave. The best way to elicit them is with repetitive, bright full-field flashes with a constant stimulus interval. Figure 56–2 shows the oscillatory potentials superimposed on the a- and the b-wave of the human ERG and how the various ERG components are separated by different bandpass filters. The origin of the oscillatory potentials is as yet unknown. Some of the oscillatory potentials reverse polarity at different depth of recording. The earlier OPs reverse polarity more proximally than do later ones, showing that the chain of events underlying their generation begins in the proximal retina and, then, travels distally. The current loops they reflect could be a series of feedback interactions initiated in the proximal retina, such as the feedback from amacrine cell processes onto bipolar cell terminals and other amacrine cell processes, or the feedback from the interplexiform cells onto horizontal and bipolar cells in the inner nuclear and outer plexiform layers.[11,12]

Use

Basic Technology

FACILITIES. Electroretinography is best performed in a quiet air-conditioned room that allows undisturbed dark adaptation of the patient (Fig. 56–3). A dedicated electrical circuitry should be available to isolate the recording and analyzing equipment from any outside interferences, such as the elevators or other powerful machinery, and to protect it from sudden power surges. The patient should be seated comfortably in a chair, with a sturdy head support, or reclining.

STIMULATING EQUIPMENT. The most frequently used light source is the Grass photostimulator, with adjustable flash rate and intensity, and a flash duration of 10 microseconds. Other devices are also available and, usually, include color filters to be used when separating rod and cone contributions in the recorded potentials. The ideal conditions for ERG should include a full-field dome of diffuse light stimulation, the Ganzfeld. The stimulus intensity should produce a full-field illuminance of at least 1.5–3.0 cd/m^2 measured at eye position in the Ganzfeld bowl, defined as the standard bright flash. In addition to flashes, the stimulator must be capable of producing a steady and even background illumination across the full field. In some applications, backgrounds of different wavelengths are employed. The relative and independent light adjustment of the flash and of the background must be possible. It should also be possible to attenuate the maximum flash intensity over a range of at least 3 log units, either continuously or in steps of 0.25 to 0.30 log units. The method selected must not change the wavelength composition of the light stimulus. The background illumination system needs sufficient flexibility to calibrate and recalibrate the intensity to the levels required by specific protocols of testing. The color temperature of the background must remain constant over the range of the intensity changes. The total quantity of light falling on the eye from each flash must be documented after measurement with an integrating photometer placed at eye distance. In most commercially available instruments, the light output per flash, unfortunately, varies with the repetition rate, so that separate calibrations for single and repeti-

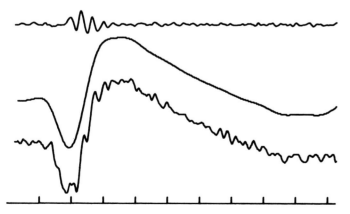

FIGURE 56–2. ERG traces with different bandpass characteristics recorded in response to "standard" white flash after 30 min of dark adaptation repeated three times and averaged. With bandpass of 1–1000 Hz, the record includes a- and b-waves and the superimposed oscillatory potentials (*bottom*); with bandpass of 1–40 Hz, the high-frequency components are eliminated and only a- and b-waves remain (*middle*); with bandpass of 100–1000 Hz, the slow components are eliminated and only the high-frequency oscillatory potentials remain (*top*).

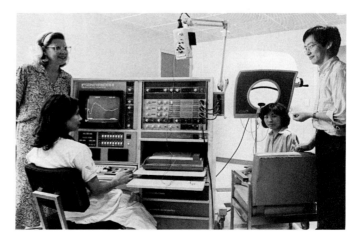

FIGURE 56–3. Pathfinder II microprocessor and the Ganzfeld visual stimulator. (Courtesy of Nicolet Biomedical, Madison, Wisconsin)

tive stimuli are advisable. Photometer measurements should be provided by the manufacturer. Recalibration of the light output from the dome is advised occasionally, especially if it includes incandescent sources. The self-calibrating units are the best choice.

Electrodes

The active electrodes in current use are of different types: hard contact lens electrodes, some disposable and others custom designed for specific purpose and type of recording, some made of gold foil, silver-coated nylon threads or polyvinyl immersed carbon fibers.

HARD CONTACT LENS ELECTRODES. Several different types of hard contact lens electrodes are in current use, sharing a similar design (Burian–Allen, Riggs, Henkes, and the disposable jet electrode).

Henkes. (Medical Workshop, Holland): The electrode originally designed by Henkes is a 20-mm scleral hard contact lens with an optical zone of 8.5 mm and a large peripheral flange, which is used to position the electrode in the palpebral aperture, effectively eliminating lid closure. When used, the corneal surface should be protected during recording with a nonirritating and nonallergenic ionic conductive solution, such as methylcellulose. It requires the use of topical anesthesia. The electrode is very reliable and produces stable recordings. Figure 56–4 shows the Henkes ERG electrode.

Jet. (Nicolet Biomedical, Wisconsin): This is a commercially available disposable electrode. It is a 12-mm contact lens with 2-mm long prongs—to prevent lid closure at inopportune recording moments—that protrude from the monocular surface with a 5-mm optical zone. In the original design, one of the prongs contained the metal electrode; in the newer version, the conductive metal electrode appears as a circular ring around the lens. This electrode also requires the use of anesthetic. Its relatively small size causes it to slip out of position on larger eyes. Figure 56–5 shows the jet disposable ERG electrode.

DTL. The name is an acronym from the first letters of the last names of the electrode's originators.[13] This electrode consists of silver-coated nylon fibers, each 12 μm in diameter, that can be connected to conventional electrode leads. If the filament part is immersed in saline solution, it will drape over the cornea. It may be placed under the lower lid to improve the recording stability.

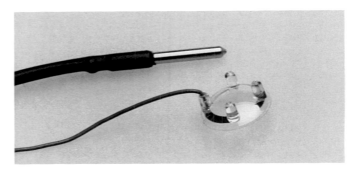

FIGURE 56–5. Jet hard contact lens disposable electrode.

This electrode does not require anesthetic or methylcellulose, does not interfere with the optical path and, therefore, is recommended for recording of averaged ERGs in response to patterned light stimulation. The electrode on the left in Figure 56–6 shows one version of the DTL electrode.

FOIL. Arden[14] advocates electrodes made of gold foil, usually hooked over the lower lid. This electrode does not require anesthetic or methylcellulose and does not interfere with the optical path, but it does not provide the recording stability of similar electrodes. With prolonged recording, its impedance is gradually reduced, and it becomes increasingly noisy. It is recommended for quick procedures, especially when corneal abrasion is at risk. It can also be used with patterned stimuli and averaged ERGs. The electrode on the right in Figure 56–6 shows one version of the foil electrode.

POLYVINYL ALCOHOL GEL. Recently an ERG electrode has been designed of polyvinyl alcohol and carbon fibers 4 to 6 μm in diameter.[15] They are stable and disposable, but are made in small quantities not readily available or in commercial use.

SKIN. With infants and small children, it may be advantageous to use skin electrodes as active electrodes, although they do not produce ERG amplitudes comparable to other electrodes.[16,17] The amplitudes recorded with skin electrodes are attenuated and will, therefore, require rigorous standardization with parametric measurements before application and averaging. They can be used with patterned stimuli.

Reference and Ground Electrodes

The reference electrodes are sometimes part of the contact lens-speculum assembly. Such ERG electrodes are referred to as bipolar electrodes. Most frequently a skin electrode is used as a refer-

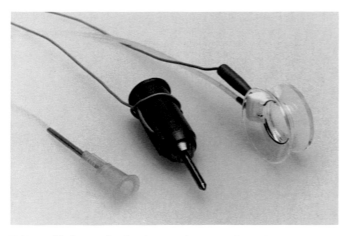

FIGURE 56–4. Henkes hard contact lens ERG electrode.

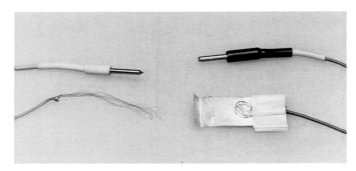

FIGURE 56–6. ERG electrodes used in research, DTL (*left*) and the foil electrode (*right*).

ence electrode, placed in the middle of the forehead or near each orbital rim as the reference for the ipsilateral eye. A skin electrode is attached to an indifferent point and connected to ground. Earclip electrodes are most often used as the ground electrodes. Occasionally, the cuff electrode will serve as the ground electrode, as is conventionally done for electrocardiography (ECG) recording.

COMMERCIALLY AVAILABLE INSTRUMENTS

Ganzfeld

The Nicolet Ganzfeld (Madison, Wisconsin) is a fully automatic, well-calibrated, sturdy visual stimulator that can be interfaced with other averaging components also developed by Nicolet Biomedical Instrument Co., such as the Pathfinder II described in some detail in Chapter 57. The Ganzfeld consists of a stimulus-controlling unit (NIC SM 600) that remotely controls the filter, strobe, and background luminance parameters and the white globe with a headrest and adjustable chin rest. The stand has an option of being tilted to accommodate various sitting arrangements. The globe is made of seamless aluminum coated with barium sulfate to assure a near-perfect diffuse reflectance of light. The light flashes are delivered by a high-intensity linear strobe (xenon) which allows selection of single flashes or variable flicker rates, from 0.1 to 35 Hz. The accompanying manual discloses the strobe's intensity–rate limitations so that one can select the intensity at which the flicker rate will not adversely affect it. The strobe has filters to absorb UV and IR radiation. Its intensities range from 0.25 to 1.5 and can be chosen in 0.25-log unit steps. Remote filter selection permits a variable strobe output over 5 log units. The filters are Kodak Wratten standard neutral-density or chromatic (no. 26 red or nos. 47, 47A, and 47B, blue) filters. Additional slots are provided for other filters. The background light is a DC-operated lamp with intensities from 1, 2, 5, 10, 15, 20, 25, and 30 ft-lamberts (0.81 to 10.02 cd/m^2) under digital control. The individual calibration data originate from National Bureau of Standards. The instrument offers a choice in fixation lights to be selected depending on the type of recording, EOG as well as ERG.

CLINICAL PROCEDURE

Despite that ERG has been performed clinically for over 40 years, no attempt at standardization of the clinical protocol has succeeded until recently. The ISCEV recently published a standard ERG protocol, which is being adopted internationally.[18] The protocol described in the following follows the ISCEV guidelines.

Patient Preparation

It is recommended that pupils be maximally dilated for ERG recording, especially for those measurements for which data are not averaged. Since one of the goals of electroretinography is to separate rod and cone responses, it is necessary to implement recording strategies to accomplish this. The most expedient way is by recording ERGs under scotopic (or dark-adapted) and photopic (or light-adapted) conditions. The amount of dark adaptation required varies for different protocols and the type of ocular disease suspected. Generally, it is recommended that dark adaptation be at least 30 minutes, although some diseases may require a longer dark adaptation. Should dark adaptation follow light-adapted ERG recording, or should the dark-adapted responses be recorded first, is a matter of arbitrary preference. Some clinicians prefer to start with photopic responses, which include responses to single flashes of light followed by the recording of 30-Hz flicker re-

sponse. This procedure will assure that most tested eyes, after a 30-Hz stimulus, will have been bleached to a similar degree from which the dark adaptation course can start; and it provides a similar light-adapted point from which deviations can be measured during the course of dark adaptation.

The contribution of the rods and cones to ERG responses is determined by retinal physiology; the contributions of rods to flashes of intense light at high background illumination will be minimized and 30-Hz flicker response under such conditions is unlikely to include any rod activity. The scotopic conditions with dim or no background light and dim single white or blue flashes will probably minimize the contribution of cones, although even with very dim backgrounds, an ERG response to an intense flash of light will have a substantial cone contribution. Color filters are often employed to improve the chances for a better rod–cone separation. Blue, dim light with dim background will optimize the rod-generated responses, while the red 30-Hz flicker superimposed on intense background will optimize the cone-generated contributions. How this is incorporated within the protocol is often an arbitrary decision and varies from laboratory to laboratory. The ISCEV standardized protocol recommends the following five measurements: (1) the maximal response in the dark-adapted eye, (2) a response developed by the rods, (3) a response developed by cones, (4) a response to flicker, and (5) oscillatory potentials.

There is a recommendation for the intensity of the *standard bright flash* (SBF), which is defined as one that produces a full-field illuminance of at least 1.5 to 3.0 cd/m^2 measured at the position of the eye in the Ganzfeld bowl. It is recommended that the *rod* response be the first signal measured after dark adaptation, since it is most sensitive to light adaptation. The ISCEV protocol recommends dark adaptation of at least 30 minutes, unless fluorescein angiography or fundus photography could not be avoided before ERG testing, when 1 hour of dark adaptation may be necessary. To measure the rod response, a dim white flash of intensity 2.5 log unit below the SBF is used. Blue light stimulus will accomplish the same, but it creates calibration problems for standardization of blue filters.

To obtain the maximal response in the dark-adapted eye, the white SBF is used, but this response, obtained under dark adaptation, is a scotopic response, not a rod response, since it is generated by both rods and cones at scotopic light levels.

The oscillatory potentials are recorded in the dark-adapted eye, using, again, the white SBF stimulus. The oscillatory potentials require special amplifier filter settings, which allow recording of very high frequency components, usually between 100 and 1000 Hz. The oscillatory potential measurements are very sensitive to the repetition rate. It is customary to ignore the first response and average only the subsequent three to four responses. The interstimulus interval of 15 seconds is considered optimal.[12]

Single flash *cone* response is best recorded in response to the white SBF superimposed on a background of 17–34 cd/m^2. It may be necessary to light-adapt the patient to the background for at least 10 minutes, if the cone response is to follow dark adaptation.

The flicker response is recorded to the same stimulus and background conditions as those described for the single cone response, flickering at 30 Hz. The response to flickering lights varies at the start, so it is routinely averaged to stabilize its amplitude. Figure 56–7 shows scotopic (on the left) and photopic (on the right) ERGs in response to single white flashes of light at two light intensities, and the averaged response to light flickering at 30 Hz.

Clinical Electroretinography Protocol

General Procedures

1. Explain procedure (contact lens to be placed *on*, not *in* the eye).

ing in age from 2 days to 16 years.[34] She has demonstrated that infants with Down syndrome and with phenylketonuria have evoked potentials with delayed latencies, as compared with normal infants. Furthermore, Marcus is able to diagnose differentially the Down's child from the phenylketonurics on the basis of the VEP alone. Additional research points to the expected result that therapeutic intervention (e.g., drug therapy and diet control) can be successfully monitored with the VEP. With effective therapeutic intervention, the change toward a more normal VEP has occurred before other, more traditional, indications. Because evoked potentials reflect neuronal activity, changes in them might be expected to occur earlier than observable behavioral improvements.

Other objective techniques for the assessment of sensory function and human development have been reported. Perhaps the most promising technique, attributed to Roy John, is a sophisticated apparatus capable of recording both EEGs and evoked potentials under about 50 different testing conditions as it monitors about 30 aspects of cortical function.[35] This test of brain function has been termed the quantitative electrophysiologic battery, and the related science has been named neurometrics. Eventual clinical use of such procedures should enable the early diagnosis of both receptor and cortical impairments in infants and, subsequently, permit treatment to be instituted before the passage of developmentally critical periods.

The VEPs have been used to test infants who were thought to be blind. The presence of pattern VEPs in such infants suggests just a delay in development and an excellent prognosis. Gittingen and Sokol[21] have reported three such infants who had only delayed development in congenital ocular motor apraxia.

VEPs have also been used as an index of recovery from behavioral blindness. Regan[2] has shown that VEPs can anticipate and parallel the progressive return of useful vision. He concluded that "both flash and pattern VEPs recorded during a period of behavioral blindness can predict recovery of useful vision in some but not all patients."

REFERENCES

1. Caton R. The electric currents of the brain. Br Med J 1875;278:28.
2. Regan D, ed. Human brain electrophysiology. In: Evoked potentials and evoked magnetic fields in science and medicine. New York: Elsevier, 1989.
3. Tyler CW, Apkarian P, Levi D, Nakayama K. Rapid assessment of visual function: an electronic sweep technique for the pattern visual evoked potential. Invest Ophthalmol Vis Sci 1979;18:703–713.
4. Fiorentini A, Maffei L, Pirchio M, Spinelli D, Porciatti V. The ERG in response to alternating gratings in patients with diseases of the peripheral visual pathway. Invest Ophthalmol Vis Sci 1981;21:490–493.
5. Sherman J. Simultaneous pattern-reversal electroretinograms and visual evoked potentials in diseases of the macula and optic nerve. Ann NY Acad Sci 1982;388:214.
6. Holder GE. Significance of abnormal pattern electroretinography in anterior visual pathway dysfunction. Br J Ophthalmol 1987;71:166–171.
7. Baker C, Hess R, Olsen B, Zrenner E. Current source density analysis of linear and non-linear components of the primate electroretinogram. J Physiol 1988;407:155–176.
8. Harter MR, White CT. Effects of contour sharpness and check size on visually evoked cortical potentials. Vis Res 1968;8:701–711.
9. Ludlam WM, Meyers RR. The use of visual evoked responses in objective refraction. Trans NY Acad Sci 1972;34:154–170.
10. Regan D. Rapid objective refraction using evoked brain potentials. Invest Ophthalmol 1973;12:669–679.
11. Marg E, et al. Visual acuity development in human infants. Invest Ophthalmol 1976;15:150–153.
12. Levi DM, Manny RE. The VEP in the diagnostic evaluation of amblyopia. In: Cracco RQ, Bodis-Wollner I, eds. Evoked potentials. New York: Alan R Liss, 1986:437–446.
13. Bartlett NR. Binocular summation and evoked cortical potential. Percept Psychophysiol 1968;3:75–76.
14. Srebro R. The visually evoked response. Arch Ophthalmol 1978;96:839–844.
15. Amigo G, et al. Binocular vision tested with visual evoked potentials in children and infants. Invest Ophthalmol 1978;17:910–915.
16. Sherman J, Bass SJ, Noble K, Nath S, Sutija V. Visual evoked potential (VEP) delays in central serous choroidopathy. Invest Ophthalmol Vis Sci 1986;27:214.
17. McAlpine D, Lumsden CE, Acheson ED. Multiple sclerosis: a reappraisal. Edinburgh: Churchill-Livingstone, 1972.
18. Bass SJ, Sherman J. Visual evoked potential (VEP) delays in tilted and/or oblique entrance of the optic nerve head. Neuro-Ophthalmol 1988;8:109–122.
19. Halliday Am, et al. The pattern-evoked potential in compression of the anterior visual pathways. Brain 1976;99:357–374.
20. Millman A, Sherman J, Della Rocca R, Eichler J. Pattern visual evoked potentials in orbital disease. Invest Ophthalmol Vis Sci ARVO Abstr 1988;29.
21. Gittinger JW Jr, Sokol S. The visual evoked potential in the diagnosis of congenital ocular motor apraxia. Am J Ophthalmol 1982;93:700–703.
22. Bodis-Wollner I, et al. Visual association cortex and vision in man: pattern evoked occipital potentials in a blind boy. Science 1977;198:629–631.
23. Davis ET, Schnider CM, Sherman J. Normative data and control studies of flash VEPs for comparison to a clinical population. Am J Optom Physiol Opt 1987;64:579–592.
24. Weinstein GW. Clinical aspects of the visually evoked potential. Ophthal Surg 1978;9:56–65.
25. Huber C. Amplitude vs. frequency of VEP to sine modulated light in optic nerve disease. Proc ISCERG Symp 13, 1976.
26. Sherman J, Richter SJ, Epstein A. The differential diagnosis of visual disorders in patients presenting with marked symptoms but with no observable ocular abnormality. Am J Optom Physiol Opt 1980;57:516–522.
27. Sherman J, Bass S, Richardson V. The differential diagnosis of retinal disease from optic nerve disease. J Am Optom Assoc 1981;52:933–937.
28. Camisa J, Mylin LN, Bodis-Wollner I. The effect of stimulus orientation of the visual evoked potential in multiple sclerosis. Ann Neurol 1981;10:532–539.
29. Kuppersmith MJ, Seiple WH, Nelson JI. Retrobulbar neuritis: loss of cortically mediated function. ARVO Suppl Invest Ophthalmol Vis Sci 1984;25:312.
30. Bodis-Wollner I, Feldman R. Old perimacular pathology causes VEP delays in man. Electroencephalogr Clin Neurophysiol 1982;53:38P–39P.
31. Vaughan HG, Katzman R. Evoked responses in visual disorders. Ann NY Acad Sci 1964;112:305–319.
32. Ikeda H, Tramain KF, Sanders MD. Neurophysiological investigation in optic nerve disease: combined assessment of the visual evoked response and electroretinogram. Br J Ophthalmol 1978;62:227–239.
33. Celesia G, Kaufman D. Pattern ERGs and visual evoked potentials in maculopathies and optic nerve diseases. Invest Ophthalmol Vis Sci 1985;26:726–735.
34. Marcus MM. The evoked cortical response: a technique for assessing development. Calif Ment Health Res Digest 1970;8:59–72.
35. John ER, et al. Neurometrics. Science 1977;196:1393–1410.

Ophthalmic Ultrasonography

Sherry J. Bass
Jerome Sherman

INTRODUCTION

Definition

Sound has been used clinically as an alternative to light in the diagnostic evaluation of a variety of conditions in many clinical settings. The advantage of sound is that it can pass through opaque tissue and afford a view of what cannot be seen with the eye alone. As the mysteries of fetal development and cardiac structure have been aided by the use of sound waves, so have the mysteries of eyes hidden by dense cataracts and opaque corneas been revealed. Sound waves expose the ominous tumor behind the globe as well as the retinal detachment that may be hiding behind the veil of a media opacity.

History

The development of ophthalmic ultrasonography as we know it today is the result of the efforts of many investigators whose work has spanned many decades.[1] In 1956, Mundt and Hughes were the first to use ultrasonography to demonstrate various ocular diseases. They used the A-scan technique, modeled after the time–amplitude method of echo display used by military radar specialists. Following their work, Oksala helped to establish the basic parameters of the pulse–echo technique, and he studied reflective properties of the globe. Howry developed a technique called compound scanning in which he "viewed" different reflecting surfaces from various angles, thus applying the B-scan technique used by military radar specialists, for the purposes of body scanning. The next phase of ophthalmic ultrasonography development came when Baum and Greenwood developed a B-scanner for the eye

and orbit. Their work set the stage for the eventual development of the immersion or water-bath technique, in which the eye is surrounded by a fluid bath.

An era of communication and interaction followed from 1965 to 1973 when, through the efforts of Nathaniel Bronson, annual conferences were sponsored by the Southhampton Hospital Association. After the 1968 conference, significant advancements occurred. Coleman and his collaborators perfected a B-scan immersion unit that incorporated both A-mode and M-mode. Bronson then developed the first commercially available hand-held contact scanner and introduced a "rapid-scanning" technique used today in ophthalmic ultrasonography. Coleman and his coworkers refined techniques for measuring axial length, anterior chamber depth, and lens thickness. These techniques made possible accurate calculations of intraocular lens implant power.

B-mode techniques continued to enjoy popularity, whereas use of the A-mode declined until Ossoinig's arrival in the United States restimulated enthusiasm for the use of A-mode technique in the diagnosis of ocular disease.

Clinical Use

Sound waves reflect the *structural* integrity of an organ. Although structure sometimes implies function, the use of sound does not provide an accurate measure of *functional* integrity. In ocular assessment, electrophysiologic tests provide an insight into function. These tests are discussed in other chapters. In addition to providing assessment of structural integrity, because of their slow speed, sound waves are used to obtain distance and thickness measurements. These measurements, referred to as *ocular biometry*, have become widely used in intraocular lens implant surgery.

INSTRUMENTATION

Theory

In ocular assessment, one makes use of ultrasound waves, rather than sound waves. An ultrasound wave exhibits frequencies above 20 kHz [1 kHz equals 1000 cycles per second (cps)] and is thus not audible to humans.[2] This differentiates the ultrasonic wave from a sonic wave, which is audible to humans. Ultrasound is an acoustic wave in which compressions and rarefactions occur because of changes in density within solid and fluid substances.[2] Ultrasonic waves can be focused, directed and reflected just like light waves. The high frequencies of ophthalmic ultrasound (about 10 MHz, or 10 million cps), in addition to the small wavelengths, make it possible to achieve detailed resolution of ocular structures. As with light, image resolution is related to the frequency or wavelength, which places a limit on resolution as a result of diffraction and interference effects.

The speed of sound in biologic tissues is approximately 1500 m/sec, and it takes only about 33 microseconds for the sound to travel to the rear of the eye and return. A cathode ray tube is used to display the ultrasonogram. Its face resembles a small television screen and is ideal for measuring such small time intervals.

In ophthalmic ultrasonography, an electrical pulse is applied to a piezoelectric crystal, which in turn generates a short pulse of ultrasound energy. This energy traverses a known path in the eye at 1500 m/sec. As the applied pulse voltage is varied in polarity, the piezoelectric crystal expands and contracts rapidly and ultrasonic vibrations result. Since electrical energy is converted into sound energy, the crystal is acting as a transducer. The ultrasonic pulse is partially reflected at various tissue boundaries because of abrupt changes in the acoustic properties of the tissues. When the re-

flected sound energy returns to the crystal, it is transformed back into electrical energy. Because the duration of a pulse is very small compared with the time between pulses, the same crystal can both transmit and receive the sound.

Use

Displaying the Ultrasonogram

Once the crystal converts electrical energy into sound energy and then back to electrical energy again, the echoes are displayed in graphic form on an oscilloscope screen. There are three display modes in ultrasonography: A-mode, B-mode, and M-mode. Each displays structural information differently, and the type of mode used is dependent on the information one is attempting to extract.

A-MODE DISPLAY. In the A-mode, also referred to as *time-amplitude ultrasonography,* each tissue boundary is displayed graphically as a function of distance along a selected axis (Fig. 58–1). It is a unidimensional display because only one axis is displayed at a time. The amplitude of the echoes on the display are proportional to the sound energy reflected at a specific tissue boundary. The A-mode display is frequently used because of the popularity of intraocular lenses. The axial length of the eye is one of the primary determinants of intraocular lens power and is best measured using the A-mode display. In ocular disease diagnosis, however, A-mode is not the preferred display because it is unidimensional. The term "A-scan" is often used to describe this mode, but it is not an appropriate term, since the transducer is fixed in one position during biometric procedures and is not scanning.

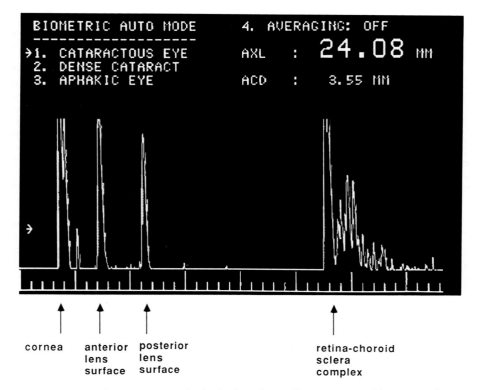

FIGURE 58–1. Characteristic A-mode display from the oscilloscope screen of the Sonomed Digital System. The left most echo is from the cornea, the next two echoes are from the anterior and posterior lens surface, respectively. At the right are echoes from the retina–choroid–sclera complex. The axial length is noted in the upper right corner of the screen. (Courtesy Sonomed, Inc.)

B-MODE DISPLAY. Unlike the unidimensional A-mode display, the B-mode display presents a cross-sectional or two-dimensional image of the eye and the orbit (Fig. 58–2). The transducer undergoes a scanning motion in various planes to produce a two-dimensional display. Since the transducer scans over the globe in this mode, the term "B-scan" is usually used. The circular structure of the globe can be visualized in this mode, unlike in the A-mode, which simply produces reflections along a single axis. The B-mode image is composed of many spots, and the greater the sound energy reflected by a particular tissue boundary, the brighter a particular spot or group of spots will be.

This type of B-mode is also called *intensity-modulated ultrasonography,* and the relative brightness of a particular area of B-scan relative to another area is referred to as the *gray scale.* In a gray scale, there are many gradations of gray, ranging from black to white. This is important, since the relative brightness of a displayed image or echo helps to identify certain tissue. More recently, some systems have capabilities of producing B-scan in color, which may enhance tissue differentiation. In the B-scan mode, the examiner mentally assembles many two-dimensional images into a three-dimensional percept, although recent advances allow computers to assemble this three-dimensional image.[3] This is considerably easier to do than to assemble all the complex unidimensional images of the A-mode to form the same three-dimensional picture.

In addition to ophthalmic ultrasonography, recent applications for B-scan have been in carotid artery testing in patients with visual disturbances[4] and in prenatal ophthalmic imaging.[5]

M-MODE DISPLAY. The M-mode or motion mode, as well as the TM or time–motion mode, are used to monitor the dilatation and constriction of blood vessels. Tissue structures that are stationary produce a display consisting of a series of parallel lines. If the tissue positions fluctuate with time, as in dilatation and constriction of blood vessels, then corresponding variations will occur in the distance between these lines so that a complete time history of the tissue position is portrayed.[6] M-mode systems are used when high-resolution data are required, such as in studies on accommodative fluctuations and vascular pulsation within ocular tumors.[7]

COMMERCIALLY AVAILABLE INSTRUMENTS

In most ultrasound systems, the examiner can perform A-mode, B-mode, and both A- and B-mode simultaneously. The system contains a vector scan dial, which can be used to select any axis on the B-mode, which then is displayed on the cathode ray tube below the B-mode display. The ultrasound is photographed using a Polaroid camera attachment that documents any desired cross-section or A-scan measurement.

Many of the newer ultrasound units utilize a paper recorder with gray scale capabilities to produce the ultrasonogram display. These newer units have microprocessors and are equipped to attach to video cameras for a dynamic display of the ultrasonogram, which can be recorded on tape for future viewing.

The most popular commercial ophthalmic ultrasound systems make use of computerized digital scanners. Others use analog presentation for theoretically better resolution. Although there are many ultrasound units on the market, only the newer, more popularly used systems will be discussed. One such unit is the Sonomed A/B-3000 Digital Scanner from Sonomed Technology, Inc. (Lake Success, New York) (Fig. 58–3). Images are processed by a computer designed to digitally enhance and to detect detail. The Digital Scanner provides real-time and processed images with simultaneous A- and B-mode display. An optional computerized color-imaging system is said to enhance tissue differentiation. Sonomed also has separate A-mode and B-mode digital scanners. There is an automatic readout in the A-mode only when the correct alignment is achieved and axial length is most accurate.

Cooper Vision Inc., (Irvine, California) also manufactures digital ultrasound systems (Fig. 58–4). This company's Ultrascan II Digital Scan Converter has a small Auditor handpiece that increases imaging angles to 50°. The Ultrascan II also employs real-time imaging video as well as photographic documentation, separate A-mode and B-mode systems, and simultaneous A- and B-mode presentations, in which a simulated three-dimensional image is displayed.

Biophysic Medical, Inc. (Pleasant Hill, California) manufactures the Ophthascan unit (Fig. 58–5A), which is capable of sepa-

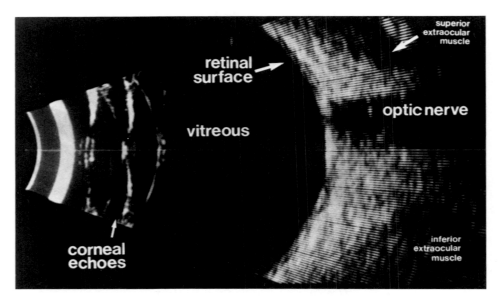

FIGURE 58–2. B-mode ultrasonogram of a normal eye. Note the corneal echo on the extreme left. The vitreous is sonolucent and appears dark. The retina–choroid–sclera complex is on the right. Note the sonolucent V-shaped optic nerve and superior and inferior extraocular muscles. (Courtesy Biophysic Medical, Inc.)

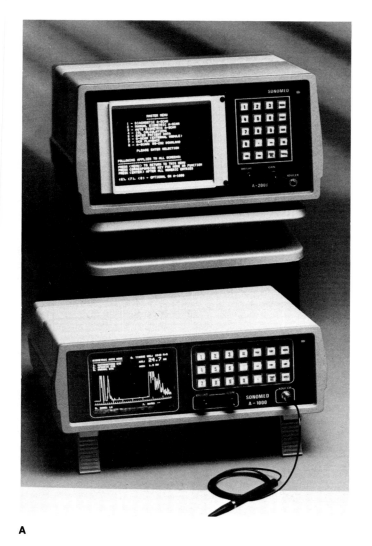

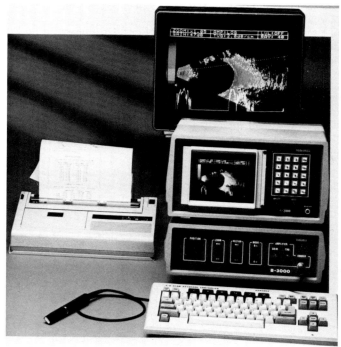

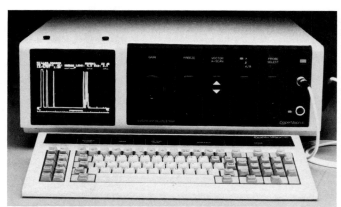

FIGURE 58–3. (*A*) Sonomed A-1000 and 2000 Digital Scanners; (*B*) Sonomed B-3000 Scanner. (Courtesy Sonomed, Inc.)

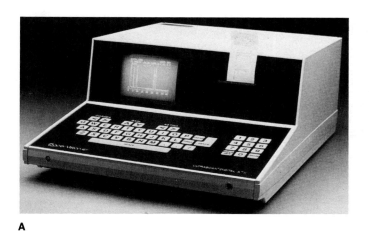

FIGURE 58–4. (*A*) Ultrascan Digital AII by Cooper Vision, Inc.; (*B*) Ultrascan Digital B1000. (Courtesy Cooper Vision, Inc.)

rate A-mode, B-mode, and simultaneous A and B mode ultrasonography. Analog presentation of the ultrasonogram is used for theoretically better resolution, rather than digital format, as other ultrasound systems use. The Ophthascan unit is the only one on the market that uses analog presentation. The Paxial unit (see Fig. 58–5*B*) is capable of performing biometry and pachymetry in either an automode, in which the instrument decides the correct alignment, or a manual mode.

The Storz Instrument Company, (St. Louis, Missouri) manufactures the Alpha II for A-mode ultrasound and intraocular lens power calculation, and the OMEGA, which can be used for A-mode measurements or pachymetry or both (Fig. 58–6).

CLINICAL PROCEDURE

The examination procedure on most ultrasound systems is fairly simple, providing no abnormalities are present. In the A-mode, the patient is seated at an instrument similar to a slit lamp, and a probe

is placed on the cornea as in Goldmann tonometry (Fig. 58–7). Some systems use a hand-held probe. Once the alignment is correct, many systems then automatically display the A-mode ultrasonogram with accurate axial length measurement (see Fig. 58–1).

In B-mode ultrasonography the patient is in a comfortable sitting or lying position with eyelids closed (Fig. 58–8). A coupling agent, such as gonioscopic methylcellulose, is applied to the scanning head or the closed lid. Since high-frequency sound waves are not transmitted through air, the probe must be coupled with the lid using a coupling agent. This causes no discomfort to the patient.

Performing B-mode ultrasonography requires that the examiner move the scanning head over the closed lid in all directions to obtain representative cross-sections of the globe. The sensitivity control should also be varied during the examination procedure. The sensitivity control allows the examiner to estimate the relative acoustic densities of various tissues. If a particular ocular structure or substance has a high acoustic density, like calcium, for example, it will reflect sound waves (and thus be visible on the screen) even at a low sensitivity setting. The initial examination is performed at the highest sensitivity, so that even weak echoes from objects with low acoustic densities will be detected.

In a typical B-scan of a normal eye (see Fig. 58–2), the ante-

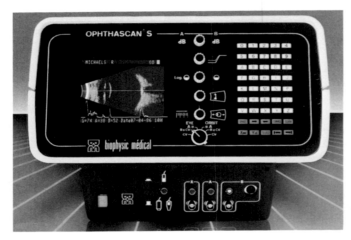

A

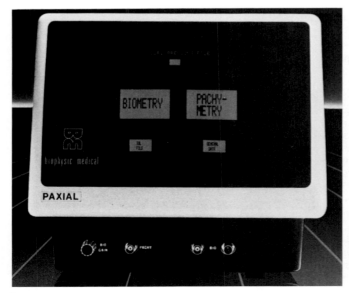

B

FIGURE 58–5. (*A*) Ophthascan B-scan unit by Biophysic Medical, Inc.; (*B*) Paxial unit for A-scan biometry and pachymetry. (Courtesy Biophysic Medical, Inc.)

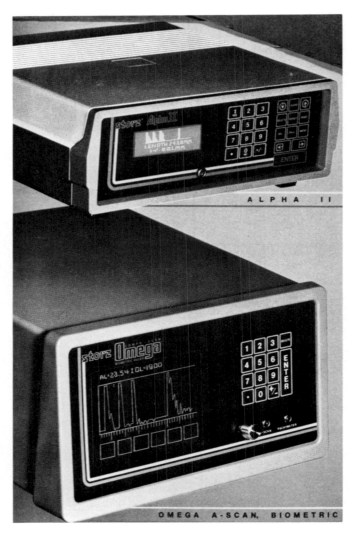

FIGURE 58–6. Storz Alpha II and OMEGA ultrasound systems. (Courtesy Storz)

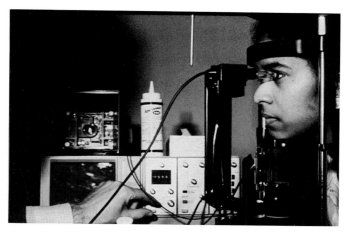

FIGURE 58–7. In the A-mode, the patient is seated in an instrument similar to a slit lamp. A probe is placed on an anesthetized cornea as in Goldmann tonometry, and the axial length is measured. The probe may also be hand-held.

rior portion of the eye is not visualized well, although there are special procedures in which the eye is immersed in a water-bath to get a better view of anterior segment structures. The posterior lens capsule may be observed behind the position of the closed lid and cornea which is at the extreme left of the screen. The vitreous and optic nerve tissue reflect sound poorly and are termed *sonolucent.* As a result, these structures appear black as opposed to structures that reflect sound well, which appear white or as shades of gray.

As mentioned previously, the better a structure or object reflects sound, the brighter the reflection will be. The black horizontal V-shaped optic nerve is an important landmark in B-mode ultrasonography. If the nerve head is elevated, this can be seen by locating the optic nerve. In the normal eye, the retina appears as a smooth concave surface with a sharp acoustic boundary on the right of the screen, which gradually disappears as the sensitivity is reduced. The echoes arising from the retina are generally indiscernible from the echoes arising from the choroid and sclera. If a white sheetlike echo is observed in the normally dark vitreous, then the sensitivity should be reduced to estimate its relative acoustic density. If the white reflection is still visible, even after the sensitivity is reduced to a low level, then the echo seen in the vitreous is likely to be retinal tissue. If the echo disappears while

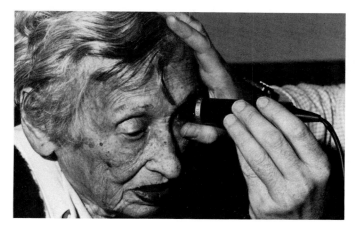

FIGURE 58–8. In B-mode ultrasonography, the patient is either seated or in a supine position. Ultrasonic gel or methylcellulose is placed on the probe or on the lid, and the probe is placed against a closed lid.

the sensitivity is still relatively high, then the echo is probably vitreal tissue. Echoes from blood disappear earlier than those from retinal tissue, but later than those from vitreal tissue.

CLINICAL IMPLICATIONS

Clinical Significance

Ultrasonography is certainly not a routine clinical procedure. It is considered a supplemental test, ordered when additional information is not readily available by routine examination procedures. In general, ultrasonography is performed when it is difficult to observe the fundus directly, as with media opacities. It is also performed when it is desirable to view the orbital tissue behind the globe—tissue also not directly observable. In addition, ultrasonography provides information about elevation and depression in certain lesions, and is invaluable in the exact determination of axial length for IOL power calculation. Ultrasonography is not used only for the detection of anomalies, but also to follow the course of a disease process that can change over time.

Clinical Interpretation

Ophthalmic ultrasonography has numerous clinical applications, some of which will be discussed here. The reader is referred to other sources for additional information.[2,8]

Vitreal Abnormalities

The vitreous is normally acoustically silent and, therefore, appears dark or clear on an ultrasonogram. Besides retinal detachments and fibroproliferative membranes, other abnormalities will result in white reflections on the screen. These include vitreous hemorrhage, vitreal membranes, asteroid hyalosis, intraocular foreign bodies, and inflammatory debris. Not all of these are easily discernible, even by the most experienced ultrasonographer. Some vitreous opacities reflect sound better than others and will still be evident even as the sensitivity is decreased. The use of gray scales is helpful in differentiating vitreous opacities of varying acoustical densities. With this scale, the whitest reflections represent the most acoustically dense opacities, which disappear late as the sensitivity is reduced. Those opacities that appear gray with this scale represent less acoustically dense opacities and disappear early with decreasing sensitivity.

Dense hemorrhage precludes funduscopic evaluation, but not ultrasonography. Dense hemorrhages appear as irregular white or gray areas on the screen. If the reflections move as the patient moves the eye, then the vitreal hemorrhage is fluid. If motion is dampened upon eye movement, then the vitreal hemorrhage is more likely to be solid. Hemorrhages can also be localized as anterior or posterior. It is prognostically helpful to determine location and density, since it has been shown that posterior hemorrhages of light density and in fluid vitreous have a greater than 50% chance of clearing, whereas denser hemorrhages into solid vitreous have only a 33% chance of clearing.[9]

Asteroid hyalosis is a vitreal condition in which calcium soaps accumulate and disperse throughout the vitreous (Fig. 58–9A). It appears similar to vitreal hemorrhage, but can be differentiated from the latter by its acoustical density. Because calcium is an excellent reflector of sound, asteroid hyalosis particles disappear late as the sensitivity is decreased (see Fig. 58–9B) and well after blood disappears, as blood is less acoustically dense than is calcium. In addition, instructing the patient to move the eye will result in movement of the calcium particles. In cases of longstanding vitreal hemorrhage, the white reflection will not move as the eye rotates. In cases of vitreal hemorrhage in a fluid vitreous, one must rely on changing the sensitivity to differentiate vitreal hemorrhage from asteroid hyalosis.

Intraocular foreign bodies can appear in the vitreous as well. However, these are often associated with inflammatory debris and vitreal hemorrhage and are sometimes difficult to discern or differentiate in ultrasonography. Intraocular foreign bodies will be discussed later in this chapter.

Retinal Abnormalities

RETINAL DETACHMENT. Normally, the retina appears on a B-mode ultrasonogram as a concave, smooth white surface, which

is indistinguishable and inseparable from the choroid and sclera (however, the resolution of some of the newer ultrasonography systems may enable differentiation of the retina from the choroid). In retinal detachment, however, the retina will appear as a thin white membrane separate from the choroid and sclera. The extent of any retinal detachment is best ascertained by performing many B-mode scans in serial, horizontal places, starting from the superior limbus and scanning toward the inferior limbus at 2-mm intervals. One can then mentally assemble all the two-dimensional scans to make a three-dimensional construct of the detachment.

The patient whose ultrasonogram is depicted in Figure 58–10 presented with reduced vision and a flat retinal detachment at the posterior pole secondary to choroidal congestion. On the ultra-

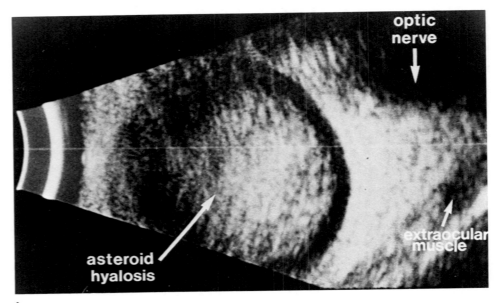

A

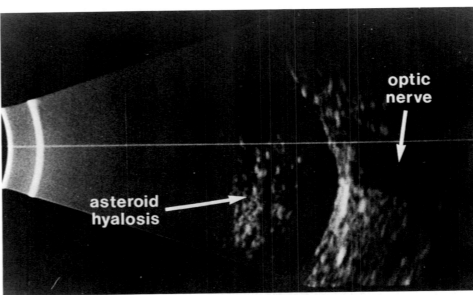

B

FIGURE 58–9. (*A*) Asteroid hyalosis or calcium soaps in the vitreous are easy to detect in B-scan ultrasonography. The reflections change position as the eye moves. (*B*) Because they are calcium particles, the reflections remain long after the sensitivity is reduced and other ocular structures disappear.

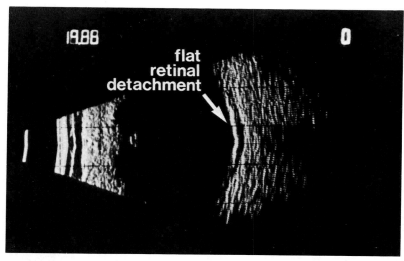

FIGURE 58–10. A flat retinal detachment appears as a thin white line (retina), separated from choroidal tissue by a dark space.

sonogram, the choroid appears to be whiter or denser in that area and thickened. The flat detachment is represented by a thin white membrane (retina), separated from the choroid tissue by a dark space.

Flat detachments can be observed by ultrasonography, but the space between the detached retina and choroid–sclera complex is narrow and may be difficult to discern by the less-experienced ultrasonographer.

On the other hand, a complete bullous retinal detachment is unmistakable in its appearance. The echoes of a highly elevated detachment appear on the ultrasonogram as a convex-shaped white reflection that extends anteriorly into the vitreous from points of attachment at the temporal and nasal ora serrata and the

optic nerve, giving the appearance of a *V*. The V-shaped appearance of the retinal detachment will be obtained only in a total retinal detachment in which the cross-sections viewed are through the optic nerve. Other cross-sections will be depicted differently. As mentioned previously, the three-dimensional picture is a sum of the two-dimensional tracings, and the examiner must mentally construct an overall picture from the two-dimensional sections (a task already being assumed by some computers).

The patient whose ultrasonogram is depicted in Figure 58–11 had a very dense cataract secondary to trauma. The patient had hand motion acuity and wanted to know if removing the cataract would noticeably improve his vision. Since ophthalmoscopy was impossible, ophthalmic ultrasonography was the tool with which

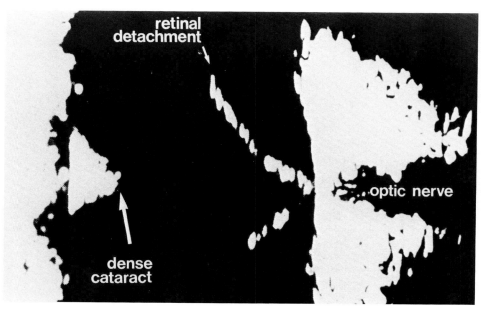

FIGURE 58–11. This patient had a dense cataract that precluded view of the fundus. A total long-standing retinal detachment is evident on the ultrasonogram. He also had flat VEPs and ERGs. Surgery (cataract removal) was not recommended. This ultrasonogram is from a Bronson–Turner unit, not commonly used today.

to assess structural integrity. The B-mode ultrasonogram showed the V-shaped appearance of a total retinal detachment. The functional integrity of the visual system in a patient such as this should be assessed by the bright flash visual-evoked potential (VEP) and the bright flash electroretinogram (ERG). Both were not recordable in this patient. The patient, therefore, could be advised that in view of the ultrasonogram, and flat VEP and ERG, surgical extraction of the cataract was not recommended.

Sometimes blood in the vitreous, as seen in a vitreal hemorrhage, adhering to the posterior vitreal face can be mistaken for a retinal detachment. The two conditions can be differentiated by lowering the sensitivity of the instrument. Since retinal tissue is a better reflector of sound than is blood, echoes from blood disappear earlier than those from retinal tissue. In addition, blood almost never appears as a thin membrane, as can the retina. Although blood may form at the face of a posterior vitreal detachment (PVD), it still appears "thicker." A dense vitreal membrane sometimes, but rarely, can also be mistaken for a retinal detachment. One way to differentiate the two conditions is to look at amplitudes of the reflections, best observed in the A-mode. Echoes from retinal tissue have a higher amplitude than echoes from vitreal membranes. Here, a simultaneous A-mode examination is a useful procedure. The two conditions can also be differentiated by using functional tests, such as an ERG and VEP, which will

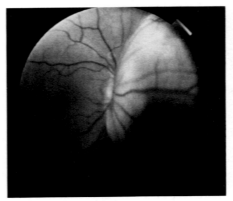 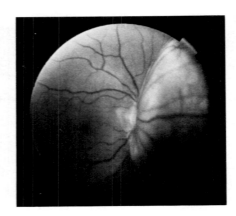

A

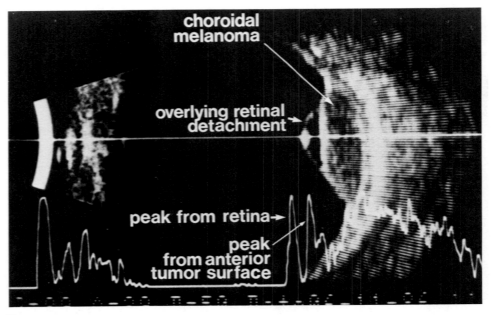

B

FIGURE 58–12. (*A*) A large nonrhegmatogenous nasal retinal detachment is evident in the right eye of this patient who had complained of cloudy vision in that eye. The elevated retina can be appreciated stereoscopically when converging on a point in front of the photographs. The cause of this detachment was not clear until ultrasonography was performed. (*B*) The ultrasonogram of the right eye shows an elevated convex mass, characteristic of malignant melanoma. Note the overlying retinal detachment with fluid separating the retina from the anterior tumor surface. The cross-vector A-mode ultrasonogram displays separate peaks for the retina and the anterior tumor surface. Because of the analog presentation of the ultrasonogram in this particular instrument, the A-mode peaks are slightly displaced to the left of the corresponding B-mode structures. (Courtesy Biophysic Medical, Inc.)

be normal or near normal when the underlying retina is normal. The exception to this is with a fresh retinal detachment in which testing results may also be nearly normal. However, a fresh retinal detachment will move or undulate as the patient moves the eye, and this can easily be observed during B-mode ultrasonography. Long-standing retinal detachments that usually have fibrous tissue proliferation will have little movement. In advanced diabetes, however, extensive fibroproliferative membranes that may exist are difficult to differentiate from such membranes that have led to traction retinal detachment.

Other retinal abnormalities that can be successfully detected by the experienced ultrasonographer include elevated macular lesions such as macular cysts and disciform macular degeneration.

Intraocular Tumors

The use of B-mode ultrasonography is invaluable in the detection of intraocular tumors, especially those that cause retinal detachment. Since an overlying detachment can hide an insidious etiology, ultrasonography should be performed to exclude the pres-

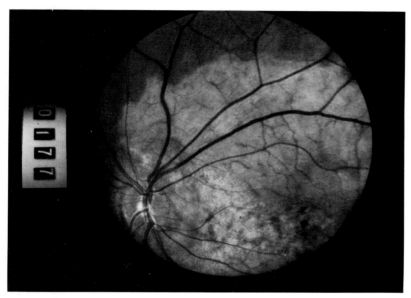

A

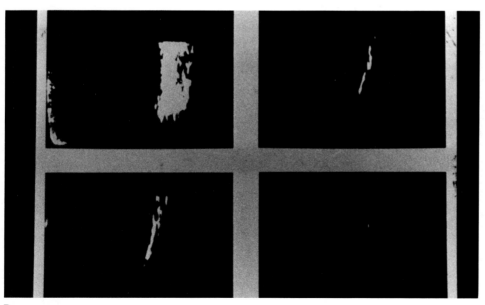

B

FIGURE 58–13. (*A*) A large juxtapapillary cream-colored lesion is evident in this fundus photograph. The appearance and location of this lesion is suggestive of an osseous choristoma, or bony tumor, of the choroid. (*B*) B-mode ultrasonography on a Bronson–Turner unit reveals an acoustically dense, flat lesion at the level of the choroid. This lesion persists at progressively lower sensitivity levels, thereby confirming the diagnosis of a bony tumor of the choroid.

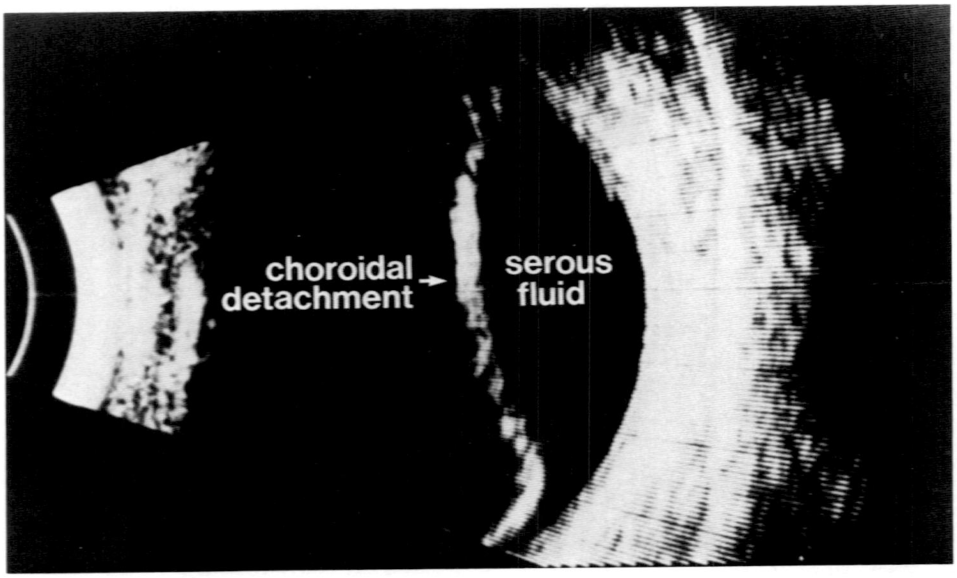

FIGURE 58–14. Serous choroidal detachment is depicted in this ultrasonogram. Note the large sonolucent area between the sclera and the retina–choroid complex. Choroidal detachments, unlike most retinal detachments, are not attached at the optic nerve head. (Courtesy Biophysic Medical, Inc.)

ence of an intraocular tumor in suggestive cases, especially in cases of nonrhegmatogenous retinal detachments (i.e., detachments without holes or tears).

RETINAL TUMORS. The most common malignant intraocular tumor in children is retinoblastoma.[10] Ultrasonography is invaluable when the tumor is concealed by an overlying retinal detachment, inflammation, or vitreal hemorrhage. Any child presenting with a retinal detachment or with blood in the vitreous should have an ultrasonogram to rule out an underlying retinoblastoma, especially in patients for whom there is a family history of such tumors. In addition, B-mode ultrasonography should be performed in cases of opaque media in children in whom the fundus cannot be visualized. B-mode ultrasonography is more valuable than A-mode in demonstrating the presence of a mass in the eye.[11]

Sterns, et al.[12] describe retinoblastomas as being either "solid" or "cystic." A *solid* mass is one that is well-defined, discrete, and touches the retina in all sections studied. A *cystic* mass, on the other hand, may or may not have discrete borders, may contain solid areas interspersed with clear spaces, and may not touch or border the retina in all sections studied.

Although the solid type may be easier to interpret, the cystic mass is very difficult to distinguish from a massive vitreal hemorrhage. However, the ultrasonic evaluation of any "mass" in the fellow eye of a patient with known retinoblastoma can still be clinically valuable if the fellow eye has opaque media. If the first eye has a retinoblastoma, the mass viewed ultrasonically in the fellow eye is most likely to be retinoblastoma as well.

CHOROIDAL TUMORS. Ultrasound is valuable in distinguishing solid choroidal tumors from those lesions that resemble choroidal tumors, but which are filled with serous fluid or blood. A-mode ultrasonography is particularly useful in differentiating an acoustically solid ocular tumor from choroidal detachment or retinal detachment with subretinal hemorrhage or fluid. Often, simultaneous A- and B-mode ultrasonography is performed in the assessment of mass lesions.

Malignant Melanoma. Malignant melanoma is the most common neoplastic choroidal tumor and ranges in size from a minimally

elevated mass to one that can extend outside the entire globe.[13] The importance of ultrasonography in the detection of tumors is highlighted in a series[14] in which eyes with clear media and suspected malignant melanomas were enucleated. In 19% of the patients, the clinical diagnosis proved to be incorrect.

Figure 58–12A is the fundus photograph of a 43-year-old man who complained of cloudy vision in the right eye of 1 week's duration. A bullous nasal nonrhegmatogenous retinal detachment was evident in that eye. The cause of the detachment was not clear until ultrasonography was performed. The morphologic and acoustic features of suspected tumors can be studied extensively by using combined A- and B-mode ultrasonography. Figure

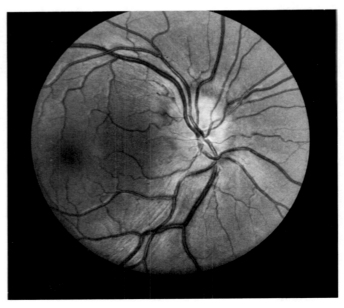

FIGURE 58–15. Note the blurred disc borders in this fundus photograph of the right eye of a 12-year-old boy.

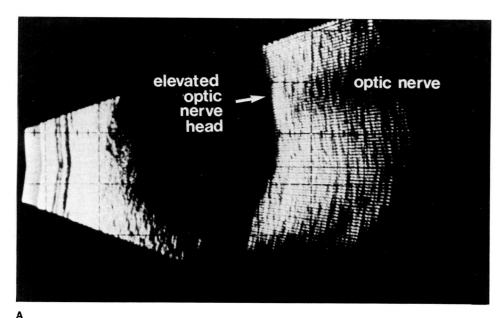

A

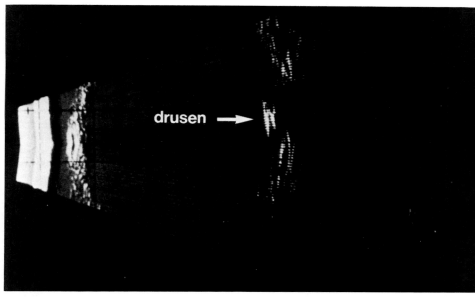

B

FIGURE 58–16. (*A*) Ultrasonography at a high-sensitivity level reveals an elevated optic nerve head. (*B*) Reducing the sensitivity, however, reveals buried calcified drusen, long after other ocular structures disappear from the screen.

58–12*B* demonstrates an elevated convex mass with overlying retinal detachment. This is a typical ultrasonographic configuration of malignant melanoma. Note the cross-vector A-mode demonstrating separate peaks for the retina and anterior tumor surface.

When Bruch's membrane is intact, this convex mass will be seen. If the tumor breaks through Bruch's membrane, then a "collar-button" shape is evident. Ultrasonography enables the clinician not only to localize the tumor, but to monitor its growth as well. Since about 10% of eyes with opaque media may harbor malignant melanoma,[15] it is especially important to perform ultrasonography in these eyes.

Malignant melanoma must be differentiated from metastatic carcinoma, hemangioma, and subretinal hemorrhage. Although the morphologic and acoustic characteristics of these differ, it is often very difficult to make the differential diagnosis by ultrasonography alone.

Osseous Choristoma of the Choroid. A bone tumor of the choroid is extremely rare, but B-scan ultrasonography can be invaluable in making the diagnosis. An 11-year-old asymptomatic girl presented with 20/25 visual acuity in the left eye. Ophthalmoscopy revealed a large, slightly elevated, well-defined creamy yellow lesion (Fig. 58–13*A*). Because of its position near and around the disc, it was thought to be an osseous choristoma or bone tumor of the choroid. Because it could have also been an amelanotic malignant melanoma, B-mode ultrasonography was performed and revealed

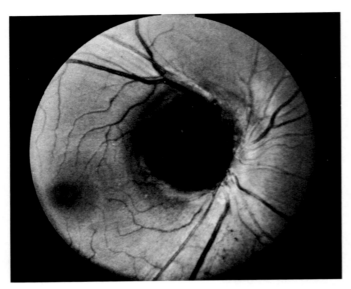

FIGURE 58–17. Melanocytomas are elevated benign collections of melanocytes that cover part or all of the optic nerve head.

a flat lesion at the level of the choroid. The persistent echoes, even at low sensitivity levels, were typical of tissue containing calcium (see Fig. 58–13*B*); hence, the diagnosis of a bone tumor of the orbit could be made.

Conditions to Be Differentiated from Choroidal Tumors. There are retinal and choroidal lesions that may simulate choroidal tumors and must be differentiated from them. Retinal detachment, retinoschisis, certain cases of chorioretinitis, and disciform macular degeneration, all show elevated vitreoretinal interface echoes. However, the acoustically sonolucent subretinal spaces distinguish these conditions from choroidal tumors. Most benign choroidal nevi do not show significant elevation on B-mode ultrasonography and, thus, can be differentiated from tumors that are elevated. Choroidal detachments present typically as a convex elevation that is attached at the ora serrata with a sonolucent area between the retina–choroid complex and sclera (Fig. 58–14). Dense reorganized vitreous hemorrhages may simulate choroidal tumors because they appear as an acoustically dense mass. However, the collar-button configuration of melanoma is not seen with vitreous hemorrhage, and the acoustic characteristics differ as well. A tumor lying within a dense vitreal hemorrhage, however (a situation more commonly occurring with retinoblastoma as opposed to melanoma[16]), is difficult to diagnose and requires repeated ultrasonic evaluations.

Abnormalities of the Optic Nerve Head

Conditions resulting in elevation of the optic nerve head can often be more greatly appreciated ultrasonically. These include papilledema, papillitis, as well as drusen and melanocytoma of the optic disc. Papillitis and papilledema are difficult to differentiate ultrasonically although a clear subretinal fluid level may be seen with papilledema.[17] In addition, the appearance of the orbital portion of the nerve may be helpful.

DRUSEN OF THE OPTIC NERVE HEAD. Drusen bodies of the optic nerve head are often visible ophthalmoscopically and can give the optic nerve head the appearance of a cluster of grapes. Buried drusen, however, are not visible to the eye and are perhaps the most common cause of pseudopapilledema. Buried drusen are

found in young individuals, and they tend to surface as the individual ages. However, when drusen are buried, ultrasonography is a useful means by which they may be detected. Although the nerve head may appear to be elevated on ultrasonography, the key to making the diagnosis is to lower the sensitivity. Since drusen usually contain calcium, they will often continue to reflect sound long after other tissues have become sonolucent at the lower sensitivity settings. Figure 58–15 is a photograph of the optic nerve head of a 12-year-old boy with normal visual acuity who presented with what appeared to be blurred disc borders in the right eye. The left optic nerve head was normal. Because he complained of headaches (although only in school and never on weekends), the decision had to be made whether an extensive neurologic evaluation was indicated. The results of ultrasonography are shown in Figure 58–16. At a high-sensitivity setting (see Fig. 58–16*A*) the nerve head appears to be slightly elevated, but no significant information is obtained. At a lower sensitivity setting (see Fig. 58–16*B*) all other ocular tissues "drop-out" because they can no longer reflect sound at that sensitivity. The only objects still reflecting sound are the calcified drusen bodies, which then become apparent.

MELANOCYTOMA. Melanocytomas are intraocular tumors that appear ophthalmoscopically as black lesions over the optic disc (Fig. 58–17). They vary in size and shape and are composed of melanocytes. They are benign lesions,[18] and as such are not likely to grow or metastasize. Elevation of melanocytoma can be appreciated ultrasonically as seen in Figure 58–18. The elevation appears to be confined to the optic nerve head and does not appear to infiltrate into the optic nerve. Sometimes a melanocytoma results in reduced visual acuity when it invades the optic nerve. In such cases, ultrasonography will reveal that the mass covering the disc is contiguous with that part of the tumor within the optic nerve itself. Therefore, ultrasonography should be considered in any patient with melanocytoma, to determine if the lesion invades the optic nerve.

PERIPAPILLARY STAPHYLOMA. Peripapillary staphyloma or scleral ectasia is a rare congenital anomaly of the optic nerve. It occurs when the most posterior portion of the sclera fails to develop during embryogenesis.[19] Patients with this condition have a normal or nearly normal optic nerve head that lies at the bottom of a deep excavation (staphyloma) and appears to be receded behind the plane of the retina. This is best appreciated when viewed stereoscopically (Fig. 58–19). The excavation of peripapillary staphyloma can be seen ultrasonically (Fig. 58–20) as a concave depression at the position of the optic nerve head. This depression might be mistaken for optic nerve cupping. However, the standard 10 MHz transducer does not have the capabilities to resolve optic nerve cupping.

Variations in Globe Shape and Size

Extremes in axial length can be easily displayed using B-mode ultrasonography. However, to get an accurate axial length measurement for correct power assessment of intraocular lenses, A-mode ultrasonography must be used.

A common finding in eyes with long axial lengths, as in high myopia, is posterior staphyloma. Although staphylomas can be detected ophthalmoscopically, they can be dramatically displayed by B-mode ultrasonography.

Staphylomas appear as a large, concave, depression in the retina–choroid–sclera complex (Fig. 58–21). If the staphyloma is present in the posterior pole, it can result in a significant increase in myopia. For every 1-mm increase in axial length, there is a 3-diopter increase in myopia. If the staphyloma involves the macula, it is not surprising to find significant increases in visual acuity once the myopia induced by the staphyloma is corrected.

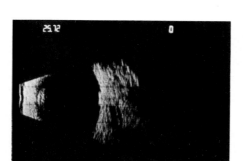
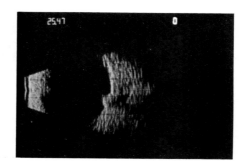
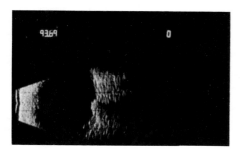
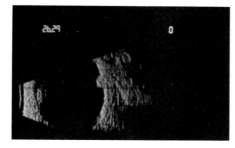

FIGURE 58–18. Ultrasonography in this patient reveals that the melanocytoma is confined to the optic nerve head and does not appear to infiltrate into the optic nerve. Although rare, some melanocytomas may infiltrate into the optic nerve and affect visual function.

Eyes with short axial lengths, as in microphthalmos, can also be displayed ultrasonically. Another condition of diagnostic importance revealed ultrasonically in phthisis bulbi, which is a shrinkage of the globe. This shrinkage results in disorganization of intraocular tissue such that an amorphous mass of tissue is seen on the ultrasonogram.

Ultrasonography becomes very important in eyes with opaque media and especially low intraocular pressures, which is suggestive of phthisis bulbi. Figure 58–22A is the anterior segment photograph of a 16-year-old girl with NLP vision, congenital cataract, and synechiae. Intraocular pressures were estimated to be very low by digital examination and measured about 1 mmHg with Goldmann tonometry. The ultrasonogram (see Fig. 58–22B) revealed no structural integrity to the globe. Surgical intervention in an eye such as this is not recommended.

Intraocular Foreign Bodies

Another clinical application of ultrasonography has been the localization of intraocular foreign bodies and the assessment of their metallic characteristics. The uses of ultrasonography in intraocular foreign body management include (1) localization, (2) axial length measurement in conjunction with x-rays for localization, (3) assessment of damage to the globe, (4) determination of magnetic properties, and (5) extraction of nonmagnetic foreign bodies.

The technique to localize foreign bodies by ultrasonography has been described in detail by Bronson.[20] The search for and identification of foreign bodies is extremely time-consuming compared with routine ocular diagnosis. Sometimes, foreign bodies are surrounded by hemorrhage. The sensitivity then has to be reduced so that the hemorrhage is not seen. Varying the sensitivity

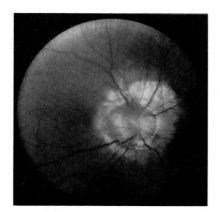
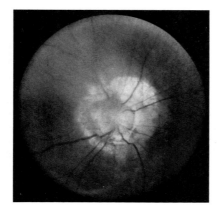

FIGURE 58–19. The optic nerve head lies at the bottom of a deep excavation in this congenital disc anomaly (peripapillary staphyloma). The depth can be appreciated stereoscopically by converging on a point in front of the photograph.

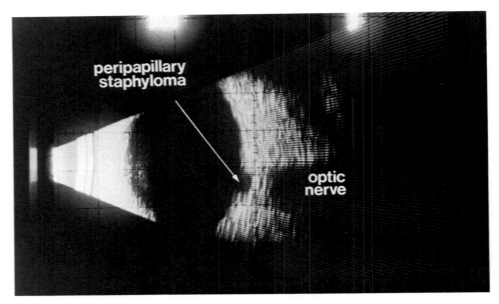

FIGURE 58–20. Peripapillary staphylomas appear on this ultrasonogram as concave depressions in the vicinity of the optic nerve head.

permits differentiation of high-amplitude echoes produced by most foreign bodies from lower-amplitude echoes emanating from the surrounding hemorrhage. The ultrasonogram shown in Figure 58–23 reveals a steel BB pellet lying underneath detached retina. Note the sonic "tail" or reduplication echo behind the BB pellet. This tail is caused by reflection of sound from the BB pellet.

Magnetic foreign bodies can be identified using an ultrasonic display of the motion of the foreign body when a magnet is applied to the globe, placed in a position over the pars plana. Foreign bodies of glass, plastic, and wood require serial sections for exact localization.

LENS DISLOCATION. Since ultrasonography is valuable in the detection and localization of intraocular foreign bodies, it is just as useful in finding a subluxated or dislocated lens. Often, subluxated or dislocated lenses, secondary to trauma or associated systemic disorders, are difficult, if not impossible to view ophthalmoscopically or biomicroscopically. In these cases, ultrasonography may

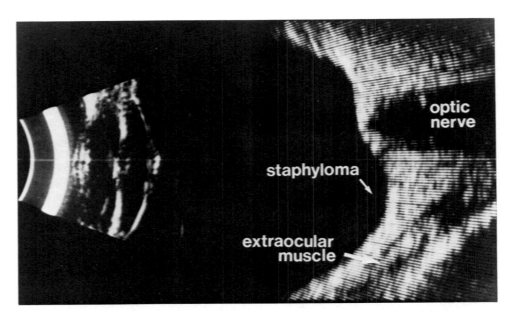

FIGURE 58–21. High myopes may have large staphylomas in the posterior pole. These appear as concave depressions in the retina–choroid–sclera complex. Accurate axial measurements are difficult if not impossible to obtain. (Courtesy Biophysic Medical, Inc.). Compare the depression in this figure with the smaller peripapillary staphyloma in Figure 58–20.

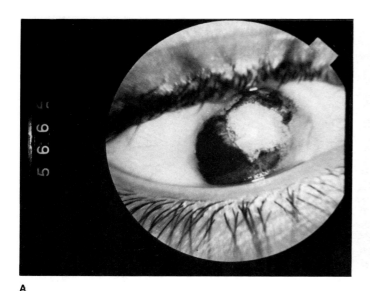 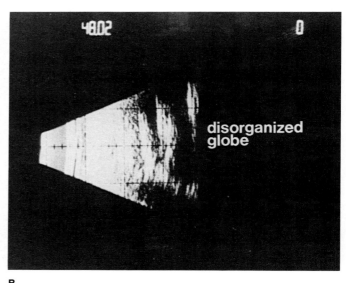

A   **B**

FIGURE 58–22. (*A*) This patient had a congenital cataract with NLP vision. (*B*) The ultrasonogram shows a shrunken disorganized globe with no structural integrity evident, a condition known as phthisis bulbi.

be the only way to locate these lenses. Figure 58–24 shows the ultrasonogram of a transverse view of a dislocated cataractous lens with a vitreous detachment.

Orbital Diagnosis

Since the orbit, unlike the retina, cannot be viewed directly, ultrasonography is invaluable in the detection of abnormalities that may be overlooked by ophthalmoscopy. In orbital diagnosis, the B-mode is ideal for the identification and delineation of orbital anomalies. A-mode analysis and dynamic scanning add information to the pattern obtained from the B-mode.

Ultrasonography of the orbit is useful in many situations including the following:

- Unilateral proptosis or bilateral exophthalmos
- Choroidal folds or retinal striae
- Unexplained optic atrophy or papilledema
- Palpation of a cyst or mass
- Microphthalmic eye
- Suspected orbital foreign body

Ultrasonography of the normal orbit will reveal a sonolucent V-shaped optic nerve. The extraocular muscles are also sonolucent

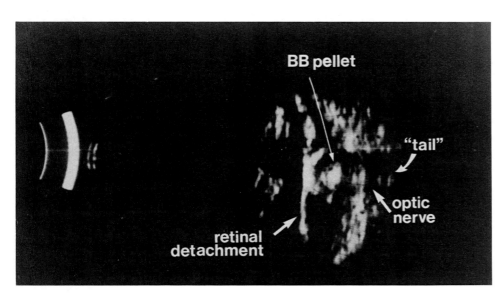

FIGURE 58–23. A steel BB pellet underlies a retinal detachment in this ultrasonogram. The "tail" or reduplication echoes, seen behind the BB are caused by reflection from the BB pellet itself. (Courtesy Biophysic Medical Inc.)

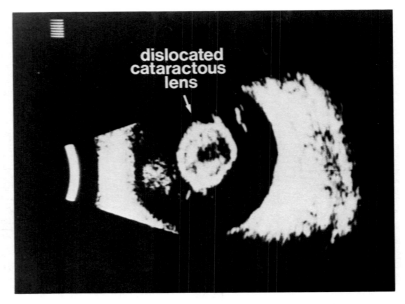

FIGURE 58–24. A transverse view of a dislocated cataractous lens. (Courtesy Biophysic Medical Inc.)

in the normal eye, whereas dense orbital fat is highly acoustic or reflective of sound.

Recall that in the *globe,* abnormalities appear *white* or *gray* against a *black* background. *Orbital* abnormalities, on the other hand, are displayed as *dark* defects against a *white* background (the acoustically dense orbital fat).

Abnormalities in the orbit are divided into three categories: (1) mass lesion, (2) foreign body, (3) inflammatory change. Mass lesions are classified as either round or irregular in shape. They are also classified by either poor transmission (posterior wall of tumor not visible), as in solid tumors and angiomatous tumors, or good transmission (visible posterior wall), as in cystic tumors and infiltrative tumors.

Solid tumors include meningioma, glioma, or neurofibroma. Angiomatous tumors include hemangioma and lymphangioma. Cystic tumors include dermoids and mucocele, whereas infiltrative tumors include lymphoma and metastatic cancer.

The patient whose ultrasonogram is pictured in Figure 58–25 complained of reduced vision in her right eye for 3 to 4 years, with lid swelling for the last 2 to 3 years. Pupillary testing revealed a

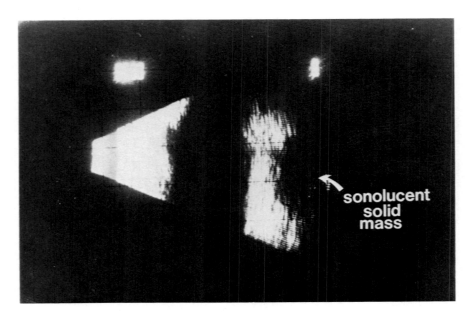

FIGURE 58–25. This is an ultrasonogram of the eye and orbit in a patient with a history of reduced vision and proptosis in the right eye. Ultrasonography reveals a probable solid tumor, since the posterior wall of the tumor is barely visible in the scan. The ultimate diagnosis was meningothelial meningioma of the optic nerve.

Marcus Gunn pupil in that eye. Motilities of the right eye were restricted in superior gaze. Visual acuity was 20/200, and the patient had proptosis of the right eye. Retinal examination revealed pigmentary changes in the posterior pole. The B-mode ultrasonogram shows a large retrobulbar mass. It was round, with little or no evidence of the posterior wall seen in the scan; hence, it fell into the category of a solid tumor. Histopathologic examination of

the mass after its removal confirmed it to be a meningothelial meningioma of the optic nerve.

An example of a rounded cystic tumor is shown in Figures 58–26 and 58–27. The patient was a 7-year-old black boy, with best-corrected visual acuity of 7/140 in the left eye. The left eye was also microphthalmic (3-mm shorter than the right eye); microcornea and an optic pit were also evident. Pupillary testing revealed a

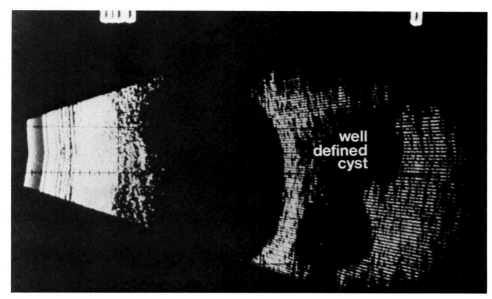

A

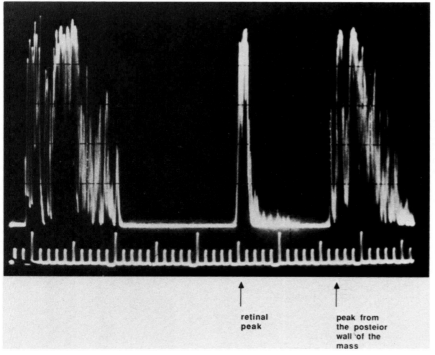

B

FIGURE 58–26. This patient had a microphthalmic eye with an optic pit and reduced vision. (*A*) The ultrasonogram revealed a rounded cystic tumor (posterior wall was visible) within the orbit. (*B*) Note the reflections on A-mode ultrasonography of the retinal peak and the posterior wall of the mass.

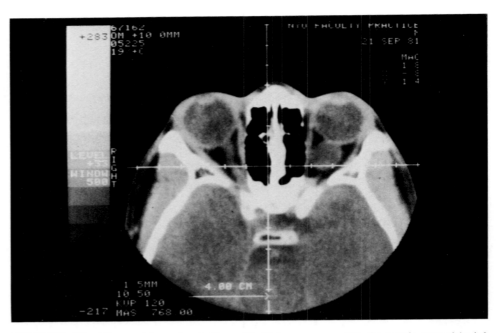

FIGURE 58–27. CT scan of the patient in Figure 58–26 shows a mass within the muscle cone of the left eye. CT is poor at differentiating a solid tumor from a cystic one.

left Marcus Gunn pupil. The ultrasonogram revealed a rounded cystic tumor (the posterior wall was visible), which is typically benign.[21] Despite the presence of the tumor, there was no proptosis and choroidal folds were not evident.

Orbital ultrasonography is also valuable in the evaluation of patients with proptosis or exophthalmos. In such patients, Graves' disease must be ruled out. Orbital ultrasonography will show ac-

centuation of the orbital walls and thickening or enlargement of the extraocular muscles. The wall of the orbit is better outlined than in normal eyes, probably because tissue is compressed against it, thereby rendering it a better reflector of sound.[22] Extraocular muscles, which are normally sonolucent, may appear as enlarged darkened areas in eyes affected by Graves' disease (Fig. 58–28).

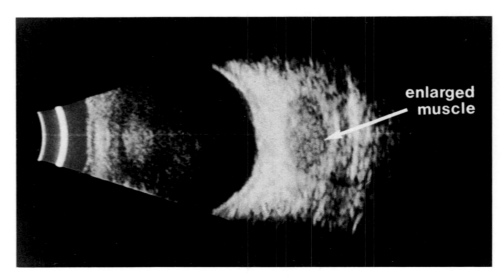

FIGURE 58–28. The extraocular muscles in Graves' disease are often thickened because of infiltration of the muscle. These muscles, which are sonolucent, appear on ultrasonography as enlarged darkened areas. In this ultrasonogram, the medial rectus muscle (*arrow*) is thickened and enlarged.

REFERENCES

1. Purnell EW, Frank KE. Development and orientation of ophthalmic ultrasonography. In: Dallow RL, ed. Ophthalmic ultrasonography: comparative techniques. Intl Ophthalmol Clin 1979;19(4):9–12.
2. Coleman DJ, Lizzi FL, Jack RL. Ultrasonography of the eye and orbit. Philadelphia: Lea & Febiger, 1977:3.
3. Coleman DJ. Advances in diagnostic and therapeutic ultrasound. Ophthalmology 1988;95(suppl 9):137.
4. Gaul JJ, Marks SJ, Weinberger J. Visual disturbance and carotid artery disease. Stroke 1986;17:393–398.
5. Rochels R, Merz E, Goldhofer W. Pranatale ophthalmologische echographie. Fortshr Ophthalmol 1986;83:240–241.
6. Coleman DJ, Lizzi FL, Jack RL. Ultrasonography of the eye and orbit. Philadelphia: Lea & Febiger, 1977:79.
7. Lowe RF. Linear A-scan ultrasonography in the measurement of intraocular distances: a stand-off technique. Trans Ophthalmol Soc Aust 1967;26:72–77.
8. Bronson NR, Fisher YL, et al. Ophthalmic contact B-scan ultrasonography for the clinician. Westport, Conn: Intercontinental Publications, 1976.
9. Coleman DJ, Franzen LA. Vitreous surgery pre-operative evaluation and prognostic value of ultrasonic display of vitreous hemorrhage. Arch Ophthalmol 1974;92:375–381.
10. Reese AB. Tumors of the Eye, 2nd ed. New York: Harper & Row, 1963:84–161.
11. Till P, Ossoinig K. Echography of retinoblastoma. Ber Dtsch Ophthalmol Ges 1969;69:203–209.
12. Sterns GK, Coleman DJ, Ellsworth RM. The ultrasonographic characteristics of retinoblastoma. Am J Ophthalmol 1974;78:606–611.
13. Sherman J. Ophthalmic ultrasonography. In: Terry JE, ed. Ocular disease—detection, diagnosis and treatment. Boston: Butterworth Publishers, 1984:539.
14. Ferry AP. Lesions mistaken for malignant melanoma of the posterior uvea: a clinico-pathologic analysis of 100 cases with ophthalmoscopically visible lesions. Arch Ophthalmol 1964;72:463–469.
15. Mackley TA, Reed RW. Unsuspected intraocular malignant melanomas. Arch Ophthalmol 1958;60:475–478.
16. Coleman DJ, Lizzi FL, Jack RL. Ultrasonography of the eye and orbit. Philadelphia: Lea & Febiger, 1977:239.
17. Coleman DJ, Lizzi FL, Jack RL. Ultrasonography of the eye and orbit. Philadelphia: Lee & Febiger, 1977:245.
18. Shields JA. Melanocytoma of the optic nerve head: a review. Int Ophthalmol 1978;1:31–37.
19. Wise JB, McClean AL, Gass JDM. Contractile peripapillary staphyloma. Arch Ophthalmol 1966;75:626.
20. Bronson NR. Management of foreign bodies. Am J Ophthalmol 1968;66:279–284.
21. Duke-Elder S. System of ophthalmology, normal and abnormal development: congenital deformities, vol 3, part 2. St Louis: CV Mosby Co, 1964.
22. Coleman DJ. Orbital Ultrasonography. In: Jones IS, Jackobies FA, eds. Diseases of the orbit. Hagerstown, Md: Harper & Row, 1979:97–98.

the liver to the body cells, and that, when elevated, are known to be associated with increased risk of coronary disease; and the high-density lipoproteins (HDL), which serve to move cholesterol from the periphery back to the liver and are the "good" lipoproteins inasmuch as they are inversely related to the risk of coronary artery disease. Therefore, although the absolute value of plasma cholesterol is valuable in a screening mode, it is often necessary to also establish HDL and LDL values to better evaluate the clinical picture.

The plasma cholesterol values and atherosclerotic risk have recently been redefined: Normal values are <200 mg/dl; values associated with intermediate risk are between 200 and 240 mg/dl; and high-risk values are those above 240 mg/dl. These are valid for all aged groups.[15]

Clinical Procedure

The patient should be instructed to have an overnight fast and abstain from alcohol for at least 24 hours before collection.

Several methods have been utilized, some of which are manual such as the Abell–Kendall method. Some of the automated methods are colorimetric. The automated method can have some limitations, although these do not prevent the use of the test for clinical decision making.[16]

Clinical Implication

Much has been written in recent years about the association between cholesterol (i.e., certain lipoproteins) and an elevated risk of atherosclerotic disease. Sedentary habits and dietary regimens have also been implicated. Consequently, there is a public awareness of the need for lower plasma cholesterol.

Elevations in cholesterol are also associated with congenital conditions: familial hypercholesterolemia, nephrotic syndrome, diabetes mellitus, hypothyroidism, pancreatitis, and others. Ocular manifestations of hypercholesterolemia are xanthomas, corneal arcus, and Hollenhorst plaques.

Medical conditions associated with low cholesterol values are hyperthyroidism, certain anemias, malabsorption syndromes, and malnutrition.

Creatinine

Definition

Creatinine is a catabolite resulting from muscle metabolism. It is excreted in the urine and is, therefore, utilized as an indication of renal function. For this purpose it is used interchangeably with the blood urea nitrogen (BUN) measurement. However, creatinine levels may provide more substantial information about the severity of the disease.[17] A number of variables affect both; therefore, interpretation must be carefully done.[2,17] Normal values are related to overall body muscle mass and are less in a child or woman and more toward the maximal values in a large muscular man. Accordingly, age, gender, and weight are important characteristics. The relationship between creatinine and creatinine clearance must also be understood.[8]

Clinical Procedure

The common method of measurement is colorimetric, in which an orange-red complex is produced when creatinine reacts with an alkaline picrate solution.[17] Because other substances may interfere, or themselves interact in the reaction, the specimen can be pretreated to ensure that only creatinine is being measured. The patient should fast for 8 hours before collection, and a record of the patient's medications should be made.[1]

Clinical Implication

Elevations in creatinine near or above 2.5 mg/dl reflect moderate to severe renal impairment and mandate further evaluations. Loss of renal function is the main reason for elevation of creatinine, with 50% or greater loss of nephrons being reflected in the elevated creatinine values.

Glucose

Definition

Glucose is the main carbohydrate used in the production of cellular energy. Blood levels are under the control of a number of hormones, primarily insulin and glucagon.

Normal serum values are between 60 and 115 mg/dl fasting, less than 200 mg/dl within a 2-hour postprandial period, and less than 140 mg/dl at the 2-hour point.[23] A National Institutes of Health study suggests less than 140 mg/dl fasting and between 140 and 200 mg/dl at the 2-hour point for plasma glucose.[18,19]

Clinical Procedure

Colorimetric methods are employed in which either Cu^{2+} or Fe^{2+} are reduced by glucose to form colored substances. Other reducing substances may be involved, thereby introducing some error into the measurement. However clear deviations from normal values are clinically indicative.

The patient should be instructed to neither eat nor drink for 12 hours before samples. A list of drugs being taken by the patient should also be recorded.

Clinical Implications

The major clinical implication of hyperglycemia is diabetes mellitus, although other endocrinologic conditions, such as Cushing's syndrome, pheochromocytoma, and hyperthyroidism, also manifest glucose intolerance. Consequently, it is important that a thorough differential process be undertaken in reaching the diagnosis. The more severe the hyperglycemia, the greater is the probability of diabetes mellitus.

The ocular implications for all of the aforementioned endocrinologic entities are well documented elsewhere. Values less than 60 mg/dl are hypoglycemic. These values are not usually detected in routine blood chemistry analyses, but are noted in glucose tolerance tests, especially in the 3- to 5-hour range. This has been attributed to a hyperinsulinemic reaction to the glucose challenge, and most clinicians consider these hypoglycemic values to be clinically important if they drop to 40 mg/dl or lower and are accompanied by symptoms.[21]

Lactate Dehydrogenase

Definition

The enzyme lactate dehydrogenase is widely distributed in the cells of the body where it participates in the glycolytic pathway. There are five isoenzymes that can be utilized in identifying diseases from different parts of the body.

Normal values are between 45 and 120 U/L according to *The Merck Index*,[5] 100–225 U/L according to Walker et al.,[6] and 100–190 U/L according to Wallach.[3] As can be seen, there is much variation, and it is thus best to refer to the range provided by the laboratory, which reflects its method of determination.

Clinical Procedure

The method of measurement is based on the absorbance of nicotinamide adenine dinucleotide (reduced) in the conversion of lactate to pyruvate.

If the test is performed by itself, the patient may eat or drink before the specimen collection, but fasting is essential if it is part of an SMA 12-like procedure.[1]

Clinical Implication

If care has been taken to prevent hemolysis in the specimen, and narcotics or intramuscular injections have not been administered to the patient within 8 hours of collection, slight elevations must be viewed cautiously. If these persist, the possibility of malignancies of one of several organs must be considered. Of more frequent importance are high elevations, which are characteristic of hemolytic and megaloblastic anemias and myocardial infarction.

Aspartate Aminotransferase

Definition

This enzyme, previously referred to as SGOT, is found in heart muscle, liver, kidney, and pancreas, and catalyzes interconversion of amino acids and α-keto acids. Normal values are 7–27 U/L.[1]

Clinical Procedure

The technique involves the formation of oxaloacetate and its conversion to malic acid and nicotinamide-adenine dinucleotide in the presence of malic dehydrogenase. Spectrophotometry is then employed in the UVA range.

Clinical Implications

This enzyme measurement is of greatest use in establishing injury. Its levels rise to a peak 24 to 36 hours after injury and, thereafter, return to normal within 5 to 7 days.

The test is utilized in the diagnosis of myocardial infarction, as well as in damage to other organs in which it is found. Since there are no isoenzymes, it should be used in conjunction with other tests.

Phosphorus

Definition

The measurement of phosphorus can be confusing in its terminology. It refers to the serum inorganic phosphate, which is ionized monobasic and dibasic phosphate, but does not involve the organic esters. The phosphorus and calcium levels are interrelated by virtue of their association with parathormone; therefore they are reviewed together. Normal levels are 2.5–4.5 mg/dl.

Clinical Procedure

Colorimetric methods are employed in which phosphomolybdate is reduced to molybdenum blue.[22]

The patient should be instructed to fast for 8 hours before collection. Water is permissible. Because of diurnal variations, the specimen should be collected in the morning.

Clinical Implications

The most common condition leading to hyperphosphatemia is chronic renal failure when the glomerular filtration rate has been significantly reduced. Other conditions are hypoparathyroidism, hyperthyroidism, and hypervitaminosis D.

Hypophosphatemia is associated with primarily hyperparathyroidism, but also with childhood rickets, rapid correction of hyperglycemia, and diabetic ketoacidosis, cirrhosis, and chronic use of certain antacids.

Total Protein and Albumin

Definition

Total plasma protein refers to albumin and the globulins found in the blood. The measurement actually also includes the serum enzymes, antibodies, and other proteins not chemically falling into the foregoing categories. The normal ranges are listed in Table 60–12.

Clinical Procedure

A colorimetric method is employed in which cupric ion interacts with protein to form a blue complex. This is called the biuret procedure. Similarly, albumin is measured colorimetrically through this procedure which involves the formation of an albumin–bromcresol green complex that absorbs at 600 nm.[23]

Clinical Implication

Although the globulin portion includes all of the α-, β-, and γ-globulins, the albumin portion is of specific importance in maintaining colloid osmotic pressure and is a carrier vehicle within the blood stream. Decreases in albumin are significant and result in a tendency to edematous states, including retinal edema, as well as reduced transport of substances. Low levels of albumin may be associated with volume expansion, the nephrotic syndrome, or others. Elevations in globulins are seen in certain chronic inflammations, granulomatous diseases, and advanced cirrhosis. Often these are accompanied by decreases in albumin or one of the globulins, whereas another is increased. The electrophoretic patterns can be used for further determinations.

Blood Urea Nitrogen

Definition

Urea is the end product of nitrogenous waste from protein degradation and is normally excreted by the kidney. In the absence of dietary factors, such as high or excessive protein intake, which would increase liver urea synthesis, this measurement basically reflects the ability of the kidney to eliminate urea. Normal values are 5–25 mg/dl.[20]

Clinical Procedure

The automated systems utilize the Fearon reaction, in which a yellow chromagen is formed.[24] The patient may be instructed to fast for 8 hours before collection.

Table 60–12
Protein and Albumin Normal Serum Values[1]

Constituent	Serum Value (g/dl)
Total protein	6.0–8.0
Albumin	3.5–5.5
Globulins	2.3–3.5

Clinical Implications

The BUN test is a good screening test for kidney function. Excessive urea production can be determined, and blood urea increases more commonly involve factors that interfere with glomerular filtration or tubular obstructions. Therefore, an elevated BUN is associated with renal failure; prerenal failure, as would occur with diminished blood supply; or postrenal failure, as with obstructive prostatic enlargement in elderly men. Elevations greater than 75 mg/dl are serious and should be aggressively pursued.[1,5]

Uric Acid

Definition

Uric acid is the purine catabolite that is excreted by the kidney. Normal values are 4.0–8.5 mg/dl in males and 2.7–7.3 mg/dl in females.[1]

Clinical Procedure

The automated measurement of uric acid is based on the production of tungsten blue by its interaction of uric acid with phosphotungstic acid.[25] This method does have some problems and can actually report levels slightly higher than true values. For the situation in which significant elevations are detected, enzymatic methods should be employed.

Clinical Implications

There are mild hyperuricemic conditions that are idiopathic. However, hyperuricemia is usually associated with gout, chronic renal failure, and a variety of other conditions. Inasmuch as gout is recognized as being involved in certain keratopathic and uveitic conditions, elevation in uric acid may be clinically significant.

VDRL and ART

Definition

The *Venereal Disease Research Laboratory test* (VDRL) and the *automated reagin test* are screening tests for the detection of reagin, a protein formed as a result of treponemal infection. The tests reflect the disease activity and, therefore, are valuable in judging the effectiveness of treatment.[26]

Clinical Procedure

The procedure involves heating serum and, thereby, flocculating the antigen cardiolipin–lecithin.[27]

Clinical Implications

Although this test is an excellent screening test for syphilis and is convenient for monitoring the effectiveness of treatment, the numerous false-positive results make it necessary to use the FTA–ABS test for confirmation.

FTA–ABS

Definition

The fluorescent treponemal antibody–absorption test (FTA–ABS) is a very specific treponemal test that is positive 3 to 4 weeks after infection.[5]

Clinical Procedure

Testing is performed on serum and involves use of *Treponema pallidum* antigen to form an antigen–antibody complex. Conjugation with fluorescein and examination with a fluorescence microscope permit detection.

Clinical Implication

This test is used as a confirmatory test, although it, too, may have a small percentage of false-positive findings associated with it.

Tuberculin

Definition

The routine screening test for tuberculosis is one that utilizes purified protein derivative (PPD) coated onto four prongs, which are then used to puncture the skin. The degree of enduration is measured at the site of puncture 48 to 72 hours thereafter.

Enduration (not reddening) equal to or greater than 10-mm diameter is positive, whereas that between 5 and 9 mm is questionable.[28]

Clinical Procedure

As noted, the test uses PPD that has been coated onto four prongs. The depression of the unit with the four prongs occurs over a cleaned area of the volar surface of the arm. This deposits the antigen at the puncture sites. The test is read 48 to 72 hours later, and the widest diameter of enduration, if any, is measured.

Clinical Implications

It must be emphasized that a positive reaction indicates previous exposure to *Mycobacterium tuberculosis* only and does not necessarily indicate an active infection. Once exposed, patients will always react positively to the test (with very few exceptions).[29] If a positive reaction occurs, the patient should be retested with the intradermal Mantoux test.

Oral Glucose Tolerance Test

Definition

The oral glucose tolerance test measures the body's ability to respond to a specific glucose load over a defined time. The criteria recommended by the National Diabetes Data Group are that an abnormal fasting level is one over 140 mg/dl, whereas a 2-hour level above 200 mg/dl with one other value above 200 mg/dl is considered clearly diagnostic. A 2-hour value between 140 and 200 mg/dl, with another level above 200 mg/dl, implies impaired glucose tolerance.[19]

Clinical Procedure

The patient is instructed to ingest a normal diet containing at least 150 g of carbohydrate for 3 days before the test and then report to the laboratory early in the morning after an overnight fast. Blood is initially drawn to measure a fasting glucose level. The patient then drinks 75 g of glucose, after which blood is repeatedly drawn at 30-minute intervals for 2 to 3 hours.

Clinical Implications

A clearly abnormal value indicating hyperglycemia suggests diabetes mellitus, although it must be emphasized that other endocrinologic disorders, such as Cushing's syndrome, pheochromocytoma, acromegaly, and use of various drugs may also cause hyperglycemia.

Kveim Test

Definition

The Kveim test, used in the diagnosis of sarcoidosis, is done with a suspension of spleenic tissue from an affected patient.

Clinical Procedure

The suspension is injected intradermally, and the skin is inspected 5 to 6 weeks thereafter for presence of a papule. A biopsy of the papule will reveal the presence of granulomas if the patient is suffering from sarcoidosis.

Clinical Implication

The test is useful in the early stages of the disease, and results will be positive for 60% to 85% of affected patients.[26,30] However, it is not used frequently and is not necessarily available. Other tests include histologic diagnosis by bronchoscopy and lung biopsy.

Thyroid Studies

Definition

Thyroid studies ascertain the levels of plasma thyroxine (T_4), plasma triiodothyronine (T_3), free thyroxine index (FTI or T_7), and can involve measurement of antithyroglobulin antibodies in the diagnosis of Graves' disease.

Clinical Use

The most common use of these tests by optometrists is in the diagnosis of Graves' disease for which proptosis may or may not be present. Certainly, any systemic signs of hyperthyroidism in addition to patient's signs and symptoms of corneal drying, stare, or lid lag indicate the need for screening for hyperthyroidism.

Clinical Procedure

There are several procedures involved. The direct measurement of T_4 and T_3 occurs by radioimmunoassay (RIA), which involves competitive binding by the endogeneous hormone and a radioactively labeled exogenous hormone for binding sites on an antibody.[31] The free thyroxine index (T_7) is actually derived from T_4 and the T_3 RU tests (T_3 resin uptake, also called thyroxine-binding globulin index). The latter test, T_3 RU, measures the availability of binding sites on thyroid-binding globulin, rather than any direct measurement of T_3. It also utilizes ^{125}I and is, therefore, a radioactive test. The measurement occurs by the addition of a resin to an incubated mixture of serum and labeled iodine, hence, its name. The T_7 test is often used as a screening test and is an estimate of the concentration of free thyroxine in the serum.[32]

The antithyroid antibody measurement consists of a hemagglutination test.

Clinical Implications

CLINICAL SIGNIFICANCE. These tests are done whenever the signs and symptoms indicate thyroid dysfunction, proptosis, or increased sympathetic activity, and are usually confirmatory.

CLINICAL INTERPRETATION. These tests allow the clinician to ascertain the circulating levels of T_4 and T_3, which are normally increased in Graves' disease. In contrast, they are decreased in hypothyroidism. Similarly, T_7 tests are elevated in hyperthyroidism and decreased in hypothyroidism. Positive antithyroid antibody tests should be interpreted with caution because they are found in 30% to 32% of individuals with Graves' disease and are also found in otherwise healthy individuals. Rives[32] suggests that these may actually be subclinical situations.

REFERENCES

1. Tilkian S, Conover M, Tilkian A. Clinical implications of laboratory tests. St Louis: CV Mosby Co, 1987.
2. Liu PI. Blue book of diagnostic tests. Philadelphia: WB Saunders Co, 1986.
3. Wallach J. Interpretation of diagnostic tests. Boston: Little, Brown, 1986.
4. Tietz NW. Clinical guide to laboratory tests. Philadelphia: WB Saunders Co, 1983.
5. Berkow R ed. The Merck manual. Rahway, NJ: Merck & Co, 1987.
6. Walker HK, Hall DW, Hurst JW. Clinical methods. Boston: Butterworth Publishers, 1980.
7. Hall, CA. Evaluation of cell numbers and morphology. In: Halsted JA, Halsted CH, eds. The laboratory in clinical medicine. Philadelphia: WB Saunders Co, 1981.
8. Epstein M, Oster JR. Renal and electrolyte disorders. In: Halsted JA, Halsted CH, eds. The laboratory in clinical medicine. Philadelphia: WB Saunders Co, 1981.
9. Rosenbaum BJ. Urinalysis: specific gravity. In: Walker HK, Hall DW, Hurst JW, eds. Clinical methods. Boston: Butterworth Publishers, 1980.
10. Popper S. Clinical nephrology. Boston: Little, Brown & Co, 1978.
11. Epstein M, Oster JR. Proteinuria. In: Halsted JA, Halsted CH, eds. The laboratory in clinical medicine. Philadelphia: WB Saunders Co, 1981.
12. Vroon DH. Alkaline phosphatase. In: Walker HK, Hall WD, Hurst JW, eds. Clinical methods. Boston: Butterworth Publications, 1980.
13. Vroon DH, Hall WD. Serum bilirubin. In: Walker HK, Hall WD, Hurst JW, eds. Clinical methods. Boston: Butterworth Publications, 1980.
14. Wells JO Jr, Hall WD, Vroon DH. Serum calcium. In: Walker HK, Hall WD, Hurst JW, eds. Clinical methods. Boston: Butterworth Publications, 1980.
15. The Expert Panel. Report of the National Cholesterol Education Program Expert Panel on Detection, Evaluation and Treatment of High Blood Cholesterol in Adults. Arch Intern Med 1988;148:36–39.
16. DiGirolamo M. Cholesterol. In: Walker HK, Hall WD, Hurst JW, eds. Clinical methods. Boston: Butterworth Publications, 1980.
17. Hall WD, Vroon DH. Creatinine. In: Walker HK, Hall WD, Hurst JW, eds. Clinical methods. Boston: Butterworth Publications, 1980.
18. Busick EJ. Natural history and diagnosis. In: Kozak GP, ed. Clinical diabetes mellitus. Philadelphia: WB Saunders Co, 1982.
19. Marble A, Ferguson BD. Diagnosis and classification of diabetes mellitus and nondiabetic melilurias. In: Marble A, Krall LP, Bradley RF, Christlieb AR, Soeldner JS, eds. Joslin's diabetes mellitus. Philadelphia: Lea & Febiger, 1985.
20. Mausolf F, Eye and systemic disease. In: The eye and systemic disease. St. Louis: CV Mosby Co, 1980.
21. Smith RJ. Hypoglycemia. In: Marble A, Krall LP, Bradley RF, Christlieb AR, Soeldner JS, eds. Joslin's diabetes mellitus. Philadelphia: Lea & Febiger, 1985.
22. Hall WD, Vroon DH. Serum inorganic phosphate. In: Walker HK, Hall WD, Hurst JW, eds. Clinical methods. Boston: Butterworth Publications, 1980.
23. Hall WD, Vroon DH. Serum total protein albumin and globulin. In: Walker HK, Hall WD, Hurst JW, eds. Clinical methods. Boston: Butterworth Publications, 1980.
24. Hall WD, Vroon DH. Blood urea nitrogen. In: Walker HK, Hall WD, Hurst JW, eds. Clinical methods. Boston: Butterworth Publications, 1980.
25. Hall WD, Vroon DH. Uric acid. In: Walker HK, Hall WD, Hurst JW, eds. Clinical methods. Boston: Butterworth Publications, 1980.
26. Zalar GL. Evaluation of specific dermatologic disorders. In: Holsted JA, Holsted CH, eds. The laboratory in clinical medicine. Philadelphia: WB Saunders Co, 1981.

27. Thompson SE III. Serologic testing for syphilis. In: Walker HK, Hall WD, Hurst JW, eds. Clinical methods. Boston: Butterworth Publications, 1980.

28. McGowan JE. PPD tuberculin skin test. In: Walker HK, Hall WD, Hurst JW, eds. Clinical methods. Boston: Butterworth Publications, 1980.

29. Goldstein E, Joye N. Laboratory diagnosis of specific bacterial and fungal diseases. In: Halsted JA, Halsted CH, eds. The laboratory in clinical medicine. Philadelphia: WB Saunders Co, 1981.

30. Barrett CR Jr. Common clinical problems in pulmonary disease. In: Halsted JA, Halsted CH, eds. The laboratory in clinical medicine. Philadelphia: WB Saunders Co, 1981.

31. Jubiz W. Endocrinology, a logical approach for clinicians. New York: McGraw-Hill Book Co, 1985.

32. Rives K. Endocrinologic diagnosis. In: Karciegliu Z, ed. Laboratory diagnoses in ophthalmology. New York: Macmillan Publishing Co, 1987.

Radiology

Leonard J. Oshinskie

INTRODUCTION

Definition

Radiology is the group of clinical procedures that use radiant energy in diagnosis and therapy. This chapter will be limited to a discussion of the main types of clinical imaging used in diagnosis of disorders of the visual system, including conventional x-ray studies, computed tomography, and magnetic resonance imaging. Other radiographic techniques that are used less frequently, but are helpful in diagnosis of the visual system, include angiography (arteriography and venography) conventional tomography, and dacryocystography. *Angiography* is the study of blood vessels by use of a contrast medium containing iodine and a series of radiographs. This is discussed in Chapter 63. A study that uses contrast medium and radiographs to image the lacrimal drainage system is called a *dacryocystogram*. Ultrasonography, a clinical imaging procedure commonly used in eye care, is discussed in Chapter 58.

An image formed through the use of x-rays is known as an *x-ray film, roentgenogram,* or *radiograph*. Conventional x-ray studies include *plain films,* which provide an image showing all layers of the body focused in a single plane. When x-rays are used to image thin sections of the body one layer at a time, a series of images result. This type of study is called *tomography* and can be done by using conventional x-ray equipment or through the use of x-rays, electronic sensors, and a computer that analyzes and displays data. This second method forms the basis for *computed tomography* (CT). Computed tomography uses computer processing to enhance detection of radiodensity differences between adjacent tissues.

Magnetic resonance imaging (MRI) relies on the detection of signals emitted by nuclei within the body, which are exposed to a strong magnetic field and radiofrequency signals. Unlike conventional x-rays and CT, this technique does not expose the patient to potentially harmful ionizing radiation to form images. Magnetic resonance imaging provides better spatial and contrast detail than CT in many instances and, therefore, provides a more sensitive tool for diagnosis.

History

Clinical imaging has been used in diagnosis of virtually every internal body system since shortly after the discovery of x-rays by Wilhelm Konrad Roentgen in 1895.[1] Since he did not understand the origin of his discovery at the time, he called it the "x-ray" (x for unknown). William James Morton, the first American radiologist, made radiographs of all parts of the body for comparison in normal and diseased states beginning in 1898.[2] The first person to publish radiographs of orbital images was an Austrian, Arthur Schuller, who did so in 1906.[3]

Hounsfield[4] and Ambrose[5] invented the technique of CT in the early 1970s, with an instrument available for whole-body imaging in 1975.[6] Many refinements to instrumentation have been made since 1975, and through this technology, CT has been used extensively to image body systems and structures in increasingly sophisticated ways, thus revolutionizing clinical imaging.

The evolution of clinical imaging continues to rapidly expand with the development of MRI. This technology has also been referred to as nuclear magnetic resonance (NMR), but because of the negative connotations of the word nuclear, it is now named MRI. Bloch and Purcell described the phenomenon of MRI in 1946. In vitro studies using MRI occurred during the following three decades.[7] Since the first human in vivo images in 1977,[8] this technology has expanded to include imaging of all body systems, as well as the nascent MRI technique of magnetic resonance spectroscopy.[9]

Clinical Use

Radiograms are used to provide skull films, allow dacryocystograms, provide the basis for arteriography, and produce chest films and spine films.

Computed tomography is particularly good at imaging bone and thus is useful in studies of the bony orbit. This technology also images certain tumors and cerebrovascular accidents particularly well.[10]

Magnetic resonance imaging has been shown to be superior to CT for imaging many brain lesions and space-occupying lesions, since it provides better spatial and contrast detail. This technology is quickly replacing CT as the procedure of choice in many conditions.

Since optometrists are members of the health care team in hospitals, outpatient clinics, and other multidisciplinary settings, it is essential that they become knowledgeable of clinical imaging techniques to allow communication with radiologists, neurologists, neuro-ophthalmologists and ophthalmologists so that the best possible health care can be rendered to patients.

INSTRUMENTATION

Theory

Radiation used in producing x-ray films and CT is of a shorter wavelength (0.5 to 0.06 A or less) than visible light and is composed of x-ray photons (Fig. 61–1). These short wavelengths allow x-rays, also known as roentgen rays, to penetrate matter.[1]

Photons are bundles of electromagnetic energy resulting from transformation of electrons. Radiography is dependent upon the ability of photons to either pass through, be deflected by, or absorbed by an object.[2] To produce a radiograph (x-ray film) x-ray photons pass selectively through body parts, depending on electron density.

The electron density of the structure studied determines how many photons penetrate a structure to form an image. Gases, such as air in sinuses, are composed of atoms with low atomic numbers and are of low electron density. Many photons can penetrate healthy sinuses and will reach the film. Therefore, sinuses that are clear appear black. Since bone is composed mostly of elements with higher atomic numbers and, as a solid, is more densely packed than gas, fewer photons find their way to the film and the radiograph appears white. Visualization of a structure on radiographs depends on the margin of two adjacent objects to be of different radiodensities and also that their edges be parallel to the

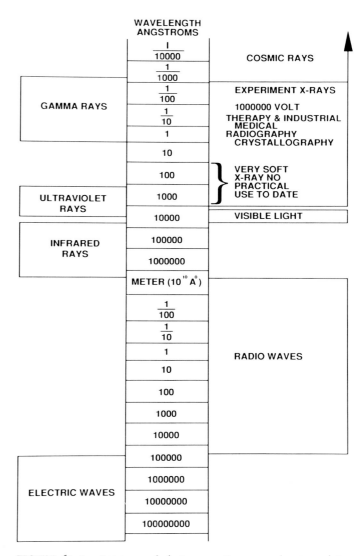

FIGURE 61–1. Spectrum of electromagnetic energy showing relative position of x-rays. (Courtesy of GE Medical Systems)

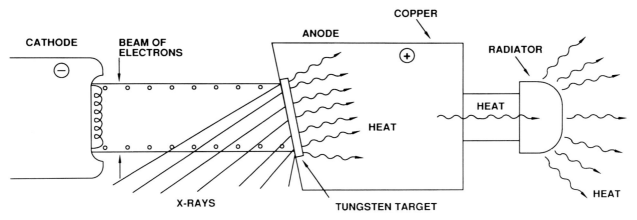

FIGURE 61–2. Basic elements of an x-ray tube. (Courtesy of GE Medical Systems)

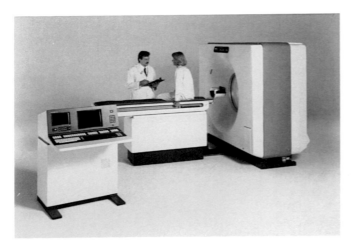

FIGURE 61-3. Computed tomography instrument. (Courtesy of GE Medical Systems)

x-ray beam. Clinicians can distinguish only five separate densities on radiographs, namely air, fat, water, bone, and metal.[2]

Photons for radiography are produced by a cathode ray tube. A very high voltage current (25,000 to 150,000 V) causes electrons to flow from a cathode toward an anode (Fig. 61-2). The electrons are then focused on a piece of tungsten which suddenly stops the electrons and thus transforms their energy into x-rays. Some of these x-rays pass through a small window in the instrument toward the patient.[11]

Because only a very small portion of the photons used to form a radiograph penetrate the subject, a high amount of radiation is needed for film to directly image the structures being studied. Indirect imaging employs phosphor screens that allow use of less radiation, are safer for the patient, and are used to produce most radiographs. These screens, held in a casette with x-ray film, are more sensitive to photons than film so that when struck by photons they generate light. This light, in turn, exposes the film adjacent to the screen. Fluoroscopy uses these types of screens to view internal structures directly and together with a contrast medium provide the basis for techniques such as carotid angiography.[11] Angiography uses contrast medium to image abnormalities in blood vessels. Contrast media are iodine-containing compounds that are radiopaque and, when injected into a structure, help define defects by increasing the radiodensity, which, in turn, changes the contrast between the structure in question and its surrounding tissues.[12]

Conventional Tomography

Plain film x-rays demonstrate all structures within the area imaged in one plane, thus causing overlap of structures and difficulty in interpreting the separation of these structures. Conventional tomography blurs out body layers in the plane on either side of the plane of interest to enhance detection in one layer. This is accomplished by moving both the film and the x-ray tube simultaneously in opposite directions about the axis of the section being studied.

Computed Tomography

Computed tomography uses x-rays like conventional tomography, but produces a series of slices of the structure studied through the use of sophisticated x-ray detectors, containing sodium iodide or xenon gas, and computer manipulation of the data received. The patient is positioned on a table that is moved into the CT gantry (Fig. 61-3). The gantry contains the x-ray tube, which produces collimated radiation and detectors. Collimation of the x-ray beam before and after passing through the body decreases the amount of radiation scatter and exposure, thereby creating an image with increased contrast resolution and density.[12] The collimated x-rays are emitted in a circular fashion around the patient by either having the x-ray tube and detectors rotate synchronously around the patient (a rotate–rotate system) or by rotating the x-ray tube in a system with stationary detectors that cover the entire circumference studied (a rotate–stationary system). Once the x-rays are detected and analyzed, they are displayed on a video monitor in a

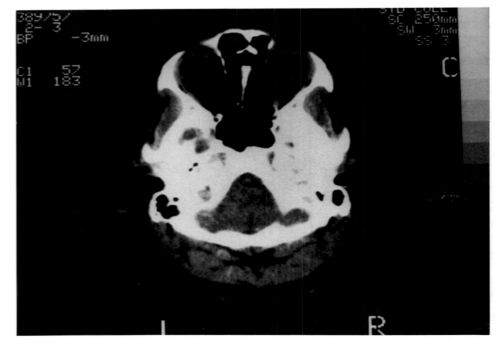

FIGURE 61-4. Axial CT through head and orbits. Note gray scale on the right of scan.

matrix composed of pixels. A *pixel* represents the linear attenuation value of x-rays at that point in the body. A *voxel* is the volume of tissue represented in 1 pixel and depends on the thickness of the slice taken.[12] In simple terms pixels and voxels are the basis for viewing contrast resolution, which is one of the characteristics that makes CT a superior technology, since it allows increased radiographic separation of structures compared with conventional radiography. A gray scale composed of CT numbers is the refer-

ence point for attenuation values of emergent x-rays (Fig. 61–4). These CT numbers are given values in Hounsfield units (HU) from −1000 to +1000, where the CT number of air is generally −1000, soft tissue +40 to +60, and fat −60 to −100.[12] Each CT instrument has its own unique gray scale; hence, these values are approximations only. This gray scale can be spread out by the use of "windowing" to change the appearance of structures. By altering the window width, contrast between two structures can be enhanced,

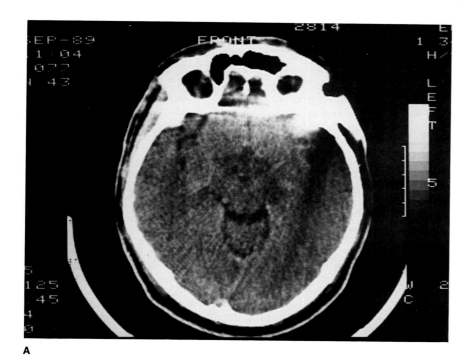

A

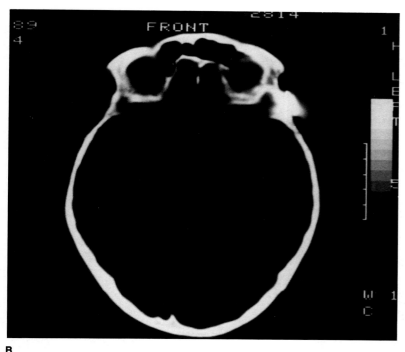

B

FIGURE 61–5. Axial CT scan of head demonstrating the same level first with soft tissue imaged (*A*) and then only bone using a "bone window" (*B*).

permitting better visualization. For example, windowing permits organ shape and contour to be examined and bone to be more easily separated from other tissue (Fig. 61–5).

Magnetic Resonance Imaging

Unlike radiographs and CT, MRI does not expose the patient to ionizing radiation. Instead, MRI depends on atoms in the body exposed to radiofrequency energy under the influence of a strong magnetic field to give off energy, which is detected and analyzed to determine characteristics of that structure. Currently, most clinical MRI scanners use the density and behavior of hydrogen nuclei (found abundantly in water of biologic tissue) as the basis for imaging.

The patient is placed on a table that is placed into the magnetic bore, housed in a gantry similar to that of a CT scanner (Fig. 61–6). A strong magnetic field (0.02 to 1.5 tesla) causes all hydrogen nuclei (as well as other nuclei such as carbon, fluorine, sodium, and phosphorus) to tilt with their axes rotating, like tops, about their z-axis (Fig. 61–7). Various hydrogen ions throughout the body will rotate differently, depending on how they are bonded in the molecule in which they exist. This rotation continues in equilibrium as long as the magnetic field is applied. By antennae built into the bore of the large magnet and surface coils or body coils placed on the patient, a radiofrequency (RF) pulse is then applied to the field, which causes the nuclei to tilt at an axis either 90° or 180° from the equilibrium state, depending on the duration of the RF pulse (resonant effect). The radiofrequency is then discontinued and, as the nuclei realign to equilibrium in the magnetic field, a radiofrequency signal is emitted by the relaxation. This signal is then detected by the antennae coils, transferred to a computer where they are analyzed, recorded, and displayed by a video monitor.[7,13]

The signal released by each hydrogen atom depends upon the local proton density, bulk motion of the hydrogen nuclei, the spin–lattice relaxation time (T1), and the spin–spin relaxation time (T2). T1, or the spin–lattice relaxation time, is the time for relaxation to the equilibrium state after removal of the RF pulse and depends on thermal interactions of adjacent protons[14] (Fig. 61–8). A second relaxation process, T2, also occurs after removal of the RF pulse, in which nuclei tilt back toward equilibrium, independently of one another. T2 depends on the "inhomogeneity in the local magnetic field"[14] (Fig. 61–9). As hydrogen nuclei differ in their environment in terms of adjacent nuclei and bonding, by measuring differences of T1, T2, and proton density, tissues can be

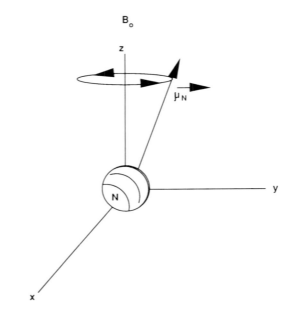

FIGURE 61–7. Diagram demonstrating nucleus within a magnetic field spinning about the z-axis. (From Kolodny NH, et al. Magnetic resonance imaging and spectroscopy of intraocular tumors. Surv Ophthalmol 1989;33:502–514, with permission)

separated on the basis of these differences, and an image is formed. The differences in proton density, T1, and T2 are accentuated by varying the time of elements of the RF pulse, namely repetition (T_R) and the time of echo (T_E). As in CT, final images in MRI are displayed in a matrix of pixels (Fig. 61–10).

Use

Optometrists are not directly involved in performing radiography, CT, or MRI in clinical practice, but a short description of the clinical methods of imaging techniques is included to facilitate the ordering of imaging studies, the various patient positioning re-

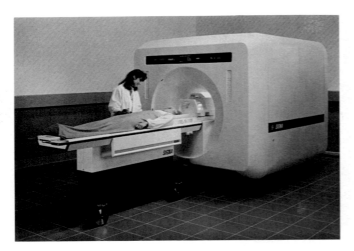

FIGURE 61–6. Magnetic resonance imaging system (Courtesy of GE Medical Systems)

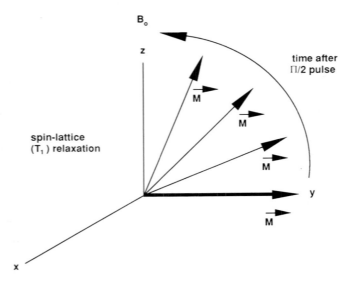

FIGURE 61–8. Diagram illustrating T1 relaxation about the x-axis. (From Kolodny NH, et al. Magnetic resonance imaging and spectroscopy of intraocular tumors. Surv Ophthalmol 1989;33:502–514, with permission)

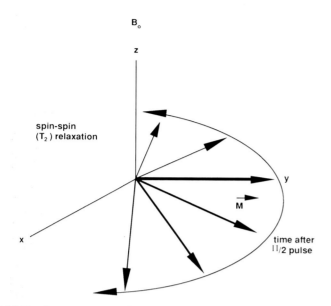

FIGURE 61–9. Diagram illustrating T2 relaxation in the *xy* plane. (From Kolodny NH, et al. Magnetic resonance imaging and spectroscopy of intraocular tumors. Surv Ophthalmol 1989;33:502–514, with permission)

quired for each type of study, and to help the optometrist educate the patient who is to undergo an imaging procedure.

Plain films that are commonly ordered in eye care include skull films, chest films, and spine films.

Skull films, typically ordered in imaging the orbits and paranasal sinuses, include posteroanterior (PA) Caldwell projection, Waters projection, lateral projection, submentovertex projection, and optic foramina views.[15] By positioning the patient and

angling the central ray of the x-ray instrument, certain structures are featured in each type of projection. Posteroanterior Caldwell projections are made by passing x-rays from the occipital region through to the face at an angle of 15° inferior to the canthomeatal line (Fig. 61–11). The PA notation indicates that the x-ray beam enters the patient at the posterior aspect of the structure being imaged and exits at the anterior aspect, which is placed closest to the film casette or x-ray table surface. A Waters projection is taken PA with the patient's chin elevated by having the patient hold the nose about 1 in. from the table surface (Fig. 61–12). During a lateral projection the patient holds his or her head with one of the ears against the surface of the film casette holder (Fig. 61–13). For a submentovertex projection the chin is hyperextended so that the canthomeatal line is perpendicular to the central ray of the x-ray instrument (Fig. 61–14). "Cone-down" views are limited to orbits and surrounding structures that improve the contrast of the films.[16]

Chest films are used in uveitis workup and include PA, lateral, and apical lordotic views (Fig. 61–15). During the apical lordotic view the patient faces the x-ray instrument and stands a few feet in front of the film casette. The patient then arcs his back toward the film just before the image is recorded.

Views of the lumbar sacral spine are very helpful in diagnosis of ankylosing spondylitis.

Conventional tomography is obtained by taking a series of images in coronal, axial, or sagittal planes. The x-ray instrument moves in a linear, circular, or hypocycloidal motion about the patient, thus blurring all planes except the one of interest.

During CT the patient is placed on a table in various positions depending on the type of study ordered. If a head scan is ordered the patient's head is immobilized in a head rest. A digital radiograph ("scout film") is taken first, so that the exact location and thickness of slices can be determined (Fig. 61–16). If a direct axial head CT study is desired, the patient lies supine so that the collimated beam can penetrate a series of axial planes. If a direct coronal scan is desired, the patient must hyperextend the chin while in the prone position. A single slice takes only 1 to 10

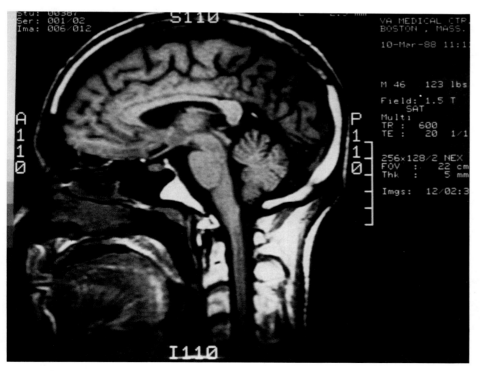

FIGURE 61–10. MRI of head in sagittal plane showing exquisite imaging of intracranial structures.

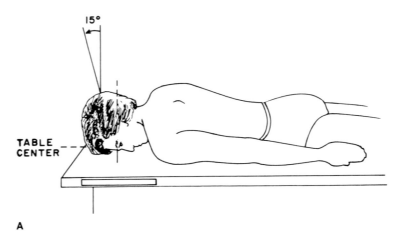

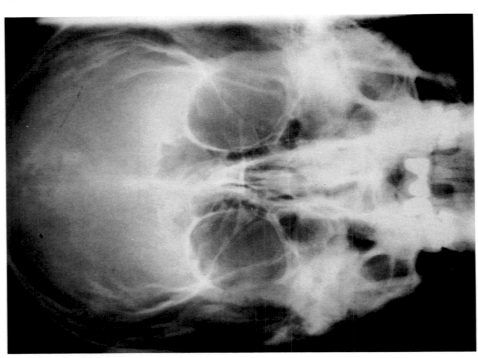

FIGURE 61–11. (*A*) Patient positioning for Caldwell projection. (From Jaeger SA. Atlas of radiographic positioning. Norwalk, Conn: Appleton and Lange, 1988, with permission) (*B*) Radiograph demonstrating the Caldwell projection.

seconds to be imaged.[12] The table moves a few millimeters into the gantry after each slice to image the next section. Generally, CT scans of the brain and orbits used in eye care are composed of between 10 and 25 slices. Slice thicknesses used in orbital imaging are generally 1.5 to 5.0 mm and, in head scans, 4 to 8 mm.[17] Computed tomography studies are often performed first with, and then without, an intravenous contrast medium during the same session.

Reconstruction is possible with CT scans, meaning that if an axial scan is performed, but a coronal or sagittal view is desired, the computer can form these images from the data collected from the axial scan. The reformatted image, however, may suffer some loss of resolution. A "hard copy" of the CT scan is made by transferring the image from the computer and monitor to x-ray film.

As with CT, during MRI, the patient is positioned on a table that is inserted into the gantry. Magnetic resonance imaging does not require repositioning of patients to obtain various section types, such as axial versus coronal. Slice thickness down to 4 mm is possible with MRI.[18,19] The MRI scans of the head generally take longer than a head CT. The duration of the study does not depend on the number of slices, but rather, on the type of study (T1 vs T2 vs proton density) performed. Reformatting is not possible with MRI, meaning that an axial slice cannot be reconstructed from a coronal study. Therefore, all slices desired must be specified before the study begins. A paramagnetic contrast agent, gadolinium–diethylenetriamine pentaacitic acid (Gd-DTPA), has been used to enhance tissue differences by increasing the T1 signal intensity.[20] Again, a hard copy of the MRI is made on x-ray film for viewing.

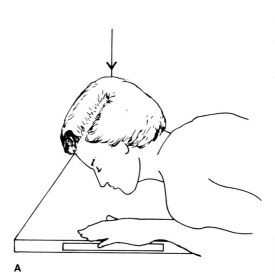

A

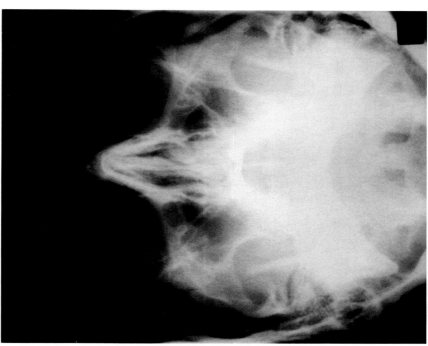

B

FIGURE 61–12. (*A*) Patient positioning for Waters projection. (From Jaeger SA. Atlas of radiographic positioning. Norwalk, Conn: Appleton and Lange, 1988, with permission) (*B*) Radiograph demonstrating the Waters projection.

COMMERCIALLY AVAILABLE INSTRUMENTS

Since optometrists will not generally purchase instruments designed to perform radiographs, CT, or MRI, the various instruments needed to do this will not be discussed.

CLINICAL PROCEDURE

As the primary eye care provider, the optometrist needs to know what imaging procedures are appropriate, given the clinical find-

ings. These indications, as well as contraindications, will be discussed.

Although CT and MRI provide superior images to plain film in many conditions, certain abnormalities can still be imaged well with conventional x-rays. Plain skull films are ordered when the patient has the possibility of an intraocular or orbital foreign body, sinus disease, or in cases of trauma to the orbit and orbital rim. Clinical signs associated with trauma, such as orbital emphysema, loss of sensation over the corresponding cheek, enophthalmos, or diplopia, are indication for plain skull films. Radiographs are also helpful in imaging orbital conditions, such as change in the orbital

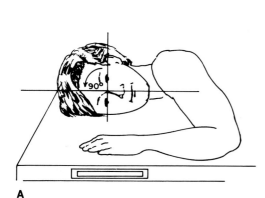

A

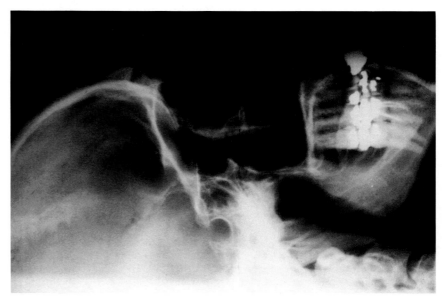

B

FIGURE 61–13. (*A*) Patient positioning for lateral projection. (From Jaeger SA. Atlas of radiographic positioning. Norwalk, Conn: Appleton and Lange, 1988, with permission) (*B*) Radiograph demonstrating the lateral projection.

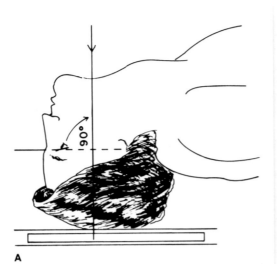

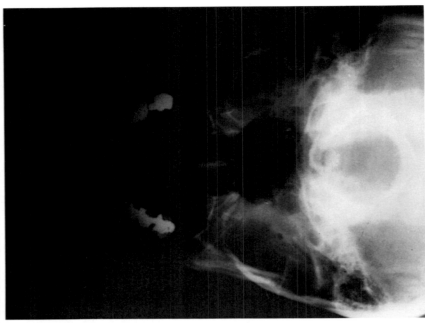

FIGURE 61–14. (*A*) Patient positioning for submentovertex projection. (From Jaeger SA. Atlas of radiographic positioning. Norwalk, Conn: Appleton and Lange, 1988, with permission) (*B*) Radiograph demonstrating submentovertex projection.

size, boney destruction, or hyperostosis. Tumors, inflammatory processes, medications, endocrinologic disorders, and radiation cause these changes.[21] Although CT has replaced plain films in imaging blowout fractures (especially if surgical intervention is planned), plain films are indicated if CT is not readily available.[22] The expense of plain films is also much less than CT or MRI. For medicolegal reasons, even cases of minor orbital trauma should have plain skull films ordered.

Four basic projections are ordered as part of the radiographic

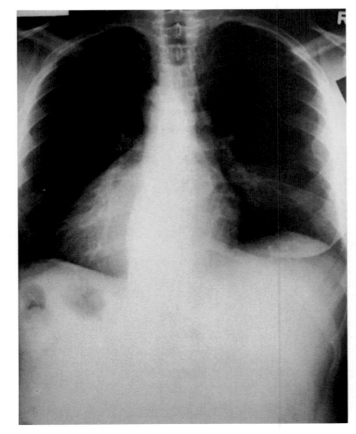

FIGURE 61–15. PA projection of chest.

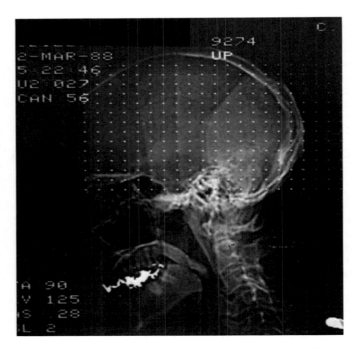

FIGURE 61–16. Scout film used to position slices before sagittal CT scan.

evaluation of the orbit and paranasal sinuses. A PA Caldwell projection is used to image the floor of the sella turcica, the superior orbital fissure, and the ethmoid and frontal sinuses. If a view of the orbital rim, orbital roof, or maxillary sinuses is desired, a Waters projection is ordered. Lateral projection demonstrates the anterior clinoid processes, the sella turcica, and the sphenoid sinuses. A submentovertex projection may be helpful in examining the maxillary sinuses and the posterolateral wall of the orbit.[15] In addition to these four basic plain films, optic foramina views can be obtained by angling the patient's head so the central ray passes through the foramina without striking a maze of other bony structures first.

Other conditions that indicate plain film radiography include uveitis and Horner's syndrome. Anteroposterior lumbar–sacral films, with views of the sacroiliac joints should be ordered whenever ankylosing spondylitis is considered in the differential diagnosis. Reiter's syndrome also causes radiographic detectable changes in the spine and lower limbs.[23] Conditions associated with uveitis, such as tuberculosis, sarcoidosis, and histoplasmosis, can show chest lesions and, therefore, chest films (PA and lateral) are ordered in the diagnostic workup of anterior and posterior uveitis.

A preganglionic Horner's syndrome is an indication for a PA and lateral chest film to screen for an apical lung lesion. If a lesion is found, the patient may need additional studies, such as apical lordotic views or CT of the chest.

Conventional tomography has been used to study the orbits and optic canals; however, CT and MRI are quickly replacing this procedure. In certain cases of less severe trauma, plain films and tomography may be indicated.[24]

Indications for CT are changing as MRI techniques become more sophisticated. Occasionally, the two techniques are complementary, but ideally, for cost-effectiveness reasons, only one study should be ordered for diagnosis. Generally, CT is still used to image bone and calcification, thus providing good detail of the bony orbit and paranasal sinuses in trauma.[22,24]

Other ocular conditions that may indicate the need for CT include unilateral exophthalmos; progressive, unilateral vision loss that cannot be explained on the basis of clinical examination; unexplained ophthalmoplegia; unilateral disc swelling; palpebal orbital masses; and when conventional films indicate changes in bony orbital structures.[25] Computed tomography images acute hemorrhagic stroke better than MRI[26] and is the procedure of choice if a meningioma of the posterior visual pathway is suspected.[10] Generally, a full CT scan of the head is much shorter (10 minutes) compared with a head MRI (40 minutes), thus may be useful in patients who are restless. It is also more readily available and less expensive. Contrast media is appropriate when soft-tissue disease, especially a vascular tumor or metastatic disease, is suspected.

The MRI images soft-tissue disease extremely well, compared with CT and, therefore, has replaced CT in the evaluation of neurogenic tumors and small infarcts.[27] Because the dense cortical bone of the posterior fossa causes artifacts on CT, MRI is the test of choice in imaging most lesions of the posterior fossa.[27] Tumors of the posterior visual system, except meningiomas, and the brain stem (except acoustic neuromas) are imaged better with MRI than with CT. Pituitary tumors and intracranial extension of an orbital mass are imaged well with MRI.[21,28] An MRI scan can demonstrate white plaques appearing in the gray matter of patients suspected of having multiple sclerosis and can help confirm the diagnosis.[29]

Once an indication for use of an imaging procedure is established, the optometrist will need to take a careful history to determine if the patient has any contraindications to the procedures before they are ordered.

In plain films and conventional tomography the contraindications are few. Excessive exposure to radiation is a concern because

of its possible genetic, leukemogenic, and carcinogenic effects.[30] Because cumulative effects can occur in patients undergoing repeated studies, a patient should not be exposed to more than 10 rad during the first 30 years of life. After age 30, 5 rad per decade should not be exceeded.[1] A typical chest film delivers about 45 mrad.[30] A head CT may deliver up to 5 rad per slice, but since the radiation is collimated, adjacent tissues receive little radiation.[31] Ionizing radiation can cause cataracts, so patients receiving serial CT procedures in follow-up need to be monitored for the amount of radiation received.

Pregnancy contraindicates use of ionizing radiation at any stage, unless a life-threatening condition necessitates radiographs or CT.[30]

Other contraindications to CT are claustrophobia (since the aperture the patient is placed into is confining) and, if contrast material is to be used, decreased kidney function.[32] Since contrast media are cleared through the kidneys, the clinician ordering the test must ascertain that renal function is normal through the use of a blood urea nitrogen (BUN) and creatinine test. If renal function is abnormal, the patient may develop an adverse effect. Fatal reactions occur in approximately 1:40,000 studies.[33] Since shellfish contain iodine, any patient with a history of shellfish allergy should not be given iodine-containing contrast medium. The use of a contrast medium is also not appropriate in a patient suspected of a hemorrhagic stroke or immediately following head trauma because it may compromise the appearance of extravascular blood and, thereby, alter diagnosis and treatment inappropriately.[2] The additional radiation received during a contrast scan must also be considered in the total radiation the patient has received.

Because MRI uses a very strong magnetic field as the basis for imaging, contraindications include a history of metallic foreign body, aneurysm clips, hip prosthesis, stapes prosthesis, cochlear implant, respiratory equipment, and IV poles. These objects may be displaced by the strong magnetic field, which may also cause tissue surrounding these structures to increase in temperature. It is also important to elicit a history of metallic foreign body, and if positive, a plain film taken to rule out its existence. The RF pulse may also alter a pacemaker's signal.[26] The National Institutes of Health suggest that MRI "should be used during the first trimester of pregnancy only when there are clear medical indications and it offers a definite advantage over other tests."[34] Again, claustrophobia may contraindicate MRI, because the aperture of the magnetic bore is small. The procedure takes approximately 40 minutes, so any patient anticipated to be unable to remain quiet for that period (children, hyperactive patients, patients with dyspnea, or involuntary movement disorders) may not be a good candidate or may need sedation. Artifacts caused by dental fillings during CT are not present in an MRI study and do not contraindicate MRI.[26]

Once contraindications are considered, the tests are ordered by completing a form indicating which procedures are desired. Computed tomography or MRI is ordered in the axial (most common), coronal, or sagittal view of the head, orbits, or both. If views of the chiasm are desired the radiologist should be informed, so that coronal views can be obtained. The order should also indicate whether the scan is to be performed with or without contrast medium. Previous exposure to ionizing radiation, major surgery, region to be imaged, and suspected location of lesion or process should be recorded on the order form.

CLINICAL IMPLICATIONS

Clinical Significance

Radiographs, CT, and MRI are a cornerstone of medical diagnosis. The imaging techniques discussed in this chapter are noninvasive

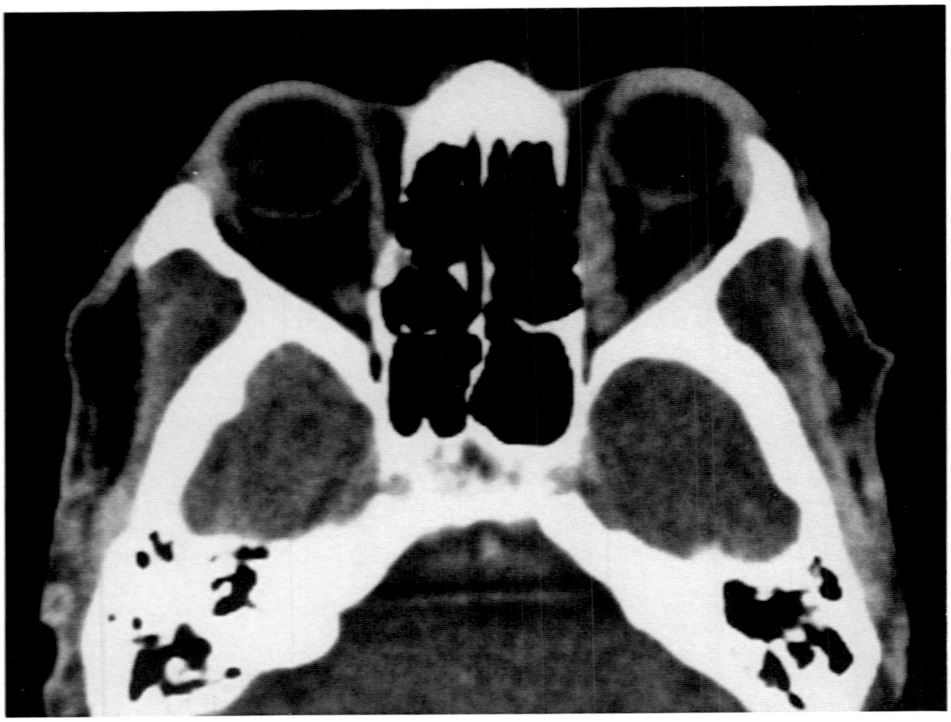

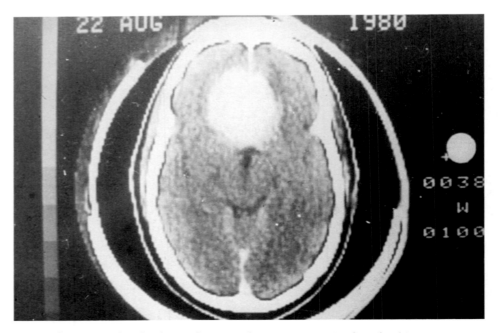

FIGURE 61–17. Orbital CT (axial view) demonstrating thickened left medial rectus in a patient with Graves' disease.

methods of examining internal body structures, contrary to exploratory surgery, insertion of catheters, or lighted scopes. Diagnostic and therapeutic decisions depend, in large part, on the diagnosis reached through the use of radiologic techniques. Progression or regression of a condition can also be monitored through the use of these modalities. Patient education can be assisted when an image of the condition being managed is available.

Specifically in eye care, radiographs are used to diagnose conditions associated with uveitis, such as tuberculosis, sarcoidosis, ankylosing spondylitis, and Reiter's syndrome. The workup of Horner's syndrome includes a chest film. Orbital diagnosis has been advanced dramatically by CT and MRI, since soft tissue can now be imaged. Trauma evaluation often includes radiography and CT. Evaluation of the paranasal sinuses also depends on radio-

FIGURE 61–18. Axial CT head scan of patient with meningioma arising from the chiasm.

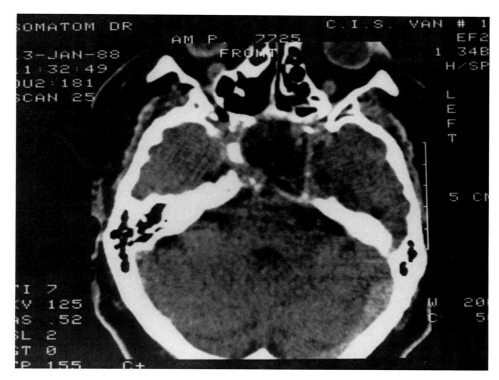

FIGURE 61–19. Axial CT head scan showing erosion of bone in the sellae and left petrous bone in a patient with a pituitary tumor.

graphic techniques. Tumors, strokes, vascular abnormalities, and other neurologic abnormalities can all be imaged with CT or MRI. As MRI technology advances, differential diagnosis will be made more accurate so appropriate therapy can be initiated.

Clinical Interpretation

Detailed interpretation of imaging techniques requires a vast amount of knowledge and experience that few health care practi-

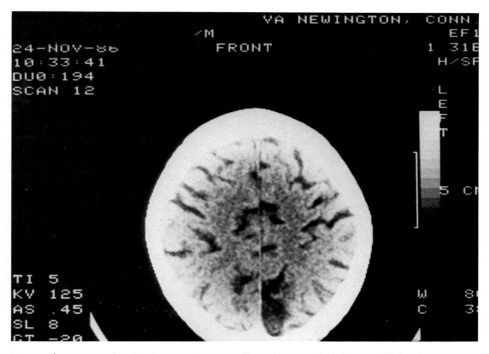

FIGURE 61–20. Axial CT head scan with an area of hypodensity in the left occipital lobe, characteristic of an old stroke. (From Tower H, Oshinski IJ. An introduction to computer tomography and magnetic resonance imaging of the head and visual pathways. J Am Opthom Assoc 1989;60:619–628, with permission)

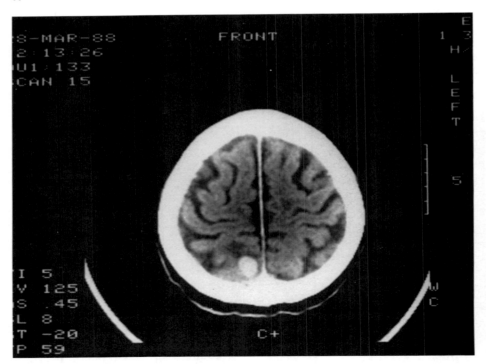

FIGURE 61–21. (*A*) Axial CT head scan, without contrast, showing an area of hypodensity in the right occipital lobe. (*B*) Axial CT head scan, with contrast, of same patient, demonstrating a metastatic lesion in the right occipital lobe. (From Tower H, Oshinski LJ. An introduction to computer tomography and magnetic resonance imaging of the head and visual pathways. J Am Opthom Assoc 1989;60:619–628, with permission)

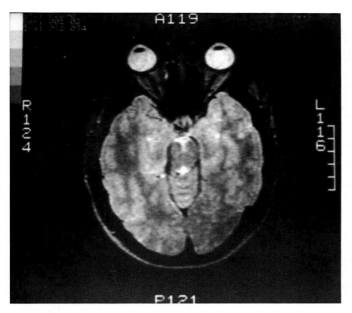

FIGURE 61–22. Axial MRI head scan through orbits (T2-weighted). (From Tower H, Oshinski LJ. An introduction to computer tomography and magnetic resonance imaging of the head and visual pathways. J Am Opthom Assoc 1989;60:619–628, with permission)

tioners, other than the radiologist, possess. However, optometrists should be familiar with basic interpretation of radiographs, CT, and MRI, so communication between other health care providers and between clinician and patient can occur.

Radiographs

Comparison of size, shape, density, and position are all considered during interpretation. Change in any of these characteristics over time is also noted. Since the skull is symmetric relative to the central sagittal plane, comparison of one sinus, orbit, or other structure with its fellow structure on the opposite side is very helpful in interpretation. Most changes in soft tissue are made by inference using radiographs because soft tissue does not image well in conventional radiography. For example, changes in bone structure may indicate a space-occupying lesion that is not otherwise apparent.[30]

Description of certain abnormal conditions are presented to illustrate the interpretation of radiographs:

- Blowout fractures are often seen as radiolucencies in the floor of the orbit in which soft tissue is entrapped. The maxillary sinus on the involved side may be relatively radiodense owing to blood.
- Plain film radiographs in a patient with sinusitis may show the sinus to be hazy, have thickened mucosa, or reveal an air–fluid line.[2]
- The sacroiliac joints are always affected in ankylosing spondylitis (AS). A faint radiopaque line of the sacroiliac joint is characteristic of this sclerosed joint of the AS patient.

Computed Tomography

Several normal CT scans are presented in the following. As with conventional x-rays, familiarity with normal structures imaged with CT is vital before subtle abnormalities can be assessed. Bone is imaged as a very hyperdense structure, so it appears white. Air, having little radiodensity, appears black. Other structures are of intermediate densities on the gray scale. (See Figure 61–4 for examples of normal orbital and intracranial structures.) Note that

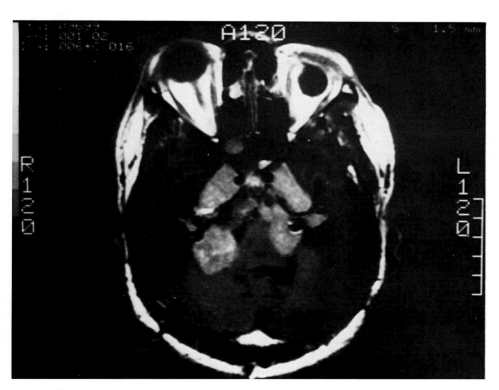

FIGURE 61–23. Axial MRI head scan through orbits of a patient with a right-sided acoustic neuroma (T1-weighted).

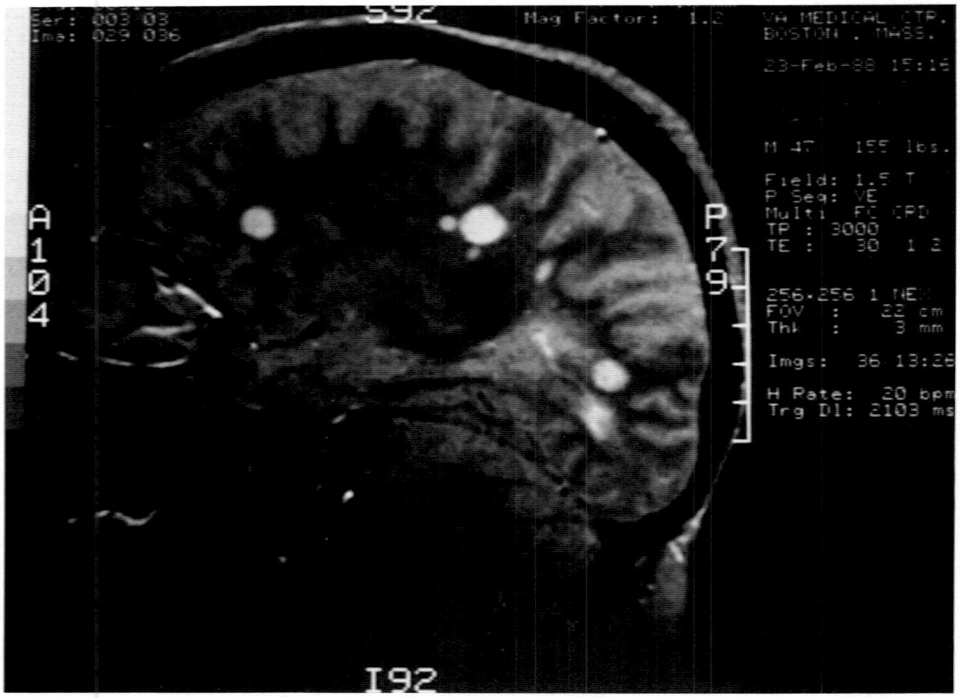

FIGURE 61–24. Sagittal MRI head scan showing white plaques characteristically found in multiple sclerosis. (From Tower H, Oshinski LJ. An introduction to computer tomography and magnetic resonance imaging of the head and visual pathways. J Am Opthom Assoc 1989;60:619–628, with permission)

CT images are viewed from an inferior aspect; accordingly, it is important to use the right–left orientation label provided on the film to gain proper perspective.

To illustrate abnormalities imaged with this technology, examples of CT studies are presented in the following:

- Computed tomography can be used in diagnosis of ocular masses, particularly if they contain calcium. These include retinoblastoma, certain metastatic tumors, hamartomas, and choroidal osteoma.[17]
- Orbital abnormalities such as tumors of the optic nerve or extraocular muscles can be examined by CT. A patient who presented with lid retraction had a CT to confirm a diagnosis of Graves' disease (Fig. 61–17). Note the enlargement of the medial rectus muscle in the left orbit, which is a characteristic finding in patients with thyroid ophthalmopathy.
- Blowout fractures are imaged very well with coronal and saggital CT of the orbits.
- Figure 61–18 shows a 56-year-old black man who complained of slightly decreased vision. A visual field suggested a chiasmal lesion, and the CT scan demonstrated a large hyperdense mass arising from the chiasmal region. The diagnosis was a meningioma.
- Bone erosion is seen in Figure 61–19. A pituitary tumor was the cause of superior temporal field defects, and bone loss, secondary to this tumor, is seen along the patient's left petrous bone. Again, since CT images bone better than MRI, processes causing calcification and bone loss are appropriately imaged with CT.
- A hypodensity characteristic of old stroke is demonstrated in Figure 61–20. This CT was performed because the patient had a right homonymous inferior quadrantanopia.
- Metastatic disease from the lung to the occipital lobe is seen as a diffuse mass without contrast (Fig. 61–21A) and as a hyperdensity following contrast enhancement (Fig. 61–21B).

Magnetic Resonance Imaging

Three types of clinical studies with various T_R and T_E are used most often to study images in MRI. These studies are T1-weighted, T2-weighted, and proton density. By accentuating the differences in tissues in each of these studies, structures both normal and abnormal can be identified.

In general, tissues with relatively high numbers of hydrogen nuclei per unit volume give a stronger signal intensity.[14] Liquids appear hyperintense on T2 studies, whereas soft tissue appears hypointense (Fig. 61–22). The opposite tends to hold for T1 studies so that vitreous appears hypointense on a T1 study (Fig. 61–23). Muscle and optic nerve are intermediate density on both types of studies. Bone, air, and circulating blood, all appear black in T1 and T2 studies.[14] Note that orbital fat is very bright (hyperintense) in a T1-weighted study.

Differential diagnosis of lesions can be aided by knowing the characteristic appearance of various abnormalities in T1 and T2 studies. The reader is referred to references 14 and 28 for detailed descriptions of T1 and T2 appearances of various ocular and orbital abnormalities.

Magnetic resonance images lesions of demyelination in multiple sclerosis much better than CT can and can help to confirm the diagnosis. An example of these hyperintense plaques is demonstrated in Figure 61–24.

Figure 61–23 demonstrates the ability of MRI to image intracranial tumors. Noted in this T1-weighted study are shifting of midline structures and an area of hyperdensity in the right cerebellarpontine angle of this patient with neurofibromatosis. This is an acoustic neuroma. The left orbit contains a silicon implant following enucleation for a neurilemoma of the ciliary body.

As of this writing, MRI technology is rapidly expanding. Research using ^{23}Na MRI and ^{31}P scanners, as well as MRI spectroscopy, show potential for clinical applications in assessment of the visual system.[13]

REFERENCES

1. Thompson TT. Primer of clinical radiology. Boston: Little, Brown & Co, 1980.
2. Freedman M. Clinical imaging: an introduction to the role of imaging in clinical practice. Edinburgh: Churchill-Livingston, 1988.
3. Hammerschlag SB, Hesselink JR, Weber AL. Computed tomography of the eye and orbit. Norwalk, Conn: Appleton–Century–Crofts, 1983.
4. Hounsfield GN. Computerized transverse axial scanning (tomography) part 1: description of system. Br J Radiol 1973;46:1016–1022.
5. Ambrose J. Computerized transverse axial scanning (tomography) part 2: clinical applications. Br J Radiol 1973;46:1023–1047.
6. Grainger RG. Techniques and imaging modalities. In: Grainger RG, Alison DJ, eds. Diagnostic radiology, vol 1. New York: Churchill-Livingston, 1986.
7. Bydder GM, Steiner RE, Worthington BS. Magnetic resonance imaging. In: Grainger RG, Alison DJ, eds. Diagnostic radiology, vol 1. New York: Churchill-Livingston, 1986.
8. Hinshaw WB, Bottomley PA, Holland GN. Radiographic thin section of the human wrist by nuclear magnetic resonance. Nature 1977;270:722–723.
9. Weiner M. The promise of magnetic resonance spectroscopy for medical diagnosis. Invest Radiol 1988;23:253–261.
10. Rubenfeld M, Wirtschafter J. The role of medical imaging in the practice of neuro-ophthalmology. Radiol Clin North Am 1987;25:863–876.
11. Juhl JH. Essentials of roentgen interpretation. Philadelphia: Harper & Row, 1985.
12. Husband JE. Whole body computed tomography. In: Grainger RG, Alison DJ, eds. Diagnostic radiology, vol 1. Edinburgh: Churchill-Livingston, 1986.
13. Kolodny NH, Gragoudas E, D'Amico DJ, Albert DM. Magnetic resonance imaging and spectroscopy of intraocular tumors. Surv Ophthalmol 1989;33:502–514.
14. Saint-Louis LA, Haik BG. Magnetic resonance imaging of the globe. In: Haik BG, ed. Advanced imaging techniques in opthalmology. Int Ophthalmol Clin 1986;26(3):151–167.
15. Huckman MS, Grainer LS. Radiology in ophthalmic diagnosis. In: Peyman GA, Sanders DR, Goldberg MF, eds. Principles and practice of ophthalmology. Philadelphia: WB Saunders Co, 1980.
16. Trokel SL. Radiology of the orbit: In: Duane TD, Jaeger EA, eds. Clinical ophthalmology, vol 2. Philadelphia: JB Lippincott Co, 1988.
17. Haik BG, Saint-Louis LA, Smith ME. Computed tomography in ocular disease. In: Haik BG, ed. Int Ophthalmol Clin 1986;26(3):77–101.
18. Bilaniuk LT, Schruck JF, Zimmerman RA, et al. Ocular and orbital lesions: surface coil MR imaging. Radiology 1985;156:669–674.
19. Shenck JF, Hart H, Foster T, et al. Improved MR imaging of the orbit at 1.5 T with surface coils. AJNR 1985;6:193–196.
20. Brant-Zawadzki M, Berry I, Osaki L, et al. Gadolinium–DPTA in clinical MR of the brain: intraaxial lesions. AJNR 1986;7:781–788.
21. Weiss RA, Haik BG, Smith ME. Introduction to diagnostic imaging techniques in ophthalmology. In: Haik BG, ed. Advanced imaging techniques in ophthalmology. Int Ophthalmol Clin 1986;26(3):1–24.
22. Koornneef L, Zonneveld FW. The role of direct multiplanar high resolution CT in the assessment and management of orbital trauma. Radiol Clin North Am 1987;25:753–766.
23. Gold RH, Bassett LW, Seeger LL. The other arthritides. In: Weinstein AS, Kattan KR, eds. Arthritis and other arthropathies. Radiol Clin North Am 1988;26:1195–1212.
24. Kassel EE. Traumatic injuries of the paranasal sinuses. Otolaryngol Clin North Am 1988;21:455–493.
25. Davis DO, Alper MG. Computerized tomography of the orbit and orbital lesions. In: Arger PH, ed. Orbit roentgenology. New York: John Wiley & Sons, 1977.
26. Anderson RE. Magnetic resonance imaging versus computed tomography—which one? Postgrad Med 1989;85(3):79–87.
27. Mafee MF, Campos M, Raju S, et al. Head and neck: high field magnetic resonance imaging versus computed tomography. Otolarygol Clin North Am 1988;21:513–546.
28. Saint-Louis LA, Haik BG, Amster JL. Magnetic resonance imaging of the orbit and optic pathways. In: Haik BG, ed. Advanced imaging techniques in ophthalmology. Int Ophthal Clin 1986;26(3):169–185.
29. Rosenblatt MA, Behrens MM, Zweifach PH, et al. Magnetic resonance imaging of optic tract involvement in multiple sclerosis. Am J Ophthalmol 1987;104:74–79.
30. Meschan I, Ott DJ. Introduction to diagnostic radiology. Philadelphia: WB Saunders Co, 1984.
31. Maue-Dickson W, Trefler M, Dickson DR. Comparison of dosimetry and image quality in computed and conventional tomography. Radiology 1979;131:509–514.
32. Tower H, Oshinskie LJ. An introduction to computed tomography and magnetic resonance imaging of the head and visual pathways. J Am Optom Assoc 1989;60:619–628.
33. Shehadi WH, Toniol G. Adverse reactions to contrast media. Radiology 1980;137:299.
34. Abrams H, Berne A, Dodd G, et al. Magnetic resonance imaging. Natl Inst Health Consensus Dev Conf Statement 1987;6(14):1–9.

Carotid Artery Assessment

Barbara J. Jennings

INTRODUCTION

Definition

Examination and diagnosis of ocular problems frequently necessitates consideration of the patient's general health status. One of the most important systemic conditions that directly affects the eye is carotid artery occlusive disease caused by atherosclerosis. Because of the potential for significant morbidity and mortality associated with atherosclerosis of the carotid arteries,[1-9] it is prudent to routinely evaluate carotid pulses and auscultate the neck for carotid artery bruits on asymptomatic older patients, as well as those who are symptomatic. This simple, rapid examination procedure could be the key to saving the patient's life, or preventing him or her from suffering through a long, difficult, and generally imperfect recuperative period.

Any reduction in blood flow through the extracranial carotid arteries will result in a concomitant reduction in blood flow through the vasculature nourishing the eye and orbit. Therefore, it is essential to rule out carotid artery occlusive disease when assessing the vascular status of the eye. Analysis of the carotid pulses is an important part of that evaluation. Palpation of the carotid arterial pulse gives the examiner an indication about the strength of blood flow through the carotid arteries. The carotid pulse reflects the aortic pulsation. If the pulsation is decreased, it may be due to either decreased stroke volume or localized factors, such as stenosis caused by atherosclerosis.

The use of a stethoscope to listen for physical signs is called *auscultation*. When listening to sounds produced within the body by placing the unaided ear directly on it, one performs *immediate auscultation;* conversely, the use of a stethoscope to hear sound is termed *mediate auscultation.*[10]

The French word *bruit* means noise. When auscultating the carotid arteries, a swishing noise may be heard in a partially oc-cluded vessel, and a bruit is diagnosed. Patients presenting with unilateral, pulsating exophthalmos may demonstrate an orbital bruit, and auscultation of the orbit is performed to rule out that finding.

History

The ancient Egyptians recognized the importance of palpation and inspection of the patient, as well as direct auscultation. The Ebers Papyrus, which dates to approximately 2850 BC, indicates that the physicians of that era had a knowledge of auscultation and contains the phrase "Here the ear hears beneath . . ."[11] Later, the Hippocratic doctrines mandated auscultation as an aid in diagnosis in the fifth century BC.[12] The physician was to shake the patient's chest, and the physician then placed his ear on the patient's thorax to hear the specific sounds produced by various diseases; however, the Greeks did not pursue this diagnostic aid because they did not recognize disease as being a result of pathologic anatomy. It was in the middle of the 18th century that Leopold Auenbrugger laid the foundation for diagnosis, based on pathologic anatomy, when he published his experiments on percussion of the thorax with the fingertips, which allowed recognition of specific sounds resulting from specific diseases.[13] Since Auenbrugger was the son of an innkeeper, he was aware of the use of tapping on a barrel to determine whether it is full or empty. The same method of tapping on the chest to elicit sounds characteristic of various diseases became a mainstay in differential diagnosis.

One of the great clinicians of all time,[11,13,14] René Théophile Hyacinthe Laënnec, invented the stethoscope in 1816. Thomas Addison, a well-known physician after whom Addison's disease is named, credits Laënnec with contributing more toward the advancement of the medical art than any other single individual.[11]

The previous experience of the Greeks with direct auscultation of the chest indicated that some patients had specific noises produced in their chests. In 1816, Laënnec had an obese female patient suffering from heart disease. Modesty and the patient's size prevented his putting his ear on her chest to detect the heart sounds.[15] One day as Laënnec passed the Louvre, he noticed some urchin children playing with long beams of wood. One child had his ear on the end of a beam, and another tapped a signal on the opposite end. This game reminded Laënnec that sounds are magnified when passing through a hollow tube. When Laënnec reached his patient, he fashioned a tube from a piece of paper, and listened to the heart and breath sounds more clearly than he had previously ever heard. Later, Laënnec devised a hollow wooden tube to be used for mediate auscultation of the heart and lungs. In 1819, when Laënnec's book *De l'Auscultation* was published, a stethoscope was included with each copy of the book.

Clinical Use

Physical examination of a patient should include palpation of the carotid pulses, as well as auscultation of the extracranial carotid arteries. These procedures yield objective information on whether or not these vessels are patent or are partially occluded or stenosed. Auscultation for orbital bruits provides objective evidence of significant vascular malformation, and is performed on any patient in whom such malformation is expected, such as those patients presenting with intermittent or pulsating exophthalmos.

INSTRUMENTATION

Theory

The common carotid artery originates somewhat differently on the left and right sides. Arising from the aorta, the innominate artery on the right branches off into the subclavian and common carotid arteries (see Fig. 59–1). On the left side, the common carotid artery and the subclavian artery arise directly from the aorta. The common carotid arteries will eventually bifurcate, forming an internal and an external carotid artery on each side.

The sternocleidomastoid muscles originate at the medial clavicle and the sternum and insert posteriorly at the mastoid bones on each side. Topographically, this muscle divides the neck into the anterior and the posterior cervical triangles (Fig. 62–1). Although they move deep to the sternocleidomastoid muscle on each side, the carotid arteries are auscultated in the anterior trian-

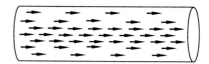

FIGURE 62–2. Blood flows progressively faster the farther away it is from the vessel wall. Maximum velocity of blood occurs at the center of the lumen.

gle of the neck. When either palpating carotid pulses or auscultating the carotid for bruits, it is essential to understand pertinent anatomy and perform the examination appropriately.

Normal blood flow through the arteries is in a laminar pattern. Blood flow is fastest at the center of the lumen, and the blood flowing closest to the vessel wall is almost stationary. Blood flows progressively faster the farther it is away from the vessel wall, reaching a maximum velocity at the center of the lumen (Fig. 62–2). When flow through vessels is in a laminar pattern, it is silent and is not heard on auscultation.

If a vessel becomes partially occluded, intrinsically as in atherosclerosis[16,17] or extrinsically as when a tumor compresses the vessel,[17,18] laminar flow through the vessel is disrupted at the point of occlusion. Turbulence develops, and swirls and vortices occur in the flow pattern. These disruptions cause vibrations in the vessel wall at the point of occlusion and the vibrations are transmitted through the skin to the stethoscope as noise. The vibrations of the vessel wall produce high-frequency sound vibrations. When heard in or around the heart or transmitted along the larger arteries from the heart, these sounds are termed *murmurs;* however, when this noise is heard in association with noncardiac vessels, it is termed a bruit. Auscultation of a carotid bruit indicates stenosis at or proximal to the site of auscultation.[19–21] If the origination of the sound is a cardiac murmur, the intensity of the sound should increase as the stethoscope is moved proximally toward the precordium. Conversely, if the sound originated at a carotid artery stenosis, the sounds will become less intense when moving proximally toward the heart.[22,23] A normal artery can transmit a systolic bruit if the artery is compressed.[24]

Both the intensity and the pitch of a bruit must be considered. Intensity of the murmur is directly proportional to the velocity of blood flow cubed (i.e., V^3). Thus, the faster the blood flow, the more intense or the louder the bruit will be.[25] After exercising, blood flow velocity is increased significantly, and the intensity of a heart murmur or a bruit is subsequently increased. High-velocity blood flow also results in higher-pitched murmurs; conversely, lower-pitched murmurs correspond to lower-velocity blood flow. The greater the occlusion, the greater the velocity is expected through the partially occluded vessel. An increased degree of occlusion will, therefore, result in a higher-pitched bruit. It has been demonstrated that a soft, early systolic bruit will result from an artery that is occluded by 50%. If the occlusion increases to 70% or 80% reduction in diameter, the bruit may be heard not only in systole, but, moreover, during early diastole. A completely occluded artery may not have an associated bruit, since blood flow is totally diminished and cannot result in transmission of audible vibrations.[16,17,19,20]

While palpating the carotid arteries, the examiner may feel vibrations, which have been likened to the throat of a purring cat.[26] These vibrations are called a *thrill* and are an indication to carefully auscultate over the vessels to detect any bruits. The same vibrations in the vessel walls that result in a bruit are the cause of a carotid thrill. After carefully palpating both extracranial carotid arteries, the examiner must auscultate the vessels to further aid in ruling out atherosclerotic disease of the carotid arteries.

The importance of owning a properly fitted and designed stethoscope cannot be overemphasized.[10,25,27] A binaural stetho-

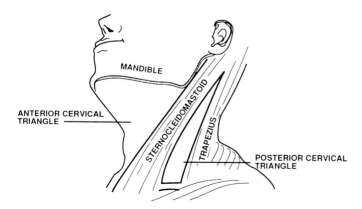

FIGURE 62–1. The sternocleidomastoid (SCM) muscle divides the neck into the anterior and posterior cervical triangles. The carotid arteries move deep to the SCM muscle on each side.

MANDIBLE

ANTERIOR CERVICAL TRIANGLE

STERNOCLEIDOMASTOID

TRAPEZIUS

POSTERIOR CERVICAL TRIANGLE

scope is intended to transmit sounds from the patient while eliminating superfluous and extraneous noise. A stethoscope that has been properly fitted to a particular examiner is an indispensable diagnostic aid.

The ear plugs must fit comfortably, but snugly, into the external auditory canals. The metal earpieces must fit to run parallel to the long axis of the external auditory canals (Fig. 62–3). The tension spring must hold the earpieces rather tightly into the auditory canal; however, care must be used to ensure that the earpieces are not held so tightly that they are uncomfortable. Extraneous noises will be blocked out by correctly fitting earpieces, whereas ear plugs that are too small or too tight may be occluded by pressing against the anterior wall of the external auditory canal.[25]

The tubing used for the stethoscope should have an internal diameter of 1/8 in.[27] A smaller inner diameter will attenuate high-frequency sounds;[25] therefore, an inner diameter of 3/16 in. (5 mm) or more has been suggested as being superior.[10] The walls of the tubing should be of either thick plastic or rubber, resulting in a relatively thick outer diameter, to reject extraneous outside noises as much as possible. For optimal transmission of sound, there should be no breaks or leaks in the tubing. Acoustically, double tubing extending to the endpiece yields better results than the Y configuration. Total length of the tubing should not exceed 12 to 15 in. (30 to 37 cm), so that the entire length of the stethoscope from the chestpiece to the ear does not exceed 20 or 21 in. (51 cm) in length.

There are two types of chestpieces found on the typical stethoscope (Fig. 62–4). The diaphragm is rigid. The diaphragm type of chestpiece naturally transmits sound at 300 cps. It therefore transmits higher-pitched sound while eliminating those that are lower pitched. For examining adults, a 1 1/2 in. (4 cm) diaphragm is most useful.

The second type of chestpiece is the trumpet bell, which is typically vaulted. Because there is no diaphragm over the bell, frequency of sounds transmitted will vary. The skin acts as a type of diaphragm, such that the amount of pressure applied to the bell will be a factor in the frequency of sounds transmitted. When light pressure is applied to the bell, the sounds transmitted are in the range of 40 cps, whereas a more firm pressure causes sounds in the range of 150 to 200 cps to be transmitted.[25] Sounds lower-pitched than 40 cps are not transmitted through the bell. A 1-in. (2.5 cm) bell is generally used to examine adult patients.

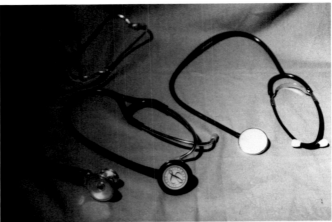

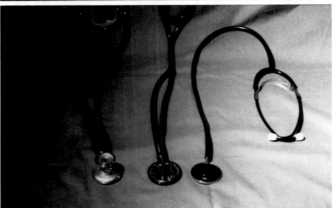

FIGURE 62–4. Several types of stethoscopes are available. The more typical stethoscope used by the optometrist (*left*) will have both a diaphragm and a trumpet bell. The Littman Master Cardiology Stethoscope (*middle*) provides only one chestpiece, but one that can alternate between low and high frequency signs by changing the pressure applied. The nurses' stethoscope (*right*) has only a diaphragm type chestpiece.

Use

Most stethoscopes employ both types of chestpieces so that a full range of sounds can be heard. For example, a lung examination is best accomplished with the diaphragm chestpiece, since the sounds transmitted tend to be higher-pitched. A low-pitched murmur is best heard with the bell of the stethoscope and a light application of pressure. A patient with aortic regurgitation is best examined with the diaphragm since the murmur is soft but relatively high-pitched. Conversely, mitral stenosis causes a deep, low-pitched rumbling sound for which the bell is better adapted for transmitting the sounds. Arterial bruits tend to be low-pitched sounds, and the bell is best suited for hearing them.

COMMERCIALLY AVAILABLE INSTRUMENTS

A stethoscope has long been used as the primary instrument for auscultation. Numerous companies manufacture binaural, double-head stethoscopes. Most of these instruments have a diaphragm chestpiece as well as a vaulted trumpet bell; however, stethoscopes are available that have only the flat diaphragm.

Tycos manufactures a Harvey stethoscope that features three chest pieces, including a bell, flat diaphragm, and a corrugated

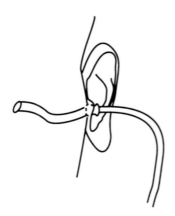

FIGURE 62–3. Correct fit of the earpieces of the stethoscope in the external auditory meatus. (Modified from Judge RD, Zuidema GD, Fitzgerald FT. Clinical diagnosis: a physiologic approach, 4th ed. Boston: Little, Brown & Co, 1982:235, with permission)

diaphragm. The three chestpieces permit a full range of sounds to be heard, from low-frequency gallops to the faint high-frequency blow characteristic of aortic insufficiency.[28]

Various stethoscopes are available specifically for cardiac auscultation. The Littmann Master Cardiology stethoscope made by 3M allows the examiner to hear both high- and low-frequency sounds through one chestpiece, since the traditional bell and diaphragm have been incorporated into a single-sided master chestpiece.[28]

Many different adaptations of stethoscopes are available, such as a Doppler stethoscope or even diplomicrophones for microvascular auscultation.[29,30] Technological advances in instrumentation continue to be devised, and the amount of use a particular instrument will receive must be considered before making a major financial investment. For most optometric practices, a high-quality binaural stethoscope will be sufficient to adequately diagnose ocular and related systemic problems.

CLINICAL PROCEDURE

Evaluation of Carotid Pulses

A reduction of blood flow through the extracranial carotid arteries will result in a concomitant reduction in blood flow through the vasculature nourishing the eye and orbit. It is essential to rule out carotid artery occlusive disease when assessing the vascular status of the eye. Analysis of the carotid pulses is an important part of that evaluation.

Gross inspection of the patient's neck should reveal any significant prominent pulsations. If severe kinking of the common carotid artery has occurred secondary to lengthening and tortuosity of the aorta,[26,31] a bulging, pulsatile mass may be noted in the proximal portion of the neck and may be mistaken for a carotid aneurysm. Older, hypertensive women tend to demonstrate this finding, and it most commonly occurs on the right side. A true carotid aneurysm, however, will also present as a pulsatile mass upon gross inspection, and a patient with this sign must be referred for correct differential diagnosis. Both carotid arteries may demonstrate dramatic pulsations in association with any high-output state, such as fever, thyrotoxicosis, or aortic insufficiency.[25]

Although some practitioners prefer to auscultate the carotid arteries for bruits first, many feel that the evaluation of carotid pulses initially gives clues to the need for careful and diligent auscultation of the extracranial carotid arteries. Regardless of the order of examination, there are two methods of performing the carotid pulse examination.

Determine the hand dominance of the patient, and examine the ipsilateral carotid system first. These carotid vessels will circulate blood to the ipsilateral cerebral hemisphere, which will be the nondominant hemisphere. Should the examination procedures result in precipitation of a stroke by embolization to the brain, or vascular occlusion, the nondominant hemisphere would be affected. Although this complication is extremely rare, it can occur with vigorous examination techniques, especially in older patients. Consequently, care should be taken to avoid excessive pressure on the carotid vessels.

The carotid pulses are palpated in the anterior triangle of the neck. If using the thumb, the examiner stands in front of the patient and uses the left thumb to palpate the right carotid pulse, and the right thumb to palpate the left carotid pulse. The appropriate thumb is gently placed medial to the sternocleidomastoid muscle on the neck, at approximately the level of the cricoid cartilage (Fig. 62–5). Pressure on the artery is slowly increased until maximum pulsations are felt, and the pressure is subsequently slowly released. If the examiner palpates the vessels too high on the neck, he or she may press directly on the carotid sinus. This structure is

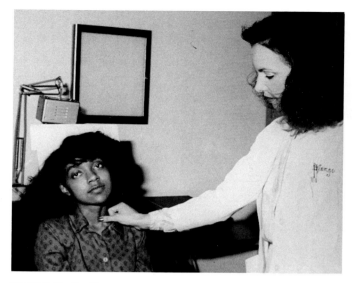

FIGURE 62–5. The examiner is using her thumb placed on the carotid artery to check pulsations. The carotid artery is palpated medial to the sternocleidomastoid muscle, at the level of the cricoid cartilage.

located at the level of the top of the thyroid cartilage. Excessive pressure on the carotid sinus, in a sensitive patient, may result in an increase in vagal tone and a subsequent reflex bradycardia, a reduction in blood pressure, and even a substantial enough vagal response to result in syncope. Extreme bradycardia and cardiac standstill may occur, although rarely.[25] Because of the possibility of an increased vagal response and the greater potential to cause embolization from carotid atheromas, much caution should be used to palpate the carotid pulse correctly at a point proximal to the carotid sinus. Palpation of one carotid pulse should be performed at a time, and bilateral evaluation of the pulses should never be attempted.[32]

A second method for palpation of the carotid pulses employs the three middle fingers. The examiner may stand either to the side or behind the patient (Fig. 62–6). The fingers are again placed at the medial edge of the sternocleidomastoid muscle at the level of the cricoid cartilage. When standing behind the patient, the examiner uses the right hand to palpate the right carotid vessels, and vice versa; however, when standing next to the patient, the examiner uses the hand opposite the side to be evaluated.

Palpation of the arterial pulse allows the examiner to compare the findings with what the examiner knows to be "normal" and to compare the findings between the right and left sides. Any tenderness should be noted. The amplitude of the pulse or the pulse pressure is compared between sides, and should be equal. The contour of the pulse should be evaluated. A smooth upstroke of approximately 0.10 seconds duration should occur, with the rounded crest adding another 0.08 to 0.12 seconds.[25] The initial percussion wave corresponds to the systolic component of the heart beat, whereas the dicrotic notch, which separates the systolic and diastolic components of the pulse, corresponds to closure of the aortic valve (Fig. 62–7). The dicrotic wave is not felt in a normal patient. Table 62–1 summarizes the findings to assess while palpating the carotid arteries.

The examiner must be certain that he or she is, in fact, feeling the carotid pulses and not the internal jugular vein pulsations,[24] although they are not frequently palpable. When palpable, these pulsations are generally found in the suprasternal notch, between the insertion of the sternocleidomastoid at the sternum and at the clavicle. The internal jugular vein can also be palpated in the poste-

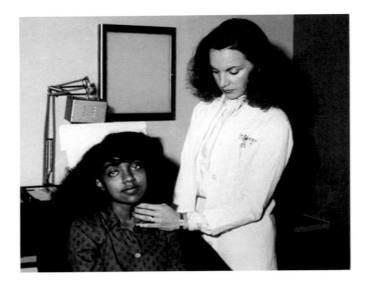

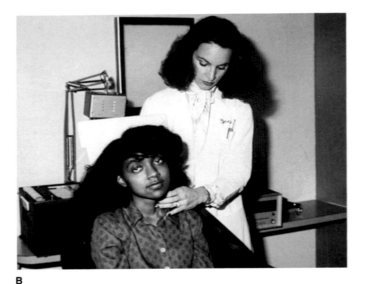

B

FIGURE 62–6. With the three-finger method of checking carotid pulsations, the examiner may stand either to the side of the patient (*A*) or behind the patient (*B*).

rior triangle immediately posterior to the sternocleidomastoid muscle in some patients. Differentiation of these pulses should not be difficult, as shown in Table 62–2.[26]

Auscultation for Carotid Arterial Bruits

When auscultating the carotid vessels, the examiner should place the chestpiece lightly on the neck, beginning at a position in the supraclavicular fossa to auscultate the subclavian artery (Fig. 62–8). If too much pressure is applied, iatrogenic bruits may be heard owing to compression of the vessels by the stethoscope.[21,33] The examiner must be careful not to move the stethoscope over the skin while listening to the sounds, since the friction noises produced will result in extraneous sounds. Care must also be taken not to move the fingers on the chestpiece or even breathe on the tubing, because confusing sounds can also be produced. Nor-

---

Table 62–1
Assessment of the Carotid Pulse

Rule out visible pulsations
Rule out tenderness, pain
Compare sides for equality of pulsations
Evaluate amplitude of pulsations
Evaluate contour of pulsations
Rule out variations in amplitude of beats
Rule out variations with respirations

---

mal children and adolescents may demonstrate supraclavicular systolic arterial murmurs, which are usually quite brief.[34,35]

After auscultating the subclavian artery, the examiner should then listen to the carotid arteries at three positions in the neck (Fig. 62–9). In the low position, the examiner will be auscultating the common carotid artery. At approximately the midlevel position, the examiner will be listening over the point of carotid bifurcation into the internal and external vessels. The examiner will auscultate the internal carotid artery at a position high in the neck. Any bruit discovered may be auscultated either at the site of stenosis or distally, following the direction of the blood flow.[19,21]

At each point of auscultation, the examiner should ask the patient to stop breathing. By doing so, the breath sounds will not obscure sounds produced within the vessel. Closing your eyes and assuming a relaxed position while listening is also important.[25] It is best to listen to one sound at a time. The systolic sounds should be identified, and the diastolic sound should then become familiar. Lastly, the presence of any bruit should be detected. In analyzing a bruit, it should be determined whether the bruit becomes softer and less pronounced or louder and more pronounced as the stethoscope is moved up the neck. Arterial bruits tend to be relatively low-pitched sounds (Fig. 62–10) of less than 100 cps; therefore, the bell of the stethoscope will be best adapted for hearing them.[33,36] Because some bruits are high-frequency sounds, however, some examiners believe that auscultation of the carotid arteries should be performed with the diaphragm chestpiece.[25,37,38] Considering the high-frequency sounds that can be produced with a near-total occlusion,[39] it is best to auscultate the carotid system first using the bell and then using the diaphragm chestpiece. The

---

Table 62–2
Differentiation of Internal Jugular and Carotid Pulsations

Internal Jugular Pulsations	Carotid Pulsations
Rarely palpable	Palpable
Soft undulating quality, usually with two elevations and two troughs	A more vigorous thrust with a single outward component
Pulsations eliminated by light pressure on the vein(s) just above the sternal end of the clavicle	Pulsation not eliminated by this pressure
Level of the pulsations usually descends with inspiration	Level of the pulsation not affected by inspiration
Level of the pulsations changes with position, dropping as patient becomes more upright	Level of the pulsation unchanged by position

(From Bates B. A guide to physical examination and history taking, 4th ed. Philadelphia: JB Lippincott Co, 1987:277, with permission)

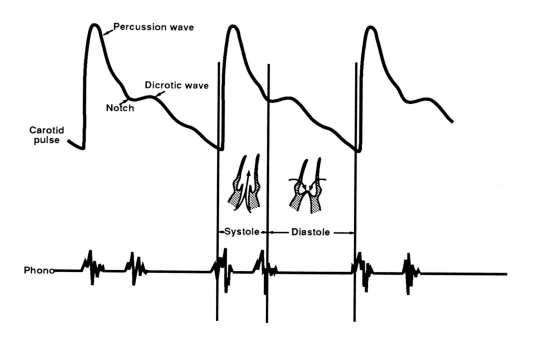
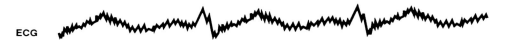

FIGURE 62–7. Normal carotid pulse. Pulse contour is shown as related to the timing of aortic valve motion, phonocardiogram, and electrocardiogram. (From Judge RD, Zuidema GD, Fitzgerald FT. Clinical diagnosis: a physiologic approach, 4th ed. Boston: Little, Brown & Co, 1982:214, with permission)

extra minute that it may take to perform this examination is certainly worth the possibility of detecting a high-frequency bruit for which a patient could be treated.

A bruit will be heard a fraction of a second after the cardiac apical impulse,[27] and is systolic in timing. As such, the bruit will be heard a fraction of a second after the carotid pulse is palpated, if

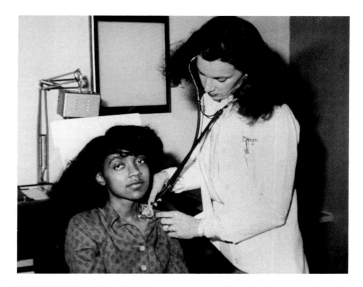

FIGURE 62–8. The subclavian artery is auscultated in the supraclavicular fossa.

the examiner were able to palpate the vessels and auscultate simultaneously.

It has been recognized that maneuvers performed that alter cardiovascular sounds in predictable ways can frequently aid the practitioner in making a correct differential diagnosis.[25,40–43] Maneuvers that change the pitch, intensity, or duration of a bruit can be very helpful to the clinician attempting to isolate carotid arterial bruits. For example, the vasodilatory effects of increased carbon dioxide tension[44] in the arteries result in subsequent increases in blood flow through the extracranial internal carotid vessel. Because of the increased demand and consequent rush of more blood through the stenotic vessels, an increase in the pitch, intensity, and duration of a bruit at the carotid bifurcation or internal carotid artery will be noted. Thus, if the patient were to either hold his breath or breathe 5% CO_2 in air, an increase in bruit sounds will be noted (Fig. 62–11). Conversely, hyperventilation would be expected to decrease the bruit, since the arterial carbon dioxide tension will result in constriction of the arterioles and, therefore, a decrease in blood flow through the internal carotid arteries.

After performing carotid auscultation with normal respiration, the patient may be instructed to take a deep breathe and hold it for 40 to 60 seconds while the examiner continues to auscultate the carotid vessels. Beasley and associates[45] have demonstrated a 30% increase in internal carotid bruit intensity by using this procedure, as long as the patient does not concomitantly perform a Valsalva maneuver, which may decrease the bruit for up to the first 10 seconds of the procedure.[45,46] If facilities are available to have the patient breathe a mixture of 5% CO_2 in air, a significant increase in bruit sounds may be noted, since as much as a 75% increase in internal carotid blood flow has been demonstrated with use of this procedure.[47]

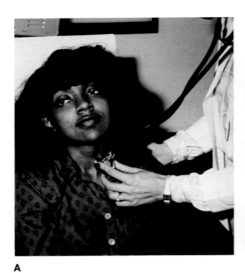
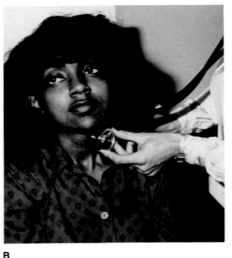
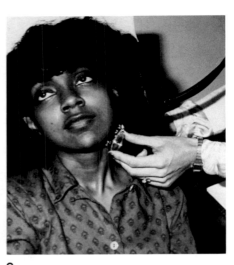

A　　　　　　　　　　　B　　　　　　　　　　　C

FIGURE 62–9. Auscultation of the carotid artery is performed in three positions. In the low position (*A*), the examiner is auscultating the common carotid artery. At the midlevel position (*B*), the stethoscope is placed over the carotid bifurcation. The internal carotid artery is auscultated at the high position in the neck (*C*).

By compression of specific arteries, internal carotid artery bruits may be intensified. For example, the practitioner can manually compress both the ipsilateral superficial temporal, and facial arteries (Fig. 62–12). Since the latter two vessels arise from the ipsilateral external carotid artery and compressing them will decrease blood flow through that artery, a decrease in a bruit originating in the external carotid artery will be noted, whereas an increase in flow through the internal carotid artery will result in an increase in bruit sounds if a stenosis is present in that vessel.[46,48] If a bruit emanates from both the internal and external ipsilateral vessels, however, differential diagnosis may not be confirmed with this procedure.[48]

If blood flow through the circle of Willis can be decreased by compression of the contralateral common carotid artery, external carotid bruit sounds will be decreased, and an internal carotid bruit will become more prolonged[49] as well as more intense.[50]

In examining the carotid arteries, the practitioner must be cautious not to confuse a jugular venous hum with carotid arterial sounds. If the bell chestpiece is placed in the supraclavicular fossa and the posterior triangles of the neck, a low-pitched hum will be detected that extends throughout the cardiac cycle (Fig. 62–13). Frequently, the hum is augmented during diastole.[31,51] A jugular venous hum is quite commonly heard in children[52] and, less frequently, in young adults; however, most healthy adults do not demonstrate this sound. Patients with marked anemia or patients with hyperthyroid conditions do, in fact, present with this low-pitched venous hum. If the patient demonstrates both a venous hum and an intracranial bruit, intracranial malformations must be ruled out. To aid in differential diagnosis, the examiner should attempt to abolish the sound by placing light pressure with a finger beside the trachea to occlude the venous flow through the jugular veins[22,31,34] (Fig. 62–14).

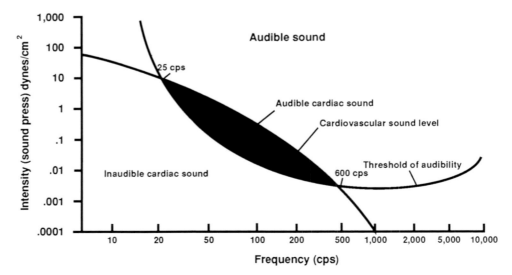

FIGURE 62–10. Ranges of audible and inaudible sound. Only a narrow range of sound generated in the heart may be heard on auscultation. (From Judge RD, Zuidema GD, Fitzgerald FT. Clinical diagnosis: a physiologic approach, 4th ed. Boston: Little, Brown & Co, 1982:237, with permission)

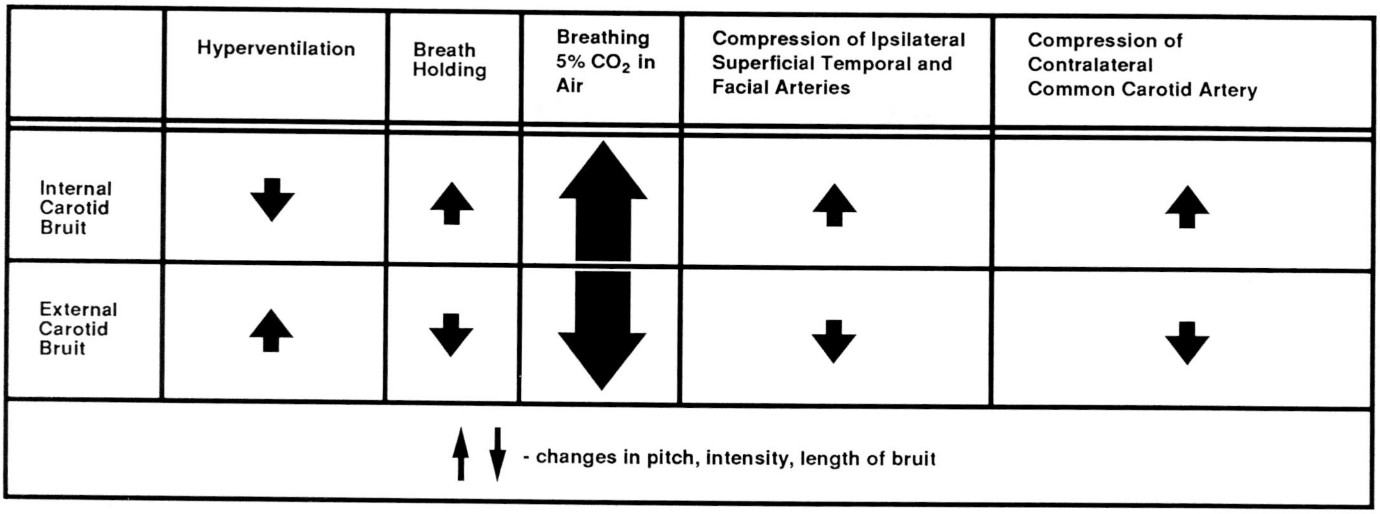

	Hyperventilation	Breath Holding	Breathing 5% CO₂ in Air	Compression of Ipsilateral Superficial Temporal and Facial Arteries	Compression of Contralateral Common Carotid Artery
Internal Carotid Bruit	↓	↑	⬆ (large)	↑	↑
External Carotid Bruit	↑	↓	⬇ (large)	↓	↓
↑ ↓ - changes in pitch, intensity, length of bruit					

FIGURE 62–11. Dynamic maneuvers useful in auscultation of carotid artery bruits. CO_2 = carbon dioxide. (From Kurtz KJ. Dynamic vascular auscultation. Am J Med 1984;76:1066–1074, with permission)

Auscultation for Orbital Bruits

When a patient presents with a unilateral, pulsating exophthalmos, auscultation should be performed to detect a bruit if it is present. The bell chestpiece is used for auscultation of orbital bruits.

The bell is held just as it is to perform carotid auscultation. It should be placed on the forehead at the midline, as well as above the eyebrow and at the temple (Fig. 62–15). If a bruit is not heard in these positions, it may be audible if the orbit is auscultated for a bruit.[53] To do so, first ask the patient to gently close his or her eyes, then the examiner places the bell over the superior eyelid (Fig. 62–16). Some examiners prefer the patient to keep both eyes closed; however, others ask the patient to open the opposite eye once the bell of the stethoscope is in place[25] (Fig. 62–17). Ausculta-

tion should be performed with the patient seated, lying on his or her back, and lying on each side.[54]

Occasionally, an orbital bruit may be difficult to hear. By having the patient bend forward or by lowering his head, the sounds produced will increase in intensity.[54] Conversely, compression of the ipsilateral carotid artery will decrease the intensity of the bruit.

Trauma patients present special requirements when auscultating for orbital bruits. Certainly, care must be taken not to produce greater tissue damage by applying excessive pressure to the eyelid and the globe indirectly when listening for orbital bruits. An additional technique, however, may be added to the examination while listening for orbital bruits. The patient is instructed to speak while the examiner applies the stethoscope first to the closed eyelid of the injured eye and secondly to the closed eyelid of the uninjured

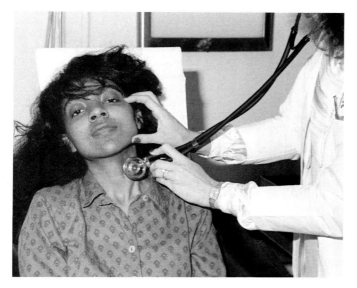

FIGURE 62–12. Compression of the superficial temporal and facial arteries can increase internal carotid artery bruit sounds if a stenosis is present.

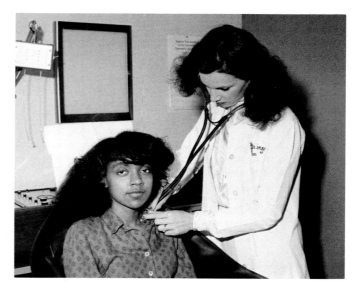

FIGURE 62–13. The bell chestpiece can be placed in the supraclavicular fossa to detect a low-pitched hum, extending throughout the cardiac cycle. This sound is a jugular venous hum.

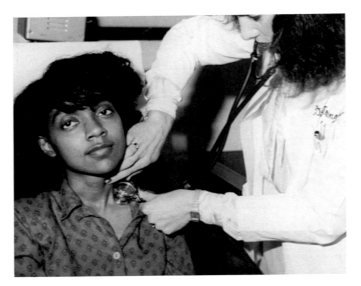

FIGURE 62–14. The venous hum can be abolished by applying pressure lateral to the trachea.

eye. Increased vocal resonance when auscultating the injured eye suggests the presence of a foreign body in the orbit.[54]

CLINICAL IMPLICATIONS

Clinical Significance

Carotid artery occlusive disease frequently has associated ocular signs and symptoms. Auscultation of the carotid arteries is an easy, rapid method to aid in the diagnosis of significant carotid occlusions. With a properly fitting stethoscope and routine auscultation for carotid bruits, early detection of hemodynamically significant lesions can prevent the morbidity and possible mortality associated with stroke. Furthermore, auscultation for orbital bruits can be essential in diagnosing critical vascular malformations that also may have fatal implications.

The primary care practitioner must routinely incorporate the measurement of certain vital signs into his or her examination of all patients. All middle-aged and elderly patients not only should have brachial blood pressures checked but, moreover, should undergo palpation of carotid pulses and auscultation for carotid bruits. As many as 4% of patients over 45 years of age have cervical bruits, and it has been estimated that 8 million adults in the United States have carotid bruits.[3] If the carotid examination is systematically incorporated into the routine evaluation, it takes very little time and can have great benefits in detecting hemodynamically significant carotid occlusive disease. With practice, the ear can be trained to hear carotid bruits, just as it is trained to hear heart sounds. By routinely listening to expectedly normal carotid arteries, the practitioner will find abnormal sounds to be much more easily detected when they do occur. As such, it would behoove the practitioner to choose an age over which all patients will undergo carotid palpation and auscultation. If, for example, the practitioner listens to the carotids of all patients who are over 40 years of age, numerous nondiseased arteries will be heard; therefore, when a patient does appear with major carotid occlusive disease, that finding will be far more apparent to the practitioner.

Clinical Interpretation

In a normal patient, the carotid arterial pulses will be equal, and all the assessed characteristics of the pulse will be within normal limits. Some patients, however, will demonstrate a markedly reduced or completely absent carotid pulse. This finding may be secondary to a partial or a complete occlusion of the carotid arteries, or to decreased stroke volume. Conversely, occluded carotid arteries may not demonstrate changes in arterial pulsations. Consequently, although assessment of carotid artery pulsation may be helpful in making a differential diagnosis, the findings must be taken in the appropriate context, and other more exact testing measurements must be added to the examination to arrive at a correct diagnosis.

Whether or not a carotid bruit that is auscultated is of any importance depends on several factors. Since the examiner auscultates for carotid bruits at several locations on the neck, it is possible to compare the loudness or intensity of the bruit at each location. A bruit in the supraclavicular space corresponds to a partial or

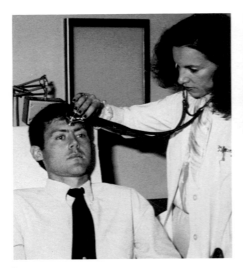
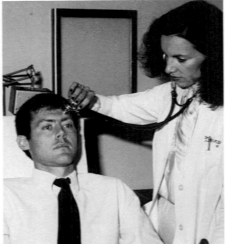
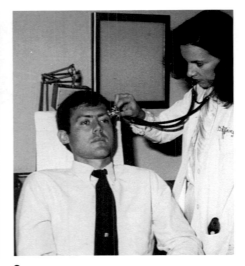

A   **B**   **C**

FIGURE 62–15. The bell of the chestpiece is placed on the forehead at the midline (*A*), as well as above the eyebrow (*B*), and at the temple (*C*) to auscultate for orbital bruits.

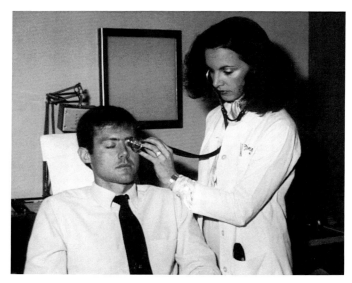

FIGURE 62–16. An orbital bruit can be auscultated with the patient's eyes closed, and the bell of the stethoscope is held over the superior eyelid.

complete occlusion of the subclavian artery. Patients may concomitantly complain of findings typical of the subclavian steal syndrome, in which proximal obstruction of the subclavian artery results in a decrease in arterial pressure in that artery at the point of bifurcation of the vertebral artery. Blood pressure in the affected arm may be decreased by more than 20 mmHg, and the radial pulse may be delayed or unequal, when compared with the contralateral pulse. If sufficient occlusion should occur, blood flow in the vertebral artery may be reversed and may be drained from the basilar artery through the vertebral artery to the subclavian and tributary vessels to the arm, especially when that arm is exercised in any way. The patient subsequently complains of symptoms of transient vertebrobasilar ischemia, including dizziness or vertigo, possible bilateral blackouts or grayouts of vision and impairment or loss of consciousness with exercise of that arm.[55,56]

If the examiner hears a bruit low in the neck that becomes progressively softer moving distally up the carotid vessels, trans-

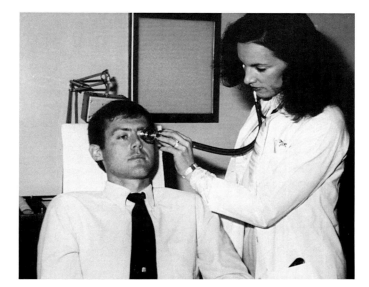

FIGURE 62–17. Some examiners prefer to have the patient open the opposite eye during auscultation for an orbital bruit.

mission of an aortic murmur must be considered in the differential diagnosis. In this event, a thrill may or may not be palpated. When an aortic murmur is suspected, auscultation should be performed both below and above the clavicle, as well as over the innominate and subclavian arteries, and over the common carotid artery, carotid bifurcation, and the internal carotid artery.

When a very soft bruit is heard in the proximal common carotid and increases in intensity when moving distally to the carotid bifurcation and the internal carotid artery, an atheromatous plaque at the carotid bulb is the most suspect cause. This plaque results in turbulent blood flow at the point of obstruction, as discussed earlier. The bruit may be heard in both the systolic and diastolic components, or just during systole.

Certainly, the patient's age must be a consideration in diagnosing the significance of a bruit. A middle-aged or elderly patient demonstrating a cervical bruit most likely has some degree of arterial narrowing; however, a cervical bruit can be detected in almost nine of every ten children under 5 years of age.[24,57] Furthermore, a systolic or a continuous bruit may be heard over the temporal areas in children younger than 5 years of age.[30] By adolescence, approximately one in three patients present with asymptomatic bruits and less than one in ten adults in middle age will demonstrate bruits.

All patients presenting with amaurosis fugax should be carefully examined, including a thorough dilated fundus examination and palpation of carotid pulses with auscultation for carotid bruits. A frequent cause of this type of monocular transient ischemic attack is embolization of plaque material from atheromas, either at the carotid bifurcation or at the origin of the internal carotid.[58] Among these patients, the incidence of carotid atheromatous disease is very high,[59,60] and, consequently, early detection with prophylactic management is essential. In many patients, the diagnosis of amaurosis fugax and its concomitant carotid atheromatous disease can be made solely on the signs and symptoms presented (Table 62–3);[30] however, careful evaluation of the hemodynamic status of the carotid system and an evaluation of the retinal blood vessels for Hollenhorst plaques must be performed, owing to the potential adverse consequences of such lesions. Should embolization occur that occludes a smaller vessel in the brain, the patient will suffer a cerebrovascular accident, or stroke, which is the third leading cause of death in the United States.[61] Before the actual stroke, more than 75% of these patients experience some type of transient ischemic neurologic symptoms.[62] Furthermore, in about three-fourths of patients with symptoms of ischemic cerebrovascular insufficiency, the lesions were surgically accessible, as dem-

Table 62–3
Symptoms and Signs of Carotid Atheromatous Disease

Transient Symptoms	***Chronic Ocular Hypoxia***
Amaurosis fugax	Dilated episcleral veins
Photopsias	Edematous cornea
Orbital and ocular pain	Anterior chamber reaction
	Rubeosis and iris atrophy
Ophthalmoscopic Signs	Synechiae
Arteriosclerotic retinopathy	Cataract
Hypertensive retinopathy	Glaucoma (or hypotony)
Bright plaques	Retinal venous dilation
Occluded arteries	Microaneurysms, hemorrhages
Optic atrophy	Neovascularization
	Arterial occlusions

(From Glaser JS. Topical diagnosis: prechiasmal visual pathways. In: Duane TD, Jaeger EA, eds. Clinical ophthalmology. vol 2. Philadelphia: Harper & Row, 1987:7, with permission)

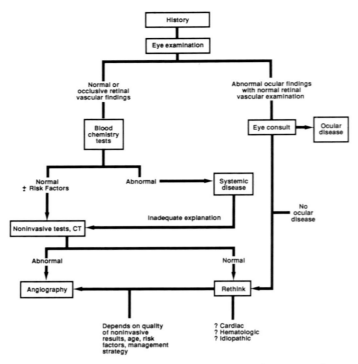

FIGURE 62–18. Scheme for workup of patients with amaurosis fugax. (From Barnett HJM, Bernstein EF, Callow AD, et al. The Amaurosis Fugax Study Group. Amaurosis fugax (transient monocular blindness): a consensus statement. In: Bernstein EF, ed. Amaurosis fugax. New York: Springer-Verlag, 1988:290, with permission)

Table 62–4
Laboratory Workup to Rule Out Bruits Caused by Anemia or Hyperthyroidism

Anemia	Hyperthyroidism
Complete blood count, including:	Serum total T_3
Hemoglobin	Serum total T_4
Red blood cell count (RBC)	T_3 resin uptake
Hematocrit (PCV)	Thyrotropin-releasing hormone stimulation test (TRH test)
Mean corpuscular hemoglobin (MCH)	Thyroid radioiodine uptake (RAIU)
Mean corpuscular volume (MCV)	Plasma thyroglobulin
Mean corpuscular hemoglobin concentration (MCHC)	Plasma iodide
White blood cell count (WBC) and differential	
Platelet count	
Reticulocyte count	
Serum ferritin levels	
Serum iron levels	
Total iron-binding capacity (TIBC)	

onstrated by contrast arteriography.[63] If a patient experiences transient cerebral ischemic attacks, reduced ophthalmic artery pressures, retinal arterial occlusions, chronic hypoxic retinopathy, cholesterol emboli, or a carotid bruit, in addition to amaurosis fugax, it has been determined that there is a greater risk of the patient suffering permanent cerebral deficits.[59] Thus, it is clear that many of these patients present with signs and symptoms indicative of carotid atheromatous lesions, and that many cases of fatal stroke or significant debilitation secondary to a cerebrovascular accident can be avoided if the primary care examiner pursues appropriate referrals. The Amaurosis Fugax Study Group[64] has suggested an

Table 62–5
Major Pathophysiologic and Clinical Features of Arteriovenous Shunts and Venous Anomalies

Lesion	Site of Shunt	Principal Orbital Hemodynamic Pathology	Principal Symptoms
Arteriovenous Shunts			
AVM (arteriovenous malformation)	Intraorbital	Hyperdynamic antegrade shunt with mass effect	Proptosis, faint orbital pulsations, bruit
	Extraorbital	Collateral flow to extraorbital shunt	Epibulbar vascular congestion
Posttraumatic carotid cavernous fistulas	Cavernous sinus	High-flow shunt with pulsatile retrograde flow into orbital veins	Bruit, prominent orbital pulsation, orbital congestion with elevated venous pressure
Dural arteriovenous fistulas of cavernous sinus	Cavernous sinus	Low-flow shunt with faintly pulsatile or nonpulsatile retrograde flow in orbital veins	Same as above but to a lesser degree
Venous Anomalies			
Nondistensible	No shunt	Spontaneous hemorrhage	Episodic hemorrhages with frequent spontaneous resolution
Distensible	No shunt	Enlargement with elevation of systemic venous pressure	Intermittent proptosis

(From Rootman J, Graeb DA. Vascular lesions. In: Rootman J, ed. Diseases of the orbit: a multidisciplinary approach. Philadelphia: JB Lippincott Co, 1988:546, with permission)

PART 3

Contact Lens Procedures

Contact Lens Evaluation

Gerald E. Lowther

INTRODUCTION

Definition

The dimensions and quality of contact lenses are measured and evaluated to determine whether they meet the specifications ordered from the laboratory or to determine the specifications and suitability of lenses being worn by the patient.

History

Since the early use of scleral lenses, manufacturers and clinicians have used various techniques to measure the different lens parameters to determine their dimensions. Some early techniques consisted of only qualitative estimates of lens curvatures, for example, by matching the lens to known curvature templates or using devices similar to lens clocks used for spectacle lenses. Because of the small dimensions and high tolerances required of contact lenses, more sophisticated measuring techniques are often required. Instruments utilizing optical, mechanical, electrical, and ultrasound principles have been developed and used. Some have withstood the test of time and are generally used in laboratories and clinical practice, whereas others either lacked accuracy or have proved too difficult or time-consuming to be practical.

Clinical Use

Contact lenses must be manufactured and fit to close tolerances, usually to the 0.1 or 0.01 mm. It is difficult to consistently fabricate contact lenses to such tolerances because of the variability in lens material and equipment. Therefore, it is mandatory that the manu-facturer be able to measure the lens after fabrication to determine the dimensions.

The clinician must be able to verify several dimensions of the contact lens received from the contact lens laboratory to determine if the parameters are within the tolerance of what was ordered. Due to mass production of contact lenses and the inevitable mistakes that will occasionally occur, such inspection is necessary to prevent an improper lens from being dispensed to the patient.[1–5]

INSTRUMENTATION

Theory and Use

V-Gauge

A V-gauge is used to measure the diameter of rigid lenses. It consists of a piece of metal or plastic with a V-shaped channel cut into it with a scale along the side of the gauge indicating the width of the channel at that point (Fig. 64–1). The lens is placed in the wide end of the channel, the gauge tilted up at this end and the lens allowed to slide down the gauge until it stops. The value on the scale corresponding to the center of the lens is the diameter.

Measuring Magnifier

The measuring magnifier, often called a hand-held magnifier, can be used to measure overall diameter, optic zone diameters, and peripheral curve widths. It consists of an eyepiece with a face plate at a fixed distance from the eyepiece (Fig. 64–2). There is a scale on the face plate used to measure linear distances. The eyepiece can be rotated to obtain sharp focus on the scale. Looking through

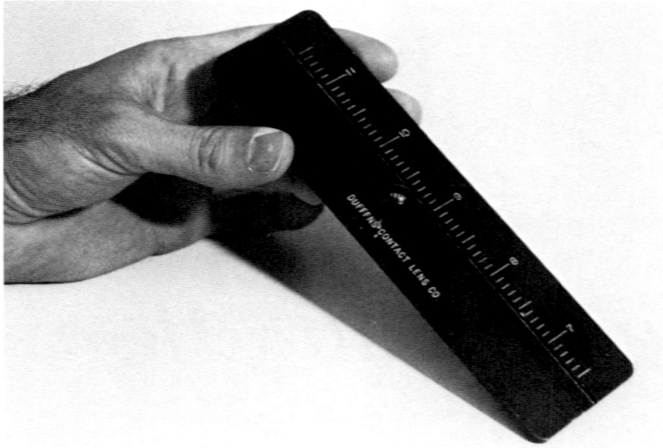

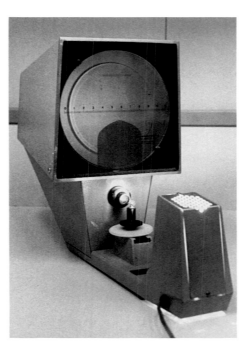

FIGURE 64–3. Projection magnifier used to measure the overall diameter, optical zone diameter, peripheral curve widths, edge shape, and surface defects of a rigid lens.

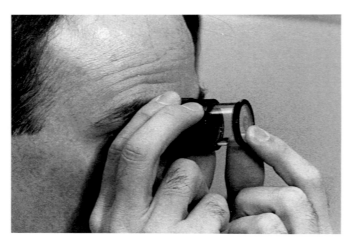

FIGURE 64–1. V-gauge used to measure the overall diameter of a rigid contact lens with the lens in place.

the instrument toward an uniformly illuminated background, the eye piece should be rotated outward, counterclockwise, until the scale is blurred. Then the eye piece is rotated clockwise until the scale comes into sharp focus. The lens can then be held on the face of the magnifier and the desired linear dimension measured.

Shadowgraph

The shadowgraph (projection magnifier, comparator) (Fig. 64–3) consists of a collimated light beam in which the contact lens is placed. The shadow of the lens is projected onto a screen that can have a scale for measurement. This instrument can be used to measure and inspect lens diameter, optic zone diameter, peripheral curve widths, surface quality, and lens edge shapes.

Radiuscope

The radiuscope (radiusgauge) is used primarily for measuring the base curve radius of rigid contact lenses; however, it can also be used to measure the front radius and center thickness of lenses. The radiuscope (Figs. 64–4 and 64–5) is a modified microscope that has an illumination system that projects a spoke pattern down

the axis of the instrument through the objective by a beam splitter. By placing the contact lens on the stage of the instrument under the objective, one can focus on the lens surface. Then by changing the plane of focus by racking the microscope upward (or the stage

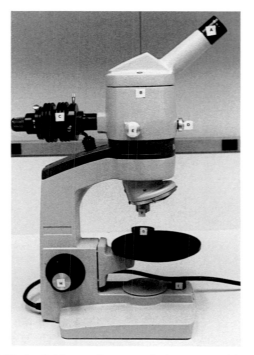

FIGURE 64–4. Reichert radiuscope with the eyepiece (*A*), main body (*B*), light source (*C*), scale focus (*D*), adjustment for the reference line (*E*), objective (*F*), and stage (*G*) where the lens is mounted, focusing knobs (*H*), and light control (*I*).

FIGURE 64–2. Rigid contact lens being held on the face of a hand magnifier to measure overall diameter, optical zone diameter, or peripheral curve widths.

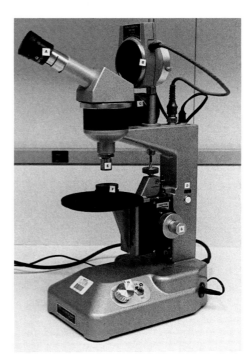

FIGURE 64–5. R H Burton Digital Radiusgauge with the eyepiece (*A*), digital scale (*B*), light source (*C*), adjustment for zeroing the digital scale (*D*), objective (*E*) and stage where the lens is mounted (*F*), focusing knobs (*G*), and light control (*H*).

down, depending on the instrument), the aerial (reflected) image of the pattern can be brought into view. The contact lens is used as a concave mirror. The distance from the surface image to the aerial image is the radius of the base curve. A scale, either a dial externally or one in the field of view of the eyepiece, is provided to determine the radius.

Lensometer

Lensometers are used to measure the power of contact lenses with procedures very similar to those used for spectacle lenses (see Chap. 30). Because of the greater sagittal depth of a contact lens, compared with spectacles, special stops are commonly supplied with lensometers to use when measuring contact lenses. Their use is especially important with higher prescription lenses.

Thickness Gauges

Thickness gauges for rigid lenses have a pedestal (rounded post) on which the lens is placed and then a movable top post that is brought down on the lens surface (Fig. 64–6). The circular scale indicates the thickness of the contact lens in millimeters. Gauges with round posts or ball-bearings on the posts, which prevent lens scratching or damage, should be used.

A method for measuring center thickness of hydrogel lenses is to use the lens as an electrical switch, since the water-laden lens will transmit electricity.[6,7] Devices that use this principle have some means of bringing an electrode in contact with the back surface and a second one in contact with the front surface with a scale indicating the separation of the two. An example is shown in Figure 64–7 in which the lower dome has an electrical wire (electrode) in the center of it. With the contact lens on the lower dome, the upper dome, which also has an electrode in the center, is brought down until it touches the lens. At this time the light on the

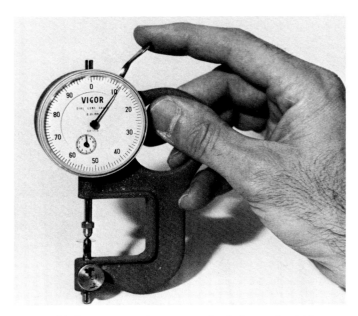

FIGURE 64–6. Gauge used to measure the thickness of a rigid contact lens.

base comes on indicating the electrical circuit is closed. The lens thickness is read from the gauge.

Refractometer

The water content of hydrogel lenses can be measured using a refractometer, since the water content is directly related to the

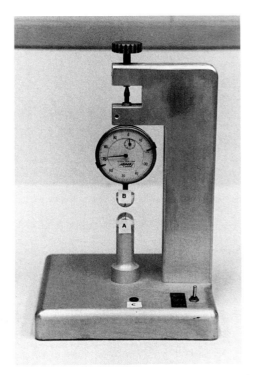

FIGURE 64–7. Redher electronic center thickness gauge with hydrogel lens in place to be measured. Dome on which lens is placed (*A*), upper dome brought down on lens (*B*), light (*C*) that illuminates when upper dome touches lens.

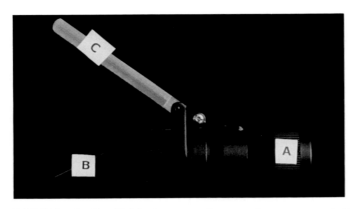

FIGURE 64–8. Hand-held refractometer for measuring water content of hydrogel lenses. Eyepiece (*A*), measuring prism (*B*), and plate to flatten lens on prism (*C*).

refractive index. A hand-held refractometer (Fig. 64–8) has been designed specifically for this purpose.[8] The lens is placed on the prism of the refractometer after blotting, flattened onto the prism with a cover, and the refractive index read from the scale seen internally.

COMMERCIALLY AVAILABLE INSTRUMENTS

V-Gauges

V-gauges are available from most contact lens laboratories and are manufactured using either plastic or metal material.

Measuring Magnifiers

Numerous measuring magnifiers are available from most contact lens laboratories with either 7× or 10× magnification. Either magnification is sufficient.

Radiuscopes (Radiusgauges)

Reichert (Formerly American Optical) Radiuscope

The Reichert radiuscope (see Fig. 64–4) consists of an eyepiece (*A*), main body (*B*), light source attached to the side of the body (*C*), objective (*F*), and stage (*G*). There is a small slide in the tube between the light source (*C*) and the body of the instrument that has two different aperture sizes to control the area of the lens illuminated. If this slide is moved so that it is half way between the two apertures, light will not enter the instrument. Normally, the large aperture is used. The scale is seen in the eyepiece and is focused by the small knob (*D*) on the side of the instrument. The reference line seen on the scale is moved by the small knob (*E*) on the front of the instrument body below the eyepiece. The objective (*F*), not the stage, moves on this instrument when the different images are brought into focus by using the coarse and fine focus knobs (*H*) near the base of the instrument. This instrument is available with either a single eyepiece or as a binocular instrument, both are equally accurate, with the binocular instrument being more comfortable for those spending long hours using it.

R H Burton Digital Radiusgauge

The R H Burton instrument (see Fig. 64–5) uses the same principle as the Reichert radiuscope except it has a digital readout (*B*) in-

stead of an internal scale. The R H Burton radiusgauge is also available with an external clock dial-type scale, instead of the digital readout. In addition the stage (*F*) moves to change focus instead of the objective.

Neitz Radiusgauge

This instrument is very similar to the R H Burton instrument, except that it has a clock-type external dial gauge.

Thickness Gauge

Mechanical Gauge

Numerous mechanical thickness gauges for measuring center thickness of rigid contact lenses are available from contact lens laboratories. They are all similar. The Vigor gauge (see Fig. 64–6) is an example showing the mechanical gauge (*A*), a movable post (*B*), and a pedestal or stage on which the lens rests (*C*).

Redher Gauge

This gauge (see Fig. 64–7) uses an electrical circuit to determine when the movable portion of the gauge touches the lens surface. The lens is placed on the lower dome (*A*), the upper dome (*B*) is brought down by using the knob until it touches the lens surface. When it touches, the light on the base (*C*) lights up and the thickness can be read from the dial (*D*).

Refractometer

Atago Model CL-1

The Atago refractometer (see Fig. 64–8) is the only one specifically made for use in measuring water content of hydrogel contact lenses. The lens surface is blotted and placed on the measuring prism (*B*) and flatten with the flat plate (*C*) that comes down against the prism. The measurement is made by the location of the line seen on the scale when viewing through the eye piece (*A*).

CLINICAL PROCEDURE

Rigid Lenses

Lens Diameter

The linear dimension across the largest portion of the lens is the lens diameter, also called the overall diameter (OAD) or overall size.

An accurate and simple method to measure the lens diameter is with the V-gauge. The procedure for using the V-gauge is the following:

1. The lens and gauge should be cleaned and dried with a soft tissue.
2. The contact lens is placed in the wide end of the gauge and allowed to slide down the channel by lifting the wide end of the gauge upward and allowing the lens to slide down by gravity until it stops. The lens should not be pushed down the channel, since it may flex and, thereby, give an erroneous reading.
3. The diameter is read by noting the mark on the scale corresponding to the center of the lens.
4. The lens should be slid up the scale, rotated slightly, and measured again to assure the lens is round. If the lens is not round, or if it is truncated, the largest and smallest diameters should be recorded.

Another method of measuring the diameter is to use a hand-held magnifier of approximately 7× to 10× magnification. The magnifier has a millimeter scale on the flat face. To use the hand magnifier:

1. The lens and scale is cleaned and dried with a soft tissue.
2. The lens is placed concave side down on the flat surface and held in place by the tip of the finger (see Fig. 64–2).
3. The magnifier is held up toward a light source.
4. The lens is positioned on the scale and the diameter read.
5. The diameter is read in more than one meridian, and if the lens is not round the narrow and wide dimensions are recorded.

A projection magnifier (shadowgraph) can also be used to measure overall diameter. To use the projection magnifier

1. The lens is cleaned and dried with a soft tissue.
2. The lens is placed on the stage in the light beam and the image of the lens is projected on the screen (see Fig. 64–3).
3. The lens diameter is read from the scale on the screen.
4. The diameter is read in more than one meridian, and if the lens is not round, the narrowest and widest dimensions are recorded.

Posterior Optical Zone Diameter

The posterior optical zone diameter (POZD), also called back optical zone diameter, back central optic diameter, or very commonly, just optical zone diameter (OZD), is the back central portion of the lens corresponding to the base curve of the lens. This is the portion that contains the lens power required to correct the patient's refractive error. Peripheral to this region is the secondary curve, which has a longer (flatter) radius than the base curve. The junction between the base curve and secondary curve forms the outer limit of the posterior optical zone.

To use the hand-held magnifier:

1. The lens and scale are cleaned and dried with a soft tissue.
2. The lens is placed on the flat face as before, being held in place by the tip of the finger and held up toward a light source.
3. The magnifier may have to be moved or aimed in different positions toward the light source to discern the junction, particularly if there is little difference between the base curve radius and secondary curve radius or if the lens is blended.
4. The lens is positioned such that one edge of the posterior optical zone is at zero on the scale and the value directly across from the widest part of the optical zone that corresponds to the junction between the curves is measured.
5. The lens should be rotated to measure different chords to be sure the optical zone is round. If it is not, the widest and narrowest dimensions should be recorded.

The projection magnifier can also be used to measure the posterior optical zone diameter by placing the lens in the beam of the instrument and using the scale and the screen to measure the posterior optical zone in the same fashion as with the hand-held magnifier.

Posterior Peripheral Curve Widths

There may be one or multiple curves peripheral to the base curve. Each successive curve from the base curve toward the edge of the lens is longer (flatter). The first curve beyond the base curve is often called the posterior secondary curve, the next one the posterior tertiary curve. Sometimes the most peripheral curve, the one nearest the edge, is narrow (0.1 to 0.2 mm) and a relative long

radius and is called the bevel. If there are more than two peripheral curves, they can be specified by numbering them beginning with the curve adjacent to the optical zone.

The width of the posterior peripheral curves can be measured with the hand magnifier or projection magnifier as described in the foregoing for the posterior optical zone diameter, except the width of each curve is determined with the scale on the instrument.

The sum of the posterior optical zone diameter plus two times the widths of the peripheral curves must equal the overall lens diameter. For example, if the optical zone is 8.0 mm, secondary curve width 0.4 mm, and the bevel is 0.2 mm, the overall lens diameter is 9.20 mm.

Blends

The transition between the base curve radius and secondary curve is often blended by polishing this junction slightly with an intermediate-radius polishing tool. This blurs the junction making it more difficult to discern the optical zone diameter. As it is not possible to measure the amount of blending, blends are usually specified as light, medium, or heavy. Some laboratories will use 1, 2 or 3 or a, b, or c in place of the light, medium, or heavy notation. A light blend means the junction is still fairly distinct, whereas a heavy blend makes it practically impossible to determine where the junction occurs. With experience, the degree of blending can easily be determined viewing lenses with the hand-held magnifier or projection magnifier.

Posterior Central Curve Radius

The radius of the curve that makes up the posterior optical zone diameter of the lens is called the posterior central curve radius (PCCR), base curve radius (BCR), or back central optic radius (BCOR). It is the primary curve of the lens and the portion containing the optical portion of the lens that the patient will be looking through.

The most common instrument used to measure the posterior central radius is the radiuscope (also called a radiusgauge or optical microspherometer).

To use the radiuscope the following procedure is used:

1. The contact lens should be dried and cleaned with a soft tissue. If the lens is not clean, all of the spokes may not come into focus at the same time giving a false impression of a toric surface. One must be careful not to handle the lens roughly or flex it before measurement, as this can produce erroneous readings.
2. The lens is placed on the holder, convex surface down, on a small drop of water (Fig. 64–9). The water is used to eliminate the confusing reflection of light from the front (convex) lens surface, since only the back (concave) surface reading is desired. Excessive water should not be used under the lens, as the lens may move during the measurement giving erroneous values.
3. The contact lens is positioned under the objective by looking outside the instrument and moving the stage until the spot of light is seen in the center of the lens.
4. Then looking into the instrument, focus the reflected (upper) image of the spoke pattern.
5. Adjust the stage until the spoke pattern is in the center of the field of view and the oblique spokes are aligned with the diagonal reference lines.
6. Next focus down on the surface image (lower spoke image—below the image of the filament). Small surface debris and scratches that were not seen with the upper reflected image should be seen in this image. One must be sure the spoke pattern is in sharp focus when zeroing and

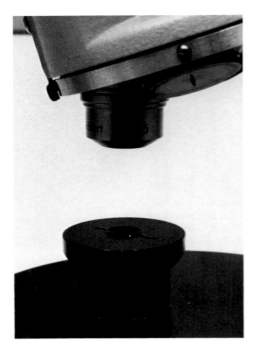

FIGURE 64–9. Lens positioned on a drop of water on the stage of the microscope.

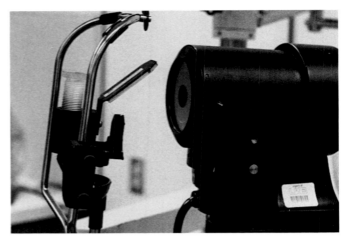

FIGURE 64–10. Holder attached to the keratometer for measuring the posterior central curve radius of a rigid lens. The lens is placed on a drop of water on the pedestal under the front surface mirror, which is used to reflect the image of the lens into the axis of the keratometer.

making the measurement. This is best done by concentrating on one spoke near the center and being sure the edges of the spoke are in as sharp a focus as possible. Do not try to view the entire pattern at once.

7. Depending on the manufacturer, the instrument has a scale either in the field of view through the ocular or on an external gauge. This gauge should be zeroed or placed on a reference number by using the appropriate knob.
8. The scope is focused upward to the aerial spoke pattern again.
9. With this image in sharp focus the posterior central curve radius is read from the millimeter scale or dial.

If a toric posterior central curve lens is being measured the procedure is the same as above, except when focusing on the aerial (top) image, only one of the spokes can be focused at a time. The first spoke brought into focus when moving upward from the surface image is the radius of curvature of the steeper meridian. By focusing farther upward, the spoke 90° from the first, the flat meridian, is brought into focus. If a single spoke cannot be focused, the lens must be rotated, while viewing the aerial image and rotating the lens holder, until a single spoke is in focus.

The keratometer or ophthalmometer may also be used to measure the posterior central curve radius. A special holder is attached to the instrument on which the contact lens can be mounted (Fig. 64–10). To use the keratometer:

1. The lens is cleaned and dried with a soft tissue.
2. The lens is floated on a small drop of water, which is placed in a holding device.
3. The keratometer mires are aligned on the lens with the aid of a front surface mirror. The keratometer is used to measure the radius in the same fashion as one would use the instrument to measure the cornea (see Chap. 15).
4. The drum reading, if given only in diopters, can be converted to radius of curvature using the same charts that are used for measuring cornea curvature. Since the contact lens surface is concave and the instrument is designed to

measure a convex surface, the lens central posterior curve will be slightly flatter than the drum reading by 0.02 to 0.04 mm, depending on the radius range. Conversion tables are available with the instruments or in standard contact lens textbooks.

Lens Power

The power of a rigid contact lens is measured using the same procedures as used for spectacle lenses (see Chap. 30).

1. The contact lens should be cleaned and dried with a soft tissue.
2. The special contact lens stop is placed on the lensometer if one has been supplied with the instrument.
3. The lens is held centered over the stop, with the tip of the finger on the bottom edge of the lens. With lensometers that are vertical, or can be tilted to the vertical position, the contact lens does not need to be held in position.
4. The lens power is read using the same procedures as used with a spectacle lens.

If a bitoric or toric posterior curve lens is being measured, the power in both of the major meridians must be measured as with a cylindrical spectacle lens. However, the axis does not need to be specified, since there is no reference for the vertical meridian of the lens. Therefore, the total power in both meridians is recorded, for example −2.00/−5.00 D. In the case of a prism ballast, front surface cylinder lens, the lens is placed on the stop and rotated until the prism is read as base-down. The sphere, cylinder and axis is then read as one would read a spectacle cylindrical lens. The base–apex line is used as the vertical reference.

Optical Quality

If a contact lens surface has not been cut or polished properly, the surface may be distorted. Improperly manufactured lenses may also warp. When measuring the power with the lensometer, one may notice some mild distortion of the image if the lens has poor optics, but often this is not noticeable. Clinically one can attain a better estimation of the optical quality by holding the lens up between the fingers at arms length and viewing a line or grid pattern (a fluorescent light fixture, for example) through the lens. If the lines are wavy or distorted, the lens has poor optics.

Center Thickness

The center thickness can be measured by using hand-held thickness gauges as follows:

1. The scale should read zero without the lens in place. If not, the scale should be adjusted with the outside ring until it reads zero.
2. The movable post should be lifted, the lens positioned in place, and the post gently brought down onto the lens. The lens should be positioned such that the reading is being taken at the center of the lens to determine center thickness.
3. The thickness is read from the scale.

The thickness at different points on the lens can be measured if one wishes to determine the variation in thickness across the lens. For example, with a lenticular design it may be used to verify that a lenticular lens is being worn or has been fabricated.

Edge Contour

The edge shape and thickness of a rigid contact lens are very important for comfort. Because of the shape of an edge, it is not clinically feasible to measure the edge thickness of a finished lens. Before shaping, the edge should be about 0.10 mm thick. If the edge is too thick or the peak of the edge is too far toward the front of the lens, the superior lid will hit the thick edge causing discomfort. If the edge is too thin or the peak at the back surface, discomfort from the cornea or lid will result. A thin edge can easily chip or crack, also causing discomfort. A good edge should have the peak of the edge about two-thirds of the distance from the front surface and one-third from the back.[9,10]

A stereomicroscope with approximately 40× magnification with a high-intensity external source can be used to inspect the edge (Fig. 64–11) as described in the following:

1. The lens is cleaned and dried with a soft tissue.
2. The lens is gently held against the index finger as if the finger is the cornea.
3. The light source is positioned such that there is maximum intensity on the lens.
4. The edge is viewed at the top with the view being the same as the superior eyelid would have coming downward on a blink. Do not try to view the edge in cross section by looking at what would be the 3- or 9-o'clock positions on the lens.

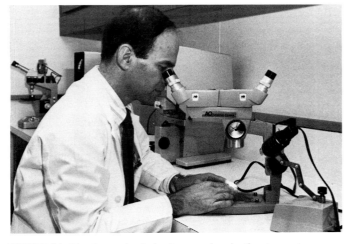

FIGURE 64–11. Lens edge being inspected under the stereomicroscope.

5. Note the shape of the edge and the position of the peak. Usually there is a bright light reflex from the peak.
6. The thickness of the edge is estimated by the distance of the peak from the finger.

It takes time and effort to learn to hold and position the lens properly under the microscope, but the time saved later in inspection and the ability to see the edge shape are worth the effort.

The biomicroscope or hand-held loupe[11] can be used to inspect the lens edge, using the same procedure described for the stereomicroscope.

The projection magnifier is also used to inspect lens edges. This instrument is easy to learn to use; however, it has the disadvantage of making some poor-quality edges appear as good-quality edges. Since a shadow of the lens is seen on the screen, any edge detail on the inside portion of the edge is obscured. If the inside portion of the edge is tapered from the front toward the back, causing the peak to be near the front surface, the edge will appear well shaped even though it may be thick. The forward positioned peak will result in discomfort to the patient.

Tints

Contact lenses are often tinted for ease of handling and locating the lens. They may also be tinted to enhance or change eye color. The tint should be inspected to determine if it is the color and density ordered. Tint density is usually specified as light, medium, or dark (1, 2, or 3). Most lenses have only light tints. The tint can also be inspected under the stereomicroscope to determine whether the tint is uniform, without clumps or irregularities.

Hydrogel Lenses

Lens Diameter

With hydrogel lenses, it is often necessary only to approximate the lens diameter to decide whether a lens is in the wrong vial. For example, one may want to determine whether a lens is 14.00 or 14.50 mm in diameter. This measurement can be made with a hand magnifier in this manner:

1. Remove the lens from the solution with soft lens tweezers.
2. Hold the lens with soft lens tweezers and shake off any excess water.
3. Place the lens in a lint-free tissue. Gently blot the surface with a lint-free tissue by lightly pressing the folded tissue against the lens.
4. Move the lens to a dry spot on the tissue and blot it again.
5. Place the lens gently on the flat face of the hand magnifier (as previously described for rigid lenses) being careful not to bend or distort the lens.

If a more accurate diameter determination is desired the lens can be placed in a wet cell to keep it fully hydrated (Fig. 64–12). The wet cell can be held against the hand magnifier and the diameter measured. This method is usually sufficiently accurate for clinical measurements.

A projection magnifier may also be used, with the lens either blotted or in a wet cell. The lens diameter can be measured by using the scale on the screen as with rigid lenses.

The posterior and anterior optical zone diameters, as well as the peripheral curve widths, can be measured using the same techniques as described previously.

Power

The easiest clinical method for measuring lens power is to blot the lens and place it on the stop of the lensometer,[12] as described

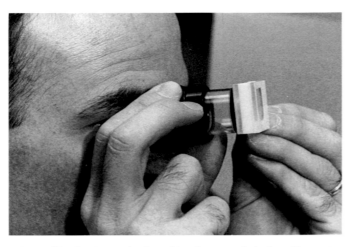

FIGURE 64–12. Determination of the diameter of a hydrogel lens using a hand magnifier with the lens in a wet cell.

below:

1. Remove the lens from the solution with soft lens tweezers.
2. Hold the lens with the tweezers and shake off any excess water.
3. Place the lens on a lint-free tissue. Gently blot the surface with a lint-free tissue by lightly pressing the folded tissue against the lens.
4. Move the lens to a dry spot on the tissue and blot it again.
5. Place the lens on the lensometer stop (Fig. 64–13) taking care not to distort the lens. The lens may be positioned on the stop used for spectacles.
6. If the mires are distorted sufficiently to prevent a good reading, the lens should be rehydrated and the foregoing steps repeated.

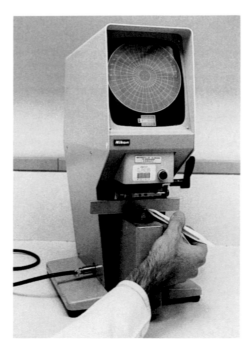

FIGURE 64–13. Placing a lens, after the surface moisture has been blotted off, on the stop of the lensometer for power measurement.

The power should be read within a few minutes of placing the lens on the stop because the refractive index of the lens will change as the lens dehydrates.

If the lens is a toric design, the procedure just given can be used, except that once placed on the lensometer stop

1. The stop should be rotated so the prism power reads base down. If the lens is a double-thinned zone lens and marked with horizontal reference lines, the reference lines should be positioned in the horizontal meridian.
2. The lens sphere, cylinder, and axis may then be measured in the same manner as a spectacle lens is measured.
3. If the lens is prism ballast, in addition to the power, the position of the mark indicating the base should be noted. Most lenses are marked with a line or dot at the base of the lens, but sometimes the mark may be incorrectly located. In such cases, when the lens is rotated to read base down, the mark will be in some position other than 6 o'clock. This position should be noted because when evaluating the fit of the lens on the eye this dot or line is used as a reference, and its position in relation to the base–apex line must be known. Special holders have been devised to help hold and orientate the lens while making the power measurement.[13]

Hydrogel lens power has been measured with the lens in a wet cell to keep it hydrated.[14–16] The wet cell is placed against the stop of the lensometer. There are several problems using this technique. First, one cannot position the lens in the plane of the stop. More importantly, with the lens in saline the power read on the lensometer is not the true lens power. The power read must be multiplied by a correction factor. The correction factor is the index of the lens minus 1.0 (index of air) divided by the index of the lens minus 1.336 (index of saline). For most hydrogel materials, this means that the power read must be multiplied by 4.57. This magnifies any error in measurement, for example, a reading error of 0.12 D means an error in the judgment of lens power of over 0.50 D. Therefore, this method is not accurate unless specifically designed lensometers are used.

Center Thickness

The center thickness of hydrogel lenses is important with respect to the amount of oxygen the lens will transmit. If the lens is too thick, the corneal edema may occur.

The center thickness can be measured with a radiuscope[17–20] using the following procedure:

1. Blot the lens as described before.
2. Place the lens concave side down on the radiuscope holder with the pedestal designed to measure the front radius of rigid lenses (Fig. 64–14). Water should not be placed under the lens.
3. Focus on the back surface image of the lens.
4. Zero or place the reference line on a number on the scale of the instrument.
5. With only the fine focus control, focus upward to the front surface of the lens. The surface images are very close together and will appear to be overlapping.
6. The difference in these readings multiplied by the refractive index of the lens, often 1.43 for hydrogel lenses, will give the lens thickness.

This technique works well for relatively thick lenses, 0.10 mm or thicker, but the two images are too close together for use with many of the thinner lenses.

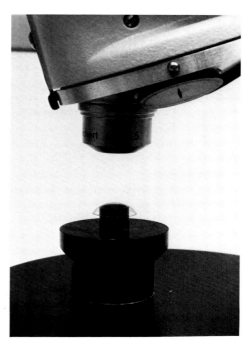

FIGURE 64–14. Hydrogel lens positioned on the pedestal for center thickness measurement with the radiuscope.

An alternative method of thickness measurement using the radiuscope is as follows:

1. Place a flat sheet of glass, such as a glass microscope slide, on the stage of the radiuscope.
2. Focus the spoke pattern on the glass surface.
3. Place the radiuscope reference light on zero or some number.
4. Blot the lens as previously described.
5. Place the blotted lens, convex surface down, on the glass surface with the center of the lens directly under the objective, being careful not to move the glass surface.
6. Focus on the surface of the lens.
7. The difference between the scale value for the reading on the glass surface and on the lens surface is the lens thickness.

The difficulty with this technique is that the lens must be centered under the objective so the exact center is being measured.

The lens thickness may also be measured by using the Redher gauge as follows:

1. Turn the instrument on.
2. Slowly bring the upper dome down to touch the lower dome watching the light on the base of the instrument. When the light comes on the two have touched. The dial should be read zero, if not, adjust the dial to read zero.
3. Move the top dome upward away from the lower dome.
4. Blot the lens as described before.
5. Place the lens on the lower dome which has a small electrode (wire) in the center. Place the center of the lens over the electrode.
6. The top dome is slowly brought down until it contacts the lens surface, at which point the circuit is closed and the small light on the base comes on.
7. Read the thickness of the lens from the gauge dial.

Surface and Edge Inspection

If the surface of the lens is coated with residue from compounds from manufacturing, foreign material or tear film components, comfort and vision may be adversely affected. Likewise, if there are tears in the lens or chips out of the edge of the lens, the lens will be uncomfortable.

The lens can be inspected under a stereomicroscope or held before the light beam of the biomicroscope. However, it is difficult to detect many problems, other than major tears or chips, in this manner because of surface drying.

A projection magnifier may be used in conjunction with a wet cell. By projecting the lens image on the screen, a number of lens defects, such as the tears, chips, lathe marks, and major surface coatings, can be visualized.

Surface coatings, such as the common protein deposits, can be easily detected by blotting the lens surface dry and holding the lens at arms length and viewing with illumination from the side. The lens must be viewed against a dark background. The coatings will show up as a white haze or patches on the lens.

Posterior Central Curve Radius

There have been numerous methods used to measure the posterior central curve radius of hydrogel lenses.[21–32] However, most are either inaccurate or are quite time-consuming. Therefore, most clinicians do not have in-office methods for measuring this dimension. The lens is examined on the eye for proper movement and position. If it is not the same as the diagnostic lens or the patient's previous lens, the assumption is made that the base curve or other lens parameter is incorrect and another lens tried. A more practical method would be of great clinical value.

Water Content

The water content of a hydrogel lens is important, for oxygen transmissibility is related to water content, and some care systems are not compatible with high water content lenses. It can also be used to help identify lenses. A Trago Refractometer can be used to measure water content by

1. Blotting the lens as previously described.
2. The lens is placed on the prism of the instrument.
3. The lens is flattened against the prism of the refractometer by the cover.
4. The water content is determined by noting the position of the boundary on the scale while looking through the instrument.

Tints

The lens tint should be inspected for proper color, density, and uniformity as ordered. Clinically, this is usually accomplished by gross inspection or under low magnification with the stereomicroscope or biomicroscope to determine if the tint is uniform without patches of missing tint or areas of excessive tint. Density is inspected by comparison with diagnostic or standard lenses. It is best to view the lens against a white background.

CLINICAL IMPLICATIONS

Contact lenses of patients new to a practice must be measured to determine the dimensions of the lenses being worn. This is necessary to ascertain if the lenses are correct for the patient as well as for the purpose of recording damaged or lost lenses. In addition, contact lens dimensions may change over time. Since contact lenses are made of polymers (plastics), they may warp or change dimensions from exposure to heat, chemicals, or rough handling by the patient. Patients also interchange lenses right for left or new lenses with previous lenses, requiring the clinician to measure the lens parameters to establish which lenses are worn. A patient may, unknown to the clinician, obtain a new pair of contact lenses from another source and not be wearing the lenses indicated in the patient's record. For these reasons, it may be necessary to verify lens parameters at routine contact lens examinations.

Because of the difficulty when measuring some lens parameters, particularly with soft lenses, not all parameters are commonly measured in clinical practice. Only those techniques that have proved practical and are in common use in private practice have been covered in this chapter. For the more complicated, time-consuming, or advanced techniques, the reader may consult standard contact lens textbooks[9,33-36] or other literature.

REFERENCES

1. Barr JT, Lowther GE. Measured and laboratory-stated parameters of hydrophilic contact lenses. Am J Optom Physiol Opt 1977;54:809–820.
2. Davis HE, Anderson DJ. An investigation of the reliability of hydrogel lens parameters. Int Contact Lens Clin 1979;6:136–142.
3. Schoessler JP, Barr JT. Measured and stated parameters of hydrophilic contact lenses from six different manufacturers. Int Contact Lens Clin 1980;7:168–185.
4. Molinari JF, Semes LP. The validity of labeled lenses. Am J Optom Physiol Opt 1982;59:680–685.
5. Seibel EJ, Trilsch WR, Lee D. Evaluation of soft contact lens quality: a manufacturer's perspective. Am J Optom Physiol Opt 1988;65:298–307.
6. Fatt I. A simple electrical device for measuring thickness and sagittal height of gel contact lenses. Optician 1977;173:23–24.
7. Pollack SL. A contact lens sagittal height and thickness gauge. Am J Optom Physiol Opt 1981;58:640–642.
8. Brennen NA. A simple instrument for measuring the water content of hydrogel lenses. Int Contact Lens Clin 1983;10:357–362.
9. Mandell RB. Contact lens practice, 4th ed. Springfield, Ill. Charles C Thomas, 1988;352–387, 554–567.
10. Morris S, Lowther GE. A comparison of different rigid contact lenses: edge thickness and coutours. J Am Optom Assoc 1981;52:247–249.
11. McMonnies CW. Assessment of hard lens edges. Int Eyecare 1986;2:532–538.
12. Saver MD, Harris MG, Mandell RB, et al. Power of Bausch and Lomb Soflens contact lenses. Am J Optom Physiol Opt 1973;50:195–199.
13. Wodis M. Manufacturer's report: checking toric power. Contact Lens Forum 1987;12:52–54.
14. Poster MG. Hydrated method of determining dioptral power of a hydrophilic lens. J Am Optom Assoc 1971;50:546–552.
15. Yumori RW, Mandell RB. Optical power calculation for contact lens wet cells. Am J Optom Physiol Opt 1981;58:637–639.
16. Campbell CE. Converting wet cell measured soft lens power to vertex power in air. Int Contact Lens Clin 1984;11:168–171.
17. Harris MG, Hall K, Oye R. The measurement and stability of hydrophilic lens dimensions. Am J Optom Physiol Opt 1973;50:546–552.
18. Port M. New methods of measuring hydrophilic lenses. Ophthal Optician 1976;16:1079–1082.
19. Paramore J, Wechsler S. Reliability and repeatability study of a technique for measuring the center thickness of a hydrogel lens. J Am Optom Assoc 1978;49:272–274.
20. Malin AH, Pizzo C. Measuring soft lens center thickness. Contact Lens Forum 1983;8:77–83.
21. Loran DFC. Determination of hydrogel contact lens radii by projection. Ophthal Optician 1974;14:980–985.
22. Holden BA. An accurate and reliable method of measuring soft contact lens curvature. Aust J Optom 1975;58:443–449.
23. Huyler JC, Johansen CP, Peterson JE. Soft lens base curve measurements. J Am Optom Assoc 1980;51:259–263.
24. Goldberg JB, Lebow KA. Soft lens base curves and the BC Tronic F. Int Contact Lens Clin 1980;7:145–151.
25. Garner LF. A comparison of two methods for measurement of the sagittal height of soft contact lenses. Int Contact Lens Clin 1981;8:19–23.
26. McDonald R. Clinical applications of the Soft Lens Analyzer. Am J Optom Physiol Opt 1981;58:626–630.
27. Koetting RA. Clinical use of the Medicornea BC Tronic unit for measuring soft lenses. Am J Optom Physiol Opt 1981;58:631–632.
28. Koetting RA. Clinical use of the Sohnges Kontr-Mess System for measuring contact lenses. Am J Optom Physiol Opt 1981;58:633–634.
29. Chaston J, Fatt I. Optical measurement of front and back radius of soft contact lenses in saline. Int Contact Lens Clin 1982;9:11–19.
30. Patella VM, Harris MG, Wong VA, et al. Ultrasonic measurement of soft contact lens base curves. Int Contact Lens Clin 1982;9:41–53.
31. Pearson R. BCOR measurement of soft lenses: A review of instrumentation. Contact Lens J 1983;11(3):2–5.
32. Lowther GE, Palardy AM. Betron soft contact lens analyzer. Int Eyecare 1986;2:481–485.
33. Lowther GE. Contact lenses: procedures and techniques. Boston: Butterworth Publishers, 1982:153–213.
34. Stone J, Phillips AJ. Contact lenses. London: Butterworth Publishers, 1980:282–301, 469–495.
35. Dabezies OH. Contact lenses: the CLAO guide to basic science and clinical practice. Orlando: Grune & Stratton, 1984; chaps 18–20.
36. Mandell RB. Contact lens practice. 4th ed. Springfield, Ill: Charles C Thomas, 1988.

Evaluation of Contact Lens Fit

Gerald E. Lowther

INTRODUCTION

Definition

The fit of a contact lens consists of the relationship between the lens and certain ocular structures (e.g., cornea, limbus, bulbar and palpebral conjunctiva and lids) as well as the position and movement of the contact lens.

History

The method of evaluating the lens fit of rigid contact lenses, with sodium fluorescein started in the late 1930s when Obrig discovered the value of using blue light to excite fluorescein, a water-soluble compound, which was placed in solution under scleral lenses.[1] With the introduction of corneal contact lenses in the late 1940s,[2,3] fluorescein was naturally used to evaluate the fit of the lenses. Today fluorescein is supplied impregnated in filter paper strips for convenient instillation. It is routinely used with all rigid lenses. The fluorescein is usually excited with either a blue filter in the slit-lamp or by a hand-held lamp (often called a "black light" or "Burton lamp") with bulbs emitting near ultraviolet (UV) and blue light.

Fluorescein cannot be used in the fitting of hydrogel (soft) lenses because it will be absorbed into the lenses. Therefore, the fit of hydrogel lenses is evaluated using a slit lamp biomicroscope. By observing the position and movement of the lenses the clinical fitting relationship is determined. A high molecular weight fluorescein (Fluorexon) has been developed and used with hydrogel lenses.[4,5] However, it has not been found to be of general value for routine evaluation of the fitting characteristics of hydrogel lenses.

Clinical Use

Proper procedure must be used to evaluate the fit of a contact lens. For rigid contact lenses this means proper diagnostic lenses, lens placement, fluorescein instillation, and appropriate viewing conditions are required. With hydrogel lenses this requires selecting appropriate diagnostic lenses, placement of the lens on the eye and proper use of the biomicroscope. In this chapter only examination procedures will be discussed. For more indepth information on contact lens fitting procedures reference should be made to those standard books mentioned in the general reference section.

INSTRUMENTATION

Theory and Use

Rigid Lens Evaluation

FLUORESCEIN PATTERN. Rigid lenses are normally evaluated using the dye sodium fluorescein to stain the tear film to determine the relationship between the lens and the cornea. If illuminated with an ultraviolet source the dye-stained tears will fluoresce a bright green. The goal is to stain the normal tear film without significantly increasing the tear volume. Fluorescein stain allows visualization of the tear thickness under the lens. It is used to determine if the central curve (base curve radius) is steeper (shorter radius) than the cornea, thus giving a green central pool of tears, or if flatter (longer radius) giving a central dark area void of tears. If the central radius of the lens matches the corneal curvature a uniform dark area relatively void of the stained tears will be present under the central portion (optical zone) of the lens. In addition to the central region, the peripheral portion of the lens must be evaluated. A proper fit will result in a green fluorescence under the periphery of the lens corresponding to the lens peripheral curve area. If the staining (tear depth) in this area is insufficient, there will not be adequate tear exchange on blinking. If the peripheral tear pool is too great the lens may move excessively, the lens edge will stand excessively off the cornea producing lid discomfort and increased likelihood of lens loss. The lens may also not center well and bubbles may form at the lens edge becoming trapped under the lens.

Fluorescein also allows the clinician to easily evaluate lens position and movement, since the lens is very visible as a result of the pooling of tears at the edge. The dynamic positioning as well as the amount of lens movement on blinking will help determine long-term lens comfort and visual performance. A lens that positions high on the cornea or drops down and positions low will often result in both physiologic and visual problems. Excessive movement of the lens will result in more discomfort than a more stable lens. It will cause visual disturbance due to the lens periphery impinging over the pupillary area, giving rise to blurred vision and what is often referred to as flare. *Flare* is the subjective complaint of streaks visible around objects, particularly lights at night, and ghost images around objects.

DIAGNOSTIC LENSES. The type and condition of the contact lenses used as diagnostic (also termed fitting or trial) lenses, or the patient's lenses when they are being evaluated, may be very important to the assessment of the fit. It is best that the lenses are clear because tinted lenses can both absorb the UV light used to illuminate the fluorescein as well as absorb the fluorescence of the dye passing back through the lens. If one evaluates a brown-tinted lens and then a clear one the fit will appear quite different. Light blue tints have the least effect, whereas brown tints have the greatest. Therefore, diagnostic lenses should be clear to avoid the effects of a tint. Of course, a patient's lens may be tinted and the clinician must be aware of any tint when determining the fit of lenses.

Some manufacturers are now adding compounds with UV-absorbing properties to some lens materials.[6] Such materials effectively absorb all the UV from most lamps (black light) used to excite the fluorescein. Therefore, when one attempts to evaluate the fit of such lenses, they appear black because of the absorption of the UV. To overcome this, the clinician needs to use a light source with a predominance of longer wavelengths. Often cobalt blue filters used in slit lamps pass the longer wavelengths. One can also substitute the normal fluorescent bulbs in the hand-held lamps with standard white bulbs and then cover the bulbs with a blue Kodak Wratten No. 47 filter and then place a yellow Kodak Wratten No. 12 or No. 15, or Tiffen Yellow No. 2, filter over the viewing lens of the lamp. Such filters are available from photographic supply stores.

Diagnostic lenses must be of good quality to be of value. The curves and other dimensions must be exact and known to accomplish an orderly fitting procedure and to ascertain what lens parameters to order for a patient. Diagnostic lens sets should have as many constant parameters as possible. When changing from one diagnostic lens parameter to another, for example, the base curve, the overall diameter and optical zone should not change so the effect of changing only the base curve can be evaluated. Usually diagnostic sets consisting of two or three diameters, with base curve steps of 0.1 mm (0.50 D) in each diameter, are sufficient.

A very important factor is the lens edge. Most of the sensation the patient experiences with rigid contact lenses is the result of the lid margin. A patient who has not worn lenses will have very sensitive lid margins. When a lens is placed on a patient's eye for the first time if the lids are held away from the eye the patient will have little or no sensation from the lens, but will become immediately aware of it on blinking. Therefore, the edge must be thin and

well contoured. If the edge is thick or its peak is toward the front of the lens it will cause lid irritation on each blink resulting in excessive tearing. It is impossible to adequately evaluate the fit of a lens with excessive tearing.

The method of lens placement on the eye can also be important to the proper assessment of the fit. Obviously the lens must be clean and in good condition. A wetting solution that is not too viscous should be used, because a viscous solution will remain on the lens for some time after lens placement. This causes the fluorescein to collect on the lens surface and obscures the view of the fluorescein pooling under the lens. Many wetting or conditioning solutions are too viscous; therefore, it is a good idea to rinse the lens with a saline solution formulated for hydrogel lenses before placing the rigid lens on the cornea.

The lens should be placed on the eye without causing any excess irritation, particularly for the new patient. The clinician must have good control of the lids to prevent the patient from blinking during lens placement. The lens should be placed gently on the cornea and the patient asked to look down in the reading position. This decreases lid sensation and prevents excessive discomfort and tearing. After a few minutes the patient may gradually look up and the fit evaluated.

FLUORESCEIN INSTILLATION. Fluorescein strips, strips of filter paper impregnated with sodium fluorescein, are the most common form of fluorescein used in contact lens practice. They come in a variety of designs from different manufacturers. The easiest strips to use are moderately stiff, with the impregnated filter paper being only a few millimeters at the end of the strip. Strips that have a long section of filter paper are difficult to handle, since they become very floppy when wet and difficult to properly place on the eye.

The fluorescein strips should be moistened with a sterile saline or irrigating solution. The solution should not be viscous or preserved with benzalkonium chloride because benzalkonium chloride will precipitate the fluorescein. A saline solution used with hydrogel lenses works well for wetting a strip. Fluorescein strips should never be placed on the eye dry, as this will irritate the eye and cause excessive tearing.

Before placing the strip against the eye, any excess solution should be shaken off the strip. The clinician wants to add stain to the eye, but not any greater quantity solution than required. After properly preparing the strip, the clinician should have the patient either look down or up and firmly grip the lids (Fig. 65–1). The flat

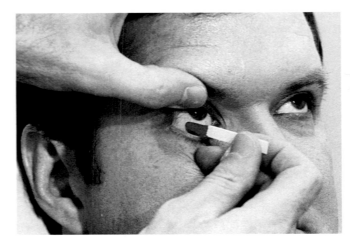

FIGURE 65–1. Illustrating the proper grip of the lids with fingers extended over the lashes so the lids are under control and away from fluorescein strip. The fluorescein strip, without excess solution, is placed against the bulbar conjunctiva and lifted away without any rubbing action.

side of the moistened strip should be touched against the bulbar conjunctiva and then lifted away. The strip should not be wiped or rubbed against the eye, since this is unnecessary and irritates the eye. The strip should never be touched to the patient's cornea, as this is not only irritating but will result in epithelial staining. The area at which the strip touches the conjunctiva will also show epithelial uptake of the stain but is of no consequence.

If the patient is apprehensive, it is best to have the patient look up and touch the strip to the inferior bulbar conjunctiva. This will prevent the strip from touching the cornea if the patient makes a sudden eye or lid movement as the stain is being instilled. With an experienced wearer or nonapprehensive patient, the patient may be instructed to look down and the fluorescein strip placed on the superior bulbar conjunctiva.

CLINICAL PROCEDURES

Rigid Contact Lenses

1. Once the fluorescein has been instilled, the patient should be instructed to blink several times and the lens fit viewed immediately in a darkened room. The fluorescein will usually be diluted relatively quickly.
2. The best manner in which to evaluate the fit of a rigid lens is to use a hand-held ultraviolet lamp, often called a "Burton lamp" after one of the major manufacturers of such lamps. These lamps usually consist of two tube UV sources with a magnifying lens (Fig. 65–2). The lamp is held in front of the patient and the contact lens viewed through the magnifying lens of the lamp. This gives an overall view of the contact lens, cornea, and lids; therefore, not only the relationship of the back of the contact lens to the cornea can be evaluated, but the effect of the lids on lens movement and position is easily determined. Many clinicians find it more convenient to use one of the small lamps, as it is easier to hold and manipulate.
3. Some clinicians use the slit lamp biomicroscope to evaluate the fluorescein pattern. By using the cobalt blue filter provided in the illumination system, the fluorescein pattern can be viewed through the instrument. This has the limitation that an area of usually less than the corneal diameter is illuminated making it more difficult to evaluate the effect of the lids, lens movement, and positioning.
4. Once fluorescein has been instilled and the patient has blinked several times, fluorescein should be pumped under the contact lens. This may also be accomplished by gently pushing the inferior lid against the lower edge of

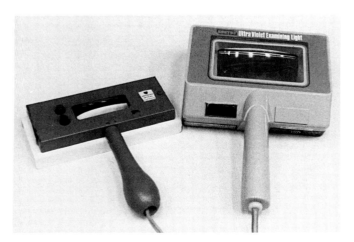

FIGURE 65–2. Ultraviolet sources used to evaluate fluorescein patterns.

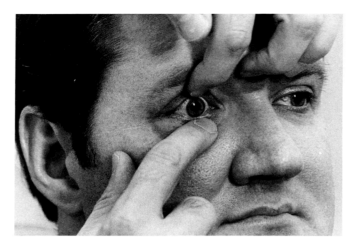

FIGURE 65–3. Centering the contact lens using the lid margins so the relationship of the lens to the cornea can be determined with the lens centered on the cornea.

the lens. The lens is lifted up slightly so the stained tears can flow under the lens. This prevents the clinician from interpreting the contact lens as matching the corneal contour when the lens base curve is actually steep and sealing off tear flow, thereby preventing stain from getting under the lens. With contact lens curves that match the corneal shape, the fluorescein will immediately flow out from under the lens.

5. The contact lens should be viewed in both static and dynamic situations. If a contact lens is decentered, due to the aspheric shape of the cornea and flatter limbal area, the relationship of the contact lens to the eye can not be determined. A lens flatter than the cornea may have fluorescein pooling under the lens in the decentered position because the lens is bridging the area between the steeper apex of the cornea and the limbal area. However, if the lens is centered, it will appear flat as the center of the lens will be resting on the steeper corneal apex. Therefore, not only should contact lens movement and position with lid movement be evaluated, but the lens must also be viewed in the centered position. The lens can be centered by placing one finger on the superior lid margin and another on the inferior lid margin using the lid margins to hold the lens in a centered position (Fig. 65–3).
6. The clinician should not mistake the natural fluorescence of the crystalline lens seen in the pupil for fluorescein in the tears under the contact lens. The amount of crystalline lens fluorescence varies with individuals and has a more blue appearance than fluorescein. Likewise, one must not mistake fluorescein in the tear film on the lens front surface for fluorescein under the lens. Often if the fluorescein is on the lens it will be seen to flow on the surface. The patient should be asked to blink if the clinician suspects fluorescein is on the front surface of the lens.

Hydrogel Contact Lenses

Standard fluorescein cannot be used with hydrogel lenses because it is absorbed by the lens. A large molecular weight fluorescein has been developed and used with hydrogel lenses. Since most hydrogel lenses are very flexible and thin, they conform to the cornea with little or no tear pooling under the lens to evaluate. Thus, the use of dyes to evaluate the fit of hydrogel contact lenses is not routinely used.

1. When a hydrogel lens is placed on the eye, just before evaluating the fit, the clinician should be sure the lens is comfortable. If a foreign body, such as a small piece of lint or mascara, is under the lens it will be uncomfortable. A new lens that has never been on an eye may also be uncomfortable. In each case, just sliding the lens off the cornea and moving it around on the conjunctiva before recentering will often eliminate the problem.

2. Before evaluating the fit, the clinician should allow a few minutes for tearing to subside and the contact lens to settle. At this point, the initial evaluation may be made. If the lens appears as though it is reasonably fit, the patient should be allowed to wear the lens for at least 15 to 20 minutes before a final evaluation is made. With time, the lens tends to dehydrate and lens movement often decreases. The greatest water loss occurs in the first 15 to 20 minutes of lens wear. High-water-content lenses usually dehydrate more than low-water-content lenses. Therefore, the clinician wants more movement initially than desired, rather than less.

3. Hydrogel lenses are evaluated by using the biomicroscope to determine lens positioning and the amount of lens movement. A well-fitted hydrogel lens will reveal approximately 0.25 to 1.0 mm of movement with each blink on straight-ahead gaze. Thick lenses show more movement than thin lenses. Commonly more movement is desired with extended wear than daily wear lenses. On up gaze, hydrogel contact lenses will usually show slightly more movement than on straight-ahead gaze. The lens should be centered or nearly centered on the cornea. The lens should never be decentered to the point that the edge of the lens impinges on the cornea. A lens that is too flat ("loose") will show more than the desired movement on straight-ahead gaze as well as with up gaze and will not center as well as a properly fitting lens. A steep ("tight") lens will show very little movement and will usually be centered on the cornea.

4. The amount of lens movement is determined by examining the lower edge of the lens using moderate magnification (10× to 20×) and direct illumination with the biomicroscope. A reticule may be placed in the eyepiece of the biomicroscope to measure the movement. Most clinicians do not have such a reticule, however, if the slit lamp has a scale for the height or width of the slit, a slit 1 mm high or square may be used. The amount of movement relative to this 1-mm scale can be accurately gauged. If just an estimate of movement is made, it will commonly be graded as more movement than actually exists, since it is being observed with magnification. Similarly, the amount of movement with the patient looking in upgaze can also be determined.

5. The lens position is also determined with the biomicroscope by observing the position of the lens edge relative to the limbus.

6. The keratometer can be a secondary aid in evaluating lens fit. By performing keratometry readings over the surface of the lens one can determine if the mires are clear or distorted. Distorted or fluctuating mires may indicate an improper lens fit.

AFTERCARE EVALUATION PROCEDURES

To appropriately evaluate the performance and effect of contact lenses on the eye after a period of wear, there are several procedures that should be performed on each visit in addition to the case history and visual acuity measurement. These include (1) refraction with the patient wearing the contact lenses, called the over refraction; (2) slit lamp evaluation with the contact lenses on the eye; (3) slit lamp examination with sodium fluorescein instillation after lens removal, (4) corneal curvature measurement (keratometry); and (5) spectacle refraction with lenses removed, often called the spectacle blur refraction.

Case History

The case history will vary if and when the patient was last seen by the clinician, but should include questions relative to patient complaints, type of lenses worn, how long contact lenses have been worn, how many hours the lenses have been worn at the time of the examination, and average wearing time per day. The patient should be questioned about all solutions used with the contact lenses, such as daily cleaners, rinsing solutions, disinfection system, and enzymatic cleaners.

Over Refraction

The over refraction is performed to determine if the contact lens power is correct. Normal refractive procedures are used as the patient wears the lenses. If, for example, the patient requires more minus power over the contact lens to obtain best visual acuity, then the lens must be modified to obtain more minus power or a new lens ordered. Another useful aspect of the over refraction is in those situations for which visual acuity can not be improved with the over refraction. No improvement in visual acuity with over refraction may mean that the lens is badly coated with tear film materials or foreign matter, the optics of the lens are distorted, the surface is scratched, or some other damage has occurred. Patients often accidentally switch lenses from right to left eyes, and the over refraction may indicate this if the contact lens powers are different.

Slit Lamp Evaluation with the Contact Lenses

In addition to evaluating the lens fit, examining the contact lens on the eye is useful in detecting surface deposits, lens tears or chips, debris collection under the lenses, and other problems.

Slit Lamp Evaluation with the Contact Lenses Removed

After the contact lenses are removed the cornea and conjunctiva should be examined for any adverse effects of lens wear. Sodium fluorescein should be instilled as previously described. The cornea and conjunctiva should be examined with and without the cobalt filter in place. Many different types of epithelial staining of the cornea can occur. There may be superficial punctate keratitis caused by a poor lens fit, dirty lens, toxic or allergic reaction to solutions, drying because of interruption of the normal blink, or dehydration of hydrogel lenses. Conjunctival staining may occur due to the edge of the lens or drying. There may be corneal edema causing a cloudy cornea, corneal striae, and epithelial microcysts. The limbal area must be examined for new blood vessel growth and infiltrates. The superior area of the cornea must be examined by having the patient look down and lifting the superior lid. Likewise, the lid margins should be examined for irritation and infection. The superior lid should be everted and examined for papillary changes. With hydrogel lenses, the residual fluorescein should be irrigated out of the cul-de-sac before placing the lens on the cornea. This is a simple procedure, and even if a small amount of fluorescein is absorbed into the lenses, it will eventually leach out without causing a problem.

Keratometry After Lens Removal

After the cornea has been examined with the slit lamp, the corneal curvature should be measured with the same instrumentation used to measure the baseline corneal curvature. Changes in corneal curvature may indicate possible adverse effects of contact lens wear, such as corneal edema, irregular astigmatism, or corneal distortion.

Spectacle Blur Refraction

Measurement of the refraction after lens removal is another procedure used to determine if there are any adverse effects of contact lens wear. If the refraction changes this is a possible indication of an improper fit that is causing corneal edema or undue mechanical pressure on the cornea. Any change in refraction of 0.50 D or more from the prefitting baseline should be cause for further investigation into the reason for the difference.

Sequence of Tests

The sequence of testing for a patient coming into the office wearing contact lenses should be as follows:

1. Case history
2. Visual acuity
3. Over refraction
4. Slit lamp examination with the lenses on
5. Slit lamp examination with the lenses off
6. Keratometer (K) readings
7. Spectacle blur refraction
8. Lens inspection

The sequence is important not only for efficient use of time, but also to gather accurate data. One must examine the eye immediately after lens removal with the biomicroscope, since some conditions such as corneal edema resolve rapidly. Keratometric and refractive values do not change significantly over the time of the examination.

CLINICAL IMPLICATIONS

Clinical Significance

It is important to obtain the proper physical fit of a contact lens on the eye to maintain normal corneal physiology, comfort, and good visual performance. If contact lenses are fit such that there is not adequate movement (too "tight"), tears will stagnate under the lens. The buildup of debris and metabolic waste products, inadequate oxygen supply (hypoxia), a drop in the pH, and other changes will result in corneal epithelial edema, breakdown and sloughing, ulceration, conjunctival injection, and ocular discomfort.

If contact lenses are fit with excessive movement (too "flat"), the lenses may not be comfortable and visual disturbance is common. Flat-fit rigid lenses may also cause central corneal staining as well as corneal distortion.

Clinical Interpretation

When fitting a rigid contact lens with the aid of fluorescein, one must evaluate the relationship of the base curve radius of the lens to the cornea, the peripheral clearance, and lens positioning and movement. If in the central portion of the lens there are no tears (a dark area), this indicates that the center of the lens is touching (bearing) on the center of the cornea. In this case the base curve radius of the lens is too long (too flat) for the eye, and a shorter radius must be tried. On the other hand, if there is a significant amount of green (pooling) in the center of the lens, this indicates the base curve radius is too short (steep), and a longer radius must be tried.

There should be pooling of tears around the edge of a rigid lens because it is important that the lens edge stand off the cornea. Therefore, a reasonably bright green band should be visible around the lens edge. The width of this band depends on the width of the lens peripheral curves. If there is insufficient peripheral pooling, tear exchange with blinking will be inhibited with the same results as a steep base curve. If the peripheral curve clearance is inadequate, longer peripheral curve radii or a wider peripheral curve is needed. With excessive peripheral curve clearance, one will see very deep pooling at the lens edge with possible bubble formation, especially with blinking. With too much edge clearance, there will be excessive lens movement and possible lens decentration. In this event, steeper peripheral radii must be ordered to decrease the clearance.

Rigid lens centration, movement, and comfort are affected by the choice of lens diameter. If the superior lid holds a lens up following a blink, there will be less discomfort because the patient does not feel the edge of the lens with each blink or eye movement. However, if following a blink the lens drops from under the superior lid and rides low, discomfort and physiologic problems may develop. If the lens falls from under the superior lid a larger overall lens diameter may prevent this downward movement, assuming the superior lid covers enough of the cornea to remain over the contact lens. For a high superior lid that cannot hold the lens up, a small lens diameter may perform better, since a lighter, smaller lens usually centers because of surface tension of the tear film. Therefore, watching the lens movement and positioning while evaluation the fluorescein pattern gives the clinician valuable information.

With hydrogel lenses the lens movement and positioning must be evaluated to deduce the lens fit. If there is very little or no movement with blinking on straight-ahead or up gaze, the lens is too steep (tight). A lens with a longer base curve radius (or smaller diameter with the same base curve radius) must be used. If the movement is excessive, then the lens base curve is too long (flat), and a shorter radius must be used. A flat lens also may not center well over the cornea.

REFERENCES

1. Obrig TE. A cobalt blue filter for observation of the fit of contact lenses. Arch Ophthalmol 1938;20:657–658.
2. Muth EP. Kevin Michael Tuohy Optician, The father of modern contact lenses. Opt Prism Sept/Oct 1987;42–48.
3. Touhy proclaimed "Father of modern contact lenses." Contact Lens Spect 1987;2:62.
4. Refojo MF, Korb DR, Silverman HI. Clinical evaluation of a new fluorescent dye for hydrogel lenses. J Am Optom Assoc 1972;43:321–326.
5. Refojo MF, Miller D, Fiore AS. A new fluorescent stain for soft hydrophilic lens fitting. Arch Ophthalmol 1972;87:275–577.
6. Lebow, KA. Clinical evaluation of the Boston Equalens for cosmetic extended wear. Contact Lens Spect 1987;2:47–52.

SUGGESTED GENERAL REFERENCES

1. Bennett ES, Grohe, RM. Rigid gas-permeable contact lenses. New York: Professional Press, 1986.
2. Bier N, Lowther GE. Contact lens correction. Boston: Butterworth Publishers, 1977.
3. Lowther GE. Contant lenses: procedures and techniques. Boston: Butterworth Publishers, 1982.
4. Mandell, RB. Contact lens practice. Springfield, Ill: Charles C Thomas, 1988.

PART 4

Pediatric Procedures

Pediatric Visual Acuity

Mitchell Scheiman

INTRODUCTION

Definition

Visual acuity testing is the clinical procedure used to assess the ability of an individual to discriminate detail or distinguish form. It can be evaluated in many ways using different tasks. The various forms have been described by Riggs[1] as

- *Detection*—in which the actual presence or absence of a target is determined
- *Recognition*—in which letters or pictures or orientation of symbols are identified
- *Resolution*—in which gratings, checkerboards require discrimination of the separation between elements
- *Localization*—in which differences in spatial position of segments of a test target are determined

Clinically, the methods used most often are recognition and resolution. Clinical tests such as the Snellen chart, Landolt C's, picture charts, and Tumbling E's are examples of recognition tasks. The use of gratings in preferential-looking procedures is an example of a resolution task.

History

Visual acuity testing has always been a very important part of any vision evaluation and has a long historical development. Snellen introduced his chart in 1862, and an attempt at standardization was made in 1903 by the American Ophthalmological Society, in which they established the use of capital letters of 5 minutes of arc with a 1 minute of arc width.[2] Specific attempts to develop acuity testing techniques for children were not reported until the mid-1950s, with the establishment of the Allen cards.[3] Since that time, particu-larly the last decade, there has been a major research effort to develop reliable, valid, testing procedures for infants and preverbal children.

Clinical Use

As with adults, visual acuity is of extreme importance when examining a child. In the clinical reasoning process used by most clinicians, hypotheses are generated very early in the interview and examination process. The ability to successfully gather data about visual acuity is important in this process because it helps to deny or confirm certain hypotheses and, thereby, provides direction for the remainder of the examination. For example, a unilateral reduction in visual acuity should alert a clinician to the possibility of several hypotheses, including optical disturbances, optic nerve or chiasmal lesions, optic neuropathy, macula disorders, or functional amblyopia. A finding of 20/20 acuity in each eye, on the other hand, enables the clinician to eliminate many vision and ocular disorders.

Visual acuity, therefore, is a test that is routinely utilized to initially set the direction for the rest of the examination. Acuity testing in children should be used in this same manner.

It has been recognized, for some time, that visual acuity testing has three different components or variables that affect the obtained result. The acuity that we obtain from a patient on any given task is affected by the optical components of the eye, the underlying physiologic capabilities of the patient, and a behavioral or psychological component.[3] It is this last variable that necessitates unique tests for children. Because standard, subjective, visual acuity testing requires verbal communication and sustained attention and concentration on the task, such testing cannot be used with preverbal children and is often difficult to use with preschool children.

As a result, many visual acuity tests have been designed to be used with preschool children. These tests are far too numerous to include a description and detailed clinical procedure for all of them. Rather, an attempt has been made to select a test that is unique because it satisfies a specific need, is readily available, or is currently a test frequently used by optometrists.

In a recent review of visual acuity testing in preschool children, Fern and Manny[4] divided these tests into four different categories, including

- Tests that use pictures of objects
- Tests that use the Landolt C, or variations
- Tests that use the Tumbling E, or variations
- Tests that use Snellen letters

For this chapter at least one test from each of these four categories was selected.

The particular visual acuity test selected by an optometrist to assess any specific child will depend upon factors such as test availability, age of the child, and responsiveness of the child. Generally, once a child reaches the developmental age of 6 to 7, standard Snellen acuity charts can be utilized with slight modification in technique. For children younger than this, it is important to keep in mind that certain designs are more desirable and more likely to yield valid, reliable data. For instance, Fern and Manny[4] recommended the following as being desirable characteristics for a preschool visual acuity test.

1. Use of the Landolt C format
2. Use of single, isolated optotypes, rather than a full line or chart
3. A two-alternative forced choice paradigm or a matching response
4. Avoidance of the need for a verbal response or a directional response
5. A short test distance such as 3 m, rather than traditional 6-m distance
6. Borders or contour surrounding the test optotypes to control for contour interaction

INSTRUMENTATION

10-Prism Diopter Fixation Test

Theory and Use

This procedure is used with infants and preverbal children from birth to about 3 years of age. This is an indirect means of assessing whether there might be a difference in acuity between the right and left eyes of a particular patient. It is based upon the observation that a constant, unilateral strabismic patient will prefer to fixate with either the right or left eye. In patients who can respond to traditional acuity testing, we find that if there is a constant, unilateral strabismus, the visual acuity will be lower in the eye that is not used for fixation. On the other hand, if a strabismus is alternating the visual acuity is generally equal in the two eyes.

This forms the basis for the use of the observation referred to as binocular fixation pattern.[5] In a preverbal child, if a unilateral strabismus is present, we assume that the eye being used for fixation has better acuity. In nonstrabismics, to assess fixation preference, vertical prism can be used to cause dissociation.[6] Presumably, the vertical prism should induce diplopia, and if both eyes have equal visual acuity, the clinician will observe the infant switching back and forth from the right to left eye. Thus, fixation preference is applicable to anisometropic amblyopia and nonfunctional loss of visual acuity, as well as strabismic amblyopia. In addition to general assumptions about acuity level, specific guidelines have been developed for clinical use to estimate the acuity level based upon the strength of the fixation preference.[7]

Before the advent of behavioral and electrophysiologic procedures for assessing visual acuity in preverbal children, fixation preference was essentially the only procedure available to clinicians. As more direct assessment procedures became available, it has become evident that fixation preference is not always an accurate predictor of acuity level. Mayer et al.[7] and Jacobson et al.[8] have both documented cases in which preferential looking acuity and fixation preference did not show a strong association. For example, Mayer reported an infant with congenital esotropia in which an inequality was found in preferential looking although no fixation preference was present. Another problem reported with this test is that with small angle strabismics a strong fixation preference may be present, even in the presence of equal visual acuity.[5]

Other potential sources of error include:

1. Poor fixation
2. Poor attention or lack of interest in the target

COMMERCIALLY AVAILABLE INSTRUMENTS

The only equipment necessary to perform this test is a fixation target, a 10-prism diopter prism, and a cover paddle. The fixation target should be one that is interesting to an infant or young child. Examples of such targets are shown in Figure 66–1.

CLINICAL PROCEDURE

The clinical procedure involved in assessing visual acuity with the 10-prism diopter fixation test is as follows:

1. With the child sitting comfortably, the examiner selects a fixation target. The 10-diopter prism is placed before the right eye to dissociate the patient (Fig. 66–2).
2. Once the eyes are dissociated, the examiner must observe whether the child alternates from one eye to the other, or tends to fixate with one eye.
3. If the child spontaneously alternates from one eye to another, this is recorded as "alternates." The assumption in this situation is that visual acuity is equal in the two eyes.
4. If a fixation preference appears to be present, the degree of preference is quantified by momentarily covering the fixing eye to force refixation of the nonpreferred eye. The following criteria are used to grade the fixation preference:

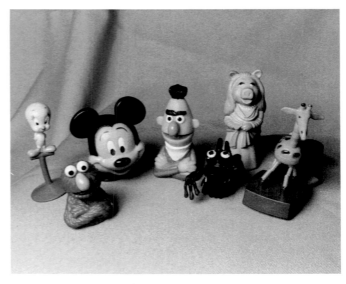

FIGURE 66–1. Examples of fixation targets for young children.

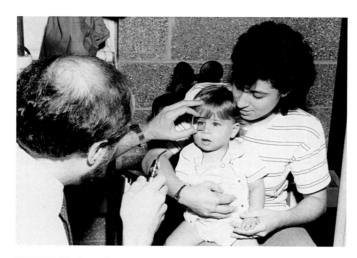

FIGURE 66–2. Administration of 10-prism diopter fixation test.

Table 66–1
Visual Acuity Norms for Teller Preferential Looking Cards

Age	Normal Acuity Range	
	Binocular Acuity	*Monocular Acuity*
1 month	20/400–20/1200	24/400–20/1600
4 months	20/80–20/300	20/100–20/400
12 months	20/50–20/200	20/80–20/300
18 months	20/40–20/100	20/50–20/150
24 months	20/30–20/80	20/40–20/100
30 months	20/20–20/50	20/20–20/50

A. *Spontaneously Alternates:* The patient freely alternates without any intervention on the part of the examiner.
B. *Holds Well:* The nonpreferred eye can hold fixation for at least 5 seconds, through a smooth pursuit movement, or through a blink.
C. *Holds Momentarily:* The nonpreferred eye holds fixation for less than 3 seconds, but not through a blink, or a smooth pursuit movement.
D. *Will Not Hold:* The nonpreferred eye will not hold fixation at all, and there is immediate refixation with the dominant eye.
5. Categories A and B are considered normal, suggesting equal acuity in the two eyes. Categories C and D are considered indications that a difference in acuity or amblyopia exists.

If a patient falls into the abnormal categories, at least a two-line difference in acuity should be suspected.

INSTRUMENTATION

Preferential Looking Acuity (Teller Acuity Cards)

Theory and Use

The preferential looking technique was first described by Fantz.[9] In these early research studies he found that infants prefer to fixate high-contrast, bold stripes rather than homogeneous fields of light. By using this principle, one can find the finest striped field that the infant will consistently fixate in preference to a uniform field. This can be used as a measure of grating acuity.

Many researchers have used this principle over the past decade to investigate the development of visual acuity in infants. These investigations have been very successful and have provided us with visual acuity norms for infants that can be used clinically when using preferential looking procedures (Table 66–1). Generally, however, the equipment used was not readily available, and the procedure itself is somewhat time-consuming. More recently, attempts have been made to refine the procedure so that it can be used in routine clinical care of preverbal children.

This process has led to the development of the Teller Acuity Cards. Recent studies[10–12] have demonstrated that the Teller cards can be used quite successfully in children between the ages of 1 and 12 months, and that acuity can be assessed in both right and left eyes in less than 15 minutes. Dobson et al.[11] reported that they were able to successfully test 90% of children in the aged group 2

months to 12 months, but only 56% of children younger than 2 months, and 74% of children older than 12 months. After the age of approximately 12 months, children become more active, and no longer seem to be absorbed by the preferential looking task. It is still important, however, to assess acuity in the preverbal child that is older than 12 months. To deal with this population, a modification of forced choice preferential looking has been developed, called operant preferential looking (OPL). This procedure utilizes the same targets as FPL. Instead of observing the child's preference by observation of their fixation, the child is encouraged to actually point or touch the field with the stripes. If the child responds correctly, his response is reinforced with a Cheerio or some other object that might be of interest, such as a cartoon.[13] This technique has been demonstrated to be quite effective in assessing acuity from aged 18 months to 3 years.[14]

Preferential looking acuity, which is a form of grating acuity, is not necessarily equivalent to Snellen or recognition acuity. Mayer et al.[15] reported that acuities obtained from grating tests, such as preferential looking, generally yield better visual acuity than recognition acuity tests, such as the Snellen Chart. Particularly in cases of dense amblyopia or foveal abnormalities, the discrepancy between grating and recognition acuity is greatest. In such cases, preferential looking acuity would provide more optimistic data than recognition acuity tests. Studies have also indicated that, although grating acuity may be sensitive to refractive amblyopia, it tends to overestimate the acuity in strabismic amblyopia. Thus, the data obtained from preferential looking must be interpreted with an understanding that it may represent an overestimate of acuity compared with Snellen acuity. Particular caution is necessary in cases of strabismus.

Other potential sources of error include the following:

Poor fixation
Poor attention
Lack of interest in looking at the grating
A preference for looking to one side
Holding the child off center and closer to one side

COMMERCIALLY AVAILABLE INSTRUMENTS

A set of Teller cards consists of visual acuity cards, and each card is constructed of gray cardboard. One card is blank and the other 15 contain a square wave grating (vertical black and white stripes) ranging in steps from 38.0 to 0.32 cycles/cm. This grating is located to the left or right of an aperture that is located in the middle of the card (Fig. 66–3). Each card is labeled on the back with the grating size.

The cards are supposed to be used with a screen (Fig. 66–4). This screen, however, is not commercially available. Rather, the Teller Card manual includes directions for construction of the screen. The cardboard used for this screen is identical with that used for the cards.

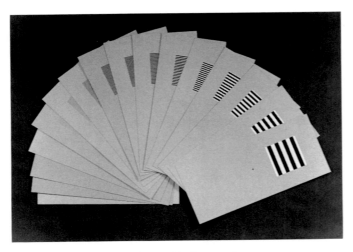

FIGURE 66–3. Teller preferential looking cards.

CLINICAL PROCEDURE

The clinical procedure involved in assessing visual acuity with the Teller Acuity Cards is as follows:

1. The child is held in front of a gray cardboard screen that shields his or her view of the room (see Fig. 66–4). The test distance can be selected by the examiner, although the manual provides conversion of cycles per centimeter to equivalent Snellen values for 38, 55, and 84 cm. For infants the 38-cm distance is recommended, whereas the 55-cm distance is recommended for toddlers.
2. The examiner then holds an acuity card with very wide stripes up to the opening, and then one with no stripes to become familiar with the infant's looking style in the presence and absence of a visible stimulus.
3. To test acuity, the examiner displays a series of cards, each containing a black-and-white grating of a different spatial frequency (stripe width), located to the left or right of the central peephole (see Fig. 66–3).
4. The examiner observes the child through the peephole and, on the basis of the child's eye movements or visual responsiveness, decides which card contains the finest stripe that the child can see.

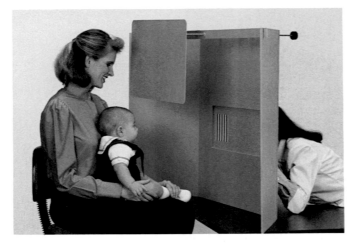

FIGURE 66–4. Teller preferential looking cards being used with screen.

5. Generally it is best to begin with a stripe width that is wider than the threshold predicted for the age of the infant. Refer to Table 66–1 for acuity norms for different ages. If it is clear that the child can see the stripes, the examiner presents the card with the next finest stripe width.
6. Testing continues until the examiner feels confident enough about the child's responses to make a judgment concerning the finest grating that the child can detect.
7. The spatial frequency of this grating is taken as an estimate of that child's visual acuity.
8. To eliminate the possibility of a side preference for a particular child, the examiner should position the cards so that the side with the stripes varies from right to left in a random fashion.
9. The test is conducted first with the right eye only and then with the left eye.
10. The test can also be conducted without the cardboard shield. This is sometimes necessary when the child has a motor handicap and cannot sit or be held in an upright position. In this format the child is seated on the parent's lap and the examiner holds the cards in front of the child and then proceed with steps 3 through 9.

INSTRUMENTATION

Broken Wheel Acuity

Theory and Use

The broken wheel acuity procedure is used with children about 2½ to 5 years of age. Developed by Richman et al.,[16] these cards are an excellent technique for children within this age range. Very little verbal communication is necessary, and the cards utilize a picture of a car which, of course, is very recognizable to children in this age group. The underlying theory is quite ingenious, as can be seen from Figure 66–5. Two cards are held before the child and he simply has to identify which one has broken wheels. As Figure 66–5 illustrates, the car with the "broken wheels" has Landolt C targets instead of circles for the wheels. Thus, if the child can distinguish which car has the broken wheels, it indicates that he can resolve the gap size of the Landolt C for that particular card. Recently, the Committee on Vision of the National Academy of Sciences' National Research Council defined the Landolt C as the optimum visual acuity test type.[17]

Of the six recommendations made by Fern and Manny[4] for an ideal preschool acuity chart, the broken wheel test accomplishes all six. There appear to be no sources of error specific to this test. It meets all of the requirements researchers have suggested for a preschool visual acuity test.

Sources of error that would effect any preschool visual acuity test include the following:

Poor attention and concentration on the task
Peeking around the patch
Incorrect working distance

COMMERCIALLY AVAILABLE INSTRUMENTS

The Broken Wheel test consists of eight pair of test cards and one sample pair of cards. The sample card is equivalent to a 20/120 acuity level at 3 m. There is a pair of test cards at each of the following acuity levels: 20/20, 20/25, 20/30, 20/40, 20/60, 20/80, 20/100, 20/120. Each card has a black line drawing of a car on a white background, one with solid wheels, the other with broken wheels (see Fig. 66–5).

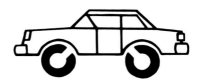
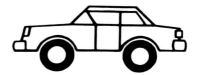
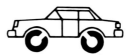
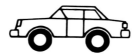
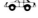

FIGURE 66–5. Broken wheel cards.

CLINICAL PROCEDURE

The clinical procedure involved in assessing visual acuity with the broken wheel cards is as follows:

1. The lighting level is important. The testing manual suggests that the use of a goose-neck lamp and a 75-W bulb provides adequate light (40 footcandles). Care must be taken to avoid reflections or glare. It is also useful to use tape on the floor or some other marking to indicate the appropriate testing distance.
2. The administration of the test is divided into three steps:
   - A pretest to teach and check the child's reliability in responding to the test
   - A test to assure that the child's responses are reliable at 10 ft (3 m)
   - Actual measurement of acuity level at 10 ft (3 m)
3. For the *pretest* hold the sample cards at a distance of about 50 cm from the child with the cards held about 30 cm apart. The cards should be held at eye level and under binocular viewing conditions. Now the examiner says, "Here are two cars. One has wheels that are broken, the other one has wheels that are okay, or not broken." Point to the appropriate card as you describe them. Then say, "I want you to point at the car with the broken wheels." This is referred to as the *forced choice procedure.* If the child points correctly, place the cards behind your back, randomly change them from hand to hand, then present them to the child to make a choice. Usually, after two or three trials, the examiner can tell whether or not the child understands the task. If you are unsure, it is important to have four of four trials correct in succession to proceed to the next step.
4. To assure that the child's responses are reliable at the testing distance move to a distance of 3 m and repeat the forced choice procedure, as in step 3, under binocular viewing conditions. The developers of this test stress the importance of requiring the child to look at both cards and to slow down when making responses. A recommended modification is having the child use a small flashlight as a pointer. To be sure the child understands the task, correct responses on four of four trials is recommended.

If the acuity is less than 20/120, repeat this step at 1.5 m, and if necessary at closer distances.

5. Once the child demonstrates that he understands the task by correctly identifying the car with the broken wheels on four of four presentations you can begin to assess visual acuity. Place an elastic eye patch over the left eye of the child. It is important to observe the child at all times to make certain that he or she is not peeking through the eye that is occluded. Move to a distance of 3 m. Select the pair of 20/200 cards and present them to the child with one card in your right hand and the other in your left hand. Ask the child to point to the car with the broken wheels. If the child is able to successfully point to the car with the broken wheels on four of four presentations, proceed to the next pair of cards. Richman[16] recommends beginning with the 20/20 cards and then decreasing accordingly (20/30, the 20/40, and so on) if necessary.

   Another way to proceed is to begin with targets that the child can easily see (20/120, 20/100) and proceed with targets that become more difficult (20/30, 20/20).
6. The visual acuity is recorded as the last set of cards at which the child is able to correctly respond on four of four presentations.
7. Repeat the procedure with the right eye occluded and then with both eyes open.
8. If the testing distance is modified from the 3-m distance for which the cards were calibrated, the resulting visual acuity level must be adjusted.

INSTRUMENTATION

Lighthouse Cards

Theory and Use

This procedure is used with children about 2½ to 5 years of age. The New York Lighthouse Flash Card Test was developed as a visual acuity test for the visually handicapped preschool child, the nonreader of any age, and the multiply impaired person of any age.[18] Instead of the use of optotypes the Lighthouse test utilizes three stylized pictures. Snellen equivalents were obtained by measurement and clinical testing.

Although picturelike optotypes, such as the Lighthouse Cards, have been developed to improve testability of young children, they suffer from the drawbacks of any picture recognition task.

1. They are affected by the child's familiarity with the pictured object. Cultural and social factors influence responses to such tests, increasing variability and decreasing reliability.
2. They require a naming response rather than a nonverbal pointing response.
3. The results from picture-type tests are difficult to correlate, except in an approximate way, with those obtained from standard optotype tests.

COMMERCIALLY AVAILABLE INSTRUMENTS

The Lighthouse test consists of 12 reversible 4 × 5-in. flashcards with one symbol on each side (Fig. 66–6). Snellen acuity notation is printed on every card, and there are three symbols for each acuity level from 20/200 to 20/10. The reverse side of the 20/200 symbols are paired with the 20/100 symbols, the 20/50 with the 20/40, the 20/30 with the 20/20, and the 20/15 with the 20/10 symbols.

CLINICAL PROCEDURE

The clinical procedure involved in using the New York Lighthouse Flash Card Test is as follows:

1. Use the cards with the largest-size pictures and hold them at a distance of about 50 cm from the patient. Ask the patient the name of each of the three cards. If he does not know the names, spend several minutes teaching the names of the three pictures.
2. Once you feel the child knows the names of the pictures, present one card at a time at the same distance and ask the child "What is the name of this picture?" If the child is able to correctly identify the three pictures you can proceed to assess acuity as suggested in steps 4 through 6. If not, spend additional time teaching the names of the pictures, try a different test or step 3.
3. If the child will not verbalize the names of the pictures you can try to use the following procedure instead. Place one card with each of the three pictures before the child and simply ask the child to point to the card that matches the one you are holding up. If this procedure is also not successful, try a different test. If this method is successful uti-

lize this approach in steps 4 through 6, instead of asking for the name of the picture.

4. Place an elastic eye patch over the left eye of the child. It is important to observe the child at all times to make certain that he or she is not peeking through the eye that is occluded.
5. Move to a distance of 3 m and present the 20/200 cards, one at a time. Ask the child to name the card being presented. If the child can correctly identify the three pictures, present the set of cards with the next best acuity value until you reach a point at which the child is unable to name all three pictures at a given acuity level.
6. Record the acuity as the last level at which the child could name all three pictures.
7. Repeat steps 4 to 6 with the right eye occluded and then with both eyes open.

INSTRUMENTATION

Allen Chart

Theory and Use

This procedure is used with children about 2½ to 5 years of age. The Allen Picture Chart is a modification of the original test design[19] in which eight individual picture cards were available for testing. Today a projected chart using six of the eight original pictures is available (Reichert and Marco). With use of this projector chart, six pictures can be projected from an AO or Marco projector. Like the Lighthouse Cards, the Allen chart is made up of pictures instead of optotypes, which theoretically should be easier for a young child to identify than letters or numbers. Six pictures (horse, birthday cake, hand, telephone, bird, car) are used and acuity values of 20/200, 20/100, 20/70, 20/50, 20/40, and 20/30 are available. Because a full chart is available, multiple targets can be present at once or targets can be isolated. Therefore, both single-line and single-letter acuity can be evaluated by this procedure.

One limitation of this test is that the best acuity obtainable is 20/30. A recent study[20] found that in a sample of 33 known amblyopes, 13 of the 33 had equal vision with the Allen chart. Thus, this procedure missed almost 40% of the amblyopes in this sample. This same study also indicated that in comparison with the illiterate E and HOTV tests, the Allen chart tended to yield better acuities. When using this technique one should, therefore, be aware that the acuities obtained may be an overestimate. In addition, because the Allen chart uses pictures, it suffers from the drawbacks of all picture recognition tasks (refer back to the discussion of the sources of error with the Lighthouse cards).

COMMERCIALLY AVAILABLE INSTRUMENTS

For this procedure a projector, and slide with the Allen chart must be available. These are manufactured by Reichert and Marco (Fig. 66–7). Similar charts are available for visual acuity testing at near distances (Fig. 66–8).

CLINICAL PROCEDURE

The clinical procedure involved in using the Allen Projected Picture Chart is as follows:

1. The projector slide is inserted into the projector that has been calibrated for the room length to simulate optical infinity.

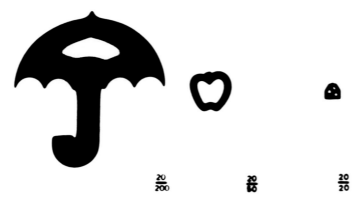

FIGURE 66–6. Lighthouse cards.

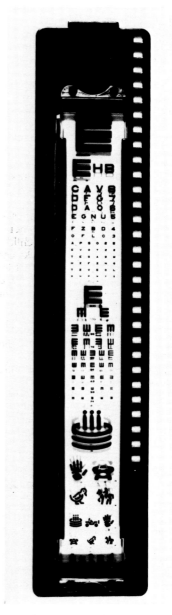

FIGURE 66–7. Sample of projector slide with Allen chart and illiterate E chart.

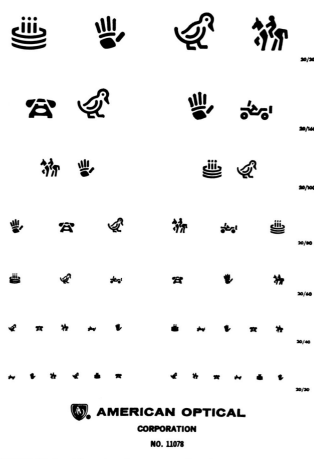

CHILDS RECOGNITION AND NEAR POINT TEST
TEST DISTANCE 13 INCHES

FIGURE 66–8. Allen chart for near visual acuity testing.

2. To be sure that the child knows the names of the pictures hold the nearpoint Allen card at 10 in. (25.5 cm) from the child. With the largest line of pictures, review the different pictures with the child until it is clear that he or she knows their names.
3. Place an elastic eye patch over the left eye of the child. It is important to observe the child at all times to make certain that he or she is not peeking through the eye that is occluded.
4. Isolate the chart, line by line, and ask the child to call off the names of the pictures he sees.
5. If the child is calling off the pictures, but the order appears to be out of sequence, it is often helpful to isolate each picture. This also helps prevent memorization.
6. Repeat steps 3 and 4 with the right eye occluded.

7. Repeat step 4 with both eyes open.
8. If the child is nonverbal, or refuses to call off the letters, it is sometimes helpful to just have the child point to the pictures on the near point Allen card.
9. Record single-line acuity for OD, OS, and OU. Record the acuity as the smallest line for which not more than one picture is read incorrectly. If a child reads incorrectly one picture on the 20/40 line, record the aquity as 20/40 − 1. If the child reads three of the five pictures on the 20/30 line, record the acuity as 20/40 + 3.
10. If amblyopia is suspected, record isolated acuity as well. This should be recorded using the same convention as described in step 9.

INSTRUMENTATION

Tumbling E

Theory and Use

The tumbling E procedure is used with children about 2½ to 5 years of age. The tumbling E or illiterate E test is designed so that the only response necessary is for the child to point in the direction the E is pointing. Theoretically, the absence of the need for identification of the optotype or for any verbal response should make this an ideal test for preverbal and preschool children. In addition, because a letter optotype is used the results from this test should correlate well with Snellen acuity.

However, studies[21,22] have demonstrated that there is a major drawback with the tumbling E test. Young children have difficulty with the directional concepts necessary to respond to this test. Although up–down discrimination is usually not a problem even in 3-year-old children, the left and right discrimination does present difficulty. Even when the child is given a plastic "E" to hold and is merely asked to turn it in the direction the E is facing, some children experience confusion with the task. Simons[23] has suggested a simple solution to this problem. He suggests changing the test from a four- to a three-alternative test format. In this proposed format possible responses would be up, down, or sideways. The removal of the left–right discrimination would still allow less than a 5% chance of guessing correctly for the recommended three repetition test trial.

As explained in the foregoing the major drawback of this test is the problem of discrimination of direction. Young children often experience directional confusion, making the results of this test difficult to interpret.

COMMERCIALLY AVAILABLE INSTRUMENTS

The tumbling E test is available in many formats. These include

- Graduated E cards
- The E box
- A simple cardboard chart
- A plastic chart that fits into the Goodlite Professional Eye Chart Cabinet, which is rear illuminated
- A projected eye chart for both Reichert and Marco for use in the AO type Project-O-Chart

See Figures 66–7 and 66–9 for an illustration of some of these different formats.

CLINICAL PROCEDURE

The exact procedure varies depending on the particular format being used. The Goodlite version, graduated cards, and "E" box use a 3-m testing distance, whereas the projected chart uses the distance at which the projector is calibrated.

1. The tumbling E chart is projected on the distance screen. The projector must be calibrated for the length of the room.

2. The first task is to ensure that the child understands the nature of the task. Isolate an E on the chart that is pointing up and ask the child which way the E is pointing. Alternatively, the child can be asked which way the "legs" of the E are pointing. The child can respond verbally or simply point in the appropriate direction.

3. Now isolate an E that is pointing down and ask the child which way it is pointing.

4. Next isolate an E that is pointing either right or left. To simplify the task and improve the chance of successfully using this test, tell the child that this one is pointing "sideways." It is, therefore, not necessary for the child to distinguish between right and left.

5. To be certain that the child understands the task, he or she should be able to successfully identify the direction in three out of three trials.

6. Once the child has successfully completed steps 1 to 5, you can begin the visual acuity assessment. Place an elastic eye patch over the left eye of the child. It is important to observe the child at all times to make certain that he or she is not peeking through the eye that is occluded.

7. Isolate the chart, line by line, and ask the child to call off the direction, up, down, sideways, or to point in the direction the E is pointing.

8. If the child appears to be confused by the number of Es on the line and calls out the direction of the Es out of sequence, it is often helpful to isolate the Es. This also helps prevent memorization.

9. Repeat steps 3 and 4 with the right eye occluded.

10. Repeat step 4 with both eyes open.

11. Record single-line acuity for OD, OS, and OU. Record the acuity as the smallest line for which not more than one E is read incorrectly. If a child reads incorrectly one E on the 20/40 line, record the acuity as 20/40 − 1. If the child reads three of the Es on the 20/30 line, record the acuity as 20/40 + 3.

12. If amblyopia is suspected, record isolated acuity as well. This should be recorded using the same convention as described in step 11.

INSTRUMENTATION

HOTV Subtest of STYCAR Test

Theory and Use

This procedure is used with children about 2½ to 5 years of age. The HOTV Test is part of the Sheridan STYCAR battery of tests.[24] STYCAR is an acronym for *screening test for young children and retardates*. Like the tumbling E test, the HOTV test utilizes letter

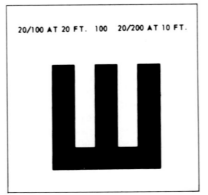
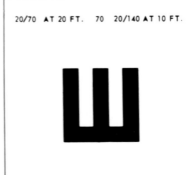
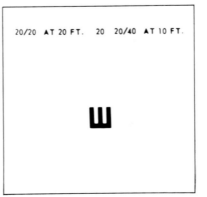

FIGURE 66–9. Illiterate E chart.

optotypes, which is a desirable characteristic, making the results more easily correlated with Snellen acuity values. The unique aspect of this test is that it requires no verbal response. Instead, the child must simply point to the appropriate letter on a nearby key card when the examiner holds up a letter at the testing distance. The letters *H, O, T, V* were selected because they are symmetrical around the vertical, axis and this avoids right–left confusion.

Several studies[24–26] have demonstrated that a significant number of young children, aged 4 and under are untestable with this procedure. Kastenbaum[25] found 52% of his population of 2 to 5 year olds untestable with the HOTV test. Savitz[26] reported that 56% of his sample could not respond to this test.

COMMERCIALLY AVAILABLE INSTRUMENTS

The HOTV test chart is available in several different formats. The original chart, which is a subtest of the STYCAR battery, is a cardboard chart that is set up at a distance of 3 m. It comes with a near-response panel which the child can point to to indicate his response. The HOTV test is also available as a plastic chart that slides into the Goodlite Professional Eye Chart Cabinet to be rear illuminated (Fig. 66–10). With the Goodlite device, testing also takes place at 3 m.

Finally, the HOTV format is now available as a projector chart from both Reichert and Marco. In the Reichert version the slide comes with a response panel. The Marco slide also includes the Allen-type picture chart and the tumbling E chart on the same slide (Fig. 66–11).

CLINICAL PROCEDURE

1. The HOTV chart is set up at a 3-m distance if the cardboard version or Goodlite version is being used. If the projector chart test is utilized, the child is seated at the standard distance for which the projector is set up. A

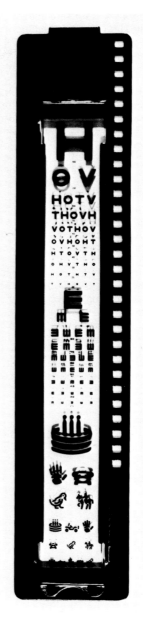

FIGURE 66–11. Projector slide with HOTV chart.

separate card with the letters *H, O, T, V* is placed within close range of the child.

2. The first task is to ensure that the child understands the nature of the task. Point to one of the four letters on the chart and ask the child to point to the same letter on the nearby chart.

3. To be certain that the child understands the task, he or she should be able to successfully identify the letter in four out of four trials.

4. Once the child has successfully completed steps 1 through 3, you can begin the visual acuity assessment. Place an elastic eye patch over the left eye of the child. It is important to observe the child at all times, to make certain that he or she is not peeking through the eye that is occluded.

5. Isolate the chart, line by line, and ask the child to point to the letter on the nearby chart that corresponds to the letter on the distance chart.

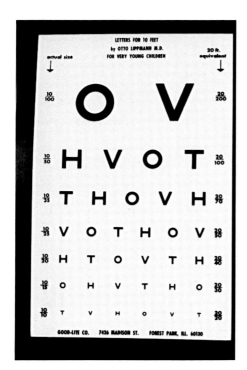

FIGURE 66–10. HOTV chart that can be used in the Goodlite Professional Cabinet.

6. If the child appears to be confused by the number of letters on the line and going out of sequence, it is often helpful to isolate the letters. This also helps prevent memorization.
7. Repeat steps 4 and 5 with the right eye occluded.
8. Repeat with both eyes open.
9. Record single-line acuity for OD, OS, and OU. Record the acuity as the smallest line for which not more than one letter is read incorrectly. If a child incorrectly reads one letter on the 20/40 line, record the acuity as 20/40 − 1. If the child reads three of the five letters on the 20/30 line, record the acuity as 20/40 + 3.
10. If amblyopia is suspected, record isolated acuity as well. This should be recorded using the same convention as described in step 9.

CLINICAL IMPLICATIONS

Clinical Significance

Visual acuity results from young children are important for several reasons. As with adults, normal acuity in infants and young children can help the clinician rule out a number of disorders, including significant refractive error, amblyopia, and ocular disease. Reduced visual acuity can be used to help confirm a suspicion of strabismus, anisometropia, or bilateral refractive error. Visual acuity data in infants probably has its greatest value in the management of amblyopia, strabismus, and refractive error. In the past, before clinicians could obtain reliable visual acuity information in this age group, it was more difficult to assess the efficacy of any implemented treatment. By using the techniques described in this section, the effectiveness of amblyopia therapy can be more easily monitored.

Clinical Interpretation

For older children and adults, the visual acuity data obtained are compared with the standard visual acuity of 20/20. For infants, the visual acuity data obtained are compared with the visual acuity expected for the particular age of the infant (see Table 66–1).

REFERENCES

1. Riggs LA. In: Graham CH, ed. Visual acuity in vision and visual perception. New York: John Wiley & Sons, 1965:321–349.
2. Bennett AG. Ophthalmic test types. Br J Physiol Opt 1965;22:238–271.
3. Weymouth FW. Visual acuity of children. In: Hirsch MJ, Wick RE, eds. Vision of children. Philadelphia: Chilton Books, 1963:119–143.
4. Fern KD, Manny RE. Visual acuity of the pre-school child: a review. Am J Optom Physiol Opt 1986;63:319–345.
5. Zipf RF. Binocular fixation pattern. Arch Ophthalmol 1976;94:401–405.
6. Wright KW, Walonker F, Edelman P. 10-Diopter fixation test for amblyopia. Arch Ophthalmol 1981;99:1242–1246.
7. Mayer DL, Fulton AB, Hansen RM. Preferential looking acuity obtained with a staircase procedure in pediatric patients. Invest Ophthalmol Vis Sci 1982;23:538–543.
8. Jacobson SG, Mohindra I, Held R. Visual acuity of infants with ocular diseases. Am J Ophthalmol 1982;93:198–209.
9. Fantz RI, Ordy JM, Udelf MS. Maturation of pattern vision in infants during the first six months. J Comp Physiol Psychol 1962;55:907–917.
10. McDonald M, Dobson V, Sebris SL, Baitch L, Varner D, Teller D. The acuity card procedure: a rapid test of infant acuity. Invest Ophthalmol Vis Sci 1985;26:1158–1162.
11. Dobson V, Mcdonald M, Kohl P, Stern N, Samek M, Preston K. Visual acuity screening of infants and young children with the acuity card procedure. J Am Optom Assoc 1986;57:285–289.
12. Kohl P, Rolen RD, Bedford AK, Samek M, Stern N. Refractive error and preferential looking visual acuity in human infants: a pilot study. J Am Optom Assoc 1986;57:290–296.
13. Birch EE, Naegele J, Bauer JA, Held R. Visual acuity of toddlers. Invest Ophthalmol Vis Sci 1980;20(suppl):210.
14. Birch EE, Gwiazda JA, Bauer J, Naegele J, Held R. Visual acuity and its meridional variation in children aged 7–60 months. Vis Res 1983;23:1019–1024.
15. Mayer DL, Fulton AB, Rodier D. Grating and recognition acuities of pediatric patients. Ophthalmology 1984;91:947–953.
16. Richman JE, Petito GT, Cron MT. Broken wheel acuity test: a new and valid test for preschool and exceptional children. J Am Optom Assoc 1984;55:561–565.
17. Committee on Vision, Assembly of Behavioral and Social Sciences, National Academy of Sciences. Recommended standard procedures for the clinical measurement and specification of visual acuity. Report of working group 39. Adv Ophthalmol 1980;41:103–148.
18. Faye EE. A new visual acuity test for partially sighted nonreaders. J Pediatr Ophthalmol 1968;5:210–212.
19. Allen HF. A new picture series for preschool vision testing. Am J Ophthalmol 1957;44:38–41.
20. De Young–Smith MA, Baker JD. A comparative study of visual acuity tests. Am Orthop J 1986;36:160–164.
21. Friendly DS. Preschool visual acuity screening tests. Trans Am Acad Ophthalmol 1980;76:383–480.
22. Lippmann O. Vision screening of young children. Am J Public Health 1971;61:1586–1601.
23. Simons K. Visual acuity norms in young children. Surv Ophthalmol 1983;28:84–92.
24. Sheridan MD, Gardiner PA. Sheridan–Gardiner test for visual acuity. Br Med J 1970;2:108–109.
25. Kastenbaum SM, Kepford KL, Holmstrom ET. Comparison of the STYCAR and Lighthouse acuity tests. Am J Optom Physiol Opt 1977;54:458–463.
26. Savitz RA, Reed RB, Valadin I. Vision screening of the preschool child. Washington, DC: Dept. of Health, Education, and Welfare, Children's Bureau, Publ. No. 414, 1964:55.

Hirschberg, Krimsky, Bruckner Tests

Mitchell Scheiman

INTRODUCTION

Definition

Pediatric binocular alignment testing refers to the clinical techniques designed to detect the presence of a heterotropia and to evaluate the frequency, direction, and magnitude of the deviation. The cover test is generally used, but with pediatric patients it is sometimes necessary to use the Hirschberg test, the Krimsky test, or the Bruckner test.

History

Historically, the assessment of binocular alignment has been a key part of an optometric evaluation. For children, objective techniques are most important. The cover test is considered the most important procedure in the objective assessment of binocular alignment. The Hirschberg method of assessing the amount of heterotropia was first described in 1885[1] and in the 1940s Krimsky reported a modification of the procedure to make measurement more accurate.[2] Most recently, Bruckner described a test in 1962 called the "transillumination" test, which also represents a modification of the original Hirschberg procedure.[3] This original paper was in German, and it was not until Tongue and Cibis[4] reported on the procedure in 1981 in the English language that the test began to gain popularity in the United States.

Clinical Use

The clinical use of binocular alignment testing is to detect the presence of a significant heterophoria or heterotropia. This is particularly important in children because binocular vision anomalies during the preschool years can cause amblyopia and reduced binocular function.

INSTRUMENTATION

Hirschberg Test

Theory and Use

This procedure is used with infants and preverbal children from birth to about 3 years of age. The test is based upon the assumption that if central fixation and binocular alignment are present the corneal reflection of a light being fixated by the patient will be in identical positions in the two eyes. If a strabismus is present there will be a relative difference in the position of the corneal reflection between the two eyes.

Although the Hirschberg test is an objective test, it does depend upon the child attending and fixating long enough for the examiner to make the necessary observations. Very young infants, younger than the age of 6 months, are usually easy to evaluate with this technique because they are very attracted to the light source. As infants approach the age of 12 months, however, they become more active and are less likely to attend to a light source. If a child does not attend well, it becomes extremely difficult to make the observations that are necessary with this test. For instance, a misalignment of $1/2$ mm represents a deviation of approximately 10 prism diopters, a misalignment of $1/4$ mm represents a deviation of 5 prism diopters. Although such an observation may be possible with an attentive, cooperative patient, such fine differences are difficult to observe in inattentive, active children. Thus, a significant deviation can easily be missed with this procedure.

Another potential source of error is lack of attention to angle lambda.

COMMERCIALLY AVAILABLE INSTRUMENTS

The only equipment needed to perform the Hirschberg test is a penlight or transilluminator.

CLINICAL PROCEDURE

The clinical procedure involved with performing the Hirschberg test is as follows:

1. A transilluminator or penlight is held 50 cm from the child's face in the midplane, and the patient is encouraged to fixate the light (Fig. 67–1).
2. The examiner observes the position of the corneal reflection of the light in each cornea when the other eye is covered. This position is a measurement of angle lambda. *Angle lambda* is the angle subtended at the center of the entrance pupil of the eye by the intersection of the pupillary axis and the line of sight. Most individuals have a small positive angle lambda, meaning that the corneal light reflection is displaced slightly nasalward relative to the center of the pupil (Fig. 67–2A). This is referred to as a positive angle lambda. A negative angle lambda refers to the situation in which the corneal light reflection is displaced temporalward (see Fig. 67–2B).

    The examiner should determine the location of the corneal reflection in each cornea relative to the center of the pupil. The displacement of the corneal reflection from the center of the pupil (angle lambda) should be estimated in millimeters.
3. Hold the light source about 50 cm in front of the child's eyes with both eyes open and observe the displacement of the corneal reflection from the center of the pupil in millimeters in both the right and left eyes. If the displacement is identical for the two eyes record this observation as "aligned." If one reflection is displaced relative to the other it is important to determine the fixating eye.
4. Determine the fixating eye by observing which eye has the

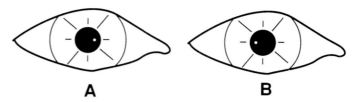

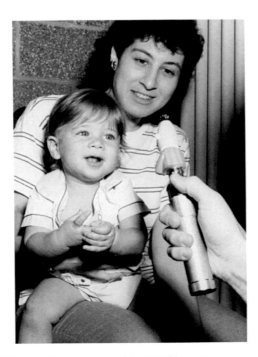

FIGURE 67–1. Administration of the Hirschberg test.

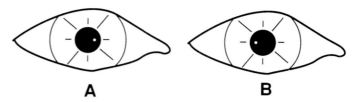

FIGURE 67–2. (*A*) Positive angle lambda: Corneal light reflection is displaced slightly nasalward. (*B*) Negative angle lambda: Corneal light reflection is displaced temporalward.

corneal reflection in the identical position observed during the angle lambda measurement.
5. The other eye is the misaligned or deviated eye and the magnitude of the deviation is determined by observing the displacement of the corneal reflection in the deviated eye from its angle lambda position. For example, if angle lambda was measured at +1.0 mm for both eyes, and under binocular viewing conditions, you observe that the corneal reflection in the right eye is 1-mm nasal to the center of the pupil, whereas the corneal reflection in the left eye is 1-mm temporal to the center of the pupil, this would indicate that the right eye is the fixating eye and the corneal reflection in the left eye is displaced 2 mm from its angle lambda position.
6. The amount of displacement of the corneal reflection from the angle lambda position is a measurement of the heterotropia and should be recorded in millimeters.

CLINICAL IMPLICATIONS

Clinical Significance and Interpretation

The results from the Hirschberg test can be used to make a diagnosis of the presence or absence of a strabismus. If strabismus is present, the magnitude of the deviation can be estimated based upon the relative displacement of the reflexes. A relative difference in position between the right and left eye reflexes of one 1 mm, has been reported to equal 22 prism diopters.[5,6]

If a patient has an angle lambda in each eye of +0.5 mm, but under binocular viewing conditions, the reflex in the right eye is +0.5 mm and the reflex in the left eye is +2.0 mm, the patient would have a left exotropia of 33^Δ ($1.5 \times 22^\Delta$).

INSTRUMENTATION

Krimsky Test

Theory and Use

This procedure is a modification of the Hirschberg test in an attempt to make a more accurate measurement of the amount of strabismus. Like the Hirschberg test, there is minimal communication necessary, making this test useful with infants and preschool children. Unlike the Hirschberg test, instead of simply observing the relative difference in the position of the corneal reflections of the two eyes, prism is used to change the position of the corneal reflection in the deviating eye. The amount of prism needed to reposition the corneal reflection in the deviating eye to the angle lambda position is the measurement of the magnitude of the strabismus.

Good attention and fixation are necessary for an accurate measurement, and the procedure does require the examiner to place a loose prism or a prism bar in front of the dominant eye.

Although very young infants will often not object to this, children between the ages of 12 months and 3 years often resist having anything placed before their eyes.

COMMERCIALLY AVAILABLE INSTRUMENTS

The equipment needed to perform the Krimsky test is penlight or transilluminator and a prism bar or loose prisms.

CLINICAL PROCEDURE

The clinical procedure involved with performing the Krimsky test is as follows:

1. A transilluminator or penlight is held 50 cm from the child's face in the midplane.
2. The examiner observes the corneal reflection of the light in each cornea while the other eye is covered (angle lambda).
3. The examiner determines which eye is the fixating eye and places a prism bar or loose prism in front of this eye (Fig. 67–3). If esotropia is present, base-out prism is used, if exotropia is present, base-in prism is used. The amount of prism is increased until the corneal reflection in the deviating eye moves to the angle lambda position. The amount of prism to accomplish this is a measure of the magnitude of the strabismus.

CLINICAL IMPLICATIONS

Clinical Significance and Interpretation

The Krimsky test provides a measurement of the amount of the strabismus in prism diopters for a given fixation distance.

INSTRUMENTATION

Bruckner Test

Theory and Use

The Bruckner test utilizes an ophthalmoscope to compare the red reflexes of the two eyes. Both eyes are simultaneously illuminated with the ophthalmoscope beam at a distance of 100 cm. If a difference in the brightness of the pupil area is noticed, the eye with the brighter, whiter pupil area may be strabismic or amblyopic. The test is, therefore, objective, and can be used to provide useful information about an infant or preschool child's visual status.

Bruckner believed that a difference in the nature of the appearance of the pupil area in the two eyes could be attributed to the differences between pigmentation in the macula and peripheral retina. Roe and Guyton[7] more recently proposed another theory. They demonstrated that the difference in the brightness can be explained by the principle of conjugacy between the light source of the ophthalmoscope and the retina. The fundus reflex will appear darker in an eye that is fixating and focused on the ophthalmoscope light because the light and the retina are conjugate to each other. If an eye is deviated, off axis optical aberrations decreases conjugacy and the pupil area will appear brighter and whiter.

Griffin and Cotter[8] have evaluated the clinical usefulness of the Bruckner test. They reported that the test should serve as an adjunct to Hirschberg and the cover tests in the clinical evaluation of microstrabismus and other types of strabismus, particularly in infants and uncooperative patients.

Although Griffin and Cotter[8] suggested that the Bruckner test is a useful procedure, they did suggest two potential problems that should be considered when using this procedure.

1. In a visual screening, the presence of uncorrected refractive error would make the procedure less reliable.
2. The use of the Bruckner test alone in a screening process might result in many false-positive results.

COMMERCIALLY AVAILABLE INSTRUMENTS

The equipment needed to perform the Bruckner test is an ophthalmoscope.

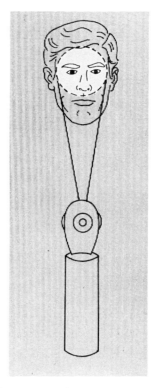

FIGURE 67–4. Administration of Bruckner test.

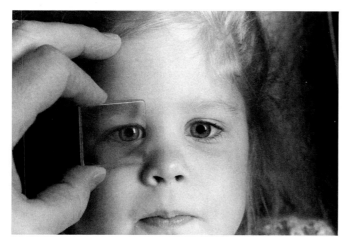

FIGURE 67–3. Administration of Krimsky test.

Accommodative Response

Kent M. Daum

INTRODUCTION

Definition

The *accommodative response* is a measure of the actual amount of accommodation that is present. The difference between the accommodative stimulus and the accommodative response is called the *lead* or *lag of accommodation*. Because of the depth of focus of the eye, and other factors, the accommodative response is generally less than the accommodative stimulus.

History

Clinically, the accommodative response is determined from dynamic retinoscopy. Although a form of static retinoscopy was described in 1862 by Bowman,[1] it was further developed by Cuignet, Parent, and Leroy.[1,2] Techniques describing dynamic retinoscopy followed soon after. Most authorities credit Cross[3] for its initial description in 1901.[4-11] In this early period when the relationship between accommodation, convergence, and refraction was still being studied, there were a number of slightly different techniques proposed to determine the accommodative response.[3,5-7,10-14] The objective of these techniques varied somewhat; however, most were concerned with the determination of the "true" refractive error or an appropriate near point correction.[13] Among these early descriptions, Sheard[5] and Nott[7] had a clear and surprisingly modern understanding of the theory of dynamic retinoscopy, particularly the relationship between accommodation and vergence.

The binocular cross cylinder test has been used as a measure of the lag of accommodation. Fry[15] and others[16] have concluded that this is not the preferred technique for this purpose.

Clinical Use

Dynamic retinoscopy is used to objectively determine the point that is conjugate to the retina when the patient is viewing a particular target. This conjugate point is affected by the patient's accommodation, refractive correction, and binocularity. It also is dependent on the nature of the target. A lag of accommodation of about 0.50 D to 0.75 D is usually found for a target positioned 40 cm away from the patient. Lesser lags (1.00 D or greater) imply an accommodative insufficiency, presbyopia, significant esophoria, or uncorrected hyperopia. A reduced lag or a lead of accommodation suggests an accommodative spasm, significant exophoria, or an overminused refraction.

INSTRUMENTATION

Theory

The objective of this clinical procedure is to determine the correlation between the accommodative stimulus and the accommodative response. This correlation is obtained by determining the dioptric difference between the target of regard and the point in space that is conjugate to the retina.

The point in space that is conjugate to the retina is generally determined in one of two ways: by briefly interposing additional lenses into the line of sight to achieve neutrality or by moving the retinoscope in space to the point that is conjugate to the retina. Although these techniques produce equivalent results, there are reasons why each may be the method of choice in particular circumstances. Briefly interposing additional lenses is the *monocular estimation method* (MEM).[17-19] Moving the retinoscope to find the neutral point is called the *Nott method*.[7]

Table 71–1
Potential Sources of Error in Dynamic Retinoscopy

Unknown or mistaken variables
  Power of correction
  Power of neutralizing lenses
  Uncorrected astigmatism
  Unknown disease
  Distance estimation (placement of the target and point of neutrality)
  Estimate of neutrality
Changes in fixation or accommodative level
  Poor cooperation
  Poor motivation
  Poor understanding
Inadequate visibility
  Target (by patient)
    Contrast
    Illumination
    Size
    Spatial frequency
  Retinoscopic reflex (by clinician)
Retinoscopy errors
  Small pupils, cataracts, error
Adaptation to measuring lens

Sources of Error

Sources of error for this clinical procedure include unknown or mistaken variables, changes in fixation or accommodative level, failure to understand or cooperate, inadequate visibility of either the target (by the patient) or the retinoscopic reflex (by the clinician), other retinoscopy errors, and adaptation to the measuring lens (Table 71–1).

A great many types of errors can occur because of unknown or mistaken variables. Assumptions about the power of the habitual correction may be incorrect. Uncorrected astigmatism may cause an error. Any time the patient is not wearing a known correction, there is the possibility of error. A frequent clue to this error is apparently unequal lags of accommodation. Barring some abnormality, such as Adie's syndrome, amblyopia, cataracts, or third cranial nerve dysfunction, the lags of accommodation should be equal, regardless of which eye is fixating and controlling the accommodative response. This assumes that different eyes control the base of accommodation during the process. Frequently, with an unknown refractive cause, there is a difference.

Other "mistaken" variables causing error include distance estimation or measurement errors in placing the target, in determining the distance to neutrality in the Nott technique, or in the power of the lenses used to neutralize the reflex with the MEM method. Frequently, the target distance is initially estimated correctly, but it is moved closer over time. This tends to occur regardless of whether the clinician or the patient holds the target.

Changes in fixation or accommodative response are often related to a failure of the patient to understand the task or to cooperate with the clinician. The attention and full cooperation of the patient are essential for this clinical procedure. An error can result if the patient looks at a different fixation distance than the one requested by the clinician. In this event, the clinician relates the lag to an incorrect fixation distance. The lag changes as a function of fixation distance, increasing as the fixation distance is reduced. Erratic changes in fixation may simulate a variable lag. If marked, such changes may make dynamic retinoscopy impossible to complete.

The characteristics of the target and the degree of illumination are important factors in causing both the target and the retinoscopic reflex to be visible. Clear, detailed, high-contrast targets allow the accommodation system to work efficiently.[20] At low levels of illumination and contrast, the accommodative system tends to adopt a rest point that is about a meter in front of the patient.[21]

The high level of illumination that provides the best stimulus for accommodation can interfere with retinoscopy. Since very high levels of light make it difficult to see the reflex, a compromise must be reached so that retinoscopy can be completed satisfactorily. Directed light onto the target and away from the patient may be useful for this.

Darkness tends to mask accommodative aftereffects.[22] Schor et al.[22] show that the effects of previous accommodation are often masked under the reduced illumination conditions that are often used to assess the lag of accommodation (Figs. 71–1 and 71–2; Tables 71–2 and 71–3). Currently, the implications of these data have not been fully understood by clinicians. Schor suggests that adaptation of accommodation probably serves to reduce and sustain the accommodative response. This is similar to the function of prism adaptation with vergences.

Dynamic retinoscopy is subject to all of the errors that affect static retinoscopy. Scissors motion, small pupils, and dim media, if present, may critically affect the clinician's ability to perform the task.

Adaptation of the accommodative system to the measuring lens is an error that could occur with the MEM technique. Within certain limits, the accommodative system will relax to accommodate plus lenses and become activated in response to minus lenses. The latency of the accommodation system is about 250 to

Table 71–2
Duration of Accommodative Aftereffects (secs)*

| | Open Loop Conditions | | | | | | | | | | | |
| | 5-sec Stimulus Duration | | | | | | 1-min Stimulus Duration | | | | | |
	1	2	3	4	5	6	1	2	3	4	5	6
Maxwellian view	5.3	7.5	16	12	4.7	6.4	58	120	94	108	78	68
Empty field	4.0	6.4	14	10	4.5	4.8	45	115	85	105	71	54
Darkness	2.2	2.5	3	6	3.5	4.2	7	6	5	11	5	5

* The mean durations of aftereffects of monocular accommodation, for six subjects, to a 2-D step stimulus, presented for 5 or 60 sec, are shown for three open-loop conditions.

(Modified from Schor CM, et al. Adaptation of tonic accommodation reduces accommodative lag and is masked in darkness. Invest Ophthalmol Vis Sci 1983;27:820–827)

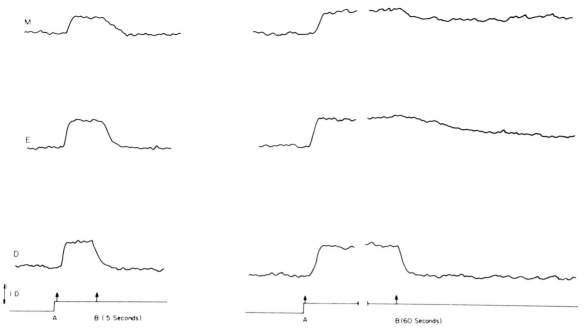

M

E

D

I D

A   B (5 Seconds)   A   B (60 Seconds)

FIGURE 71–1. Different time constants for relaxation of accommodation under three different open-loop conditions [Maxwellian view (M), empty field (E), and darkness (D)] after stimulating accommodation monocularly for either 5 or 60 seconds. Arrows marked *A* and *B* beneath the recordings indicate when accommodation was stimulated and when the loop was opened, respectively. Incomplete relaxation of accommodation after long-term stimulation demonstrates a tonic aftereffect of accommodation. (Modified from Schor CM, et al. Adaptation of tonic accommodation reduces accommodative lag and is masked in darkness. Invest Ophthalmol Vis Sci 1986;27:820–827)

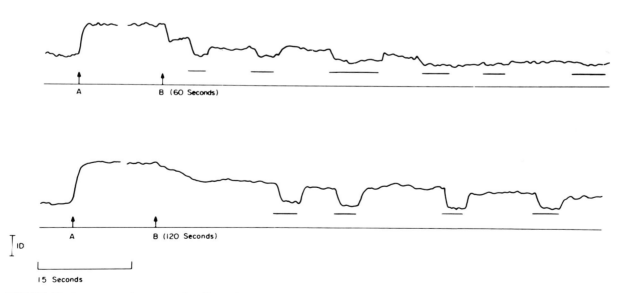

A   B (60 Seconds)

A   B (120 Seconds)

ID

15 Seconds

FIGURE 71–2. Decay of a tonic aftereffect of accommodation shown during open-loop (Maxwellian view) conditions interrupted by brief periods of darkness (*underlined segments*). Adaptation was for 1 minute to a 2-D stimulus (*top*) or for 2 minutes to a 3-D stimulus (*bottom*). During dark periods accommodation went to its resting level, but it returned to the adapted state when the Maxwellian view condition was reinstated. This illustrates that tonic adaptation did not decay more rapidly in darkness, but rather, it was masked by darkness. (Modified from Schor CM, et al. Adaptation of tonic accommodation reduces accommodative lag and is masked in darkness. Invest Ophthalmol Vis Sci 1986;27:820–827)

Table 71–3
Gain of Tonic Accommodation*

Stimulus Amplitude (D)	Subjects	
	2	1
1	0.89	0.52
2	0.95	0.54
4	0.94	0.48
6	0.51	

* Gain of tonic accommodation (open-loop aftereffect/ closed-loop response amplitude) is shown for two subjects as a function of accommodative stimulus amplitude. Accommodation was stimulated for 2 min, and then the accommodative loop was opened using a Maxwellian view. Amplitude of the aftereffect was measured 45 sec after opening the loop.

(Modified from Schor CM, et al. Adaptation of tonic accommodation reduces accommodative lag and is masked by darkness. Invest Ophthalmol Vis Sci 1983;27:820–827)

500 milliseconds (0.25 to 0.5 second).[23] Lenses inserted into the line of sight and removed within the latency period will not cause significant changes in the accommodation. Lenses inserted for longer than that latency may cause changes in the accommodative level, decreasing the level with plus lenses and increasing the level with minus.

There are, therefore, several factors that must be dealt with for dynamic retinoscopy to provide an accurate estimate of the lag of accommodation (Table 71–4). These factors concern (1) the physical arrangement for the measurement; (2) the instructions given to the patient; and (3) the patient's cooperation.

COMMERCIALLY AVAILABLE INSTRUMENTS

Equipment necessary to assess the accommodative response includes the following:

1. A retinoscope: These are available from a variety of optical equipment manufacturers (see Chap. 16).
2. Fixation stimuli: Various near point material is suitable and readily available.
3. Loose lenses: These are typically taken from a trial lens set for the MEM technique.
4. Measuring tape or near point rod: Many types are in use (for the Nott technique).

Table 71–4
Prerequisites for Dynamic Retinoscopy

1. The physical arrangement
   a. Slightly dim lighting to enable retinoscopy, but still allow adequate stimulus visibility
   b. High-contrast, detailed stimulus (Snellen letters between 20/20 and 20/200)
   c. Known (and correct) correction
   d. Known stimulus distance
   e. Retinoscopy near the line of sight of the patient
   f. Accurate measurements of distance (Nott) or lenses (MEM)
2. The instructions given to the patient clear, simple, understandable
3. The patient's cooperation stable, accurate fixation and accommodation

Table 71–5
Clinical Procedure for the MEM Technique

1. Position the patient a known distance away from a detailed, high-contrast target.
2. Place a known correction on the patient.
3. Arrange the lighting so that the patient can see the target and the retinoscopic reflex is visible.
4. Move so that the retinoscope and the target are 40 cm from the spectacle plane.
5. Instruct the patient.
6. Perform retinoscopy. Estimate the lag.
7. Assess the estimate of the lag. Repeat to bracket and determine the endpoint.
8. Record the results.

CLINICAL PROCEDURE

Monocular Estimation Method (MEM) (Table 71–5)

1. Position the patient a known distance away from a well-detailed, high-contrast target (often letters in the 20/20 to 20/30 range). These are small enough that the individual must accommodate to resolve the letters. Lovasik et al.[24] and Tan and O'Leary[25] have shown that there is little difference in accommodative response for letters between 1 and 10 minutes of arc (20/20 to 20/200) at the nearpoint (40 cm; Fig. 71–3). Letters, however, are not required for the technique. Many times with children, it is best to use some interesting and brightly colored figure, such as a small animal character.
2. The patient should wear a known correction. Generally, it is of little importance whether the patient wears his own

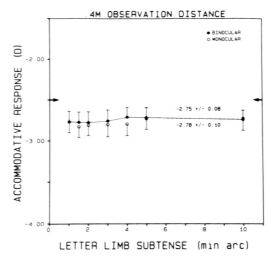

FIGURE 71–3. Group-averaged accommodative responses as a function of letter limb subtense for binocular and monocular viewing conditions for the 0.4-m observation distance. Accommodative responses were independent of letter limb subtense for both monocular and binocular testing. The numbers beside each data set correspond to their respective average response and group standard deviation values. The small *horizontal arrows* indicate the accommodative demand for the observation distance. (Modified from Lovasik JV, et al. The influence of letter size on the focusing response of the eye. J Am Optom Assoc 1987;58:631–639)

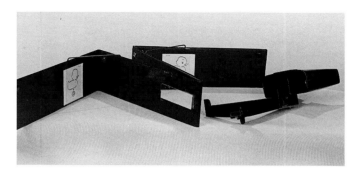

FIGURE 73–1. The various types of stereoscopes use either mirrors or septums to separate the targets presented to each eye.

Use

Targets are presented to the patient in a clinical situation using various types of instruments to assess the use of both eyes under binocular-viewing conditions at different distances and directions of gaze. Because of the nature of suppression, subjective responses are required from the patient. Any type of subjective testing requires patient responses for the examiner to detect and quantify suppression. This can pose problems with interpretation of the responses when the patient is uncooperative or too young to give accurate responses.

COMMERCIALLY AVAILABLE INSTRUMENTS

Basic Design

Stereoscopes

There are three main classes of stereoscopes (Wheatstone, Brewster, and haploscope), with several variations of each available. The primary purpose of stereoscopes is for testing and training binocular fusion. Since the use of both eyes is needed for fusion, stereoscopes can be conveniently used to test for suppression.

A major criticism of stereoscopes for examination of suppression is that they change the conditions of natural vision. This can be a major source of error. Stereoscopes will detect suppression at a different level than that experienced in everyday life.

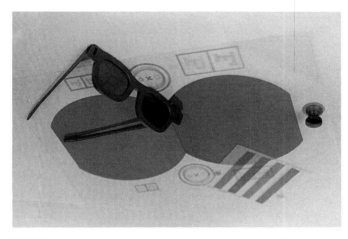

FIGURE 73–2. Anaglyphic and polaroid techniques use filters to separate target details presented to each eye.

WHEATSTONE STEREOSCOPE. The first class of stereoscope was designed by Charles Wheatstone in 1838.[1] It is shaped like a large W with mirrors placed on each side of the center apex as it is pointed toward the nose. The apex acts as a septum and each eye sees a separate image of a target placed on the outside arms reflected from each mirror. By varying the angle the targets make with the mirrors, different vergence demands are placed on the visual system. Fusion can be achieved only when each eye sees its respective target, and suppression is evident when a target, or a portion of a target, is missing.

Commercial examples of the Wheatstone stereoscope are the Pigeon–Cantonnet stereoscope, and the Bernell mirror stereoscope.

Changing target size, brightness levels, movement of a target, or flashing the lights can help evaluate the depth of suppression. These techniques can also provide a starting point for training if fusion cannot be obtained without them.

BERNELL STEREOSCOPE. A Bernell stereoscope is a common Wheatstone type (Fig. 73–3). It is W-shaped with a separate mirror on each side. Separate targets for each eye are placed on each arm. The patient is asked to fuse the targets. If they report that they can only see one target or only one of the different parts of the target, they are suppressing. Various target parameters can be used to quantify suppression.

BREWSTER (REFRACTING) STEREOSCOPE. The refracting stereoscope was invented by Brewster in 1844.[9] It uses a septum to dissociate the targets and two plus lenses that are decentered to create base-out prism.[10] The design allows this device to test, as well as treat, suppression.[11] As with mirror stereoscopes, suppression can eliminate the ability to fuse the two targets.

The Brewster stereoscope is designed so that at a distance of 0.2 m a separation between the targets of 2 mm equals 1 prism diopter of vergence demand. This fixation distance represents a "distance" measurement because of the +5.00-diopter (D) lenses used in the instrument. For near-point measurements the targets are moved to 0.133 m. Since the dioptric value of 0.133 m is 7.50 diopters, the difference between this and the +5.00-diopter lenses creates 2.5 diopters of accommodative demand (Fig. 73–4). Changing the target distance and using stereograms with different separation between targets allows varying accommodative and prismatic demands to be placed on the visual system. Suppression testing can be done at any of these positions. When an inability to see one of the targets (suppression) is found, the examiner can change the separation between the targets to evaluate the suppression.

When using stereoscopes, giving accurate directions for its use is as important as the accuracy of the patient's responses is

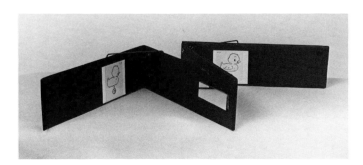

FIGURE 73–3. The Bernell stereoscope is a common Wheatstone type. It is W-shaped with a separate mirror on each side. Targets visible to each eye are placed on each arm. The patient fuses the targets and reports the presence or absence of suppression checks.

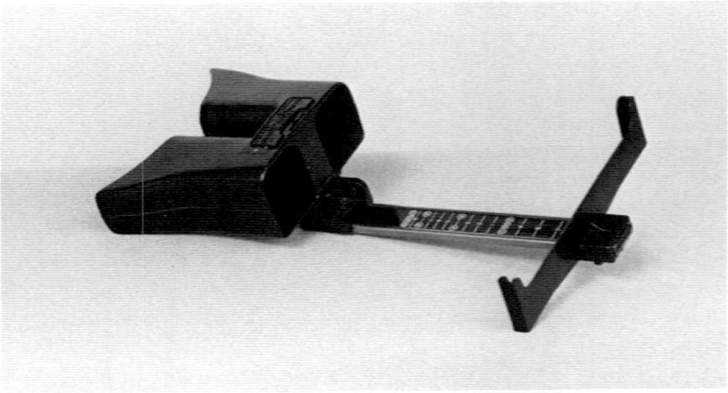

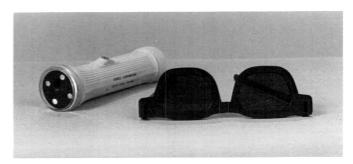

FIGURE 73–4. When using a Brewster stereoscope, a 0.20-m fixation distance represents a "distance" measurement because of the +5.00-diopter lenses used in the instrument. The targets are moved to 0.133 m for near measurements. Since the dioptric value of 0.133 m is 7.50 diopters, the difference between this and the +5.00-diopter lenses creates 2.5 diopters of accommodative demand. (Adapted from Eskridge JB. Accommodation and vergence with the Brewster stereoscope. J Am Optom Assoc 1976; 47:919–924)

critical in eliminating errors. It can be helpful to phrase questions to inquire what the patient sees, rather than asking if they see what you would like them to see.

Anaglyphic Tests

Targets are viewed while the patient wears a red filter over one eye and a green filter over the other eye. The color of the target and the filter should match as closely as possible to ensure that perception of the target is totally extinguished by the filter.[12] Anaglyphic targets consist of anything that is red and green, such as print, toys, lights, or even food. When the target is on a white background, the eye with the red filter sees *only* the green target, and the eye behind the green filter sees *only* the red target. When the background color is black, the eye behind the red filter sees *only* the red target and the eye behind the green filter sees *only* the green target. The reverse is true when red and green *lights* are used.

A major source of error may arise when the color of the filters does not match that of the targets. When this happens the target is not completely extinguished by the filter, and it is seen by both eyes, thus suppression cannot be accurately determined. Another source of error might arise when the patient rapidly alternates fixation; they may never report any portion of the diagram missing.

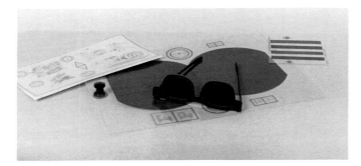

FIGURE 73–5. Anaglyphic tests, in addition to the Worth dot test, include the three-figure test, the Keystone Basic Binocular Test Set, root rings, Brock posture board, red–green bar reader, and red–green TV trainer.

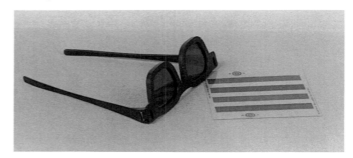

FIGURE 73–6. The Worth dot test consists of a lighted stimulus with four holes of 2 to 3 cm diameter. Classically, the upper opening is red, transmitting only red wavelengths, the lateral openings are green, transmitting only green wavelengths, and the bottom opening is white, transmitting all wavelengths.

There are numerous anaglyphic devices. The usual clinical test is the Worth dot test. Others include the three-figure test, and the Keystone Basic Binocular Test Set. Also available are root rings, Brock posture board, red–green bar reader, and red–green TV trainer (Fig. 73–5). The list of anaglyphic targets is limited only by the examiner's ingenuity and imagination.

Worth Dot Test

The Worth dot test, an adaptation of Snellen's colored glasses, consists of a lighted stimulus with four holes of 2- to 3-cm diameter. Classically, the upper opening is red, which transmits only red wavelengths, the lateral openings are green, which transmits only green wavelengths, and the bottom opening is white, transmitting all wavelengths (Fig. 73–6).

The patient wears a pair of spectacles with a red filter (usually over the right eye) and a green filter (over the left eye). When looking through the red filter, the patient sees only the red dots and, through the green filter, only the green dots. Both eyes see the white dot, which may appear red or green.

Javal Grid Bar Reader

The Javal Grid Bar Reader consists of five vertical bars mounted on a handle. It is a septum test for suppression, which is designed for hand-held use in detection of suppression at near distance. Modified designs, which use anaglyphic or vectographic techniques (Fig. 73–7), are discussed here. The patient starts by placing the grid on the text. The patient should be able to read the entire text, provided he is bifixating and not suppressing. If the patient is suppressing one eye, part of the corresponding text will disappear.

FIGURE 73–7. The bar reader consists of five vertical bars that use anaglyphic or vectographic material to test for suppression at near distance. The patient should be able to read the entire text with the grid placed on it.

By using multiple bar readers and septums, the clinician can create a more demanding flat fusion test and make the test more sensitive for detecting suppression.

The anaglyphic grid/bar reader may prove inaccurate in detecting suppression in a rapidly alternating strabismus (e.g., small-angle alternating esotropia). This patient is sometimes capable of switching fixation so quickly that he or she will be able to read the entire text through the bar reader even though he or she is alternately suppressing (Fig. 73–8). To overcome this error, the clinician can compare the patient's reading speed with and without the bar reader in place. If the patient shows a significantly slower reading rate with the bar reader in place, then it is likely that he or she is alternately suppressing and flat fusion is absent. Because of the design of the alternating vertical bars, a small central suppression zone may be missed if the patient fixates "just right."

Three-Figure Test

The three-figure test consists of a lighted stimulus with three figures; similar in principle to the Worth dot test. One is red, which transmits only red wavelengths, one is green, which transmits only green wavelengths, and one is white, transmitting all wavelengths. The patient wears a pair of spectacles with a red filter (usually over the right eye) and a green filter (over the left eye). Looking through the red filter the patient sees only the red target, and through the green filter only the green target. Both eyes see the white target, which may appear red or green.

Red Lens Test

The red lens test is designed to measure the depth of suppression. To conduct the red lens test for suppression, the retinal illuminance of the fixating eye must be reduced until the patient sees double. Materials required to perform the test include a small light source, such as a penlight, to serve as a fixation target and a series of red filters, ranging in various densities.

A series of red gelatine filters arranged in increasing density has been developed by Burian.[13] The patient fixates a small light source as the filters are placed before the fixating eye. The density of the filter before the fixing eye is increased until the patient recognizes diplopia (Fig. 73–9). Results recorded should include

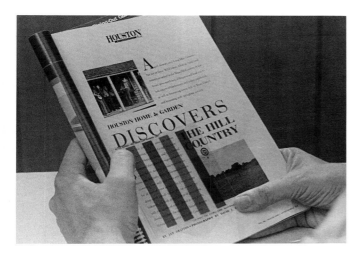

FIGURE 73–8. A bar reader may not detect suppression in patients with a rapidly alternating strabismus, who may be capable of switching fixation so quickly that they can read the entire text through the bar reader, even though alternately suppressing.

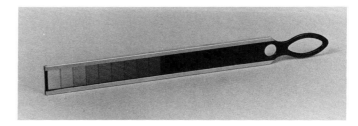

FIGURE 73–9. While using the increasing density red gelatine filters, the patient fixates a small light source as the filters are placed before the fixating eye. The darkness of the filter before the fixing eye is increased until the patient reports diplopia. Results recorded should include the test distance, light used, and density of the filter that elicits a diplopia.

the test distance, light used, and density of the first filter that elicits a diplopic response.

When conducting the red lens test, suppression may be too deep for diplopia to be noticed. In these patients, the subjective response of diplopia is further aided by reducing the room illumination and/or increasing the luminance of the lighted target.

With the red lens test, some patients require a greater density red filter in front of the fixating eye to elicit diplopia than other patients. The greater the density of red filter required to elicit diplopia, the more unnatural the conditions, and the deeper the suppression.

Keystone Basic Binocular Test

The Keystone Basic Binocular Test consists of 12 red and green print charts on a yellow background that allow first-, second-, and third-degree fusion testing. To evaluate suppression, the examiner determines if certain parts of the chart or diagram are visible while the patient wears anaglyphic filters.

Vectographic Tests

A vectographic test uses polarization to give an image to each eye while maintaining fairly natural conditions. The patient wears polarizing filters in the form of spectacles, polaroid filters in the American Optical (A/O) phoroptors, or auxiliary Polaroid analyzers for the Bausch & Lomb (B&L) phoroptor. The filter for each eye is rotated 90° from the other. In the United States, the polarizers are commonly set at 45° and 135°. The test targets are polarized so that each eye sees only a certain portion of the target.

A/O Vectographic Adult Slide

The A/O vectographic adult slide is set up for use at 20 ft (6m) in a room with moderate illumination (Fig. 73–10). Tests are included for suppression, fixation disparity, and stereopsis. The suppression test consists of a set of letters that are alternately polarized so that one letter is seen by the right and the other is seen by the left. Other sections of the slide can be used as for evaluating suppression, such as the balance portion and the cross. Each of these is also seen by one eye with a portion seen binocularly. Suppression is evident when a portion of the target seen by one eye is missing.

Vectograms

Vectograms are hand-held or used with the Polachrome Orthopter. Many different targets are available to use. Examples of targets are quoits, clown, basic fusion. Usually two vectograms, one of which is viewed by the right eye and one by the left eye, are used

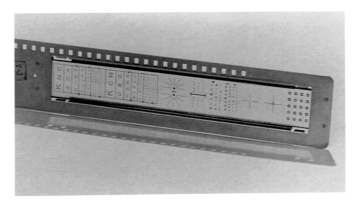

FIGURE 73–10. The vectographic adult slide includes tests for suppression, fixation disparity, and stereopsis. The suppression test is made up of letters that are polarized so that one is seen by the right eye and the other is seen by the left eye. Suppression is evident when a portion of the target seen by one eye is missing.

together with one placed on top of the other (Fig. 73–11). To evaluate suppression, two dissimilar targets can be used. An example of dissimilar targets would be the quoit for one eye and the clown for the other eye. Alternatively, most vectograms contain a small suppression clue for each eye somewhere on the target.

Pola–Mirror Test

The polaroid–mirror detection method for suppression requires the use of only two pieces of equipment: a pair of polaroid glasses and an ordinary flat mirror (Fig. 73–12). In the Pola-mirror Test the subject wears the polarizing spectacles and looks at himself in a mirror.[14] The basic design is based upon the blocking out of light by the polaroid filters placed with axes 90° apart. Thus, the right eye will appear black when viewed by the left eye and vice versa.

Vis-a-Vis Test

The Vis-a-Vis Test is a modification of the Pola–mirror Test, in which the examiner and the patient each wear polarizers. Because

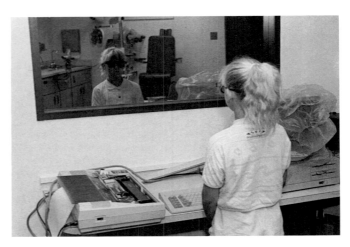

FIGURE 73–12. The polaroid–mirror detection method for suppression requires the use of a pair of polaroid glasses and an ordinary flat mirror. The subject wears the polarizing spectacles and looks at himself or herself in a mirror.

of the cross-polarization, if one eye is suppressing, the eye directly in front of the suppressing eye will be blacked out. It therefore follows that if neither eye is suppressing, each can see its own image and both eyes will be seen simultaneously.

Stereo Tests

Stereo tests (e.g., Titmus) can also be used to indirectly measure suppression. Stereo tests require that the patient wear polarizers. Each test usually has a variety of targets: a large target, such as the fly in the Titmus test for gross stereopsis (3000 seconds of arc), and a variety of smaller targets that can measure from 800 to 40 seconds of arc. The Titmus uses three rows of animals and a series of nine groups of diamonds, each with four circles (Fig. 73–13). There is a suppression check on the lower corner of the page with the fly. The Bernell stereo reindeer test is another common test. It

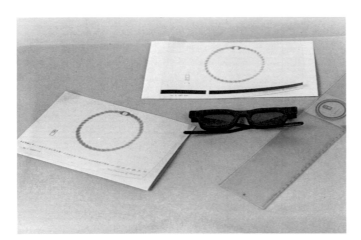

FIGURE 73–11. Many different vectograms can be hand-held or used with the Polachrome Orthopter. Usually two vectograms, one of which is viewed by the right eye and one by the left eye, are used together with one placed on top of the other. Dissimilar targets can be used to evaluate suppression.

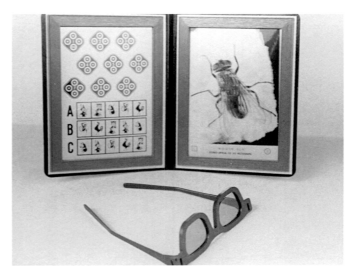

FIGURE 73–13. Stereopsis tests have a variety of targets: a large target to test for gross stereopsis and a variety of smaller targets that can measure smaller disparities. There is usually a suppression check on the lower corner of one page.

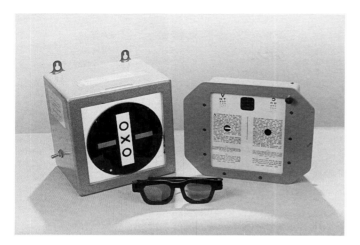

FIGURE 73–14. The Mallett near and distance unit are designed to investigate stereopsis, suppression, and binocular disorders, by using fixation disparity techniques.

also has a suppression check on both the reindeer page and the page with the six rows of circles.

Mallett Near and Distance Unit

The design of the Mallett near and distance units allows investigation of stereopsis, suppression, and binocular disorders using fixation disparity techniques. Because bright green is not easily suppressed, it was chosen as the color for the near suppression tests (Fig. 73–14), whereas the distance test uses red.

The near suppression test is designed to detect problems that the patient will have to contend with when reading or performing a similar task requiring a fine adjustment of accommodation and convergence. The test consists of a set of polarized letters with the left side seen by the left eye and the right seen by the right eye. The smallest size of the letters read indicates the size of the targets that the patient does not suppress.

The distance unit is intended to be used with fully illuminated surroundings to provide paramacular and peripheral fusion.[15] The letters target is used and the borders and the central O's form the fusion locks. The room detail surrounding the chart provides peripheral fusion.

Turville Infinity Balance

The Turville infinity balance is a far-point binocular test consisting of a 3-cm wide vertical septum placed halfway between the patient

and the Snellen chart (Fig. 73–15). Suppression can be monitored by determining which letters disappear.[16] Laterality and density of suppression can be evaluated by determining on which side the letters disappear and how small the letters must be before they disappear.

CLINICAL PROCEDURE

Bernell Stereoscope Technique

1. This type of Wheatstone stereoscope is set up in the form of a large W. The patient looks in it with their nose against the center (Fig. 73–16).
2. Targets are chosen that have different portions visible to each eye; suppression checks. The patient's responses are evaluated according to their report of which suppression check is visible under which test condition.
3. Variations can be made with lenses and different lighting on the target in front of each eye to determine how these changes affect any detected suppression.

Brewster Stereoscope Technique

1. This type of stereoscope has lenses and can be set up to test at distance or near depending on the examiner's choice. The patient looks through the lenses with their nose against the center (Fig. 73–17).
2. Targets are chosen that have different portions visible to each eye; suppression checks. The patient's responses are evaluated according to their report of which suppression check is visible under which test condition.
3. Variations can be made by using different lighting in front of each eye to determine how these changes affect any detected suppression.

Worth Dot Test Technique

The Worth dot is one of the most popular tests for diagnosing suppression. There are two models of the Worth dot test: a large type for testing at 6 m which projects a 1.25° image onto the retina and a small type for near-point testing that, when held at 33 cm, projects a 6° image onto the retina (Fig. 73–18).

1. The patient wears red and green spectacles with the red lens over the right eye and views the target at the test distance.
2. The examiner asks the patient how many dots he or she sees and what color they are.

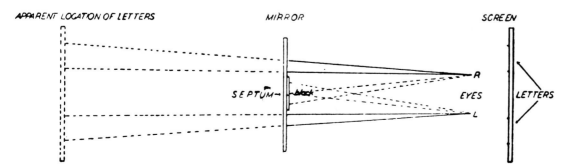

FIGURE 73–15. The Turville infinity balance is a binocular test for distance evaluation that consists of a 3-cm wide vertical septum placed halfway between the patient and the Snellen chart. (Adapted from Morgan MW. The Turville infinity binocular balance test. Am J Optom 1949;26:231–239)

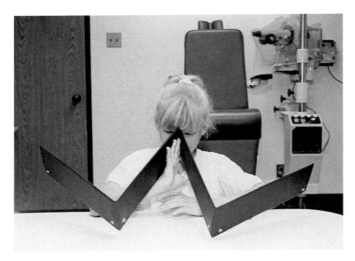

FIGURE 73–16. The Wheatstone stereoscope is set up in the form of a large W, and the patient looks in it with his or her nose against the center. Suppression checks are used (targets that have different portions visible to each eye).

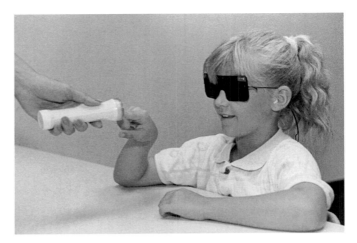

FIGURE 73–18. The Worth dot is a popular test for diagnosing suppression. There are two models of the Worth dot test; a large type for testing at 6 m, which projects a 1.25° image onto the retina, and a small type for closer testing which, when held at 33 cm, projects a 6° image onto the retina.

3. There are three responses:
   a. Four dots indicate peripheral fusion, grade I binocular vision and normal retinal correspondence when there is no angle of deviation or anomalous retinal correspondence (ARC) when there is a deviation. The white dot may alternate between red and green, because of retinal rivalry, or remain the color seen by the dominant eye.
   b. Two or three dots indicate suppression, or a cortical ignoring of visual sensations from one retina. Two dots indicate that only the eye with the red lens is being used. Three dots indicate that the eye with the green filter is being used.
   c. Five dots indicate diplopia. If the red dots are to the right of the green dots, there is uncrossed diplopia (an eso deviation). If the red dots are to the left of the green dots, there is crossed diplopia (an exo deviation).

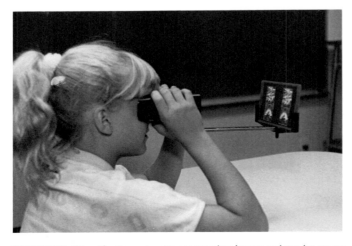

FIGURE 73–17. The Brewster stereoscope has lenses and can be set up to test at distance or near, depending on the examiner's choice. The patient looks through the lenses at targets that have suppression checks. The patient's responses are evaluated according to his or her report of which suppression check is visible under which test condition.

Red Lens Test Technique

The red lens test is useful clinically for diagnosing suppression in patients of all ages.

1. The patient wears a red lens over the right eye and views a fixation target at the test distance.
2. The examiner asks the patient how many targets he sees and what color they are.
3. There are three responses a patient can make:
   a. One "reddish" target indicates peripheral fusion, grade I binocular vision, and normal retinal correspondence when there is no angle of deviation, or ARC when there is a deviation. The reddish figure may alternate between red and white because of retinal rivalry or remain the color of the dominant eye.
   b. One red or one white figure indicates suppression, or a cortical ignoring of visual sensations from one retina, which occurs binocularly.
   c. Two lights indicate diplopia. If the red light is to the right of the white light, this represents homonymous, or uncrossed, diplopia (red lens over right eye). If the red light is to the left of the white light, this represents exotropia or crossed diplopia.

Three-Figure Test Technique

The three-figure test is very useful for diagnosing suppression in young children.

1. The patient wears red and green spectacles with the red lens over the right eye and views the target at the test distance.
2. The examiner asks the patient how many targets he sees and what color they are.
3. There are three responses a patient can make:
   a. Three targets indicate peripheral fusion, grade I binocular vision, and normal retinal correspondence when there is no angle of deviation, or ARC when there is a deviation. The white figure may alternate between red and green, because of retinal rivalry, or remains the color of the dominant eye.

b. Two figures indicate suppression, or a cortical ignoring of visual sensations from one retina, which occurs binocularly.

c. Four figures indicate diplopia. If the red figures are to the right of the green figures, this represents homonymous diplopia or esotropia (red lens over right eye). If the red figures are to the left of the green figures, there is exotropia, or heteronymous diplopia.

Keystone Basic Binocular Test Technique

The Keystone Basic Binocular Test Set consists of 12 red and green print charts on yellow background that allow first-, second-, and third-degree fusion testing.

1. The patient wears red and green filters.
2. The examiner determines through questioning if certain parts of the chart or diagram are visible. If all parts of the diagram are visible, the patient is bifixating (Fig. 73–19) or has strabismus with ARC. The unilateral cover test can be used to differentiate between the two situations, as there will be no movement on the cover test when there is bifixation. If parts of the diagram or chart are missing, the patient is suppressing. The examiner can determine which eye the patient is suppressing by figuring out what parts of the diagram are detected by the eye behind each colored filter.

Vectographic Adult Slide Technique

The vectographic adult slide has at least two areas that may be used to test suppression. These are the suppression portion of the chart and the bull's-eye target.

1. The patient views through the best refractive correction, generally in the phoropter or trial frame, and polaroid analyzers.
2. When using the suppression portion of the chart, the patient reads the letters from left to right. Begin with the 20/40 line and continue with the 20/30 line, and then the 20/25 line. A patient who is suppressing will skip some of the letters. On each line the first letter is seen by both eyes,

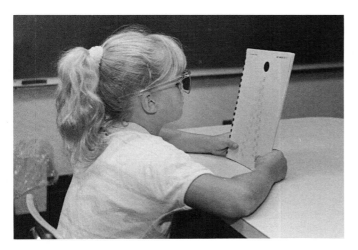

FIGURE 73–19. The Keystone Basic Binocular Test Set consists of 12 red and green print charts on white background that allow first-, second-, and third-degree fusion testing.

the second is seen by the left eye only, and the third is seen by the right eye. This pattern is repeated throughout each line. Thus, if the right eye is suppressing, the patient will not see the third and sixth letter on a line. If the bull's-eye portion of the chart is used, the central circle will be seen by both eyes. The upper vertical line and the right horizontal line will be seen by the right eye. The left eye sees the left horizon and lower vertical line.

3. To perform the test, the patient is asked to report how many lines they see and to describe the direction and end position of these lines. This chart can be used to test associated phorias as well as parafoveal suppression.

For both tests, patient cooperation and response are necessary. With the suppression chart, the patient must know letters. With the bull's-eye target, the patient must have fairly advanced verbal skills to describe what is seen. These factors may limit the usefulness of these tests. A technical problem with the distance vectographic setup is that special screens with metallic or metallic-like surfaces must be used to maintain polarization because ordinary screens break up the directionality of the light.

Pola–Mirror Technique

1. To perform the pola–mirror test the patient is instructed to put on polarizing spectacles and then look at himself or herself in a mirror that is held about 25 cm (10 in.) from his or her face.
2. The examiner then asks the patient which eye he or she can see. If one eye is blacked out, that eye is suppressing. The subject is then asked to close one eye and tell what he or she sees. This will confirm the patient's previous response, as the closed eye should be reported as appearing black.
3. The third set of instructions is to open both eyes and tell the examiner if one eye looks black.

Vis-A-Vis Test Technique

1. The vis-a-vis test requires that the subject and examiner both wear polarizing glasses.
2. Again, if the subject is suppressing, he or she will report that the examiner's eye directly in front of the suppressing eye will be blacked out. A distance of 50 cm (20 in.) should be maintained between the subject and examiner. The same questions are asked:
   a. Which of the examiner's eyes can the subject see.
   b. The subject should close one of his or her eyes and tell which of the examiner's eyes he or she sees.
3. Both the pola–mirror and the vis-a-vis can be made more sensitive for detecting central suppression if the test distance is increased.

On both the pola–mirror and vis-a-vis tests, poor illumination can lead to inaccurate results. Good illumination should be provided because the polaroid filters absorb light. If the illumination is too low, both eyes may appear too dim for valid testing. Also it is important to be very accurate in measuring and maintaining the test distance. When using the pola–mirror test the mirror is reflecting the image of the eyes and an inaccuracy in the measurement of the test distance is doubled.

The pola–mirror and the vis-a-vis are beneficial in screening for suppression in many binocular problems. Subjects who exhibit stereoacuity of 60 seconds or better generally are able to pass either of these tests,[14] which means that both eyes are seen simultaneously, no suppression.

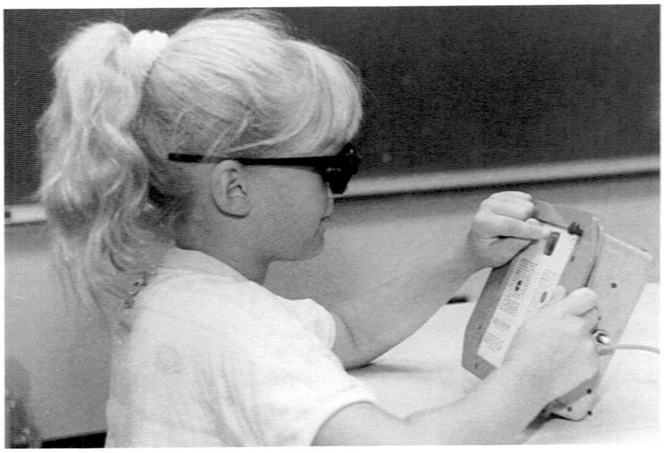

FIGURE 73–20. The Mallett unit enables the suppression of a hetero-phoric patient to be evaluated without dissociation while the patient wears the best correction. External light is often needed because the polarizers decrease the amount of light illuminating the reading target.

Mallett Unit Technique

The Mallett unit enables the suppression of a heterophoric patient to be evaluated without any form of dissociation.

1. The test is performed with the patient wearing their best correction. If an add for presbyopia is required, it should be worn during the near testing. Because the polarizers cut down on the amount of light illuminating the reading target, an external light needs to be close to ensure good results (Fig. 73–20).
2. When the polarizers are worn, the patient looks at the near suppression test target, which looks like a printed reading chart.
3. Suppression is indicated when the patient cannot see the letters on one side or the other. Because the letters subtend various sizes, the depth of suppression can be quantified and the eye that suppresses can be determined. Alternate suppression is indicated when the patient sees letters disappear on each side.

Turville Infinity Balance Test Technique

1. When using the Turville infinity balance test a septum is placed in free space at 3 m in a 6-m refracting lane. If a mirror is being used in a 3-m lane, the septum is placed directly over the mirror. Care should be taken that the right eye is seeing the right side of the chart and the left eye is seeing the left side of the chart at all times. If the septum is improperly placed (e.g., at the wrong distance) only one eye may see both sides of the chart simultaneously while the other eye is occluded.
2. The patient reports any missing lines or letters. By determining the side reported and the letter size missed, the clinician can make quantitative and qualitative determinations of suppression.

CLINICAL IMPLICATIONS

Clinical Significance

When testing for suppression, it is important to consider the conditions of the test. Generally speaking, a patient is more likely to suppress under natural conditions than when subjected to more unnatural conditions. The use of colored filters to elicit diplopia simulates moderately unnatural conditions, and indicates a greater depth of suppression than diplopia elicited in free space or using a vectographic method. Hence, the more unnatural the test required to elicit diplopia, the deeper the suppression.

The use of stereoscopes with different types of targets can give an indication of the depth or size of the suppression zone. If suppression is manifest with first-degree targets, then this indicates a deep or large area of suppression. This would be more critical than suppression seen with a second- or third-degree target. It can also be determined if the suppression seen is constant or intermittent.

One of the advantages of using these instruments is the ability to vary convergence or divergence demand, while at the same time maintaining a constant accommodative posture. This enables the clinician to isolate one aspect of the visual system and be able to measure or train it separately. This can provide a more accurate diagnosis and greater flexibility in the testing of suppression. However, the design of the instruments often means that using them for an evaluation of suppression is considered one of the more "unnatural" techniques for testing suppression. If a patient suppresses with instrument procedures, the intensity of suppression is said to be stronger than if suppression was merely noted on vectographic or septum techniques. Therefore, suppression or inability to obtain simultaneous perception with a refracting stereoscope would indicate a deep suppression and, perhaps, a decreased prognosis for a functional cure.

Children, and even some adults, may be confused by the white figure on anaglyphic tests appearing as a blend of red and green and may respond as seeing two of that figure. Thus, on the Worth dot they may report seeing five dots when they actually see four.

The Worth dot test may elicit a fusion response, from which all dots are perceived normally in the presence of macular suppression, if the suppression zone is smaller than the blank area between the four dots or when the test distance is close enough to the patient that the distance between the lights is greater than the suppression zone.

A small, central unilateral facultative scotoma can be detected by presenting the Worth dot at 6 m, then reducing the distance to 33 cm. The distance at which the suppression manifests indicates the scotoma size. For example, if the patient reports two or three dots at 6 m, then the facultative scotoma is larger than 1.25°, but if the patient reports seeing all four dots at 33 cm, then the facultative scotoma is smaller than 6°. The size can be quantified by determining at what distance the patient begins to suppress.

It is believed by some professionals that the Worth dot test is better used for heterophoria than for heterotropia because of questionable responses this test can elicit from some patients with heterotropias.

Red–green spectacles have a strong dissociating effect, which may elicit a five-dot response with the Worth dot test under the test conditions and not in everyday life. Occasionally, with the Worth dot test a heterophoric patient suppresses one eye. However, the patient can also report five dots when he or she does not have spontaneous diplopia. Thus, a patient with unstable, but functionally useful, binocular vision may elicit a suppression response.

A common cause of error during binocular testing with anaglyphs is the presence of abnormal retinal correspondence (ARC). The differential diagnosis is made with the cover test. If a patient has a strabismus and harmonious ARC, a four-dot response could be given with the Worth dot test. If the strabismus is confirmed with the cover test at the testing distance, the harmonious ARC would be confirmed.

If pseudostrabismus seems to be present in an infant, the "Worth convergence" test can be used to demonstrate single binocular vision. This is done by blinking the Worth dot flashlight on and off at a distance of 24 to 36 in. (60 mm to 90 mm) from the child while interposing a Risley rotary prism before one eye. If single binocular vision is present, a fusional convergence movement of up to 25 prism diopters may be demonstrated. Unfortunately, the infant is sometimes more interested in the Risley prism than the lights, making the test useless. This test provides only information concerning the status of peripheral binocular cooperation.

Other red green activities work in a manner similar to the foregoing. If the patient is suppressing, the examiner can determine which eye is suppressed by what the patient does not detect.

Just as for anaglyphic tests of suppression, use of polaroid lenses requires patient response and cooperation. The patient must be able to communicate to the examiner that all parts of the diagram are detected. If the patient and examiner can not communicate adequately, suppression or bifixation cannot be determined.

Clinical Interpretation

Clinical observations show conditions of strabismus and depth of suppression to be correlated in a general sense. Among these correlations are the following:

- Patients with esotropia usually have deeper suppression than patients with exotropia.
- If the strabismus is alternating, suppression is usually alternating; however, it is usually deeper in the nondominant eye.
- Depth of suppression does not correlate highly with the magnitude of the deviation.
- The more frequently the deviation is manifested, the deeper the suppression.
- Nonconcomitant strabismics may have less deep suppression than concomitant strabismics.

By isolating a specific part of the visual system at which suppression appears, it is possible to better understand when the patient is suppressing and develop a more appropriate treatment plan. By having a better understanding of the patient's suppression, a more accurate prognosis can be made.

If suppression is elicited under only very natural conditions, the suppression is of minimal depth. If a suppression is manifest under extremely unnatural conditions, a deeper suppression is present. If a patient does not elicit suppression with the vectographic slide, there may be suppression in more natural conditions, such as with Bagolini lenses. If a patient does suppress with the vectographic methods, a Worth dot test may help determine

depth, as suppression elicited on the Worth dot test reveals deeper suppression.

Measurement of the depth of suppression is useful for making judgments on the prognosis for treatment. However, other variables, such as retinal correspondence, also need to be considered. Although many clinicians believed that the deeper the suppression, the worse the prognosis, it is now known that depth of suppression is not necessarily a strong indicator of a patient's prognosis. However, information on depth of suppression is important for deciding where to begin therapy. Often antisuppression therapy may be combined with amblyopia therapy.

Methods that use polarizers provide a test environment that is very similar to the normal binocular situation. It is important to keep in mind that all the tests may not show the same depth or amount of suppression. Therefore, it can be beneficial to measure suppression with several tests.

REFERENCES

1. Wheatstone C. Contributions to the physiology of vision: part 1. On some remarkable and hitherto unobserved phenomena of binocular vision. Philos Trans 1838;128:371–394.
2. Worth C. Squint: its causes, pathology, and treatment, 5th ed. Philadelphia: P Blakiston's Son & Co. 1921:14–16.
3. Remy A. Rec Ophthalmol 1901;23:385.
4. Smith WS. Clinical orthoptic procedure, 2nd ed. St Louis: CV Mosby Co, 1954;56, 57, 65–67, 77, 81, 88.
5. Bagolini B. Diagnostic errors in the evaluation of retinal correspondence by various tests in squints. In: Arruga A, ed. International strabismus symposium. 1968:164.
6. Cuppers C. Moderne schielbehandlung. Klin Monatsbl Augenheilkd 1956;129:579–604.
7. Zellers J, Alpert T, Rouse M. A review of the literature and a normative study of accommodative infacility. J Am Optom Assoc 1984;55:31–37.
8. Duke-Elder S, Abrams D. Systems of ophthalmology, vol 4. St Louis: CV Mosby Co, 1970:700.
9. Wood CA. The American encyclopedia and dictionary of ophthalmology, vol 16. Chicago: Cleveland Press, 1920:12175.
10. Eskridge JB. Accommodation and vergence with the Brewster stereoscope. J Am Optom Assoc 1976;47:919–924.
11. Wells DW. The stereoscope in ophthalmology. Boston: EF Mahady Co, 1926.
12. Griffin JR. Binocular anomolies: procedures for vision therapy. Chicago: Professional Press, 1982:43–70.
13. Burian HM. Anomalous retinal correspondence, its essence and its significance in prognosis and treatment. Am J Ophthalmol 1951;34:237–253.
14. Griffin JR, Lee JM. The Polaroid mirror method. Optom Weekly 1970;61(40):29–30.
15. Mallett RFJ. A fixation disparity test for distance use. Optician, July 8, 1966.
16. Morgan MW. The Turville infinity binocular balance test. Am J Optom 1949;26:231–239.

Eccentric Fixation

Bruce Wick

INTRODUCTION

Definition

Eccentric fixation is a condition associated with amblyopia in which the visual axis of the amblyopic eye fails to intersect the object of regard when the other eye is occluded.[1] Clinically, eccentric fixation is associated with reduced visual acuity.[2] Eccentric fixation is found more commonly, and in larger magnitudes, in strabismic than in anisometropic amblyopia.

History

Eccentric fixation has been investigated extensively over the past 50 years. Early investigators include Worth,[3] Peckham,[4] Brock,[5] and Smith.[6] Recent investigations confirm the increased prevalence of eccentric fixation in strabismic amblyopia, especially if anomalous correspondence is also present. In addition, current research[7] suggests that spatial distortion and uncertainty may be involved in amblyopia.

Early treatment of eccentric fixation primarily involved direct occlusion. Active therapy techniques were added by Smith,[6] and these ideas were expanded and modified by Bangerter[8] and Cuppers,[9] who developed many different instruments for diagnosis and subsequent normalization of fixation patterns in patients with amblyopia. These techniques formed the basis for the pleoptic methods that were widely used in the early 1960s. However, the difficult and time-consuming nature of pleoptic techniques has led to their recent lack of use.

Clinical Use

The presence of eccentric fixation has a crucial bearing on the prognosis and the training approach that should be used during management of the amblyopic patient. Thus, it is important to test for eccentric fixation in all amblyopic patients. The clinically important characteristics of eccentric fixation include[10]

1. The location of the fixation position used and its distance from the fovea (angle of eccentric fixation)
2. The area encompassed on successive fixation attempts (fixed site versus variable site)
3. The steadiness of the response
4. Whether or not there are variations in the location of the fixation position with changes in direction of gaze

This information is useful clinically when designing therapy programs for patients with amblyopia because when eccentric fixation is unsteady, it is generally more easily treated than when it is steady. In addition, changes in perceived straight ahead also affect the considerations of therapy. When the eccentric site has gained the straight-ahead direction, more intensive therapy is generally needed for successful treatment.

INSTRUMENTATION

Theory

To determine the status of fixation, the position of the image on the retina of a fixated target needs to be known. A variety of tests may be used to evaluate eccentric fixation. Some are of value primarily when the angle of eccentric fixation is large, and some are very precise and are used for detecting and accurately quantifying small amounts of eccentric fixation. The position of the retinal image can be determined by using either objective or subjective tests.

Use

Objective testing enables the examiner to detect and quantify eccentric fixation by directly viewing the retina and noting where the shadow of a fixation target is located relative to the fovea. This can be done without depending upon patient responses. The usual objective testing technique involves use of calibrated ophthalmoscopes. Other objective techniques include comparison of angle lambda measurements between the two eyes or comparisons of measurements of the location of the blind spots.

Subjective testing requires patient responses for the examiner to detect and quantify eccentric fixation. This can pose problems with interpretation of the responses if the patient is uncooperative or too young to give accurate responses. Usual subjective testing techniques include Haidinger's brushes and afterimage transfer testing.

COMMERCIALLY AVAILABLE INSTRUMENTS

Basic Design

Objective Testing

CALIBRATED OPHTHALMOSCOPES. Calibrated ophthalmoscopes allow direct visualization of the fovea and measurement of its location relative to the image of a fixation target viewed by the amblyopic eye. Ophthalmoscopes can be used for testing fixation stability and direction by inclusion of a small opaque fixation target. The target pattern seen by the patient in the light-transmitting aperture serves as a fixation target and casts a shadow of its form onto the fundus. The size of the shadow is calibrated for the particular ophthalmoscope used. This test, originally devised by Cuppers,[12] allows the examiner to detect and quantify eccentric fixation by noting where the shadow of the fixation target is located relative to the fovea.

When using a calibrated ophthalmoscope, measurement of the magnitude of eccentric fixation can be made to within 0.5 prism diopter with concurrent assessment of steadiness and direction. Problems can arise when the foveal reflex is not well formed and, thus, is not easily visible. Poor patient cooperation or photophobia can also make the test difficult.

The Proper ophthalmoscope has a fixation target that can be used to evaluate fixation characteristics. The target has a central ring with a diameter of 1 prism diopter (Fig. 74–1). Each successive ring of the fixation target has an additional 1-prism diopter increase in diameter. By determining where the patient fixates relative to the position of the fovea, the examiner can determine the magnitude and direction of any existing eccentric fixation. Other ophthalmoscopes (e.g., Keeler Projectoscope) are calibrated in a similar manner.

When a calibrated ophthalmoscope is not available, some ophthalmoscopes with suitable optical systems can be adapted by placing a small opaque dot in the center of the green auxiliary filter.[13] Another technique for adapting an ophthalmoscope, especially one with a bright light source, is to reduce the aperture size of the instrument to produce a narrow beam or slit of light. This will furnish a small fixation target, as well as a narrow light area on the fundus. When the patient fixates the small circle of light, its

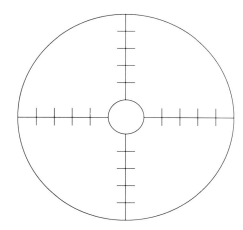

FIGURE 74–1. The fixation target in the Propper ophthalmoscope has a central ring with a diameter of 1 prism diopter. Each successive ring of the fixation target has an additional 1-prism diopter increase in diameter. By determining where the patient fixates relative to the position of the fovea, the examiner can determine the magnitude and direction of any existing eccentric fixation.

location on the fundus relative to the fovea will indicate if eccentric fixation is present. Unfortunately, it is often difficult to be certain of the magnitude with this technique.

ANGLE LAMBDA. Angle lambda testing for eccentric fixation involves comparison of the angle lambda measurements of the two eyes. *Angle lambda* (often clinically called angle kappa) is the angle between the pupillary axis (the line perpendicular to the cornea that passes through the center of the entrance pupil) and the visual axis subtended at the nodal point.[14]

When the patient fixates a light source positioned directly below the examiner's eye, the corneal light reflex is typically seen slightly nasal to the center of the image of the pupil formed by refraction through the cornea (the center of the entrance pupil). The corneal light reflex is normally displaced nasally because the fovea is located slightly temporalward from the optic axis of the eye. Thus, during fixation the pupillary axis is rotated slightly temporally because the visual axis is directed to the fixation target. This causes the corneal light reflex to be positioned approximately 0.5 mm on the nasal side of the center of the entrance pupil (Fig. 74–2). Angle lambda is designated plus when the light reflex is positioned nasally and minus when it is positioned temporally.[15]

When each eye has normal central fixation and the eyes are symmetric, the angle measured in one eye is equal in sign and magnitude to the angle measured in the other eye. If fixation in one eye is grossly eccentric, a significant difference between the

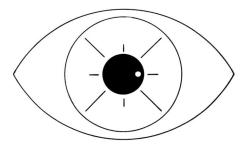

FIGURE 74–2. When the patient fixates a light source positioned below the examiner's eye, the corneal light reflex is seen displaced nasal to the center of the cornea.

two angles will be found. Thus, any difference between the angles lambda of the two eyes should be taken as presumptive evidence of eccentric fixation. This test is particularly useful for young children, who may not respond accurately otherwise. Any available penlight, or other technique for measurement, that illuminates both eyes can be used.

No matter which technique is used to measure angle lambda, this method is relatively inexact, and the results should be confirmed with more precise techniques for a positive diagnosis. Failure to detect a difference in the location of the corneal reflexes between the two eyes indicates that central fixation is present or that an eccentric fixation with an angle smaller than can be detected by this method is present. This may easily occur since a 2.5° angle of eccentric fixation results in only about a 0.12-mm difference in the locations of the corneal reflexes.

BLIND SPOT TESTING. Blind spot testing for eccentric fixation, as originally proposed by Peckham,[4] involves plotting the physiologic blind spot of each eye and then noting where the center of each blind spot is located relative to the point of fixation. Because the structure of each eye is usually symmetric, unequal displacement of the blind spots is presumptive evidence of eccentric fixation.

Obviously, the blind spot test is relatively insensitive, because plotting the boundary of the blind spot is subject to several errors. Among these are faulty patient responses, fixation inaccuracy, and examiner inaccuracy in making plot marks. Another possible source of error is the assumption that the two eyes are anatomically symmetric. When the eyes are not symmetric, this test is nearly uninterpretable, because unequal displacements of the blind spots will not necessarily indicate eccentric fixation, and there is no convenient clinical method to determine exactly where the blind spot should be. This can be a clinically important problem when a high unilateral refractive error exists.

Any available technique for measurement of visual fields can be used. These can range from a tangent screen to a fully automated visual fields device.

Subjective Testing

HAIDINGER'S BRUSHES. Haidinger's brushes are an entoptically perceived pattern of closely packed radiating lines emanating from opposite sides of a common central point.[16] They form a shape similar to an airplane propeller or bow tie (Fig. 74–3). The phenomenon of Haidinger's brushes is elicited by viewing a homogeneous field of polarized blue light, and the meridional orientation of the brushes corresponds to the axis of polarization. The entoptically perceived, brushlike, pattern is derived from the macular area with the center of the pattern corresponding to the center of the fovea.

Because the phenomenon is dependent upon the anatomical macular structure, it has been presumed that the anatomical constituents (especially the retinal receptors and fiber layer of Henle) must be normal in structure and arrangement or Haidinger's brushes will not be observed.[17] Thus, eccentric fixation and the anatomical integrity of the macular area are theoretically investigated by the use of the phenomenon.

The Haidinger brush phenomenon does not stand out boldly from the background and careful attention is sometimes necessary for the effect to be appreciated. As a result, some patients may fail to understand what they should see or may be unable to detect the brush effect. To reduce this problem, the test can initially be conducted on the normal eye. Unfortunately, this sometimes increases the number of false responses because the patient reports that the brushes are rotating about the fixation point (as was observed with the normal eye), when the brushes are really perceived elsewhere or are not perceived at all. This is especially true when testing a young patient.

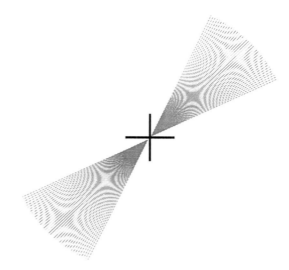

FIGURE 74–3. Haidinger's brushes, an entoptically perceived pattern of closely packed radiating lines, emanating from opposite sides of a common central point, form a shape similar to an airplane propeller or bow tie. The pattern is derived from the macular area with the center of the pattern corresponding to the center of the fovea.

An additional problem, which may occur when an existing eccentric fixation is fairly large, is that the brushes are so far away from the fixation target that they are not perceived. Inability to perceive the brushes, under these conditions, can confuse the diagnosis. The examiner cannot tell for certain if the failure to see the brushes is the result of poor observation, or if the brushes are truly absent due to an anomalous macula.

MACULA INTEGRITY TESTER–TRAINER. The most commonly used instrument for testing (or treating) eccentric fixation using Haidinger's brushes if the Macula Integrity Tester–Trainer. It is a table-mounted instrument designed for testing at a near distance and has a transilluminated motor-driven rotating polaroid filter that is viewed through a deep-blue filter (Fig. 74–4). The target plane is adjacent to, but slightly closer to, the eye than the polaroid

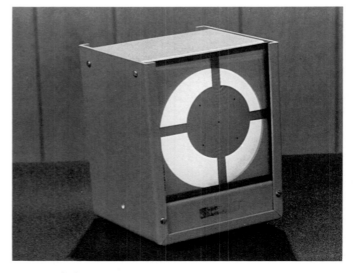

FIGURE 74–4. The Macula Integrity Tester–Trainer is a table-mounted instrument designed for near testing. It has a transilluminated motor-driven rotating Polaroid filter that is viewed through a deep-blue filter.

filter. The brushes appear as a dark blue pattern rotating against a lighter blue background.

SPACE COORDINATOR. Another instrument that produces the Haidinger's brush effect and may be adapted for testing, is the Space Coordinator. The brushes in the Space Coordinator are produced by a rotating polaroid filter closer to the eye than the target plane. Brushes are then subsequently projected in space to a more distant target plane.

COORDINATOR. An instrument similar to the Macula Integrity Tester–Trainer is the Coordinator. The Coordinator is also a table-mounted instrument designed for testing at a near distance, with a motor-driven rotating transilluminated polaroid filter that is viewed through a deep blue filter.

AFTERIMAGE TRANSFER TEST. The afterimage transfer test is based on the normally corresponding relationship of the foveae.[18] In patients with normal correspondence, stimulation of the central foveal areas of the two eyes gives rise to the same visual direction. Thus, an image falling on one fovea will be directionalized to the same spatial location as an image falling on the other fovea. The test is not useful when the patient suppresses the transferred afterimage.

Central fixation is indicated if the transferred afterimage from a target placed on the fovea of one eye appears centered on the fixation target viewed by the other eye. When eccentric fixation is present, the transferred afterimage will be projected off of the fixation target by an angular amount equal to the eccentric fixation (Fig. 74–5).

For example, if a left (nonamblyopic) eye was presented the after-image light, and then the transferred afterimage is perceived to be located 1.5 cm to the left of a fixation target viewed at 1 m by the amblyopic right eye, the diagnosis would be nasal eccentric fixation of the right eye with a magnitude of 1.5 prism diopters (the eccentric site used is nasal to the fovea, since the afterimage appeared to the left of the fixation target).

An erroneous diagnosis can be reached when the patient has anomalous correspondence[19] because, when a patient has anoma-

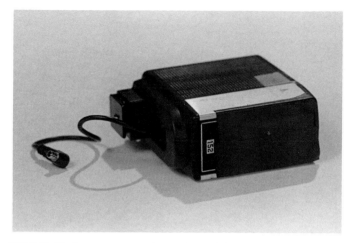

FIGURE 74–6. A camera strobe can be modified to present a line to the fixing eye so that an afterimage can be generated on the fovea of the normally fixing eye. The location of afterimage transferred to the amblyopic eye is evaluated.

lous correspondence, the foveas of the two eyes do not give rise to a common visual direction. Therefore, a perceived separation of the transferred afterimage and the fixation target would occur because of the anomalous correspondence and would confuse the detection and measurement of any existing eccentric fixation.

Any bright light source will generate an afterimage if it is fixated long enough. A light bulb, or best of all, a camera strobe, can be modified to represent a line to the fixing eye. The patient can then be "flashed" to generate an afterimage on the fovea of the normally fixing eye, and the location of afterimage transferred to the amblyopic eye can be evaluated (Fig. 74–6).

CLINICAL PROCEDURE

Objective Testing

Calibrated Ophthalmoscopes

Most foveae present a foveal reflex, a pinpoint reflex of light from the foveal center observed during ophthalmoscopy. This reflex serves as the reference point.

TECHNIQUE

1. The patient is seated comfortably in a darkened room.
2. The eye not being examined is occluded to be certain that the test is monocular. The patient is shown the ophthalmoscopic target and asked to look directly at the center of the target when it is projected in the patient's eye.
3. The examiner performs ophthalmoscopy (Fig. 74–7) with a calibrated ophthalmoscope and observes the location of the foveal reflex relative to the fixation target projected into the eye by the ophthalmoscope (Fig. 74–8).

When there is normal steady central fixation, the shadow of the fixation target surrounds or covers the fovea and is seen centered in the deeper red macular region. When eccentric fixation is present, the shadow is seen either to the side of the foveal reflex or, if no reflex can be seen, is not centered in the macular area (see Fig. 74–8). A green filter can be used in conjunction with the fixation target to facilitate observation and reduce glare. The angle of eccentric fixation is determined by the distance of the fixation target features from the foveal center. All the examiner needs to know is the distance subtended by the vari-

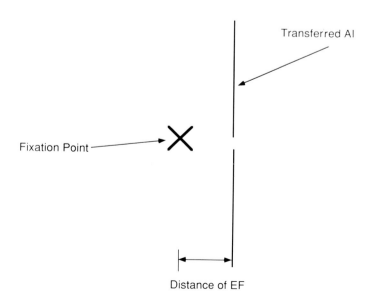

FIGURE 74–5. Central fixation is indicated when a transferred afterimage (AI) from a target placed on the fovea of one eye appears centered on the fixation target viewed by the other eye. If there is eccentric fixation (EF), the transferred afterimage will be projected off of the fixation target by an angular amount equal to the eccentric fixation.

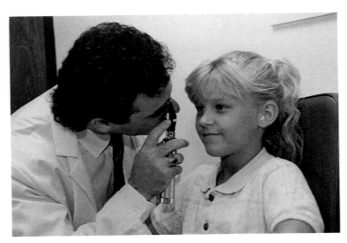

FIGURE 74–7. The examiner performs ophthalmoscopy using a calibrated ophthalmoscope and observes the location of the foveal reflex relative to the fixation target projected into the eye by the ophthalmoscope.

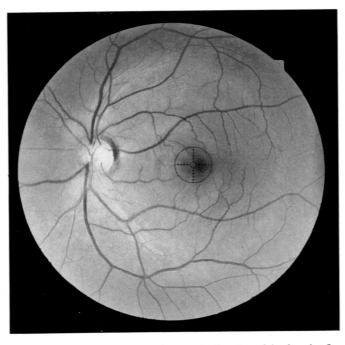

FIGURE 74–8. The examiner observes the location of the foveal reflex relative to the fixation target projected into the eye by the ophthalmoscope. Most foveae present a foveal reflex, a pinpoint reflex of light from the foveal center observed during ophthalmoscopy, which serves as the reference point.

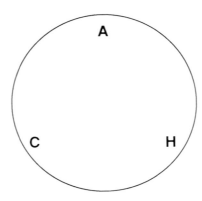

FIGURE 74–9. With some calibrated ophthalmoscopes, variations on the standard test are possible because several letters can be included as auxiliary fixation targets. Multiple fixation targets can be useful because fixation ability can be observed as fixation is directed from one letter to another.

ous target landmarks. If this is unknown, it can easily be determined by focusing the projected target on a wall at 1 m and measuring the distance in centimeters that the target features subtend. At this distance, 1 cm of target size equals 1 prism diopter.

The test should be repeated several times and in various directions of gaze. This enables the examiner to ascertain whether the same retinal location is used consistently, and if the direction of gaze influences the fixation location. The patient should be asked whether he or she feels his or her eye is aimed directly at the fixation target so that the examiner can determine whether the straight-ahead direction is subjectively associated with the eccentric site.

Each eye should be checked to compare fixation responses, even if one eye has normal vision. Evaluation of a possible central scotoma may be made by positioning a portion of the fixation target on the foveal center to determine if it disappears or becomes fainter. The test is one of the best available for investigation of eccentric fixation, because direct observation of the retinal site used for fixation is possible, and steadiness of fixation and changes in the location with different directions of gaze are easily observed.

With some calibrated ophthalmoscopes variations on the standard test are possible because several letters can be included as auxiliary fixation targets (Fig. 74–9). The presentation of multiple fixation targets can be useful because fixation ability can be observed as fixation is directed from one letter to another.

Angle Lambda

PENLIGHT TECHNIQUE

1. The patient is comfortably seated in a darkened room.
2. A penlight is held approximately 50 cm from the patient in front of the fixating eye, while the other eye is occluded.
3. The examiner sights monocularly over the penlight and determines, by estimation or measurement, the vertical and lateral displacement (in millimeters) of the corneal reflex from the center of the pupil (Fig. 74–10).
4. The procedure is repeated for the other eye and the two estimates or measurements are compared, to determine whether a significant difference exists. A difference of more than 0.12 mm implies significant eccentric fixation.

Blind Spot Technique

TECHNIQUE

1. The blind spot of each eye is plotted for each eye using the technique listed in Chapters 28 and 49.
2. The location of each blind spot is compared relative to the fixation target. Unequal displacement is presumptive evidence of eccentric fixation of the amblyopic eye.

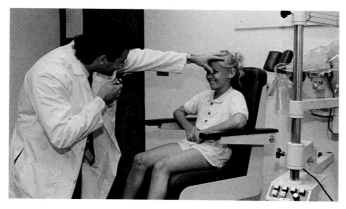

FIGURE 74–10. The examiner sights monocularly over the penlight and determines, by estimation or measurement, the vertical and lateral displacement (in millimeters) of the corneal reflex from the center of the entrance pupil. The procedure is repeated for the other eye and the two estimates or measurements are compared.

Subjective Testing

Haidinger Brushes

TECHNIQUE

1. The patient is comfortably seated in a darkened room in front of a Haidinger brush apparatus (e.g., Macular Integrity Tester–Trainer).
2. The patient wears blue filters, or a blue filter is placed in the Haidinger brush apparatus, and the unit is turned on.
3. Viewing is done monocularly with the best lens correction worn; first with the normal eye and then with the amblyopic eye (Fig. 74–11). The test is generally done using fixation distances between 40 cm and 1 m, depending on the patient and their fixation characteristics. When the test is done at 1 m, the distance in centimeters that the fixation target is seen from the rotating brushes indicates the

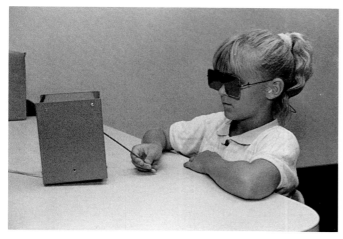

FIGURE 74–11. When evaluating with Haidinger's brushes, viewing is monocular with the best lens correction worn—first with the normal eye and then with the amblyopic eye. The test is generally done using a 1-m fixation distance because when the test is done at 1 m, the distance in centimeters that the fixation target is seen from the rotating brushes indicates the amount of eccentric fixation in prism diopters.

amount of eccentric fixation in prism diopters (pd). At closer distances, the amount of eccentric fixation is calculated from the formula

Test distance (m) × eccentricity of brushes (cm)
= eccentric fixation (pd)

4. The direction of rotation of the polaroid filter may be reversed in some instruments or the direction of rotation of the brushes may be reversed using a "quarter wave" plate. Either of these causes the brushes to appear to spin in the opposite direction. This reversal provides a means of verifying the patient's responses.

Examination of the influence of direction of gaze on the fixation response can be done by having the patient turn his or her head to the side or up or down while fixating the target such that peripheral gaze is used to view the target.

Afterimage Transfer

TECHNIQUE

1. The patient views a bright light or camera strobe with the normally fixing eye while the other is held tightly closed (Fig. 74–12A).
2. The afterimage light is constructed so that there is a fixation gap where the patient maintains fixation. With this technique, when the light has been viewed long enough, a vertical afterimage is created that brackets the fovea of the normally fixing eye.
3. Following creation of the afterimage, the stimulated eye fixates a fixation mark on a scale calibrated for the distance of fixation while the amblyopic eye remains occluded (see Fig 74–12B). As long as the same retinal area is used for the fixation of the light source and the fixation mark, the afterimage should be seen at the fixation mark. This part of the procedure enables the examiner to determine the patient's understanding of the afterimage effect and its projected localization with reference to the fixation target.
4. After the examiner is certain that the patient understands the task, the nonamblyopic eye is again stimulated to reinforce the afterimage.
5. Occlusion is then shifted to the nonamblyopic eye and the amblyopic eye is used to fixate the fixation mark. Blinking the eyelids or flashing the room lights will assist in maintaining the afterimage effect. The patient's task is to identify the location of the afterimage, transferred from the now occluded nonamblyopic eye, as he fixates the central target on the scale with the amblyopic eye. When fixation is centric, the transferred afterimage will be observed on the fixation target. When fixation is eccentric the transferred afterimage will appear to be displaced from the fixation target. The amount of displacement is a measurement of the amount of eccentric fixation.

CLINICAL IMPLICATIONS

Clinical Significance

The clinical value of determining fixation patterns in amblyopia cannot be overestimated. Patients who have eccentric fixation often have visual acuity reductions that are in direct correlation with their fixation patterns. If all or most of the reduced acuity that exists in amblyopia can be shown to be related to the fixation pattern, then a marked improvement in acuity can be expected with training, which causes fixation to become more central.

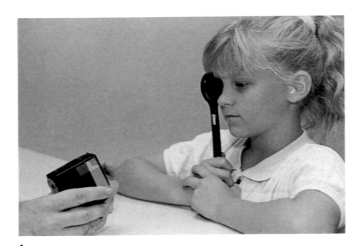

A

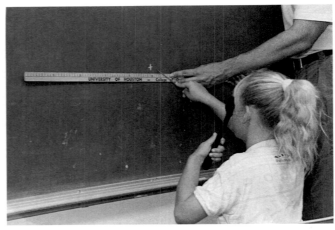

B

FIGURE 74–12. (*A*) The patient views the camera strobe with the normally fixing eye while the other is held tightly closed. A vertical afterimage is then created that brackets the fovea of the normally fixing eye. (*B*) Following creation of the afterimage, the stimulated eye fixates a fixation mark on a scale calibrated for the distance of fixation while the amblyopic eye remains occluded. As long as the same retinal area is used for the fixation of the light source and the fixation mark, the afterimage should be seen at the fixation mark.

Relation of Acuity to Eccentric Fixation

As a rule-of-thumb, fixation relates to visual acuity by the formula

$$MAR = EF + 1.$$

This means that if there is 2 prism diopters of eccentric fixation the minimum angle of resolution (MAR; visual acuity) would be expected to be about 3 minutes of arc or about 20/60 acuity.[20] Thus, if an amblyopic patient with 20/60 acuity has a 2 prism diopters of eccentric fixation, a marked improvement in acuity can be expected when fixation becomes central. However, another patient with 2 prism diopters of eccentric fixation who has visual acuity of 20/200 would not be expected to have as marked an acuity improvement with simple restoration of central fixation. Table 74–1 indicates the approximate maximum expected visual acuity for various amounts of eccentric fixation. These are only approximate because other factors, such as very unsteady fixation, can reduce the acuity found during clinical testing.

Clinical Interpretation

Most amblyopia is caused by either strabismus, anisometropia, or both. Patients who have anisometropic amblyopia with peripheral

Table 74–1
Approximate Visual Acuity for Various Amounts of Eccentric Fixation

Eccentric Fixation (prism diopters)	Expected Acuity (approximate best)
0.5	20/30
1.0	20/40
2.0	20/60
3.0	20/80
4.0	20/100
>5.0	<20/100

fusion often have unsteady central fixation and respond on many tests as if they were simply blurred,[21] whereas patients with strabismic or strabismic–anisometropic amblyopia more often have eccentric fixation associated with significant abnormalities in space perception or direction sense.[7]

During the Haidinger brush test, when eccentric fixation is indicated by localization of the perceived brushes to the side of a target that is straight ahead of the patient, the examiner can determine if the oculocentric straight ahead is associated with the eccentric area by inquiring whether the patient feels that the eye is aimed directly at, or to the side of, the fixation target. Egocentric direction (perceived direction in space of an object or image subjectively evaluated in reference to self) may be determined by inquiring if it is felt that the fixated target is located directly in front of the fixating eye. Anomalous spatial localization indicates a motor–perceptual mismatch and the possibility that incorrect motor information is being received concerning the position of the fixating eye.

Several responses are possible depending upon the retinal site possessing oculocentric (straight-ahead) direction and the retinal site possessing retinomotor zero. The patient may report that the eye is directed straight to the target that appears to be directly in front of the eye; indicating that the zero retinomotor value and the straight-ahead direction are still associated with the retinal site used for fixation. The patient may report that the eye is directed to the side of the target, but the target appears to be directly in front of the eye; indicating that the zero retinomotor value and the straight-ahead direction are still associated with the foveal center. The patient may report that the eye is directed straight to the target, but the target is not situated directly in front of the eye; indicating that incorrect motor information has been received concerning the position of the eye on fixation or that the straight-ahead direction has shifted from the fovea to the eccentric retinal site, but the zero retinomotor value has not.

The patient's response on Haidinger brush testing is verified by having them rapidly move a pointer, positioned in front of the fixating eye, to touch the fixation target as they maintain fixation on the target (Fig. 74–13). With anomalous localization, the pointer tip is moved directly to the target, although the brushes (indicating the foveal location) are observed to the side. With normal localization, the pointer tip will miss the target and be positioned in the

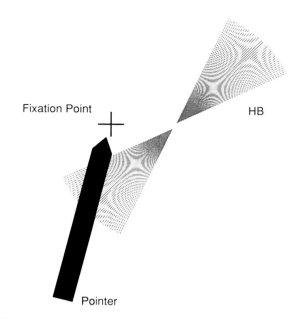

Fixation Point

HB

Pointer

FIGURE 74–13. The patient's response on Haidinger brush testing is verified by having him or her rapidly move a pointer, positioned in front of the fixating eye, to touch the fixation target as fixation is maintained on the target.

direction of the foveal projection, or corrective motions will be made in an attempt to place the pointer tip on the target. When corrective movements are made, the patient will often report that the brushes move toward or onto the fixation target. The procedure should be repeated several times to test the consistency of the response and minimize the influence of motor control of the pointer.

When an amblyopic eye, particularly one with strabismic amblyopia, attempts to monocularly fixate a stationary target, an unsteadiness is frequently demonstrated. This unsteadiness ranges from a mild exaggeration of normal micromovements to a readily observed searching nystagmoid movement. The degree of fixation unsteadiness generally varies with the type of fixation (eccentric or centric), the location of the site used for fixation, and the reduction in acuity. Unsteadiness is typically more marked when fixation is eccentric, the site used for fixation is variable, and visual acuity is

greatly reduced. Thus, steadiness of fixation should be determined during diagnosis by carefully observing the amblyopic eye as it attempts monocular fixation. These observations can and should be made while conducting monocular fixation assessment as well as other tests.

REFERENCES

1. Cline D, Hofstetter HW, Griffin JR. Dictionary of visual science. Radnor, Pa: Chilton Book Co. 1980:244.
2. Harada H, Hayashi S. Differential diagnosis of amblyopia. Jp J Ophthalmol 1958;2:268–273.
3. Worth C. Squint, its causes, pathology, and treatment, 5th ed. Philadelphia: P Blakiston's Sons & Co, 1921.
4. Peckham RM. Amblyopia, clinical research report no 2, 4th ed. Detroit: Optometric Research Institute, 1941.
5. Brock FW. Investigation of the fovea centralis in amblyopia. Am J Ophthalmol 1962;54:821–827.
6. Smith WS. Clinical orthoptic procedure, 2nd ed. St Louis: CV Mosby Co, 1954.
7. Flom MC, Bedell HE, Barbeito R. Spatial uncertainty and acuity in anisometropic amblyopia. Invest Ophthalmol Vis Sci 1984;26(suppl):80.
8. Bangerter A. Amblyopiebehandlung, 2nd ed. Basel: S Karger, 1955.
9. Cuppers C. Orthoptic and pleoptic problems in Germany, lecture before the North of England Ophthalmological Society, June 12 and 13, 1958. Printed by W Foster & Sons, Ltd.
10. von Norden GK. Pathogenesis of eccentric fixation. Am J Ophthalmol 1966;61:399–422.
11. Flom MC, Wick B, Cotter SA. Eccentric fixation in each eye: a documented case and underlying explanation [abstr, poster no 18]. Am Acad Optom Meeting, 1982.
12. Schapero M. Amblyopia. Radnor, Pa: Chilton Book Co, 1971:134.
13. Tsujimoto EY, Calorosso E. Visual field screening with an ophthalmoscope. Am J Optom Am Acad Optom 1970;47:496–498.
14. Cline D, Hofstetter HW, Griffin JR. Dictionary of visual science. Radnor, Pa: Chilton Book Co, 1980:30.
15. Borish I. Clinical refraction. Chicago: Professional Press 1970.
16. Hallden U. An explanation of Haidinger's brushes. Arch Ophthalmol 1957;57:393–399.
17. Gording EJ. A report on Haidinger's brushes. Am J Optom Arch Am Acad Optom 1950;27:604–610.
18. Brock FW, Givner I. Fixation anomalies in amblyopia. Arch Ophthalmol 1952;47:775–786.
19. Wick B. Anomalous afterimage transfer, an analysis and suggested method of elimination. Am J Optom Physiol Opt 1974;51:862–871.
20. Flom MC, Weymouth FC. Centricity of Maxwel's spot in strabismus and amblyopia. Arch Opthalmol 1961;66:260–268.
21. Barbeito R, Bedell HE, Flom MC, Simpson TL. Effects of luminance on the visual acuity of strabismic and anisometropic amblyopes and optically blurred normals. Vis Res 1987;27:1543–1549.

CHAPTER

75

Fixation Disparity

David A. Goss

INTRODUCTION

Definitions

Fixation disparity is the condition in which the images of a binocularly fixated object are not imaged on exactly corresponding retinal points but are still within Panum's fusional areas.[1] Therefore, a fixation disparity may be present when a patient has single binocular vision. If the lines of sight intersect closer to the patient than the object of regard, an *eso fixation disparity* exists. If they intersect farther away from the patient, an *exo fixation disparity* exists.

An *associated phoria* is the amount of prism required to reduce fixation disparity to zero.[1] The associated phoria should be distinguished from the dissociated phoria, in which binocular fusion is disrupted.

A *fixation disparity curve* is an *x, y* coordinate plot of the angular amount of the fixation disparity in minutes of arc as a function of the amount of prism through which the patient views.[2–10] Fixation disparity is plotted on the ordinate with eso above the *x*-axis and exo below it. Prism is plotted on the abscissa with base-in to the left of the *y*-axis and base-out to the right of it. An example of a fixation disparity curve (FDC) and its parameters is given in Figure 75–1. The primary parameters of a FDC are curve type, slope, *y*-intercept, and *x*-intercept or associated phoria, and the center of symmetry (Table 75–1). In the commonly used classification system of Ogle et al., FDCs are categorized as types I, II, III, or IV, as shown in Figure 75–2.[3] A *type I* FDC has vertically ascending and descending segments that asymptote on the base-in and base-out sides and a relatively flat central portion. A *type II* curve is flat on the base-out side and ascends on the base-in side. A *type III* curve is flat on the base-in side and descends on the base-out side. A *type IV* FDC is flat on the base-in (BI) and base-out (BO) sides and has a higher slope in its central portion. The slope of an

FDC is expressed in minutes of arc per prism diopter. It is usually determined using points at 3^ΔBI, 0^Δ, and 3^ΔBO. The *y-intercept* is the amount of fixation disparity with no prism in place. The *x-intercept* is the associated phoria, the amount of prism power that reduces fixation disparity to zero. The *center of symmetry* is the flattest central portion of the curve.

History

Apparently the first description of fixation disparity was made by Hofmann and Bielshowsky in 1900.[3] They called it "residual disparity." In 1928, Ames and Glidden reported that fixation disparity was correlated with (dissociated) heterophoria.[3] They referred to fixation disparity as "retinal slip," a term popularly used for many years. The term "fixation disparity" appears to have originated with Ogle and his colleagues.[2,11]

Clinical Use

One source of eyestrain or asthenopia is oculomotor imbalance or, more specifically, strain on fusional vergence. Traditionally, this has been assessed by measurement of the amount of fusional vergence required for single vision (the dissociated phoria) and of the fusional vergence ranges (negative relative convergence and positive relative convergence).[9,12–14] Fixation disparity and associated phorias are measured under conditions of binocular vision, and are thought to be related to the strain on fusional vergence.[2,4,5] In fact, a fixation disparity curve itself demonstrates that the amount of fixation disparity is dependent upon the amount of fusional vergence required for single vision. Several studies have shown weak correlation of dissociated phorias with fixation dis-

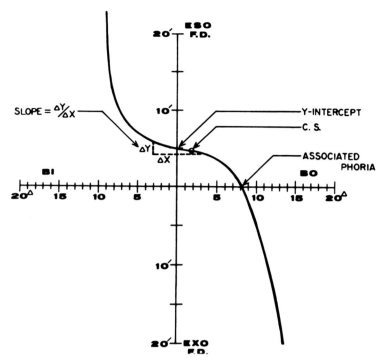

FIGURE 75–1. Example of a fixation disparity curve with the major parameters labeled.

parity and associated phorias.[3,15,16] Fixation disparity is also related to prism adaptation, a high level of which is associated with lack of ocular symptoms.[5,17–19]

Sheedy and Saladin performed two studies of the relationship between asthenopia and various diagnostic criteria for horizontal imbalances.[20,21] They confirmed the validity of traditional measures such as Sheard's criterion, Percival's criterion, and the amount of the dissociated phoria. They found that fixation disparity curve parameters were also valid predictors of the presence of ocular symptoms. Studies by Eskridge and Rutstein have shown vertical-associated phorias to be a useful method for the prescription of vertical prism.[22,23] These studies and the collective experience of a number of clinicians have shown its usefulness in the diagnosis of motor anomalies of binocular vision.[9,24–26]

INSTRUMENTATION

Theory

Test targets for fixation disparity or associated phoria contain an area that is binocularly fixated and an area in which binocular vision is excluded. The latter area contains marks for patient judg-

Table 75–1
Parameters of Fixation Disparity Curves

Curve type
Slope
y-Intercept
x-Intercept (associated phoria)
Center of symmetry

ment of alignment. Commercially produced instruments use polarization to make some of these marks seen only by the right eye and some seen only by the left eye. Some targets, like that one illustrated in Figure 75–3, allow only a measurement of the associated phoria. Prism is added until the patient reports that the marks are perfectly aligned. A target such as that in Figure 75–4 could be used for a measurement of fixation disparity. The patient identifies the upper line to which the arrow is pointing. The angular separation on the test target of the arrow and that line is the amount of the fixation disparity.

Fixation disparity measurements are influenced by several target design and testing variables. The amount of fixation disparity and the slope of the curve decrease as the size of the area in which binocular vision is excluded is decreased.[3,11,27,28] It has been proposed that this occurs primarily in symptomatic persons.[29] Variability of fixation disparity measurements decreases with the addition of a central fusion lock.[30,31] An increase in the prism power through which a patient views will change fixation disparity owing to the change in fusional vergence effort. Base-in prism stimulates negative fusional convergence and results in a shift toward eso fixation disparity. Base-out prism induces positive fusional convergence, and fixation disparity shifts in the exo direction. Since prism adaptation reduces fusional vergence effort and fixation disparity, an increase in the time the patient is allowed to view through the prism will decrease the amount of fixation disparity.[5,27,28] In patients with greater prism adaptation, curve slope and amount of fixation disparity are less.[32,33] Spherical lens adds that are over the correction for refractive error change the relative amounts of accommodative convergence and fusional vergence, resulting in a change in fixation disparity.[3,11,34] Plus lenses decrease accommodative convergence, thereby either increasing positive fusional vergence or decreasing negative fusional vergence, causing a shift toward exo fixation disparity. Minus lenses increase accommodative convergence, and either decrease positive fusional vergence or increase negative fusional vergence, thus leading to a shift in fixation disparity in the eso direction.

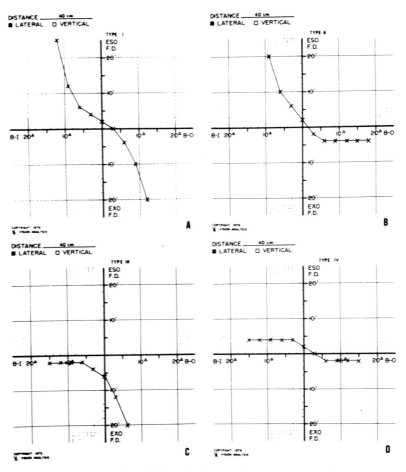

FIGURE 75–2. Examples of Ogle's four fixation disparity curve types.

Ogle reported that fixation disparity curves were repeatable with some variability associated with fatigue, prior use of the eyes, and with interest level.[2] Cooper et al. found fixation disparity to be repeatable over a 10-week period, with an increase in variability at prism powers approaching the limits of fusional vergence.[35] Over a 5-month time span, Daum found the curve type to be repeatable, with less variability on the base-in side than on the base-out side, and some change in the *y*-intercept over time.[36]

Use

Current clinical methods for fixation disparity measurement are all subjective. That is, they require a response from the patient. Laboratory studies have generally found subjective measurements of fixation disparity to be less than objectively measured binocular fixation misalignment.[37–39] The meaning of this fact is presently unknown. Therefore, in the interest of simplification, the following description of the use of subjective vernier alignment for fixation disparity will be based on the assumption that subjective measures will be the same as the physical misalignment of the eyes.

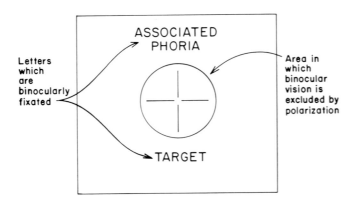

FIGURE 75–3. Illustration of a target for measurement of associated phorias. Typically the upper and right-hand lines are seen by the right eye, lower and left are seen by the left eye.

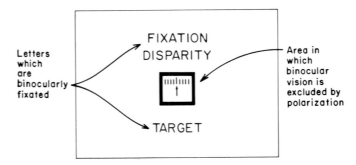

FIGURE 75–4. Illustration of a target for measurement of lateral fixation disparity. Typically the upper lines are seen by the right eye and the lower mark by the left eye.

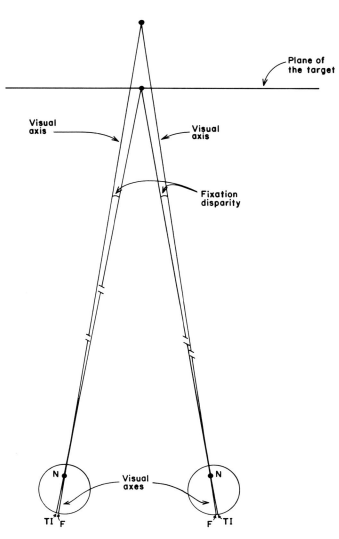

FIGURE 75–5. Illustration of exo fixation disparity. The visual axes cross behind the plane of the target. Legend: N, nodal point; F, fovea; TI, retinal image of the target. See text for further explanation.

Figure 75–5 is an illustration of exo fixation disparity. The visual axes cross behind the plane of the target. The amount of fixation disparity is the sum of the right eye and left eye angles between the visual axes and the line from the target feature used for alignment to the respective nodal points (see Fig. 75–5). For an associated phoria target, as in Figure 75–3, the images of the target lines fall on temporal retina. They are thus each seen in the nasal visual field, so the right eye target is seen to the left and the left eye target is seen to the right. For a measurement of the angular amount of fixation disparity, a target such as in Figure 75–4 is necessary. The patient reports to which of the upper lines seen by the right eye the arrow seen by the left eye is pointing. Referring once again to Figure 75–5, the physical separation of the arrow from the upper line identified by the patient would be equal to the separation of the points at which the visual axes of the two eyes intersect the plane of the target. The amount of fixation disparity is the angle subtended at the eye between those two points. In exo fixation disparity, the upper line identified by the patient as aligned with the arrow would appear to the examiner without polaroid goggles to be to the left of the arrow.

Table 75–2
Instruments for the Measurement of Associated Phorias

Distance
  American Optical vectographic slide
  Bernell lantern far point target
  Mallett far point unit

Near
  Borish card
  Bernell lantern near point target
  Mallett near point unit
  RMS rotary near point card

COMMERCIALLY AVAILABLE INSTRUMENTS

Table 75–2 lists the targets available for the measurement of associated phorias. The clinical procedures are basically the same on all of these instruments. The targets all have the basic features of the schematic in Figure 75–3.

Instruments that yield measurements of the angle of the fixation disparity, rather than just associated phorias, are the Sheedy disparometer and the Wesson fixation disparity card (Table 75–3). Both of these will allow the generation of an entire FDC.

Instruments for Measurement of Associated Phorias at Distance

American Optical (AO) Vectographic Slide

The AO vectographic slide, illustrated in Figure 75–6, is placed in a standard AO projector. The projected chart is viewed with polaroid goggles or the polaroid setting on the phoropter. It was designed for use in binocular refraction as well as for the measurement of horizontal and vertical associated phorias.[40–42]

Bernell Test Lantern

The Bernell test lantern consists of an incandescent bulb in a plastic housing back illuminating targets that can be slid into place. Included are targets for both distance (Fig. 75–7) and near associated phorias. The upper line is seen by the right eye, the lower by the left, and other features by both eyes. The target can be rotated for vertical-associated phorias. A target for the Worth four-dot test is built into the side of the lantern.

Mallett Unit

The Mallett unit for distance-associated phorias (Fig. 75–8) is also a back-illuminated target.[43] As with all of these instruments, viewing must be done through polaroïd goggles or the phoropter polaroid setting. The upper line is seen only by the right eye, and the lower line only by the left eye. Other features are seen binocularly. The target is rotated for vertical-associated phorias. The distance Mallett unit can be purchased with targets for other tests, as shown in Figure 75–8.

Table 75–3
Instruments for the Determination of Near Point Fixation Disparity Curves

Sheedy disparometer
Wesson fixation disparity card

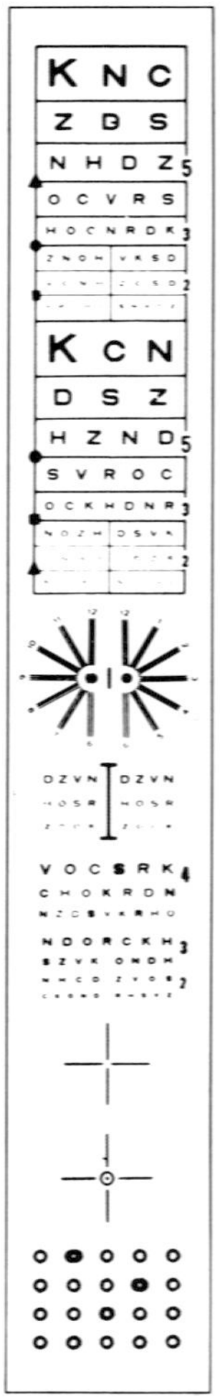

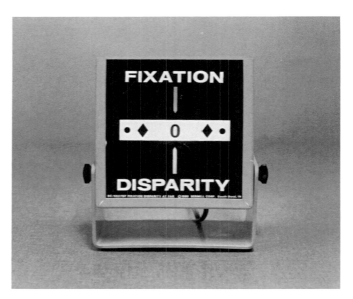

FIGURE 75–7. Bernell test lantern with the distance associated phoria target inserted.

phorias are measured by using the bottom middle portion of the slide.

Mallett Unit

A Mallett unit for near point-associated phoria testing, a separate instrument from the distance Mallett unit, is illustrated in Figure 75–11.[45] The instrument is hand-held.

RMS Rotary Near Point Card

The associated phoria target on the RMS rotary near point card is shown in Figure 75–12. This card can be either hand-held or mounted on a reading rod. The associated phoria targets are at the top of one side of the card (see Fig. 75–12).

FIGURE 75–6. Vectographic slide. Some features are seen only by the right eye, some only by the left eye, and some are viewed binocularly. In the associated phoria target toward the bottom, the upper and right lines are seen by the right eye, and the lower and left lines are viewed by the left eye.

Instruments for Measurement of Associated Phorias at Near

Borish Near Point Card

The Borish near point card is a two-sided near point test card that can be either hand-held or mounted on a reading rod.[44] It contains reduced visual acuity charts for OD, OS, and OU with polaroid lenses in place, grid patterns for near point cross cylinder, a diamond-shaped figure for dissociated phoria testing, and the typical crosslike array of lines for associated phoria testing. The side of the card with the associated phoria target is shown in Figure 75–9. In this target the lines are seen monocularly. The *x* and the circles are seen binocularly, serving as a fusion lock.

Bernell Test Lantern

The Bernell test lantern near point-associated phoria target is shown in Figure 75–10. In the center of the plate the two vertical lines are used for horizontal-associated phorias. Vertical-associated

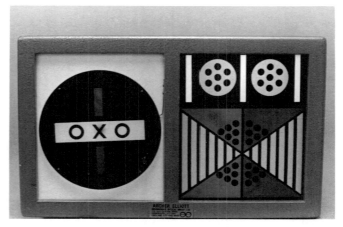

Figure 75–8. Mallett unit for distance-associated phoria testing. The associated phoria target is on the left side of this version of the Mallett unit. Also included are targets for Jackson cross cylinder testing for astigmatism (in the *upper right*) and for the bichrome test (in the *lower right*).

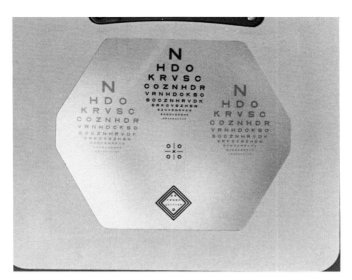

FIGURE 75–9. Borish near point card with associated phoria target.

Instruments for the Determination of Near Point Fixation Disparity Curves

Sheedy Disparometer

The Sheedy disparometer (Figs. 75–13 to 75–15) is made of hard plastic.[23,46] It can be hand-held or mounted on a reading rod. The patient's side of the disparometer is shown in Figure 75–13. Pairs of targets with different angular separations (see Fig. 75–14) are rotated through the window until the patient notes that a pair appear to be aligned. Bracketing is used to arrive at the fixation disparity measurement. There is one window for horizontal fixation disparity, and one for vertical fixation disparity. The examiner's side of the disparometer is shown in Figure 75–15. The clear plastic loops are fiber optic tubes that back illuminate the vernier

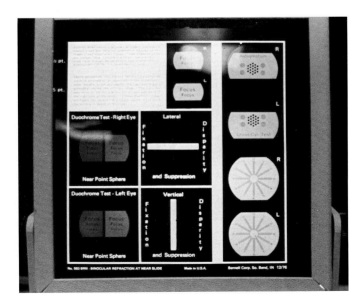

FIGURE 75–10. Bernell test lantern with the near point target inserted.

lines seen by the patient. These tubes originate on the patient's side of the target, where they should be adequately illuminated. Also seen on the examiner's side of the disparometer are the knob for rotating the pairs of nonius lines and windows through which the examiner can read the amount of fixation disparity corresponding to the angular separation of the lines seen by the patient. These values are calibrated for a working distance of 40 cm.

Wesson Fixation Disparity Card

The Wesson fixation disparity card, made of laminated posterboard, is illustrated in Figure 75–16.[47] The card is calibrated for use at either 25 cm or 40 cm. The patient should be asked if he sees both the black arrow and the colored lines above it to rule out suppression. The examiner should then ask the patient to identify the colored line to which the arrow points. For instance, if the patient identifies the green line to the right of the central red line, then the fixation disparity is 8.6 minutes of arc exo. When communication is difficult, the patient can point to the appropriate line with an object that will not mark or damage the card. However, this can potentially shift fixation disparity in an eso direction because of the proximal convergence associated with kinesthetic input. The card can be rotated 90° for vertical fixation disparity measurements.

CLINICAL PROCEDURE

Measurement of Associated Phorias

The basic procedures for the measurement of associated phorias are the same for each of the instruments listed in Table 75–2.

1. The instrument is readied for use. If the AO vectographic slide is being used, it is placed in a standard AO projector and the projector is turned on. If the Bernell lantern far point target is to be used, the target is slid into place in the Bernell lantern, and the Bernell lantern is placed on a table or other surface at distance and it is turned on. If the Mallett far point unit is used, the target lines are oriented vertically, and the illumination system is turned on. The Borish card and RMS rotary near point card are near point targets that can be either placed on the phoropter reading rod or hand-held. They should be illuminated by the near point reading lamp in the examination room. The Mallett near point unit is typically hand-held. The Bernell lantern when used for near point is usually placed on a table, but can be hand-held. The near point target is put in place in the Bernell lantern, and the lantern is turned on.
2. The patient wears polaroid goggles to view the target, or the examiner puts polaroid lenses in place in the phoropter, if available. The upper line and the right-hand line are seen by the right eye, with the lower and left lines seen by the left eye.
3. For the measurement of horizontal-associated phorias, the examiner asks the patient if the top line is directly above the bottom line. If so, the associated phoria is zero. If the top line is to the right of the bottom line, an eso fixation disparity exists, and base-out prism is added in increasing steps until the marks are first aligned. If the top line is to the left, base-in prism must be added to neutralize the exo fixation disparity. The associated phoria is the amount of prism necessary to eliminate the fixation disparity.
4. Vertical-associated phorias are measured by directing the patient's attention to the two horizontal lines in the target. (On the Mallett far point unit the lines must be rotated so

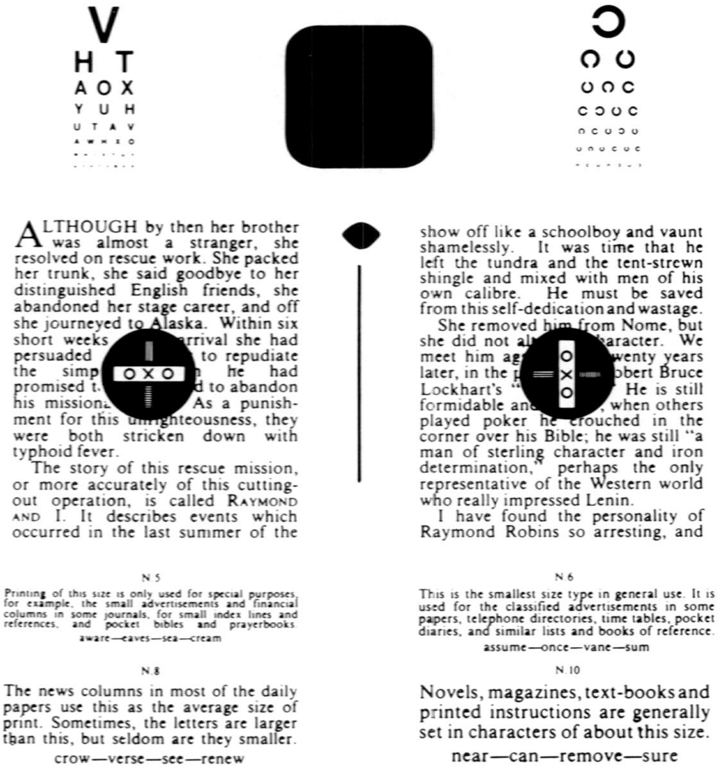

ALTHOUGH by then her brother was almost a stranger, she resolved on rescue work. She packed her trunk, she said goodbye to her distinguished English friends, she abandoned her stage career, and off she journeyed to Alaska. Within six short weeks of her arrival she had persuaded him to repudiate the simple faith he had promised to uphold to abandon his missionary zeal. As a punishment for this unrighteousness, they were both stricken down with typhoid fever.

The story of this rescue mission, or more accurately of this cutting-out operation, is called RAYMOND AND I. It describes events which occurred in the last summer of the

N 5

Printing of this size is only used for special purposes, for example, the small advertisements and financial columns in some journals, for small index lines and references, and pocket bibles and prayerbooks.
aware—eaves—sea—cream

N 8

The news columns in most of the daily papers use this as the average size of print. Sometimes, the letters are larger than this, but seldom are they smaller.
crow—verse—see—renew

show off like a schoolboy and vaunt shamelessly. It was time that he left the tundra and the tent-strewn shingle and mixed with men of his own calibre. He must be saved from this self-dedication and wastage.

She removed him from Nome, but she did not alter his character. We meet him again twenty years later, in the pages of Robert Bruce Lockhart's "_____" He is still formidable and when others played poker he crouched in the corner over his Bible; he was still "a man of sterling character and iron determination," perhaps the only representative of the Western world who really impressed Lenin.

I have found the personality of Raymond Robins so arresting, and

N 6

This is the smallest size type in general use. It is used for the classified advertisements in some papers, telephone directories, time tables, pocket diaries, and similar lists and books of reference.
assume—once—vane—sum

N 10

Novels, magazines, text-books and printed instructions are generally set in characters of about this size.
near—can—remove—sure

FIGURE 75–11. Diagram of the portion of the near point Mallett unit facing the patient. The circles inset within the reading text areas contain the marks for associated phoria measurement. The figures OXO are seen binocularly. The nearby lines are seen monocularly when polaroid lenses are in place, and are used for associated phoria determination. Targets for a polarized bichrome balance test, for stereopsis, and for suppression can be rotated into place in the square aperture at the upper-middle aspect of the unit.

that they are oriented horizontally.) A vertical fixation disparity exists if the right-hand line is higher or lower than the left-hand line. If the right line is higher, a left hyper- or right hypofixation disparity is present. The associated phoria is the amount of base-up prism OD or base-down prism OS that first aligns the two marks vertically. If the right line is lower, the right hyper- or left hypofixation disparity is neutralized by gradually increasing base-down prism OD or base-up prism OS in front of the patient. The prism necessary for vertical alignment is the vertical-associated phoria.

Measurement of Fixation Disparity and Determination of a Fixation Disparity Curve

To plot a fixation disparity curve, fixation disparity is determined at each of several different prism settings. The Sheedy disparometer and the Wesson fixation disparity card are typically placed on the phoropter reading rod, but could alternatively be hand-held.

1. The target is placed on the reading rod, and the near point reading light is directed toward it.
2. The patient wears polaroid goggles or the phoropter is set at the polaroid setting.
3. The patient is asked to look at the binocularly viewed contours and then glance at the nonius lines to make the alignment judgment. For each prism setting, the pair of

lines that appears aligned horizontally to the patient (Disparometer) is selected, or the patient indicates the upper line to which the arrow points (Wesson card). The angular separation of these marks is the amount of the fixation disparity.

4. After the fixation disparity is found at one given prism setting, the phoropter Risley prisms are then adjusted for the next prism setting. To reduce the effect of prism adaptation, the examiner can ask the patient to close his eyes between measurements, and to make a report within a few seconds after opening his eyes. Because prism adaptation affects fixation disparity, the order of prism presentation may affect the results. However, there does not seem to be a standardized order of prism presentation common to all investigators. Sheedy has recommended a measurement at zero prism, then with base-in prism starting with 3^Δ, and in 3^Δ increments to the fusional vergence limit (i.e., diplopia).[25] This is followed by base-out prism settings of 3^Δ, 6^Δ, 9^Δ, . . ., to diplopia. Wick prefers alternating base-in and base-out prism, 0, 3^ΔBI, 3^ΔBO, 6^ΔBI, 6^ΔBO, 9^ΔBI, 9^ΔBO, . . ., to diplopia.[9] Differences in the order of prism presentation may account for some of the differences in standard or mean FDC parameter values in various studies.[10]

5. For each determined fixation disparity value, a point is plotted on the FDC with the x value equal to the prism power setting, and y value equal to the amount of the

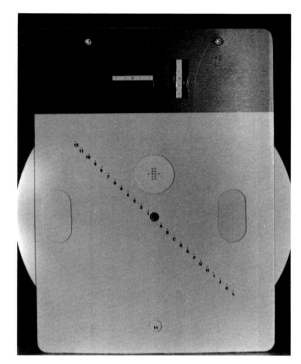

FIGURE 75–12. One side of the RMS rotary near point card. The associated phoria targets are at the top of the card.

fixation disparity. Additional details on each of these instruments follows.

CLINICAL IMPLICATIONS

Clinical Significance

Each of the horizontal FDC parameters provides diagnostic information. Studies by Sheedy and Saladin suggest that measurement of the FDC provides more useful information than determination of the associated phoria alone.[6,20,21] Curve type and slope gives information concerning the relationship between the patient's binocular vision status and extent of symptoms related to use of vision and concerning prognosis of vision training.

The measurement of associated phorias is done quicker and easier than measurement of the whole FDC. Some practitioners use the horizontal-associated phoria to prescribe prism. The vertical-associated phoria is the method of choice for the prescription of vertical prism.

Clinical Interpretation

Comparison of Results with Different Instruments

Associated phoria measurements at distance with the AO vectographic slide agree well with those obtained with the distance Mallett unit.[10] Near point-associated phorias on the Borish card are comparable with those for the near point Bernell target and for the near point Mallett unit.[10,48] The FDC *x*-intercepts using the Sheedy disparometer are greater in magnitude than the associated phorias with the Borish card, the near point Bernell target, and the near point Mallett unit.[10,49]

The FDC parameters differ somewhat in value on the Sheedy

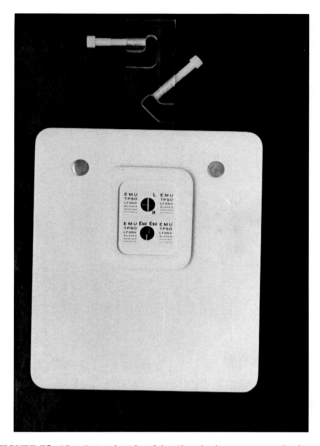

FIGURE 75–13. Patient's side of the Sheedy disparometer. The lines in the two round windows are viewed monocularly with polaroid lenses in place. All other features are seen binocularly. The upper window is used for vertical fixation disparity, and the lower window for horizontal fixation disparity.

disparometer and the Wesson fixation disparity card.[10,50] There are relatively more type I curves and fewer type II curves with the Wesson card. The Wesson card tends to result in more exo or less eso. Slopes may also be greater in magnitude with the Wesson card.

Prescription Using Horizontal-Associated Phorias

Mallett proposed that a patient with a fixation disparity in the same direction as his dissociated phoria has not adequately compensated for his phoria through fusional convergence.[43,45,51] He referred to this condition as an uncompensated phoria. For the nonpresbyopic uncompensated exophore at distance, he recommended the amount of minus add that eliminates the fixation disparity. For the uncompensated exophore at near with convergence insufficiency, he recommended orthoptics. For the elderly patient with near point uncompensated exophoria, Mallett suggested a base-in prism prescription equal to the associated phoria. For the patient with uncompensated esophoria at distance, his preferred treatment was orthoptics or the amount of base-out prism from the associated phoria. In a patient with uncompensated esophoria at near, he recommended the plus add that eliminated the fixation disparity. If a plus add equivalent in power to the reciprocal of the working distance in meters does not eliminate the fixation disparity, then base-out prism can be incorporated with the plus add.

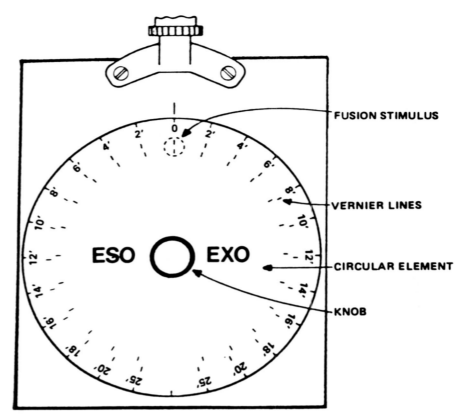

FIGURE 75–14. Schematic of the interior of Sheedy disparometer showing the pairs of lines with different angular separations.

Patient Management Using Horizontal Fixation Disparity Curves

The relative frequency of FDC types are approximately: type I, 60%; type II, 25%; type III, 10%; and type IV, 5%.[3,6,16] Patients with type I curves are usually asymptomatic.[25] When they are symptomatic, the slope of the FDC is typically steeper than the average. Sheedy and Saladin found that a slope value of approximately 1-minute arc per prism diopter discriminates between symptomatic and asymptomatic patients.[20] The patients with steeper slopes respond well to orthoptics when they are symptomatic. Success with orthoptics in patients with type I curves is correlated with a reduction in FDC slope.[21]

Most type II curves occur with esophoria.[25,46] Patients with type II curves respond better to prisms and to lens adds than to orthoptics. Type III curves are most often found in high exophoria.[9] Patients with type III curves can be trained with orthoptics, but not as easily as in type I curves.[25] These patients can also be managed with prism prescription. Sheedy and Wick recommend that prism prescriptions be based on the *x*-axis value at the flattest central portion of curve (i.e., center of symmetry), rather than the associated phoria, which is generally greater in amount.[9,25,46] There does not seem to be agreement on proper management of patients with type IV curves.

The slope of the FDC is correlated with the level of prism adaptation a patient has.[19] This appears to be why asymptomatic patients have flatter slopes than symptomatic patients. The critical slope value for distinguishing between symptomatic and asymp-tomatic patients may be steeper in exophoria than in esophoria.[6] Esophores thus may be more likely to be symptomatic with a marginal slope value than exophores. The steep slope on the base-in side and flat portion on the base-out side in type II curves may occur because these patients have better prism adaptation to convergence than to divergence.[19] Similarly, prism adaptation may be greater to divergence in patients with type III curves.[19]

The *y*-intercept is the amount of fixation disparity with no prism. Eso fixation disparity is more often associated with symptoms than exo fixation disparity.[25] A higher *y*-intercept value is correlated with the presence of symptoms, but the *y*-intercept cannot be used directly for prescribing.

An irregular FDC may be indicative of an accommodative problem.[9,25] Accommodative training results in a smoothing of the curve and relief of symptoms.

Vertical-Associated Phorias

Studies on vertical oculomotor imbalances indicate that the best method for their management is the prescription of vertical prism equal in amount to the vertical associated phoria.[22,23,52–54] Vertical associated phorias should be measured at distance and at near, with near point testing done both in primary position, as well as in downward gaze.[55] To avoid prescribing prism in patients with significant prism adaptation, prism should not be prescribed when the vertical-associated phoria is reduced after wearing a vertical prism for a few minutes.[56]

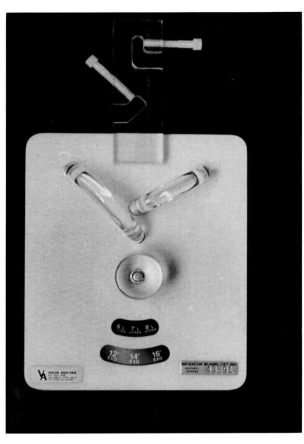

FIGURE 75–15. Examiner's side of the Sheedy disparometer. The knob in the center is used to change the pair of nonius lines being viewed by the patient. The amount of fixation disparity is displayed at the bottom of the instrument.

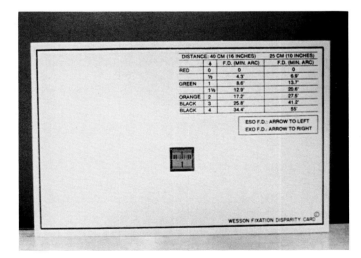

FIGURE 75–16. Wesson fixation disparity card. With polarizing filters the arrow is seen with the left eye and the lines above it are seen with the right eye.

REFERENCES

1. Cline D, Hofstetter HW, Griffin JR. Dictionary of visual science, 3rd ed. Radnor, Pa: Chilton Book Co, 1980:187, 472.
2. Ogle KN. Researches in binocular vision. New York: Hafner Publishing Co, 1950:69–93.
3. Ogle KN, Martens TG, Dyer JA. Oculomotor imbalance in binocular vision and fixation disparity. Philadelphia: Lea & Febiger, 1967.
4. Carter DB. Parameters of fixation disparity. Am J Optom Physiol Opt 1980;57:610–617.
5. Schor CM. Fixation disparity and vergence adaptation. In: Schor CM, Ciuffreda KJ, eds. Vergence eye movements: basic and clinical aspects. Boston: Butterworth Publishers, 1983:465–516.
6. Sheedy JE, Saladin JJ. Validity of diagnostic criteria and case analysis in binocular vision disorders. In: Schor CM, Ciuffreda KJ, eds. Vergence eye movements: basic and clinical aspects. Boston: Butterworth Publishers, 1983:517–540.
7. Reading RW. Binocular vision—foundations and applications. Boston: Butterworth Publishers, 1983:131–147.
8. Goss DA. Ocular accommodation, convergence, and fixation disparity: a manual of clinical analysis. New York: Professional Press, 1986:127–141.
9. Wick BC. Horizontal deviations. In: Amos JF, ed. Diagnosis and management in vision care. Boston: Butterworth Publishers, 1987:461–510.
10. Brownlee GA, Goss DA. Comparisons of commercially available devices for the measurement of fixation disparity and associated phorias. J Am Optom Assoc 1988;59:451–460.
11. Ogle KN, Mussey F, Prangen A deH. Fixation disparity and the fusional processes in binocular single vision. Am J Ophthalmol 1949;32:1069–1087.
12. Borish IM. Clinical refraction, 3rd ed. Chicago: Professional Press, 1970:861–937.
13. Fry GA. Basic concepts underlying graphical analysis. In: Schor CM, Ciuffreda KJ, eds. Vergence eye movements: basic and clinical aspects. Boston: Butterworth Publishers, 1983:403–437.
14. Goss DA. Ocular accommodation, convergence, and fixation disparity: a manual of clinical analysis. New York: Professional Press, 1986: 1–70.
15. McCullough RW. The fixation disparity–heterophoria relationship. J Am Optom Assoc 1978;49:369–372.
16. Saladin JJ, Sheedy JE. A population study of the relationships between fixation disparity, heterophorias and vergences. Am J Optom Physiol Opt 1978;55:744–750.
17. Ogle KN, Prangen A. Observations on vertical divergence and hyperphorias. Arch Ophthalmol 1953;49:313–334.
18. Carter DB. Fixation disparity and heterophoria following prolonged wearing of prism. Am J Optom 1965;42:141–151.
19. Schor CM. The influence of rapid prism adaptation upon fixation disparity. Vision Res 1979;19:757–765.
20. Sheedy JE, Saladin JJ. Phoria, vergence, and fixation disparity in oculomotor problems. Am J Optom Physiol Opt 1977;54:474–478.
21. Sheedy JE, Saladin JJ. Association of symptoms with measures of oculomotor deficiencies. Am J Optom Physiol Opt 1978;55:670–676.
22. Eskridge JB, Rutstein RP. Clinical evaluation of vertical fixation disparity. Part IV. Slope and adaptation to vertical prism of vertical heterophoria patients. Am J Optom Physiol Opt 1986;63:662–667.
23. Rutstein RP, Eskridge JB. Studies in vertical fixation disparity. Am J Optom Physiol Opt 1986;63:639–644.
24. Mallett RFJ. Fixation disparity in clinical practice. Aust J Optom 1969;52:97–109.
25. Sheedy JE. Actual measurement of fixation disparity and its use in diagnosis and treatment. J Am Optom Assoc 1980;51:1079–1084.
26. Pickwell D. Binocular vision anomalies—investigation and treatment. London: Butterworth Publishers, 1984:35–40.
27. Carter DB. Studies in fixation disparity. III. The apparent uniocular components of fixation disparity. Am J Optom 1960;37:408–419.
28. Carter DB. Fixation disparity with and without foveal fusion contours. Am J Optom 1964;41:729–736.
29. Saladin JJ, Carr LW. Fusion lock diameter and the forced vergence fixation disparity curve. Am J Optom Physiol Opt 1983;60:933–943.
30. Debysingh SJ, Orzech PL, Sheedy JE. Effect of a central fusion stimulus on fixation disparity. Am J Optom Physiol Opt 1986;63:277–280.
31. Sheedy JE. Should a central fusion stimulus be used on the disparometer? Am J Optom Physiol Opt 1986;63:627–630.

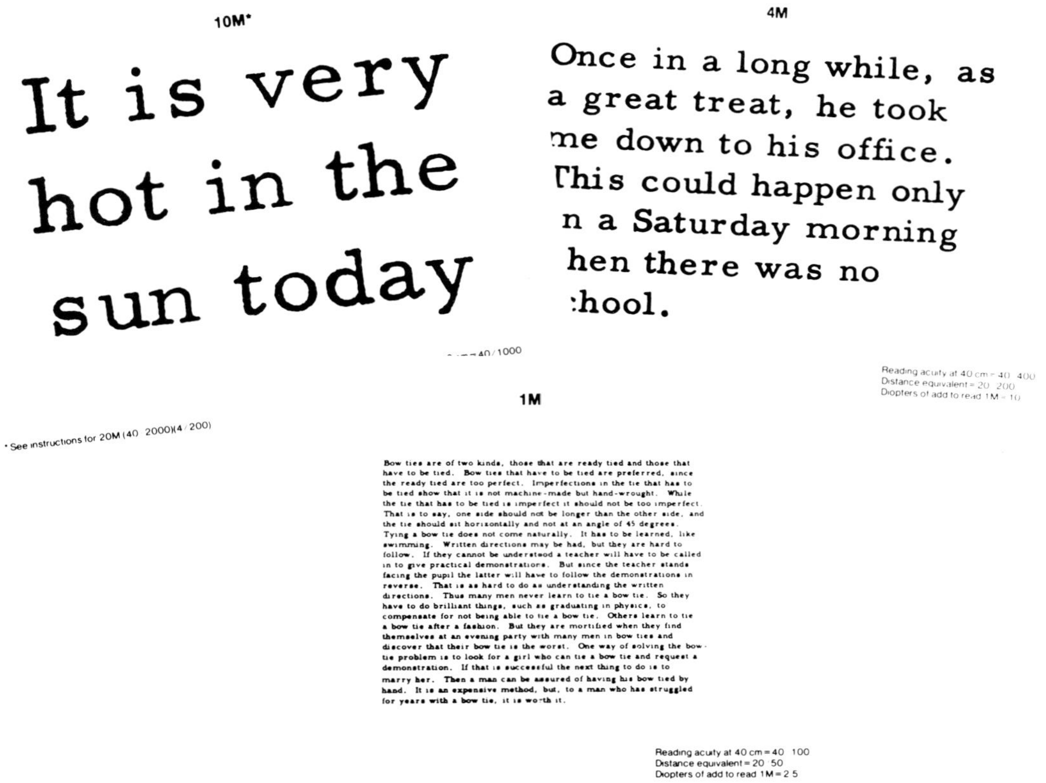

10M*

It is very
hot in the
sun today

4M

Once in a long while, as
a great treat, he took
me down to his office.
This could happen only
n a Saturday morning
hen there was no
:hool.

Reading acuity at 40 cm = 40 400
Distance equivalent = 20 200
Diopters of add to read 1M - 10

- - - 40 / 1000

1M

* See instructions for 20M (40 2000)(4 / 200)

Bow ties are of two kinds, those that are ready tied and those that
have to be tied. Bow ties that have to be tied are preferred, since
the ready tied are too perfect. Imperfections in the tie that has to
be tied show that it is not machine-made but hand-wrought. While
the tie that has to be tied is imperfect it should not be too imperfect
That is to say, one side should not be longer than the other side, and
the tie should sit horizontally and not at an angle of 45 degrees.
Tying a bow tie does not come naturally. It has to be learned, like
swimming. Written directions may be had, but they are hard to
follow. If they cannot be understood a teacher will have to be called
in to give practical demonstrations. But since the teacher stands
facing the pupil the latter will have to follow the demonstrations in
reverse. That is as hard to do as understanding the written
directions. Thus many men never learn to tie a bow tie. So they
have to do brilliant things, such as graduating in physics, to
compensate for not being able to tie a bow tie. Others learn to tie
a bow tie after a fashion. But they are mortified when they find
themselves at an evening party with many men in bow ties and
discover that their bow tie is the worst. One way of solving the bow-
tie problem is to look for a girl who can tie a bow tie and request a
demonstration. If that is successful the next thing to do is to
marry her. Then a man can be assured of having his bow tied by
hand. It is an expensive method, but, to a man who has struggled
for years with a bow tie, it is worth it.

Reading acuity at 40 cm = 40 100
Distance equivalent = 20 50
Diopters of add to read 1M = 2 5

FIGURE 80–3. Sloan reading cards. Three of nine cards are shown here. Size range extends from 10 M to 1 M.

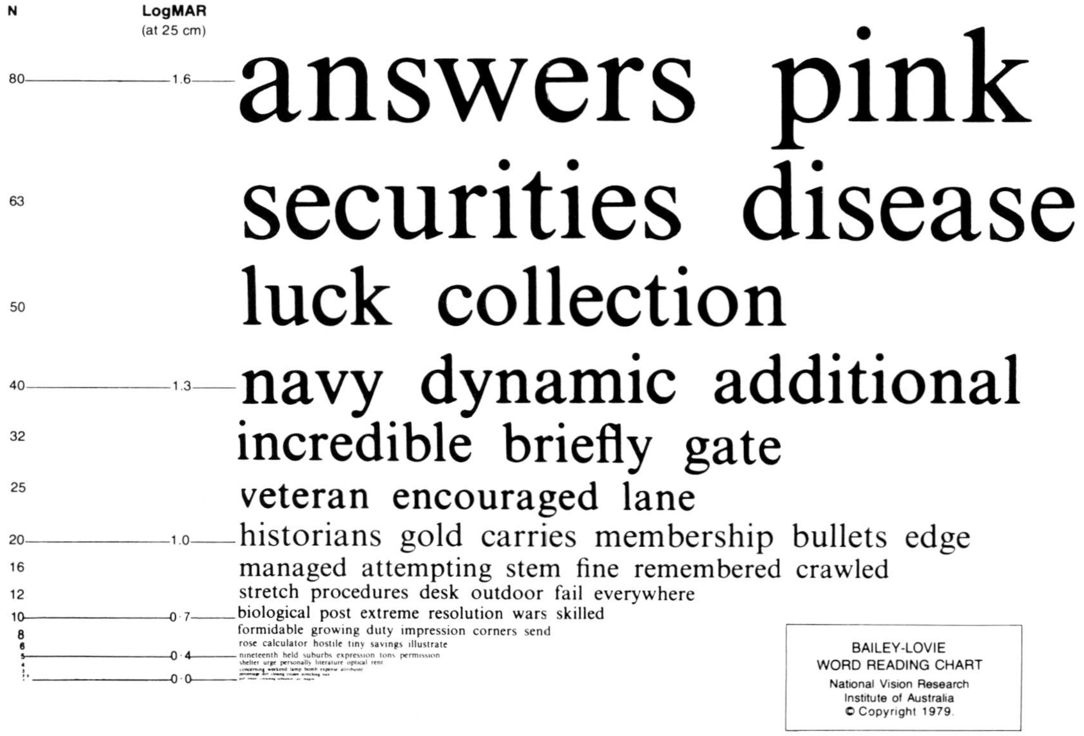

N	LogMAR (at 25 cm)	
80	1.6	**answers pink**
63		**securities disease**
50		**luck collection**
40	1.3	navy dynamic additional
32		incredible briefly gate
25		veteran encouraged lane
20	1.0	historians gold carries membership bullets edge
16		managed attempting stem fine remembered crawled
12		stretch procedures desk outdoor fail everywhere
10	0 7	biological post extreme resolution wars skilled
8		formidable growing duty impression corners send
6		rose calculator hostile tiny savings illustrate
5	0 4	nineteenth held suburbs expression ions permission
4		shelter urge personally literature optical rent
		concerning weekend lamp booth expense confront
	0 0	percentage dirt closing copier searching not
		heritage chewing adhesive or magic

BAILEY-LOVIE
WORD READING CHART
National Vision Research
Institute of Australia
© Copyright 1979.

FIGURE 80–4. Bailey–Lovie Word Reading Chart. Size range extends from 10 M to 0.25 M.

Specifying the Limit of Resolution at Near

When testing and recording measurements of near visual performance, it is important for the clinician to maintain an awareness of the distinction between visual acuities and resolution limits. Visual acuity requires both the specification of test distance and the specification of print size. It is an angular measure. The resolution limit requires only the specification of print size. From a practical perspective, the clinician's goal is usually to enable the patient to see a certain level of fine detail—that is, achieve a certain level of resolution. Consequently, the height of the smallest resolvable print becomes the critical dimension in the test of the patient's near vision performance. The angular size of that print at the viewing distance must be given, and this, with the letter height, provides a measure of visual acuity. However, the angular size is of secondary importance.

Near vision charts have their print size specified in several alternative ways, the most common of which are M units, points, N notation, reduced Snellen notation and Jaeger notation.

M Units

M units, proposed by Sloan,[12] are used to indicate print size. For a sample of print, the *M units* rating indicates a distance at which the smallest (lower-case) letters subtend 5 minutes of arc. Visual acuity can be recorded as a Snellen fraction in which the top part of the fraction represents the test distance (in meters) and the lower part represents the letter size (in M units). For example, 0.40/1 M indicates that the patient can read print that is 1 M unit in size (equivalent to newsprint) from a distance of 40 cm (0.40 m). Newsprint typically has lower-case letters that are about 1.45-mm high, and this subtends 5 min of arc at 1 m.

Points

Points are units used by printers to specify print size. Each point represents 1/72 part of an inch. Eight-point typeface has an overall height of 8/72 in. from the top of the ascending strokes to the bottom of the descenders. For most newsprint font styles, lower-case letters that have neither ascenders or descenders (e.g., a, c, m, o, x) have a height that is about half the overall height of the typeface. Thus, for 8-point newsprint, the lower-case letters are about 4/72 in.-(1.41 mm) high. For font styles such as Times or Century and others that are commonly used in newsprint, 8-point print typically has an M unit rating of 1 M. For most fonts with styles resembling the common style of newsprint, print size in points can be converted to M units by dividing by 8 (i.e., M units = points/8).

N Notation

Some charts use a British notation[19] in which the print size is labeled by an N followed by a number (e.g., N8). The N indicates that the print is standard *near* vision test type (Times Roman), and the number that follows gives the point size. Thus N8 indicates that the Times Roman font is used and the print size is 8 points. Visual acuity measurements require specification of test distance so that a visual acuity measure might be N8 at 40 cm.

Reduced Snellen Notation

So-called reduced Snellen charts are typically letter charts designed for near vision testing, but the print sizes are labeled in the Snellen fractional values that are used to express distance visual acuity. Print "20/20" on a reduced Snellen chart will demand a visual acuity that is equivalent to a distance visual acuity of 20/20, provided that the test chart is presented at the standard test distance of 40 cm.. Very few low vision practitioners use reduced

Snellen notation because test distances are usually closer than 40 cm, and then the labeled Snellen fractions become inappropriate expressions of acuity.

Jaeger Notation

On some charts print size is indicated by Jaeger notation in which the letter J is followed by a number (e.g., J3). The system has very little consistency or value. Smaller numbers denote smaller print, but there the system ends. For example, J3 on one chart may be twice the size of J3 on a similar chart from another manufacturer, and the numbers are not proportional to print size (e.g., J6 is not twice the size of J3).

Charts for Testing Infants

In the past decade, important advances have been made in visual acuity measurement in infants and multihandicapped children. The most significant development comes for the "preferential looking" techniques that were developed for research relating to the development of vision in children. Teller and associates[20] pioneered this technique. Visual acuity measurements taken with the preferential looking techniques usually are tests of grating acuity. A black-and-white striped grating target is presented against a gray background. The "gray" level of the black-and-white striped area matches the gray level of the background. A child whose resolution abilities allow the stripes to be seen is likely to be attracted to look at the stripes. Typically the area of the striped pattern may be presented in one of two positions. The examiner, observing only the infant's eyes, judges whether the child shows a preference for looking to one position or to the other. Teller's procedures developed for laboratory research must be modified to be practical for clinical application. A simpler version of the laboratory tests and less rigorous procedures have been proposed and are now often used in clinical examination of infants and handicapped children (see Chap. 66). Alternative test charts that use symbol optotypes and other tests of visual acuity have been reviewed by Fern and Manny.[21]

COMMERCIALLY AVAILABLE INSTRUMENTS

There is a wide variety of panel charts available for testing distance visual acuity. Most are letter charts, but alternative optotypes such as Landolt rings, tumbling E's or pictorial or symbol charts are available. The most commonly used letter charts are arranged on a single panel that has a large single letter at the top and below this, the letter sizes become progressively smaller, and there are progressively more letters in each successive row. Such charts are widely available from distributors of ophthalmic equipment, and they are generically referred to as "Snellen" charts (see Chap. 2).

Letter charts that have standardized the test task at each size level are available in a few different formats. The Bailey–Lovie charts are available from the Multimedia Center of the School of Optometry of the University of California at Berkeley. The print sizes range from letters that subtend 5 minutes of arc at 125 ft (38 m) down to 6.3 ft (1.9 m). These charts are printed on plastic panels, and a low-contrast (gray letters) chart is printed on the obverse side. The charts are approximately 60-cm high and 50-cm wide (24 × 21 in.). Different letter sequences are available.

The New York Lighthouse now manufactures the "Early Treatment of Diabetic Retinopathy Study" (ETDRS) charts that are similar to the Bailey–Lovie charts, except that Sloan letters are used instead of the British letters. The size range on these charts extends from 40-m to 2-m letter (131 ft to 6.5 ft), and the panels are 60 × 60 cm (25 × 25 in.). Different letter sequences are available.

Designs for Vision produces and distributes Feinbloom Distance Visual Acuity charts, which are in a book format. The optotypes are numbers and the size ranges from symbols that subtend 5 minutes of arc at 700 ft down to 10 ft. The page size is 25 × 33 cm (10 × 13 in.).

For near vision testing there are again many charts available from most ophthalmic suppliers. There are many letter charts available for near vision testing, but most near vision charts use continuous printed text or sometimes sets of printed words.

The New York Lighthouse distributes the Sloan reading charts that were designed specifically for use with low vision patients. In this set of cards, the print size ranges from 10 M to 1 M.

Keeler has its reading charts available in different languages. They use sentences or paragraphs printed in Times Roman type face, and the print size range extends from 10 M to 1 M.

The Multimedia Center of the University of California at Berkeley School of Optometry prepares Bailey–Lovie Word Reading Charts that use unrelated words printed in Times Roman typeface. The print size ranges from 10 M to 0.25 M, and different word sequences are available.

The Pepper Visual Skills Reading Test is available from the Feinbloom Center of the Pennsylvania College of Optometry.

CLINICAL PROCEDURES

Distance Visual Acuity Testing

Mehr and Mehr[22] and Mehr and Freid[23] emphasized the need to make visual acuity measurement a positive experience for the patient. The first presentation of the chart should be under conditions that permit the patient to see some of the test material. The patient should be wearing the best available refractive correction. The print size and the test distance should be chosen according to estimates that the clinician has made of the likely visual acuity score. This estimate comes from clues given by the history and prior information about the patient's visually guided behavior. Should there be doubt about whether the patient will be able to read the larger letters on the chart, the chart should be first presented at a very close distance. If this is done at 1 ft, reading the "200-ft" line of the chart would give a visual acuity score of 1/200, which is equivalent to 20/4000. If the patient performs better than expected at the very close distance, then the chart may easily be moved back toward a more conventional test distance.

Viewing Distances

The most commonly used test distances are 10 ft (3 m) and 5 ft (1.5 m), but other test distances may easily be used. Should it become necessary to test "distance visual acuity" at relatively close distances, it might appear appropriate to incorporate an addition in the spectacles to provide optimal refractive correction. This, in fact, is rarely done because at the visual acuity levels being tested, such changes in focus probably have no notable impact on the visual acuity score.

There is a facility for changing working distance that comes from the use of charts that use a logarithmic size progression. If the multiplier constant is 0.1 log units (a factor of 1.26 ×), the size progression is 200, 160, 125, 100, 80, 60, 50, 40, 32, 25, 20, 16 . . . . In meters, the equivalent values are 60, 48, 38, 30, 24, 19, 15, 12, 9.5, 7.5, 6.0, 4.8, ... This sequence of letter sizes can be used as a guide for a sequence of alternative test distances. Changing the viewing distance by one step in this sequence of numbers causes a patient's resolution limit to change by one line on the chart. Changing the viewing distance from 20 to 16 ft or from 16 to 12.5 ft, would allow the patient to read exactly one more row on the chart. Changing by two steps (20 to 12.5 ft, 16 to 10 ft) would allow

the patient to read two more rows. It may be noted that, on this scale, three steps represent a factor of two times and ten steps represent a factor of ten times.

Task Complexity

Low vision patients, especially those with disturbed macular function, often have difficulty reading with any efficiency, even when the print size is substantially above the patient's resolution limit. With charts on which letters are relatively isolated, visual acuity scores are likely to be better. Letters at the beginning and end of rows are more likely to be legible than are the letters in the middle. Patients frequently lose their place, and in such cases the clinician may need to point to the letters of immediate attention.

Eccentric Viewing

Patients with macular disorders may sometimes achieve better visual acuity by viewing eccentrically. A commonly used and simple procedure to test for this phenomenon is for the clinician to direct the patient's attention to the smallest legible letters while the patient fixates on a target (such as the clinician's hand) that is positioned, in turn, above, below, to the right, and to the left of the letters of interest. Oblique positions may also be used. The patient is instructed to observe whether the letters become any easier to read when the eye is pointed toward any one of these eccentric locations.

Illumination

Low vision patients are much more likely to have visual acuity substantially affected by changes in illumination levels. When using visual acuity charts in the form of a printed panel, an adjustable lamp should be used to illuminate the chart. Varying the position of the illumination source relative to the chart allows a wide range of task luminance. Typically, the first visual acuity measurement is made under the standard (80 to 300 cd/m²) chart luminances. Then the clinician can determine whether there is any unusually large change in acuity as a result of the chart illumination being either decreased or increased. A lamp held close to the chart and just under the smallest legible letters usually creates local chart luminances of 1000 cd/m² or more.

Performance with Telescopes

Measurement of distance visual acuity is often associated with the testing of telescopes for low vision patients. The purpose of the visual acuity measurements may be to demonstrate the advantage that the telescope offers or to confirm that the telescope actually does provide the expected resolution advantage. The clinician should ensure that the focusing adjustment of the telescope has a sufficient range to focus on the chart. When testing distance vision with telescopes, it is sometimes necessary for the clinician to simulate "optical infinity" or very distant viewing by holding a +0.25-D lens in front of the objective while the chart is placed at a distance of 4 m.

Near Visual Acuity Testing

Most testing of near visual acuity uses typeset words, sentences, or paragraphs, rather than the letter chart format that is used for distance visual acuity. Lower-case printed material presents a more congested and complex visual task than does a letter chart. Many low vision patients, especially those with macular function disorders, will have a reading chart acuity that is substantially poorer than the letter chart acuity because of the special difficulty with congested and complex resolution tasks. If the clinician really wishes to compare distance and near visual acuities, the patient should be properly focused, and the chart design features and luminances for the distant and near vision testing should be identical. Only in relatively rare cases does the smaller pupil associated with near vision cause a significant difference between the distance and near visual acuity.

Near vision test charts may be on a single card or on a series of cards. For low vision patients, it is useful to have a rather large range of print sizes available. The size of print should be labeled in M units or in points. The clinician usually records near visual acuity by specifying both the height of the smallest print read (M units or points) and the distance at which the test chart was presented.

Reading Acuity Testing

Testing of near vision in low vision patients is usually a key part of the process of enabling the patient to achieve a desired level of resolution. The resolution goal is determined by the needs of the patient. Most commonly it is the reading of print of approximately the same size as newsprint (1 M). When being tested, the patient should have an in-focus view of the test chart, and this means the power of any reading addition or accommodation should be appropriately matched to the chart presentation distance. If the patient already has reading glasses, these may be used (perhaps with some auxiliary addition), or an appropriate optical correction may be placed in a trial frame for the test of near vision. The chart presentation distance should always be one at which the chart will be in-focus, and appropriate lighting should be provided. As the patient reads the large print, note should be made of the reading efficiency, and special attention should be given to the rate at which reading efficiency decreases as smaller print is encountered and the resolution limit is approached. Patients should be encouraged to struggle to the limit of their resolution ability.

The size of the smallest-size print read and the test distance should be recorded with additional note made of the smallest print size at which the patient could read with best efficiency. For example, for a presbyopic patient it might be recorded that near visual acuity with a +4.00-D addition was 0.25/2 M (5 M with facility). For this patient to be able to just read newsprint (1 M) an 8.00-D addition would be required, and anticipated performance would be 0.12/1 M (2.5 M with facility). To achieve reading of newsprint with best efficiency a 20-D addition is indicated for this patient. With such an addition the expected near vision performance would be 0.05/0.4 M (1 M with facility). To prescribe low vision aids for this patient, optical systems that provide an equivalent viewing power of +20 D (equivalent viewing distance of 5 cm) is indicated for the efficient reading of newsprint. Spectacles, hand or stand magnifiers, near vision telescopes, or electronic enlargement systems could be considered.

Controlling Viewing Conditions

Often very close viewing distances are required for low vision patients, and many patients resist holding the test chart so close to the face. Care must be taken to ensure that the chart is in focus. A common strategy is for the clinician to first present the chart at a distance that is much too close, and to then, with the patient's help, move the chart away until it comes into clearest focus. The viewing distance should be monitored throughout the testing procedures.

Illumination on the near vision charts is usually provided by an incandescent lamp mounted on an adjustable arm. Care should be taken to avoid the patient receiving a direct view of the lamp or the inside rim of the reflector bowl. Sometimes the lamp will need to be quite close to the page to obtain high luminance levels. Specular reflections should be avoided. The illumination levels should be adjusted to meet the individual patient's needs.

Many patients benefit from a "typoscope" reading mask. This is a black card with a rectangular window through which about three lines of print may be read. This device reduces glare, and for many patients, acuity is improved. Many patients find that the typoscope makes it easier to hold the place when reading. Some patients whose vision loss causes them to lose their place may also benefit from pointing to the beginning or ends of the row or to the words as they are read. A ruler or a similar straight edge may serve as a useful line guide.

CLINICAL IMPLICATIONS

Clinical Significance

Visual acuity measurement is more important in patients who have low vision. In low vision that has been acquired from disease or trauma, there is usually a higher risk of further ocular change, and it is very important to establish a baseline visual acuity measure. Low vision patients are often considered for eligibility for special benefits or programs, and frequently visual acuity criteria must be applied. In legal cases involving compensation for loss of vision, visual acuity measures usually assume paramount importance in scaling the magnitude of the vision loss.

In prescribing optical aids for low vision patients, resolution improvement provided by various optical devices is assessed by measurement of visual acuity. Usually, the ultimate resolution goal of the clinician is expressed in terms that may be related to visual acuity measurements. Valid and reliable visual acuity measurements during the prescribing procedure allow best prediction of resolution performance when different aids are to be considered. Any failures to meet the predicted performance usually indicate that the optical aid is being used inappropriately or the optical parameters of the low vision aid are incorrectly specified.

Clinical Interpretation

The clinician should be conscious that the nature of the visual acuity chart can have a very substantial effect on visual acuity score when patients have impaired vision. In particular, patients with impaired macular function have much more difficulty resolving detail of complex and congested targets.[24] Consequently, there may be large differences between the acuities obtained with simple or isolated targets (gratings or single letters), and poorer acuity scores result when the tasks are more complex (letter charts with close spacings or reading charts). It is generally desirable that the clinician record the chart that was used for the visual acuity testing.

The visual acuity criterion for *legal blindness* is that the visual acuity should be equal to or less than 20/200. Clinicians should be aware that visual acuity chart design can significantly affect whether or not a person is deemed to be "legally blind" according to this definition. For instance, on many "Snellen" charts there is at the top a 200-ft letter, and the next row has two letters at the 100-ft size. A visual acuity score of 20/200 would be given to any patient who can read the 200-ft letter but not read either of the two letters at 100-ft size. Based on this measurement, the patient would be considered legally blind. A patient whose visual acuity was actually 20/110 would be expected to "pass" at 20/200, but fail at 20/100 and thus would receive a score of 20/200 on this chart. However, on charts that have intermediate sizes between the 100- and 200-ft levels, this patient would obtain a different score that would be better than 20/200 and, therefore, would no longer meet the definition of legal blindness. Chart design features, and the size progression ratio in particular, can have important effects on whether or not a person meets a specified visual acuity criterion. Charts on which the test task is standardized for all size levels usually minimize these difficulties.

REFERENCES

1. Snellen H. Letterproeven tot bepaling der gezigtsscherpte (P.W. van der Weijer, Utrecht, 1862), cited in Bennett, AG, Ophthalmic test types. Br J Physiol Opt 1965;22:238–271.
2. Green J. On a new series of test letters for determining the acuteness of vision. Trans Am Ophthalmol Soc 1868;1(3):68.
3. Bennett AG. Ophthalmic test types. Br J Physiol Opt 1965;22:238–271.
4. Sloan LL. New test charts for the measurement of visual acuity at far and near distances. Am J Ophthalmol 1959;48:807–813.
5. British Standard. Test charts for determining visual acuity. BS 4274: 1968. London, British Standards Institution, 1968.
6. NRC Committee on Vision. Recommended standard procedures for the clinical measurement and specification of visual acuity 1979. Adv Ophthalmol 1980;41:103–148.
7. Concilium Ophthalmologicum Universale. Visual acuity measurement standards. COU Vision Functions Committee, 1984.
8. Feinbloom W. Distance test chart for the partially sighted. New York: Designs for Vision, Inc.
9. Keeler CH. Visual aids for the pathological eye (excluding contact lenses). Trans Ophthalmol Soc UK 1956;76:605–614.
10. Bailey IL, Lovie JE. New designs principles for visual acuity letter charts. Am J Optom Physiol Opt 1976;53:740.
11. Taylor HR. Applying new design principles to the constriction of an illiterate E chart. Am J Optom Physiol Opt 1978;55:348–351.
12. Ferris FL, Kassoff A, Bresnick GH, Bailey IL. New visual acuity charts for clinical research. Am J Ophthalmol 1980;94:92–96.
13. Strong G, Woo GC. Distance visual acuity chart incorporating some new design features. Arch Ophthalmol 1985;103:44.
14. Feinbloom W. Near reading card for the partially sighted. New York: Designs for Vision, Inc.
15. Sloan LL, Brown DJ. Reading cards for selection of optical aids for the partially sighted. Am J Ophthalmol 1963;55:1187–1199.
16. Keeler CH. Keeler "A" series word chart. London: Keeler, 1958.
17. Bailey IL, Lovie JE. The design and use of a new near vision chart. Am J Optom Physiol Opt 1980;57:378.
18. Baldasare J, Watson GR, Whittaker SG, Miller-Shaffer H. The development and evaluation of a reading test for low vision macular loss patients. J Vis Impair Blind 1986;80:785–789.
19. Law FW. Standardization of reading types. Br J Ophthalmol 1951; 35:765–773.
20. Dobson V, Teller DY. Visual acuity in human infants. Vision Res 1978; 18:1469–1483.
21. Fern KD, Manny RE. Visual acuity of the preschool child. Am J Optom Physiol Opt 1986;63:319–345.
22. Mehr EB, Mehr HM. Psychological factors in work with partially sighted persons. J Am Optom Assoc 1969;40:842–846.
23. Mehr EB, Freid AN. Low vision care. Chicago: Professional Press, 1975.
24. Kitchin JE, Bailey IL. Task complexity and visual acuity in macular degeneration. Aust J Optom 1987;64:235–242.

Low Vision Refraction

Ian L. Bailey

INTRODUCTION

Definition

The determination of refractive error is a cornerstone of the optometric assessment and treatment of the low vision patient.[1] To assess properly the visual performance that a patient may be able to achieve, either with or without an optical aid, the clinician should be in a position to ensure that the image formed on the patient's eye is optimally focused. This can be done only if the clinician has a satisfactory estimate of the patient's refractive error. The refractive error of a low vision patient may be difficult to determine for several reasons:

1. There is a greater likelihood of refractive irregularities. There may be distortions or opacification of the cornea caused by trauma, dystrophy, disease, or surgery, or there may be lens irregularities caused by cataract or other changes of the lens.
2. The patient's responses are likely to be poorer; the causative disturbance of the visual system, the smallness of the pupil, or medial irregularities may render the patient less sensitive to dioptric blur.
3. There may be changes in the refractive error that are unusually large in magnitude. There may have been a recent rapid change affecting the lens, cornea, or retina, or the patient may have neglected regular eye care for a long period, or sometimes the eye care practitioner may have given insufficient attention to refractive error because either refraction seemed too difficult or too fruitless or because all efforts were directed at monitoring the ocular disease.

The clinician must begin the refraction of a low vision patient prepared to vary from the usual routine refraction procedures[2] and from having the usual expectations.

Clinical Use

Although the phoropter or refractor unit might be preferred for use in the refraction of patients with normal or near-normal vision, these instruments are not generally used for low vision patients.[3] The refraction of low vision patients should be conducted using trial lenses that may be hand-held, or placed in trial frames or in trial lens clips. There are several important reasons for preferring to use trial lenses, rather than the phoropter:

1. Many low vision patients adopt eccentric viewing strategies when performing critical visual tasks, and the clinician should be able to observe this kind of behavior.
2. Nystagmus is often present in low vision patients and the clinician should be able to observe any changes in the nystagmus with eye position, attention, or convergence, and differences depending on whether one or both eyes are being used, should be observable.
3. Unusual search behaviors, head movements, or head positions should be available to the patient and observable to the clinician.
4. Patients with special sensitivity to light may partially close their eyelids, and the clinician should be able to observe this.
5. Some patients may gain improvements in visual resolution behind a phoropter by positioning themselves so that their eye pupils are partially vignetted by the relatively small aperture of the phoropter. This rarely occurs when using trial lenses.
6. With many low vision patients, it is desirable to make abrupt changes of lens power in large steps. This is easier, and there is more freedom to change lens power in large steps when trial lenses are being used.
7. It can be important for some low vision patients to be impressed that it is their own residual vision, combined

with very simple lenses, that is achieving the improvement obtained in the clinic, and that the improvement is not a result of some mysterious effect that dwells within the imposing machine that the phoropter represents.

INSTRUMENTATION

Trial Lenses

The low vision practitioner should have a trial case, a sturdy trial frame, and a pair of trial lens clips. Full-diameter trial lenses are generally preferred, but these can present difficulties when higher-powered lenses are being used. The stronger lenses are thicker, and it can be difficult to clip or stack these into some of the trial frames or trial lens clips. Reduced-aperture trial lenses can be easier to handle, but they do restrict the clinician's observation of the patient's eye movements and eye position. For much of the refraction procedure, lenses may be held in the hand. When a reasonable estimate of the refractive error is achieved, then the appropriate lenses should be incorporated into the trial lens frame or the trial lens clip and then refinement of the refraction may proceed using low-powered hand-held lenses.

Trial Frames

Trial frames should be sturdy and adjustable and capable of holding several lenses before each eye. They should also be able to accommodate some of the telescopic and compound lens trial units, such as the Designs for Vision telescopes and microscopes, the Keeler near vision magnifying units, and similar devices that are designed to be mounted in trial rings with the standard 38-mm diameter. When adjusting the trial frame, care should be taken to create a pantoscopic tilt of the spectacle plane that will be similar to the angle anticipated in any spectacles that may eventually be prescribed. Similarly, the vertex distance of the posterior cell of the trial frame should ideally be the same as that which will be ultimately present in the patient's glasses. For larger magnitude refractive errors, the setting of the vertex distance and the pantoscopic tilt becomes more important. When the refractive error is substantial, it is advisable to have a strong lens that approximately corrects the spherical refractive error placed in the posterior cell of the trial frame. Then the fine adjustments can be achieved by low-powered lenses in the front cells. For strong lenses, the horizontal location of the optical centers should be determined by measuring from the center of the bridge to the centers of the pupil of each eye. The vertical positions of the optical centers depend on the pantoscopic tilt; the optical centers should generally be placed below the pupillary centers, allowing 1 mm of downward displacement for each 2° of pantoscopic tilt. This causes the optical axis of the lens to pass toward the center of the eye's rotation, thus minimizing aberrations.

Trial Lens Clips

Trial lens clips typically have two or three cells for trial lenses, and they are mounted to the patient's existing glasses with spring clips. Currently, the Halberg clip, the Jannelli clip, the Bernell clip, and the Bommarito clip are the most readily available trial lens clips, and some other alternatives are available (Fig. 81–1). Trial lens clips typically allow the most convenient and most accurate refraction of low vision patients. A large majority of the low vision population habitually wear glasses because this population shows high prevalences of presbyopia and high refractive error. The advantages of trial lens clips become greatest when the refractive error is

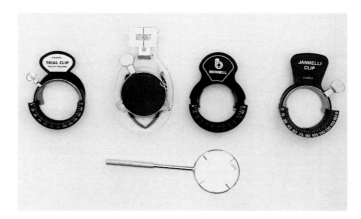

FIGURE 81–1. Trial lens clips. From left to right: Halberg clip, Bommarito clip, Bernell clip, Jannelli clip. Jackson cross cylinder is shown below.

substantial, but significant advantages still pertain to the correction of smaller refractive errors. The patient's previous glasses usually provide a more stable and secure mounting than trial frames, and the vertex distance and pantoscopic tilt of the patient's spectacles are more likely to be similar to those that will be present in any new glasses that might later be prescribed. Generally, the trial lenses required when working over the patient's old glasses will be low powered, since it is only the *change* and not the entire refractive error that is being corrected by the trial lenses used in the "overrefraction." Lower-powered lenses are usually available in finer steps of lens power and, being thinner, they are most easy to use with the trial lens clips. Of course, some care should be taken to center the trial lens clips appropriately before the patient's eyes, but, since the supplementary lenses are usually of low power, lens placement is not so highly critical.

When conducting either the subjective or objective overrefraction procedures, the refractionist should pay no heed to the spherical power, cylindric power, or cylinder axis in the patient's previous refractive correction. It is only the overrefraction that is being determined. The axis of the cylinder found in the overrefraction does not have to bear any special relationship to the cylinder axis in the existing spectacles. When the overrefraction has been determined, the existing glasses with trial lens clips with the final overcorrecting lenses in place should be taken to the lensometer and the back vertex power of the combination measured. This determines the power required in any new refractive correction. For example, a patient wears a spectacle correction of

R: $+4.00$ DS -2.00 DC $\times 30$ and   L: $+5.00$ DS -4.00 DC $\times 145$

The overrefraction in trial lens clips is

R: $+0.50$ DS -1.00 DC $\times 175$ and   L: -0.25 DS -1.00 DC $\times 30$

In the lensometer, the overrefraction lenses combined with the spectacles give readings of

R: $+4.25$ DS $-2.50 \times$ DC 19 and   L: $+4.00$ DS -3.50 DC $\times 151$

This is the lens power that should be prescribed.

This final prescription will include full compensation for any "power errors" created by the pantoscopic tilt or lens placement errors that may have been present in the previous spectacles. During the overrefraction only cylinders of moderate power are required, so that only moderate precision is required for positioning of the axis, even when the total astigmatism is high. Higher precision of axis placement is required in trial frame refractions when the entire cylindrical component is being manipulated. With trial lens clips, some care is necessary to ensure that neither the clip itself nor any cylinder lens held in the clip rotates relative to the spectacle lens, both during the refraction procedure and when en route to the lensometer.

COMMERCIALLY AVAILABLE INSTRUMENTS

Trial lens sets and trial frames, along with hand-held Jackson cross cylinders have long been standard optometric equipment for refraction of patient with low vision or high refractive error or in nonoffice environments. Low vision practitioners generally have at least one higher power (±0.75 or ±1.00 D) cross cylinder available for refracting patients with poorer discrimination of blur. Trial lens clips are designed to be attached to the patient's existing spectacles, and there are slots or clips designed to hold trial lenses. Keeler first marketed "Halberg Clips" which had three slots for holding trial lenses. Bernell Clips are similar to the Halberg clips. Jannelli Clips added a small spirit level and designed the lens holders to reduce lens rotation and these features provided improved control over the axis orientation of cylindrical lenses in the lens clip. Bommarito Clips added other new features to allow better adjustability of height (useful in testing vision through bifocals), a spacing bar to give better control of separation between the left eye and right eye units. They also have provision for incorporating auxiliary "high-plus" or "high-minus" lenses for testing patients with greater magnitudes of refractive error.

CLINICAL PROCEDURE

Objective Refraction

Retinoscopy can be a most important procedure in the examination of the low vision patient. Typically, subjective responses to dioptric change are less reliable with low vision patients, and objective refraction becomes relatively more important. When the ocular media are clear and the pupil is not especially small, standard retinoscopic procedures may be used. Special techniques and special considerations become necessary when the retinoscopic reflex is difficult to see or interpret. When the retinoscopic reflex cannot be seen, is very dull, or is moving only slowly, it is advisable to move much closer to the patient. If there is very high myopia, the image will then become brighter, faster, and easier to evaluate. A lens of appropriate minus power can be introduced and retinoscopy can then be resumed from the usual working distance. If the image remains dull and difficult to see or interpret, the cause could be high hyperopic refractive error. If this is the case, the introduction of a +10-D lens should elicit a brighter reflex that is easier to interpret. If neither moving closer nor adding a +10-D lens produce a more definitive reflex, more radical methods are called for. Moving to a very close distance or observing the reflex from substantially off-axis position might produce the only useful reflex. Of course, appropriate dioptric allowances must be made when the working distances are close. There may be errors due to difficulty estimating the working distance when it is short. Off-axis observation may also produce some inaccuracy, especially relating to the astigmatism determination. When the clinician becomes obliged to use "radical retinoscopy" techniques, almost any estimate becomes acceptable, but the practitioner should remain conscious of the potential sources and magnitudes of inaccuracies.

Lenticular or corneal irregularities, or even retinal disruptions, can cause some fragmentation of the retinoscopic reflex, and clinicians may have difficulty in deciding which component of the

fragmented image should be neutralized. In general, the brightest component should receive the emphasis.

Instrumental objective optometers are slowly gaining wider use, but currently, they do not seem to offer any special advantage for the examination of the low vision patient. These instruments rely on reflected light from the retina, and they are likely to produce erroneous results or no results at all when the media are irregular, the pupils are small, or the patient's fixation unsteady. In general, instrumental objective optometers will produce satisfactory estimates of refractive error in eyes on which retinoscopy can be performed with reasonable ease.

Keratometry

When retinoscopy does not afford a reliable measure of astigmatism, keratometry assumes more importance. Although unsteady fixation and nystagmus, both of which are more common in low vision patients, can make keratometry more difficult and less reliable, keratometry can still provide a useful estimate of astigmatism, especially when the magnitude of the astigmatism is large.

Subjective Refraction

It is expected that low vision patients will be less discriminating in the subjective judgments of relative clarity that are at the heart of the subjective refraction procedures. In general, the poorer the patient's vision, the poorer will be the ability to make discriminations, and consequently, the poorer the accuracy of the subjective refraction. This, however, is not an obligatory relationship. Some patients with very poor visual acuity will be surprisingly sensitive to refractive blur, whereas other patients with relatively good acuity will have surprisingly poor blur discrimination. Clinicians should approach the subjective refraction prepared to work initially in very large steps of dioptric power, and then reduce the size of the steps until the patient has difficulty in making the discriminations. This approach enables the clinician to tailor the accuracy of the refraction to the individual tolerances of the patient. This approach is preferred over determining the size of steps of dioptric power according to the visual acuity.[4]

Subjective refraction commences with the best estimate of the refractive error in place in the trial frame or trial lens clip. This estimate may come from retinoscopy or the patient's previous prescription. With use of a suitable visual acuity chart, the clinician should find the patient's limit of resolution. Then the patient is instructed to attend to a letter or a group of letters that are at, or near, the acuity limit, and then to report on the relative clarity and legibility of the images seen as different lens changes are made. Sometimes the patient will be asked to compare the view through two different lenses. "Which lens makes the letters clearer and blacker—lens No. 1 . . . like this . . ., or lens No. 2 . . . like this ?" And at other times the patient is asked whether the lens causes a perceptible change. "Does this lens make the letters better . . . or worse . . ., or is there no difference?

Bracketing

Bracketing is a term used to describe a strategy that is most important in low vision refractions. It involves changing from presenting "too-much-minus" and then "too-much-plus" (or vice versa), and systematically changing the midpoint of the range being bracketed and the size of the bracketing range. At the conclusion, changing from extra-plus to extra-minus in the finest discriminable steps will elicit a report that both presentations are equally and just-

PATIENT # 1 Refractive Error = +2.25 D.

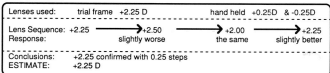

Lenses used:	trial frame 0.00 D	hand held +6.00D & -6.00D
Lens Sequence:	0.00 → +6.00 → -6.00 → 0.00	
Response:	slightly blurred, very blurred, better	
Conclusions: ESTIMATE:	Closer to 0.00 than +6.00; within +/- 6 bracket; reduce step size. Guess +1.00 to +2.50	

Lenses used:	trial frame +1.75 D	hand held +0.75D & -0.75D
Lens Sequence:	+1.75 → +2.50 → +1.00 → +1.75	
Response:	slightly better, worse, not bad	
Conclusions: ESTIMATE:	Closer to +2.50 than to 1.75; reduce step size. +2.25 or +2.50	

Lenses used:	trial frame +2.50 D	hand held +0.25D & -0.25D
Lens Sequence:	+2.50 → +2.75 → +2.25 → +2.50	
Response:	slightly worse, better, a little worse	
Conclusions: ESTIMATE:	Apears to be +2.25; should confirm. +2.25	

CONFIRMATION

Lenses used:	trial frame +2.25 D	hand held +0.25D & -0.25D
Lens Sequence:	+2.25 → +2.50 → +2.00 → +2.25	
Response:	slightly worse, the same, slightly better	
Conclusions: ESTIMATE:	+2.25 confirmed with 0.25 steps. +2.25 D	

A

PATIENT # 2 Refractive Error = +11.25 D.

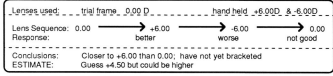

Lenses used:	trial frame 0.00 D	hand held +6.00D & -6.00D
Lens Sequence:	0.00 → +6.00 → -6.00 → 0.00	
Response:	better, worse, not good	
Conclusions: ESTIMATE:	Closer to +6.00 than 0.00; have not yet bracketed. Guess +4.50 but could be higher	

Lenses used:	trial frame +4.50 D	hand held +6.00D & -6.00D
Lens Sequence:	+4.50 → +10.50 → -1.50 → +4.50	
Response:	better, worse, not good	
Conclusions: ESTIMATE:	Closer to +10.50 than +4.50; still have not bracketed. Guess +9.00 but could be higher; greater than 8.00	

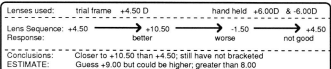

Lenses used:	trial frame +9.00 D	hand held +6.00D & -6.00D
Lens Sequence:	+9.00 → +15.00 → +3.00 → +9.00	
Response:	worse, much worse, better	
Conclusions: ESTIMATE:	Closer to +9.00 than +15.00; have now bracketed; reduce step size. Guess +10.50; probably less than +11.50, could be as low as 8.00	

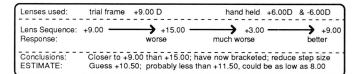

Lenses used:	trial frame +10.50 D	hand held +2.00D & -2.00D
Lens Sequence:	+10.50 → +12.50 → +8.50 → +10.50	
Response:	similar, worse, better	
Conclusions: ESTIMATE:	About midway between +10.50 and +12.50; reduce step size. Guess +11.50; almost there	

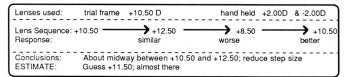

Lenses used:	trial frame +11.50 D	hand held +0.50D & -0.50D
Lens Sequence:	+11.50 → +11.00 → +12.00 → +11.50	
Response:	the same, slightly worse, better	
Conclusions: ESTIMATE:	Midway between +11.00 than +11.50; confirm with finer steps. +11.25	

CONFIRMATION

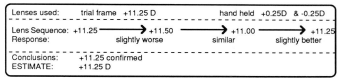

Lenses used:	trial frame +11.25 D	hand held +0.25D & -0.25D
Lens Sequence:	+11.25 → +11.50 → +11.00 → +11.25	
Response:	slightly worse, similar, slightly better	
Conclusions: ESTIMATE:	+11.25 confirmed. +11.25 D	

B

FIGURE 81–2. Examples of bracketing: (*A*) refractive error is +2.25 D; (*B*) refractive error is +11.25 D.

detectably blurred. Initially, large steps of dioptric change are made and, according to the patient's responses, the center of the bracketing range is shifted and the size of the dioptric change is reduced. The certainty or uncertainty with which the patient expresses each response should influence the refractionist's selection of lenses. The two examples shown in Figure 81–2 illustrate a series of dioptric changes made in a sequence determined by the patient's responses. In the process shown here, the patient reports on the clarity of perception as a change is made from viewing through one lens to another. Throughout the procedure, the clinician should allow the patient enough time to make decisions, especially when the decisions appear to be difficult. It is best to begin the astigmatic refraction as soon as it seems that discrimination of spherical blur has become difficult. Any uncorrected astigmatism of substantial magnitude may be contributing to the patient's difficulty in discriminating changes in spherical power.

Bichrome techniques are often used in the refraction of patients with near-normal vision, but they are less commonly applied to low vision patients. This may simply be a result of the lack of availability of suitable large-print bichrome targets.

Telescope optometers have been advocated[5] as a means of estimating spherical refraction. The patient is instructed to adjust a telescope until it is in best focus for a distant test chart. The telescope is then taken to a lensometer and the back vertex power measured. There are three problems associated with this method: (1) The vergence of light from the chart may be small (−0.25 D or less) as it reaches the telescope, but this is amplified by the telescope (by approximately the square of the magnification), and appropriate compensation must be made. (2) Lensometers often have adjustment errors that may be inconsequential when the lensometer is used to measure lenses, but when measuring telescopes, these errors in the lensometer become amplified and substantial errors in estimates of back vertex power can result. (3) Young people often accommodate by reasonably large and unpredictable amounts when they use telescopes. These three factors introduce some risk to the validity of the measurements, and there is no valid optical reason for patients being more sensitive to refractive changes when viewing through a telescope.

Some authors[6–8] have recommended performing refraction using trial lenses placed behind a fixed focus telescope that is mounted in the front cell of a trial frame. Although it is suggested that this "refines" the refraction, no rational reason has been advanced for why this technique could be of any use, nor has there been any empirical evidence advanced in its support. Given the need to consider vergence amplification effect and instrument accommodation, there are good reasons to recommend that this technique not be used.

On rare occasions, a most simple optometer can be useful.

The patient can hold a plus lens that is weaker than the required power, or a minus lens that is stronger than the required power, and then move the lens back and forth until clearest focus is found. Measuring the distance from the lens to the spectacle plane allows an estimation of the final refractive error. For example, if a +10-D lens held 2.0 cm from the spectacle plane provides a clear focus, then the refractive error (referred to the spectacle plane) will be +12.50 D. The focal plane of the lens is 8 cm (10 − 2 cm) from the spectacle plane, so the lens power required in the spectacle plane is +12.5 D.

Astigmatism

The test of choice for determining astigmatism in low vision patients is the Jackson cross cylinder test. Hand-held Jackson cross cylinders are available in a range of powers, and the selection of the power to be used for a given patient is based on the patient's sensitivity to spherical defocus. Lower powers ±0.25 D or ±0.37 D can be used for patients with good blur discrimination. For patients with poor discrimination ±0.75 D and ±1.00 D become more useful. If the clinician has no estimate of the axis or magnitude of any uncorrected astigmatism, it is advisable to start with the cross cylinder handle along or orthogonal to the 45° meridian so that the principal power meridians of the cross cylinder are at 90° and 180°. In asking the patient which presentation is clearer the clinician is, in effect, determining whether vision is clearer with a minus cylinder axis at 180° or at 90°. If the patient can make no distinction, then it may be that there is astigmatism with the principal meridians at 45° and 135°, or there is no astigmatism, or the power change is too small for the patient to distinguish. Whether or not the patient has a preference for the first two alternative views, there should be a second flip of the cross cylinder with the handle horizontal or vertical so that the principal power meridians are at 45° and 135°. If the patient's responses are valid and expressive, the axis can often be estimated at this stage to an accuracy of about 10° (Table 81–1).

Another flip of the cross cylinder might further tighten this estimate of the axis of astigmatism, but the clinician may prefer to gain some estimate of the cylinder magnitude before refining estimate of axis. With low vision patients who have already demonstrated that they can respond to, for example, a 1.00-D cross cylinder, the next step may be to introduce a moderately strong cylinder, about 2.00 D, for example, with its axis along the estimated direction. In the foregoing example, it would be −2.00 DC × 105 being held (or placed in one of the trial lens cells) in front of the previously determined spherical correction. Ideally, a +1.00-D sphere should be introduced as well to maintain the same spherical power equivalent. It is not always essential to be rigorous in maintaining spherical equivalence at this stage. With the cross cylinder held so that the principal meridians are along 105° and 15°, another flip is made and, by the patient's response, it is determined whether more cylinder is required (preference for minus axis along 105°) or less minus cylinder is required (preference for

plus axis along 105°). If the patient gives the first-mentioned response, the cylinder should be increased to a −4.00 DC × 105 and the procedure repeated. The size of the changes in cylinder power should be reduced until the patient reaches his or her own discrimination limit. Once a reasonably good estimate of cylinder power has been made, the spherical component may be rechecked or refined. If tight spherical equivalency had been maintained during the astigmatic refraction, only a small adjustment should be necessary. If a large adjustment of sphere is found to be necessary, more attention should be given to rechecking the cylinder power and perhaps even the cylinder axis. With reasonable estimates of cylinder power and with the spherical power in place, the axis determination can now be refined. If it is found there is a substantial change in axis, then it may be necessary to return to check the cylinder power and spherical power once again. Table 81–2 indicates a possible sequence in a Jackson cross cylinder test for a patient whose uncorrected astigmatism has been −4.75 DC × 55. Here the spherical component has been ignored, and it has been assumed that the refractionist has no other information about the magnitude or axis of this patient's astigmatism.

The basic process of refraction should be as efficient as possible, and it should minimize the number of difficult decisions demanded of the patient. A general model is illustrated in Table 81–3. The coarse estimate of spherical refraction should be terminated as soon as it is clear that the patient is having difficulty discriminating the changes of power as the size of the changes is reduced. For patients with better discrimination of defocus, a lower-powered cross cylinder should be used in the astigmatic determination. Generally, only two or three flips of the cross cylinder are required to obtain the coarse estimate of axis. Until the refining stages are reached, it is wasteful of time and effort to repeat a flip of the cross cylinder whenever the patient reports that it is difficult to judge which is the better. Instead, modify the conditions (cylinder axis or power) so that it should become easier for the patient to see a difference between the two presentations of the cross cylinder.

Alternative Procedures for Determining Astigmatism

When patients do not respond satisfactorily to the cross cylinder test, more desperate searching strategies may be used to identify any large magnitude astigmatism. As a test for large magnitude astigmatism, a lens of substantial power (e.g., a −5-D cylinder) can be introduced and rotated through 180°, with the patient being instructed to report when clearest vision is obtained. The rotation may be controlled by either the clinician or by the patient. If a preferred axis location is found, then cylinder power should then be varied, working in large steps and using bracketing strategies until clearest vision is obtained.

After the estimate of astigmatic error has been made, it is prudent to verify that, in fact, the astigmatism really is present and that this astigmatic correction makes a perceptible difference. A simple verification technique is to quickly rotate the correcting cylinder through 90°. If vision becomes better at any time during

---

Table 81–1

Estimating Axis of Astigmatism with Few Flips of the Jackson Cross Cylinder

Procedure	Cross Cylinder Axis	Response	Conclusions
Flip 1 Handle at 45°	a − axis at 90 b − axis at 180	Better Worse	Minus axis closer to vertical than to horizontal
Flip 2 Handle at 90°	a − axis at 45 b − axis at 135	Perhaps slightly worse Perhaps slightly better	Minus axis slightly closer to 135° than to 45° Estimated axis is 100°–105°

Table 81–2
Example of Using Jackson Cross Cylinder in Oblique Astigmatism

		Lens Added	Cross Cylinder Axis	Patient Response	Conclusion and Best Estimate
Estimate Axis					
Flip 1	a	None	− at 90	Slightly better	Closer to 90 than to 180
Handle at 45	b	None	− at 180	Slightly worse	
Flip 2	a	None	− at 45	Better	Much closer to 45 than 135 between
Handle at 180	b	None	− at 135	Worse	90 and 45; estimate 60
Estimate Cylinder Power					
Flip 3	a	−2.00×60	− at 60	Better	More cylinder required; change to 4 D
Handle at 15	b	−2.00×60	− at 150	Worse	
Flip 4	a	−4.00×60	− at 60	Better	More cylinder required; change to 6 D
Handle at 15	b	−4.00×60	− at 150	Worse	
Flip 5	a	−6.00×60	− at 60	Worse	Less cylinder required; between 4 and
Handle at 15	b	−6.00×60	− at 150	Better	6 D
Flip 6	a	−5.00×60	− at 60	Worse	Less cylinder required; between 4 D
Handle at 15	b	−5.00×60	− at 150	Better	and 5 D
Flip 7	a	−4.50×60	− at 60	Better	More cylinder required; estimate
Handle at 15	b	−4.50×60	− at 150	Worse	4.75 D
Flip 8	a	−4.75×60	− at 60	Hard to tell	About right
Handle at 15	b	−4.75×60	− at 150		
Refine Axis					
Flip 9	a	−4.75×60	− at 15	Slightly better	Shift axis towards 15; change to 50
Handle at 60	b	−4.75×60	− at 105	Slightly worse	
Flip 10	a	−4.75×50	− at 5	Slightly worse	Shift axis towards 95; change to 55
Handle at 50	b	−4.75×50	− at 95	Slightly better	
Flip 11	a	−4.75×55	− at 10	The same	Axis correct at 55
Handle at 55	b	−4.75×55	− at 100	The same	
Refine Cylinder Power					
Flip 12	a	−4.75×55	− at 55	The same	Power correct −4.75 × 55
Handle at 10	b	−4.75×55	− at 145	The same	

this rotation, or if vision is not perceptibly *worse* when the cylinder axis is perpendicular to the indicated axis direction, then the validity and value of the astigmatic correction becomes most questionable. The astigmatic determination should then be repeated in full or the astigmatic correction should be removed completely.

When objective and subjective procedures do not yield any conclusive determination of astigmatism, the clinician may consider two options—prescribe no cylindrical correction, or provide the same astigmatic correction that was present in the previous spectacles.

Table 81–3
Sequence of Steps in the Subjective Refraction of Low Vision Patients

1. Coarse sphere estimate
2. Coarse cylinder axis estimate
3. Coarse cylinder power estimate
4. Refine sphere estimate
5. Refine axis estimate
6. Refine cylinder power
7. Repeat 4 and 6 (and sometimes 5) as indicated

Stenopaic Slit Refraction

The stenopaic slit can sometimes provide a useful measure of astigmatism. A slit aperture of a width 0.5 to 2.0 mm can be introduced while the patient observes an acuity chart. The slit is rotated until clearest vision is reported. This slit orientation indicates one principal meridian. With the slit in this orientation, spherical lenses are introduced and the sphere that gives clearest vision is determined. This provides the power correction for the meridian corresponding to the slit orientation. The slit is then rotated 90° and, again, spherical lenses are introduced until the lens giving the clearest vision has been determined. This indicates the power correction required for the second meridian. Knowing the power required to correct each principal meridian, the clinician can determine the total spherocylinder refraction. For example: first, the slit gives clearest vision when at 60°; second, with the slit at 60° a +3.00-DS gives clearest vision; and then, with the slit at 150°, a +5.00-DS gives clearest vision. The refractive correction is +5.00 −2.00 × 150. The stenopaic slit technique is used infrequently. It can produce invalid results when there is significant irregularity of the optical media. Nevertheless, it is a technique that can be useful in confirming measurements of astigmatism obtained from other techniques.

There are many tests of astigmatism that rely on judgment of the relative clarity of lines in particular orientations. These include fan, clock, sunburst, cross, T, block, paraboline, and other carved or straight-line targets. Refraction techniques that use this kind of target are not often used for refracting low vision patients. With low vision patients there is more likelihood of irregularities of the cornea, lens, or retina, and this may cause lines at particular orientations to be clearer for reasons that are not related to the best estimate of overall astigmatism. Tests such as the cross cylinder procedures, which are dependent on more complex target structures, are generally preferred.

REFERENCES

1. Mehr EB, Fried AN. Low vision care. Chicago: Professional Press, 1975.
2. Borish I. Clinical refraction. Chicago: Professional Press, 1970.
3. Bailey IL. Refracting low vision patients. Optom Monthly 1978;69:131–135.
4. Freed B. Refracting the low vision patient. J Vision Rehabil 1987;1(4):57–61.
5. Woo GC. Use of low magnification telescopes as optometers in low vision. Optom Monthly 1978;69:529–533.
6. Faye EE. Clinical low vision. Boston: Little, Brown & Co, 1984.
7. Jose RT. Understanding low vision. New York: American Foundation for the Blind, 1983.
8. Newman JD. A guide to the care of low vision patients. St Louis: American Optometric Association, 1974.

Low Vision Visual Fields

Norman J. Weiss

INTRODUCTION

Definition

If one acknowledges that *visual field testing* is the mapping of those areas of the visual system that show a reduced sensitivity to visual stimuli, then there is no difference between the field testing of low vision and fully sighted patients. In low vision practice, however, we are concerned with patients whose visual abilities may be lowered, and the techniques and implications of the fields assume a greater significance.

History

From a historical standpoint, the concept of the field of vision as an island in a sea of blindness is derived from the writings of Euclid and Hieliodorus, who believed that the "island" was circular and cone shaped, beyond which there was no vision. Although the shape of the island changed some, the concept was elaborated by Roenne to include a hill of vision that incorporates the sensitivity of the visual system. Indeed, it was the work of Berry, in 1890, and then Roenne and Bjerrum some years later, who quantified the measurement of the hill of vision. Bjerrum developed the use of the tangent screen when he found that he derived more specific information on the field when he used the door of his examining room rather than the perimeters available then.[1] Originally, the intent of the field of vision was to study the advances of glaucoma by noting enlargement of the blind spot and depressions and scotoma in the central field. Field testing has progressed considerably, giving much greater detail and information on detection and management of disease. The blind spot also serves the purpose of monitoring fixation for the plot of the static visual field. Fixation shifts of only a few degrees can be detected and can provide an accurate assessment of patient fixation.[2]

Clinical Use

Clinically, use of the perimeter or tangent screen requires the patient to observe a central fixation point and to respond to a stimulus spot that is presented in various parts of the field. The stimulus may be a moving target of constant size, intensity, and color or it may be a series of stationary targets that vary in intensity. Kinetic perimetry involves the detection of a moving target as it is moved from "blind" to "seeing" areas or vice versa. Static perimetry involves the detection of a series of stationary targets that are varied in intensity or varied in size and intensity in one static field instrument.

INSTRUMENTATION

The theoretical basis and use of the various visual field testing procedures are discussed in Chapters 27, 28, and 49.

COMMERCIALLY AVAILABLE INSTRUMENTS

The instrumentation can be classified into three broad categories: (1) central field devices; (2) peripheral field devices; and (3) confrontation field devices.

Central field devices generally evaluate the central 30° or less. The tangent screen is the mainstay and basic method of plotting the central field. Variants of this device are the Auto-plot and the Amsler grid. The Auto-plot is an elaboration of the tangent screen method, which allows some freedom in recording the stimulus points and varying the fixation spots. The Amsler grid allows the qualitative recording of a central field by recording distortions on a grid. The results can be made more exact by using a 2-mm stimulus spot and quantifying the results by plotting the exact outline of the central or paracentral scotoma with greater accuracy.

The Henson 3000 is an automated device that allows plotting of the central 25° of field with static methods.

Peripheral field devices are intended to measure the most peripheral aspects of the visual field. The arc-type perimeter is an early kinetic device consisting of an arc covering a maximum of 180· in each meridian. The stimulus spots are variable in size and color. The newer devices are bowl-type perimeters, which are either kinetic or static devices or are automated. Some of the bowl-type perimeters have problems monitoring the fixation of patients with central field defects. Other problems with the bowl-type perimeter may not be obvious until the unit is used. For example, in determining the effect of a blepharoptosis using the arc-type perimeter, the operator can hold the upper lid as the points are being plotted. The bowl-type perimeters do not permit manual manipulation of the eyelid and necessitate the use of tape or some other method to temporarily open the palpebral fissure during the visual field testing.

Confrontation field devices should be kept simple, requiring a fixation object and a stimulus object consistent with the understanding of the patient. This is a screening method that is intended to give a qualitative estimate of the peripheral field. Although confrontation field methods are an approximation, they are necessary for many types of patients.

CLINICAL PROCEDURE

Diseases Involving Central Field Defects

Patients with central field defects should have mapping of the central field as well as the peripheral field. The common assumption that peripheral fields are full if there is a central field defect is often incorrect. Diseases such as macular degeneration, diabetic and hypertensive retinopathies, and central retinal hemorrhage, are examples of diseases that have central field defects, but also necessitate knowledge of the peripheral fields.

Visual fields must be plotted to

1. Map the viable areas of the retina
2. Indicate progression of the course of the disease
3. Understand the need for mobility instruction
4. Understand the need for special illumination
5. Indicate prognosis for the low vision management of the problem

A major concern of plotting the central or peripheral fields is the fixation area. Proper fixation is necessary to maintain a constant visual axis position while the plot is being done. The fixation may be maintained by encouraging the use of eccentric viewing or by using fixation targets that are large enough to see centrally with controls to be assured of central fixation.

Eccentric viewing involves the off-axis viewing of the fixation spot. Encouraging the use of eccentric viewing is not difficult. However, determining the precise amount of eccentric viewing is important to allow repeatability and accurate comparison of the results.

Measurement of eccentric viewing is easiest using the Brombach type of arc perimeter. The method is simple. The patient fixates the fixation spot using eccentric viewing. The amount of eccentric viewing is measured by finding the position on the arc at which a penlight beam is centered in the patient's pupil. The amount of eccentric viewing is read in degrees on the perimeter (Fig. 82–1).

This method has several limitations. First, it is intended to be used on an arc-type perimeter that is not readily available. The use of this method with any type of bowl perimeter or central field device is not possible. Second, as the disease underlying a central field defect progresses, the amount of eccentric viewing necessary

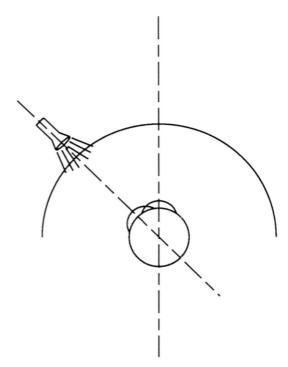

FIGURE 82–1. Schematic diagram showing the measurement of eccentric viewing using an arc perimeter. Center the corneal reflection with a muscle light and read the degree of eccentric viewing on the perimeter.

will increase. Although this may seem to be a disadvantage for direct comparison of the field, the knowledge that the amount of eccentric viewing has changed is important.

Some of the other kinetic instruments will have control on central fixation. The Haag–Streit (Goldmann) Perimeter, for example, has a telemicroscopic detection system to be sure that fixation is maintained. Other kinetic devices have other alarms to indicate when a change in fixation has occurred. However, there is no method to determine the amount of eccentric viewing when using these instruments.

Static devices often utilize the blind spot as a basis for recording deviations in fixation. Maintenance of fixation sometimes is not the major concern, but only to record deviations in fixation at the conclusion of the test so that reliability of the test can be evaluated. The Humphrey's Visual Field Analyzer has a closed-circuit viewing system so that the operator can monitor the patient's fixation.

An important principle to be followed when designing fixation targets for central field defects when the instrument will allow them to be modified is that the target must be large enough to extend beyond the central scotoma and must be designed with controls. The best object to use is an *X* with varying lengths to the extremities so that the patient can readily see four tips when fixating centrally (Figure 82–2). If the patient should change fixation, one of the tips will disappear and provide a control. This method is most readily applied to tangent screens. It is very difficult to apply this fixation method to bowl perimeters of any kind.

Once the best fixation method has been determined, testing of the field can begin. One of the oldest tests for central field defects is the tangent screen.

The Amsler grid is another method of investigating the central field. The test, when used as indicated in the instructions, is a qualitative test when investigating some central scotomas. However, slight modifications in the test will quantify the results and add precision to the test by making it more similar to a campime-

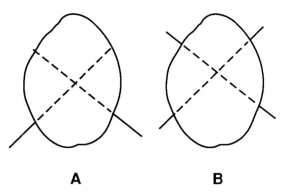

FIGURE 82–2. Schematic diagram showing (A) the incorrect use of an X for fixation for a central scotoma and (B) the correct fixation for a central scotoma, in which the equal extensions provide a control for constant fixation.

tric field study (Fig. 82–3). Rather than instructing the patient to indicate the area of scotoma in a qualitative fashion, the use of a 1-mm stimulus spot will allow specific location of the scotoma. The use of letters and numbers on the *x*- and *y*-axes of the grid enables the examiner to conveniently transfer the points at which the stimulus spot disappears. It is also helpful to reduce contrast of the lines of the Amsler grid so that the patient can notice the stimulus spot in a less-confusing field. This method permits the patient to use eccentric viewing to maintain fixation. However, it is not easy to measure the degree of eccentricity, but considering that the ultimate goal of the Amsler grid using this method is to measure the size of the central scotoma and not its position, the exact eccentric viewing position is not important.

One of the decisions to be made in plotting the peripheral fields for patients with central field defects is whether to use kinetic or static devices. Basically, the kinetic method is one in which the stimulus spot is moved in different parts of the field, recording

those areas where it is not seen. For each plot of the field, the intensity and size of the stimulus spot remains constant. Examples of instrumentation using the kinetic method are the Goldmann Perimeter or any of the arc-type perimeters.

The static method is one in which the stimulus spots have the same position and size, but are varied in intensity. Essentially, the patient responds to the intensity of the stimuli that are presented with single exposures in random fashion. The Humphrey Visual Field Analyzer allows some change in position of the stimulus spots in addition to changes in intensity and size.

Another aspect of the peripheral fields is the fixation spot. As discussed previously for the central fields, the fixation is equally important for the peripheral fields. Modification of the existing fixation spots for most of the static-type field devices is extremely difficult and may cause charges in the results. Most of these devices will record the deviations from fixation based on the position of the blind spot. This information is available after the plot has been completed and will indicate reliability of the field. Unfortunately, if the fixation is not sufficiently accurate, the visual field evaluation may have to be repeated.

Unquestionably, the arc-type perimeter allows the most inventiveness in designing fixation spots and measuring eccentric viewing for patients with a central field defect. The fixation spot can be designed with a cross using the same criteria described for the central field.

Diseases Involving Peripheral Field Defects

The innovative fixation methods are not as necessary for peripheral field defects as they are for diseases associated with central field defects. In most instances, the central visual acuity is better. For those cases of peripheral field loss that may be combined with a central field defect, the use of innovative fixation methods will enable a more accurate plotting of the field.

Generally, it is equally easy to plot constricted visual fields using a kinetic or static device. There are, however, some prob-

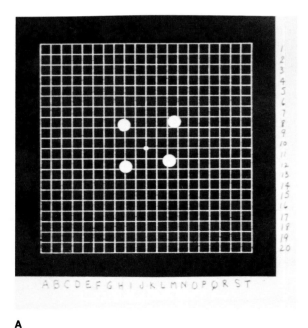

A

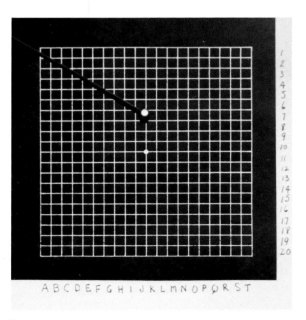

B

FIGURE 82–3. Suggested method to quantify the Amsler grid showing (A) the placement of fixation controls for a central scotoma and (B) a 1-mm stimulus spot with letters and numbers on the axes for easier recording.

lems with the static method. The static perimeters may lack sufficient stimulus points in the 5° to 8° central area to accurately plot a constricted visual field. Also, when dealing with extreme constrictions, it is important to know the changes of the field when the size and brightness of the stimulus spot are changed. This information will permit a judgment on the relative or absolute value of the field. These aspects cannot be changed with static field devices.

In addition, determining the exact dimensions of the central field is of major importance. The determination of whether an individual is "legally blind" due to visual fields or whether he or she has sufficient visual field to satisfy the Department of Motor Vehicle regulations for driving is important. This can be difficult to interpret from a static field result. A qualitative-type field such as one produced by a static field device is not sufficient in these instances, and these results are discouraged by many of the agencies requiring visual field information.

No Retinal Defects

Plotting the visual fields for defects, such as achromatopsia, albinism, and amblyopia, do not require any substantial modification of the visual field device. The anticipated results in these patients are full peripheral fields and normal blind spots with uncompromised surrounding areas, and testing of the field does not present any major difficulty. Some caution might be used on the size of the fixation spot if the distance visual acuity is poorer than 10/200. An increase in the size of the fixation spot or controlling the contrast might be of help.

Neurologic defects affecting the visual pathways may not have any associated retinal defect but may have very significant visual field changes. If there has been sparing of the macula, proper fixation can be achieved with existing fixation spots on the field device. However, when the macula has been affected, it will be necessary to provide fixation devices suitable for the defect. For hemianopias or any sector defect for which there is no macular fixation, the fixation spot must be contrived that will be large enough to fall within the seeing area. In kinetic-type devices, it may be possible to project off-center fixation areas into known seeing areas to permit control over fixation. In these devices or in static devices, it may be possible to use eccentric viewing to concentrate on the existing fixation device. In some patients, it may be possible to use a prism in front of the fixating eye to assist the off-axis fixation.

Techniques for Special Patients

It is often necessary to modify the field technique to accommodate the needs of some patients. Often the changes are very simple and relate to very basic needs.

Elderly

With the increasing aging population and the increasing incidence of age-related macular degeneration and glaucoma, we must face the problems of plotting visual fields in the elderly. One of the first things that must be done with the elderly before plotting of the visual field, is to be sure the patient understands the test. Often this will be the first time the patient has experienced visual field testing, and the patient will not have any "natural" understanding of the requirements of the test. A complete and repeated explanation of the fixation spot and the stimulus spot(s) will be necessary in a way that ensures understanding. It is helpful to avoid the use of such terms as "fixation spot" and "stimulus spot," unless the patient understands the terms. Instead, descriptions such as a "bouncing or floating ball" for a kinetic stimulus spot or "stars or twinkling lights" for static stimulus spots can be used.

By taking these precautions, the practitioner will avoid the problem of plotting a very constricted field, while expecting a full one, only to find that the patient thought it was necessary to respond when the kinetic stimulus spot, for example, was in the center of the field, rather than when it was first seen. It is helpful to use such phrases as "let me know as soon as you see this spot" or "when you have an inkling when you first see it coming in from the side, press the buzzer."

Another factor that must be assumed is that the elderly have some hearing loss. Speaking slowly, using a tone of voice slightly louder than normal conversation, and looking directly at the patient are very important aspects for giving instructions. It is inappropriate to give the initial instructions when the patient is positioned behind the instrument, particularly if the instrument is a bowl-type perimeter.

During the course of plotting the fields, it is necessary to reinforce and remind the patient of what is required. If the patient reports that the central fixation spot looks like a crystal, then periodically remind him or her to look at the "crystal" and press the buzzer when the "star" is seen as the test progresses.

Fatigue for the elderly is a very common factor. It is unreasonable to expect these patients to endure a field test without rest periods. Every field test should have several routine rest periods, whether or not the patient reports being tired.

Children

Patient cooperation is the primary need when attempting to test the visual fields of children in the early elementary school age. The results are frequently suspicious because of varying fixation and questionable subjective responses. Perhaps the best technique when using any of the static or kinetic instruments is to make the obvious resemblance to video games. Explaining the "basic rules" in these terms may help in performing the test successfully.

With younger children, this concept and the use of instrumentation does not apply. The use of variations of the confrontation field are very important in this age range. If central fixation can be achieved by having the patient look at the examiner, the use of a variety of stimulus objects can be used to determine sensitivity in the various areas of the peripheral field. Small toys, candies, pieces of breakfast foods, and small lights, all can be used. Often, the patient will respond by looking at the peripheral object. If the stimulus is introduced in that part of the field that is not sensitive, the patient will continue to fixate centrally. The use of this technique requires a great deal of practice to observe the patient's responses, but once the clinician becomes comfortable with the technique, the results will allow a very accurate *qualitative* assessment of the peripheral field. This technique will allow only the detection of depressions in the field, sector defects, or peripheral field constrictions. The amount of field defect cannot be quantified.

Another technique for judging the peripheral fields of young patients is observation of their play habits and their mobility. By having them look for coins or small toys scattered on the floor, considerable insight may be provided into their field patterns. Children with significant field constrictions will often have definite problems with mobility. Homonymous hemianopias will often be revealed as head turns and the avoidance and lack of detection of objects within the blind areas.

Multiply Handicapped Patients

Patient's who are deaf and who have visual impairments will usually not have any problems with the visual field if proper preparations are made before testing of the visual fields. The major factor is to be certain that the patient fully understands the requirements of the test before the patient is positioned behind the instrument. This requires demonstration of the fixation and stimulus spots as well as the method to respond to the stimuli. The patient should also be instructed how to stop the test for rest periods.

Depending upon the patient's abilities, instructions should be given by signing, large-print directions, or by lip reading. There should be no doubt that the patient fully understands the test.

When working with mental retardation, the patient's functional abilities must be considered very carefully. It is the basis upon which the testing procedure should be chosen. The techniques outlined for young children are often applicable to these patients. Generally, the use of any of the automated or bowl-type perimeters is contraindicated for the moderate to severe mentally retarded.

Some multiple problems are not sensory. Patients with physical handicaps, such as those who are restricted to wheel chairs or those with other physical limitations, may present a problem in positioning behind the instrument. On occasion, the patient may not be able to position himself squarely behind the instrument. These slight deviations of the patient's position may not pose a serious problem. However, when the patient's position results in an excessive distance from the fixation point or in a distorted position of the head, it may be best to abandon the peripheral field instrument and use the tangent screen for the central field as well as a precise confrontation field to investigate the peripheral field. To increase the precision of the confrontation field, a 3-mm bead at the end of a wand can be used as the stimulus spot. Portable, hand-held arc perimeters are available, which could also be used for the peripheral field.

The use of the portable, hand-held arc perimeters, refined confrontation tests, and the Amsler grid are very important for home-bound or nursing home patients when peripheral fields and central fields must be investigated. These devices are easily portable and generally adaptable to the home environment.

CLINICAL IMPLICATIONS

Clinical Interpretation

Central Field Defects

Eccentric viewing is a basic procedure that must be understood by all patients with a central scotoma. Most patients learn some form of eccentric viewing by trial and error, and many need reinforcement and support with the knowledge that this is an acceptable method to increase the quality of their vision. When eccentric viewing is not known or understood, it should be taught to the patient.

Central field defects also imply the probability of color vision defects. Reduction of the cone sensitivity will cause the color vision loss. The accurate recording and comparison of the patient's color vision can often be used as a barometer for the advancement of the scotoma.

The need to control illumination is also based upon the cone loss and the dependence upon scotopic vision. Careful attention to illumination must be given those patients who have age-related macular degeneration. Often, the older patient feels that if a little light is good, then a great deal of light is better. They, or other family members, may create problems by providing too much illumination.

The use of retinal magnification to improve the quality of vision is an obvious consideration for central field defects. Often the relationship between the size of the central scotoma and the peripheral field can indicate the success of retinal magnification.

Peripheral Field Defects

Illumination is a major consideration for patients with peripheral field constrictions. Because they lack rod function, these patients will need bright sources of illumination for work and home tasks, as well as mobility. However, attention must be given to glare situations, and tinted corrections must be considered to reduce the glare and flare. Attention must be given to the proper amount of absorption of the tinted correction, to be certain that the glare is reduced without causing the patient to use his reduced scotopic vision.

Field enhancement is another consideration for patients with visual field constrictions. It is a method to make patients with severe constrictions aware of more peripheral vision. A great deal of investigation has been done with Fresnel and spheroprisms, as well as other devices, to increase the sensitivity for more peripheral objects.[3–7]

No Field Defect

The major implication for visual fields when no defect is expected is the same as for any fully sighted patient. An indication of an abnormality in the visual field may be a potential cause for further loss of vision.

REFERENCES

1. Traquair HM. An introduction to clinical perimetry, 6th ed. St Louis: CV Mosby Co, 1949.
2. Haley MJ, ed. The field analyzer primer, 2nd ed. San Leandro: Allergan Humphrey, 1987.
3. Weiss NJ. Management of the low vision patient with peripheral field loss. J Am Optom Assoc 1969;40:830–832.
4. Weiss NJ. An application of cemented prism with severe field loss. Am J Optom 1972;49:261–264.
5. Mehr EB, Quillman RD. Field expansion by use of binocular full field reversed 1.3× telescopic spectacles: a case report. Am J Optom 1979; 56:446–449.
6. Jose RT, Smith AJ. Increasing peripheral awareness with Fresnel prisms. Opt J Rev Optom 1976;113:33–37.
7. Bailey IL. Prismatic treatment for field defects. Optom Monthly 1978; 69:1073–1078.

PART 7

Patient Care Decision Making and Reimbursement

Decision Making in Patient Care

J. Boyd Eskridge

INTRODUCTION

The essential duty and responsibility of the health care practitioner is to provide the appropriate management of patients with health care problems. This requires an appropriate patient care decision process, a method of coordinating information from the entire clinical examination to determine the appropriate management of the patient.

There are two basic health care decision-making processes involved in patient care. One is the process involved in determining the diagnosis of the patient's health care problems, and the second is the process involved in determining the management or treatment of the patient.

DIAGNOSTIC PROCESS

The diagnosis is a complete and thorough listing of all the patient's health care problems, and it is the key factor in the patient care decision process. The diagnostic process consists of developing a tentative diagnosis from the patient's history and observation, and then collecting the clinical data needed to confirm the tentative diagnosis, or developing another tentative diagnosis and repeating the cycle (Table 83–1).

The patient history is the beginning of the diagnostic process and must include the biological, psychological, and genetic aspects of the patient. The patient needs to be considered as an individual, and the personal and family health care problems, and the personal, vocational, and avocational needs and problems determined. The information obtained from the patient history can be very significant and meaningful in the diagnostic process. To be so, the clinician must know the clinical features of disease—the epidemiology, the symptoms, and signs that are highly specific for certain diseases, and other clues of distinguishing value. The his-

tory should lead to an early tentative diagnostic hypothesis that can be tested by more appropriate questions. Great skill, experience, and knowledge is often necessary to clarify the patient's symptoms and to organize questions that focus on the tentative diagnostic hypothesis.

The next phase is the selection of the appropriate clinical testing procedures and the proper evaluation of the obtained clinical data to verify or modify the tentative diagnosis. The selection of clinical testing is a function of two things: first, the selection of tests to verify the tentative diagnosis, and second, the selection of testing procedures needed to fulfill the professional responsibility and duty as a health care practitioner and primary vision and ocular health care provider. Data collection and information gathering need to use the problem-solving approach and be diagnosis oriented. The clinical data that have strong distinguishing values and that are needed to confirm or reject the tentative diagnosis— the specific and sensitive clinical data—are the most effective and critical data to obtain. Test selection is based on experience and knowledge of visual and ocular anomalies and disease. However, clinical data need to be reliable and consistent before they can be effectively used in clinical decision making. Data collection needs to terminate when it ceases to provide significant clinical direction and information.

Decisions will have to be made at certain points in the data-collection process, and checked with logical scientific understanding and knowledge. The diagnostic decision is often made with some level of uncertainty, because diagnostic certainty seldom achieves a 100% level of confidence because of ambiguous, confusing, and conflicting data. One must also consider that more than one clinical problem may be present.

The patient care decision process is concerned not only with doing those tests and procedures that will lead to a solution of the patient's stated problems and symptoms and to confirm the tentative diagnosis, but it must also include those clinical tests that

Table 83–1
The Diagnostic Process

1. Develop a tentative probable diagnosis from the patient's history and observation
2. Collect the most appropriate clinical data to confirm or reject the tentative diagnosis
3. Confirm the clinical diagnosis or develop another tentative diagnosis and repeat the cycle

are necessary to detect other anomalies that may have few or no symptoms, or to detect problems that have a low prevalence but a high risk of severe consequences. The primary vision and ocular health care provider should be able to answer the following questions at the end of the clinical examination:

1. Does this patient have any general health problems that I should have detected?
2. Does this patient have any ocular health problems?
3. Does this patient have any ocular motility problems?
4. Does this patient have any refractive anomalies?
5. Does this patient have any visual sensory or fusion problems?
6. Does this patient have any visual performance problems?

The practitioner must obtain and evaluate the data necessary to answer these questions, even though a tentative diagnosis has been selected. The practitioner must focus on the clinical data that will verify or reject the tentative or presumed diagnosis, but still be attentive and open-minded to other clinical data that may suggest other anomalies or an alternative diagnosis. This concept will assist the practitioner in the selection of the tests and clinical procedures needed and in the formulation of the sequence of the testing.

A statement of the diagnosis and the listing of all the specific problems are needed by the practitioner to formulate appropriate management and treatment procedures. The diagnostic statement also has another function in this age of third-party systems: it determines which health care services will be reimbursed and which will not.

MANAGEMENT PROCESS

Once the diagnosis is determined, the management process can begin. The diagnosis is the key factor in the management process, but two other factors must be considered—the patient character and the prognosis.

Patient Character

Before a patient can be successfully treated, it is necessary to know more than the name of the anomaly or disease. It is necessary to know the patient, what is bothering the patient, what the patient is really complaining about, what kind of person the patient is, and what are the ways that the problem(s) are disturbing this patient. We are dealing with humans, not machines. People are different physically, mentally, and emotionally. We can run through a diagnostic sequence on a machine, detect and diagnose the problem, and know what to do. We can run through a diagnostic sequence on the visual and ocular system of a patient and arrive at a diagnosis, but we must remember that the visual system is a part of a living vibrant being—and the patient's symptoms, age, mental capacity, personality, attitudes, genetic background, character, and other health problems must be considered in the selection of the recommended therapy. We must also realize that the symptoms

may be associated with the disease, or they may be fabricated. To be successful we must treat the patient, not just the anomaly. Once the diagnosis is made, we sometimes forget the patient and treat the problem or disease. What are the patient's needs and desires for visual health and performance, and how hard will the patient work to achieve them? Lack of patient compliance is a critical factor in health care and must be considered. We must also realize that we can change the diagnosis without changing the patient's symptoms or attitudes, and we can change the patient's symptoms and attitudes without changing the diagnosis.

Prognosis

Before the recommended management or treatment procedures can be selected, the prognosis of each specific clinical problem for the specific patient and the involved practitioner must be considered. The practitioner needs to ask, "What is my success rate for each specific clinical problem with this particular patient type?" The prognosis becomes more complicated when several problems or anomalies are present in the same patient. On the basis of this information, the prognosis for each clinical problem can be determined (good or poor) and used in patient care decision making.

Recommended Management

This is a statement of the treatment procedure(s) recommended for each specific problem. Careful consideration must also be given to any possible deleterious or beneficial effects of the treatment of one problem on the treatment of the other problems, and what other treatment-induced problems could result. The recommended treatment may then require modification.

This portion of the process also includes a consideration of the need for patient education. Patient education is an important aspect of health care. The patient needs to be informed and involved to promote patient compliance with therapy. To be effective, the practitioner must develop good rapport with the patient. The patient needs to feel that the practitioner cares. The development of a positive patient–doctor relationship is vital. Patient education of the problem and the involved treatment procedure, and continued patient reassurance is necessary for appropriate health care delivery.

The recording of patient care information generally follows the SOAP outline:

S (Subjective) This contains the symptoms, complaints, observations of the patient or the patient's family.

O (Objective) This contains the current and appropriate clinical or laboratory data of the patient.

A (Assessment) This contains the present assessment, evaluation, and prognosis of the patient's problem.

P (Plan) This is a statement of the current recommended therapeutic procedures, any further diagnostic testing needed, and the pertinent patient education.

PROGRESS EVALUATION

Progress evaluation is a follow-up evaluation of the patient to ascertain the effectiveness of the management. The same diagnostic and management process is utilized.

REFERENCES

1. Albert DA, Munson R, Resnick MD. Reasoning in medicine: an introduction to clinical inference. Baltimore: Johns Hopkins University Press, 1988.

2. Amos JF. Diagnosis and management in vision care. Boston: Butterworth Publishers, 1987:Chap 1.
3. Balla JI. The diagnostic process. Cambridge: Cambridge University Press, 1985.
4. Gale J, Marsden P. The role of the routine clinical history. Med Educ 1984;18:96–100.
5. Hurst JW, Walker HK. Problem-oriented system. New York: Medcom Press, 1972.
6. Lipkin M, Rogers DE. The care of patients. New Haven: Yale University Press. 1982: Chap 3.
7. Lusted LB. Introduction to medical decision making. Springfield, Ill: Charles C Thomas, 1968.
8. Weed LL. Medical records, medical education and patient care. Cleveland: Case Western Reserve University Press, 1969.
9. Weinstein MC, Fineberg HV. Clinical decision analysis. Philadelphia: WB Saunders Co, 1980.
10. Werner DL. Teaching clinical thinking. Optom Vis Sci 1989;66:788–792.
11. Wueff HR. Rational diagnosis and treatment. Oxford: Blackwell Scientific Publications, 1981.

Reimbursement

Adam Gordon

INTRODUCTION

At first glance, a chapter on reimbursement mechanisms in a book devoted to clinical procedures might seem out of place. After all, the intricacies of Medicare, Medicaid, Blue Cross/Blue Shield, managed care systems, and vision plans seem more appropriate for practice management publications than a text such as this. There are, however, compelling reasons why a discussion on reimbursement is not only appropriate, but essential, in an optometric procedures book.

What are these compelling reasons?

1. A large proportion of patients have some form of health insurance that often covers optometric care. Optometrists are often surprised to learn that many routine procedures, as well as more specialized procedures, are covered expenses under their patients' insurance plans. Different types of insurance plans cover different types of services, so knowledge of various plans is important.
2. Many experts in medicine and optometry predict that private fee-for-service income will progressively diminish to near extinction in the not-too-distant future.[1,2] Private practice physicians currently receive two-thirds of their gross income from third-party insurance plans. Ophthalmologists receive 53% of gross income from third-party plans, with Medicare payments alone providing 25% of income.[3] The various forces currently shaping medical care will very likely impact on optometry in coming years.
3. Insurance serves to remove or minimize the financial barrier to health care.[4] A patient requiring frequent monitoring and testing, as with glaucoma or diabetes, for example, is more likely to return for necessary care if it is known that all or part of the cost is covered by insurance. Thus, insurance helps improve patient compliance and indirectly improves the quality of care. The patient receives the necessary procedures or treatments that otherwise may not be performed if cost were an obstacle.
4. Health insurance is expensive and most adults are aware of the premium they pay for health coverage. Helping patients obtain their insurance benefit, therefore, is a valuable service that is greatly appreciated.
5. Practitioners knowledgeable about insurance coverage of optometric services have a distinct advantage in attracting and retaining patients. Given the choice between two identical optometry practices, patients will choose to receive care from the office where the doctor and staff are knowledgeable about insurance and help them obtain the insurance benefit in an efficient manner.

Once the clinical implications of the preceding statements are understood, the value of optometric participation in the health insurance system becomes obvious. As optometry has evolved into the primary provider of eye care services, the profession's involvement with third-party systems has greatly increased.

This chapter will provide an overview of the insurance system and detail how and when optometric care fits into the system. By necessity, the information is presented on a generic level due to the tremendous diversity of insurance plans. The goal is to provide a working knowledge of the insurance system to those with little or no prior exposure to third-party mechanisms. A working knowledge of the insurance system, along with expertise in the procedures covered throughout this book, will enable the clinician to provide high-quality, comprehensive optometric care.

OVERVIEW OF HEALTH INSURANCE SYSTEM

Insurance to cover the cost of unforeseen medical expenses originated in this country in 1847, but did not achieve notable popularity until the 1930s. Over the ensuring 50 years, health insurance gained widespread acceptance and coverage now exists for nearly every medical service.[5]

Health insurance may be broadly defined as protection against the costs of health care arising from illness or injury.[6] Individuals contract with an insurer who agrees to pay for certain services, under certain conditions, for a specified cost. The contractual agreement may be with individuals or with groups such as employees of large corporations, labor unions, and professional associations. When an approved claim is submitted, the insurer may reimburse the subscriber for out-of-pocket costs (indemnity benefit) or directly pay the provider of services such as a doctor or hospital (service benefit). With many people regularly paying premiums and a fairly predictable number filing claims, the risk of expense is shared among all the policyholders.[7]

In 1987, more than 205 million Americans, or 86% of the civilian population, had some form of private (nongovernmental) health insurance. This included over 181 million persons under age 65, or nearly 80% of this group.[8] Private health insurance is offered through over 1200 commercial insurance companies, 78 Blue Cross and Blue Shield plans, and about 600 other independent organizations including Health Maintenance Organizations (HMOs) and Preferred Provider Organizations (PPOs). In addition to private insurance, health care services are provided in a variety of public programs through federal, state, and local government. Over 207 billion dollars, or 41% of the entire national health expenditure, was spent in 1987 for health and medical care programs at all levels of government.[8] Public health programs are supported by tax revenue and are generally targeted toward six major groups: low-income individuals (Medicaid), those 65 years and older (Medicare), military personnel and their dependents (CHAMPUS), veterans (VA), federal civilian employees, and native Americans (IHS).[8]

The majority of private health insurance policies are group policies covering persons (and their dependents) sharing common employment or group membership. Group insurance is generally more comprehensive and less expensive than comparable individual policies, and employers often pay part of the premium as a benefit of employment. The portion of the premium paid by the employee is obtained by payroll deduction. The covered individual under a group plan is a subscriber, not a policyholder, and retains a certificate, not a policy. The employer or group is the insured entity.[9]

Although tremendous variation exists in the type and extent of coverage, most health insurance plans consist of four basic benefits.[6]

1. Hospital benefits, covering hospital bills for room and board.
2. Surgical benefits, covering the surgeon's fees and related care.
3. Medical benefits, covering nonsurgical physician fees both in and out of the hospital.
4. Major medical benefits, covering a broad range of services supplementing the foregoing, both in and out of the hospital. These may include medications, medical equipment, special nursing care, care for catastrophic illness, and other expenses.

A second type of major medical plan exists, called "comprehensive" major medical. Unlike the "supplemental" type, comprehensive major medical provides both basic (hospital–surgical–medical) and extended coverage integrated into one policy. This latter type of policy has become very popular in recent years and now accounts for most group major medical policies. As a result, the term "major medical" is often used synonymously with "medical" and "health" insurance.[4]

Virtually all health insurance plans have cost-sharing stipulations in addition to the premium. These include deductibles, co-

Table 84–1
Common Insurance Terms

Term	Definition
Premium	Periodic payment (usually monthly) to keep an insurance policy in force.
Deductible	Amount the insured must pay out-of-pocket before the policy benefits begin.
Copayment	Amount the insured must pay for a unit of service; the insurance pays the remainder. Example: $15 copayment per office visit.
Coinsurance	A percentage of the cost of services that the insured must pay; the insurance pays the remaining percentage. Example: insurance pays 80% of costs after deductible is met. The insured pays 20% coinsurance.

payments, coinsurance, and limitations ("ceilings" or "caps") on benefits. These terms are defined in Table 84–1.

COVERAGE OF OPTOMETRIC SERVICES[4,10]

An important feature of traditional private health insurance policies is that they specifically exclude routine and preventive care and cover only "medically necessary" care related to illness or injury. Thus, routine eye examinations and corrective eyewear, as well as annual physicals, immunizations, cosmetic surgery, dental care, and such are not covered expenses.

Although routine eye care and ophthalmic materials are typically excluded from coverage, many optometric services are nonetheless covered expenses. The key to determining whether the examination and related services are covered is the diagnosis. Refractive conditions (myopia, hyperopia, astigmatism, and presbyopia) are not considered "medical" diagnoses by the insurance industry, since they do not result from disease or injury. Examinations and treatments for refractive conditions are considered "routine" and, hence, are not covered.

When eye diseases or injuries are diagnosed, the examinations, diagnostic procedures, and treatments are covered expenses. Thus, for example, when the diagnosis is cataract, conjunctivitis, strabismus, or diabetic retinopathy, the examination fees are covered expenses. Any additional tests, procedures, or treatments that are medically necessary for the diagnosed condition are covered expenses as well. Such procedures include progress examinations, visual fields, ocular photography, gonioscopy, binocular vision evaluation, smears, and cultures, among others.

The coverage of medically necessary eye care by private health insurance essentially rewards the practitioner for diagnosing and managing medical eye conditions. In other words, these insurance policies promote primary eye care practice by optometrists! It goes without saying that insurance companies cover only those services that are within the legal scope of optometry in each particular state.

A second type of insurance covering optometric services is the vision plan. Vision plans, also known as "eyeglass" or "optical" plans, specifically cover routine eye examinations and corrective eyewear at specified intervals. In contrast, medical plans cover only medically necessary services for eye disease or injury. Again, the diagnosis (refractive versus medical) determines the applicability of insurance coverage (Fig. 84–1). If a refractive condition is diagnosed and the patient has a vision plan, the examination is covered, and many plans offer coverage or a discount on eyeglasses or contact lenses. If a patient has vision coverage, but requires more frequent monitoring or further diagnostic evaluation

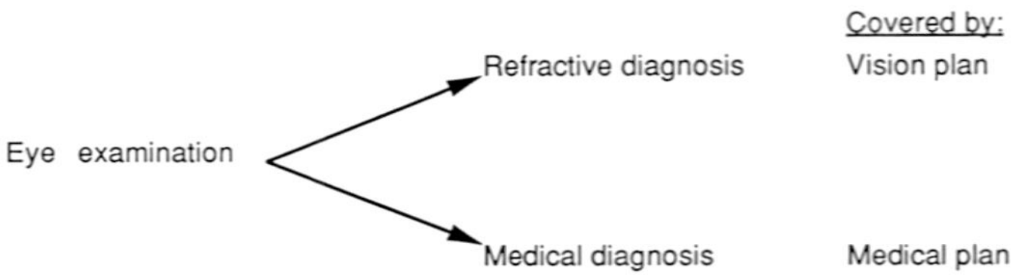

FIGURE 84–1. Diagnosis determines type of insurance coverage. (From Gordon A, Crooks CT. Optometric services and private health insurance. J Am Optom Assoc 1988;59:62–70, with permission)

for a medical eye condition, the vision plan will not pay for these services. The patient will have to pay out-of-pocket for the needed care unless he or she has medical insurance coverage. In some cases a person may have both medical insurance and vision care insurance. This individual would be covered for both routine eye care and medical eye care.

Optometrists are generally not excluded from providing covered services under private health plans. All 50 states and the District of Columbia have enacted "freedom-of-choice" laws that apply to private insurance carriers under the state insurance codes. These laws allow insured patients to select the provider of their choice for covered services, providing the practitioner is legally licensed to perform such a service. Optometrists are often defined a "physicians" for insurance purposes and, therefore, may perform physician services, as long as those services are within the state-defined scope of practice.

Some insurance plans may not be subject to freedom-of-choice laws, such as those falling under the Employee Retirement Income Security Act (ERISA). The original purpose ERISA was to protect employee pension rights, but the interpretation has now been expanded to allow large companies to self-insure and customize employee benefits. By self-insuring employee health care, a company can avoid paying premium taxes and circumvent state insurance codes and freedom-of-choice laws. Benefit plans under ERISA may have closed provider panels or different reimbursement schedules for optometrists and ophthalmologists. Private health maintenance organizations (HMOs) and preferred provider organizations (PPOs) controlled by physicians or other groups, may also form closed provider panels that exclude optometrists or limit optometric involvement to refractive and optical services. The extent to which ERISA supercedes state freedom-of-choice laws is not now clear and requires further legal clarification.

SPECIFIC INSURANCE PLANS

The preceding discussion considered two general types of insurance plans encountered by optometrists: Medical (or health or major medical) plans and vision (or eyeglass or optical) plans. For

eye care, it is possible to classify all insurance plans with these two broad categories. Some plans may have characteristics of both medical and vision plans. Medicare, for example, is a medical plan, but offers an optical benefit to aphakic patients. Some health maintenance organizations and Medicaid programs are essentially vision plans, but medical eye care is also allowed under certain conditions.

Although insurance plans differ widely on covered benefits, restrictions and cost-sharing mechanisms, it is still valuable to describe commonly encountered plans in greater detail from the eye care perspective. The major characteristics of these plans are summarized in Table 84–2.

Private Insurance Companies

Over 1200 private (commercial) insurance companies issued health insurance policies covering over 100 million people in 1985.[8] Nearly 70% of the policies issued were group policies. Major companies (or carriers) include Prudential, Equitable, Aetna, Metropolitan, and Connecticut General.

Private insurance policies provide an indemnity benefit, by which the insured is reimbursed for medical expenses according to a fixed-rate schedule. A covered patient pays the physician's fees out-of-pocket and must submit a claim to the insurance company for reimbursement. The patient also has the option to assign the insurance payment directly to the physician, if the physician agrees to "accept assignment."

The insurance payment may be less than the actual charges because of unmet deductible, coinsurance, or low reimbursement schedules. If the physician has agreed to accept assignment, he or she may then bill the patient for the remainder of the charges. If the details of the policy are known in advance, the patient may be charged for the coinsurance, noncovered services, and such, at the time of service. The chain of events associated with accepting or not accepting assignment is diagrammed in Figure 84–2.

Blue Cross and Blue Shield

"The Blues" are independent, nonprofit tax-exempt corporations providing coverage for health care services. In general, Blue Cross plans cover hospital expenses, whereas Blue Shield plans cover physician services. In 1986, there were 13 Blue Cross plans, 15 Blue Shield plans, and 50 joint Blue Cross/Blue Shield plans in the United States.[8] The Blue Shield plans developed through the efforts of state and local medical societies who helped pass state legislation that provided the authority and regulatory mechanisms. Unlike commercial insurance companies, the various Blue plans do not compete with each other so there is no overlapping of geographic areas.

Table 84–2
Characteristics of Common Insurance Plans

	Routine Examinations (refractive diagnosis)	Pathology Examinations (medical diagnosis)	Ophthalmic Materials (spectacles/contact lenses)
Vision plans	Yes	No	Yes
Medical plans	No	Yes	No
Medicare	No	Yes	Only after cataract surgery
Medicaid	Children under 21: yes Adults: varies	Yes	Varies
HMO/PPO	Generally yes	Yes	Varies

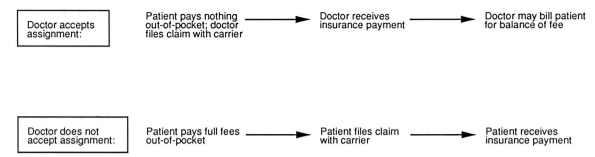

FIGURE 84–2. Assignment flow chart for private indemnity plans.

Blue Cross/Blue Shield plans pioneered the use of service benefits, whereby the provider of services (physician or hospital) receives the insurance payment rather than the insured patient.[5] This requires a contract between Blue Cross/Blue Shield and doctors wishing to participate in the plan. Participating physicians agree to accept payment according to the conditions of the contract. With most Blue plans, one must agree to accept the assigned payment as payment in full, although copayments or coinsurance may be required of the patient. If a patient with Blue Cross/Blue Shield coverage is examined by a nonparticipating physician, the claim is handled in the same manner as a commercial indemnity insurance plan.

The majority of Blue Cross/Blue shield plans reimburse physicians based on the "usual, customary, and reasonable" (UCR) system. The "usual" fee is the fee normally charged for a given service by an individual physician. If a physician's fee for a procedure varies over a given time frame, a percentile of the range is chosen (typically the 75th percentile). The "customary" fee is a percentile (usually the 90th percentile) of the usual fees charged by all doctors of the same specialty in a given area for each procedure. The "reasonable" fee or approved fee is the lowest of the usual charge, the customary charge, or the physician's submitted charge.[3,11] These fee profiles are typically collected over a 12-month period and another 12–24 months is often required to update and implement the next schedule. Thus, reimbursement under the UCR system is based upon retrospective analysis of charges submitted one to two years earlier!

Although Blue Cross/Blue Shield plans provide coverage for hospital and medical care, vision plans have recently been added to their menu of insurance products. As discussed earlier, vision plans cover routine eye examinations (including refractions) and corrective eye wear at certain intervals. The UCR mechanism is used for professional services and participating physicians accept the UCR amount as full payment. For ophthalmic materials, Blue Cross/Blue Shield usually pays on a fee-schedule basis. In some cases, the physician may charge the patient for ophthalmic material fees above the insurance payment.[11]

Medicare

Medicare is a federal health insurance program for persons 65 years of age or older and for certain disabled persons under age 65. The program is administered by the Health Care Financing Administration (HCFA) within the Social Security Administration. In 1987, over 32 million people were covered by Medicare at a cost of nearly 80 billion dollars to the federal government.[8]

The program consists of two parts: Part A is hospitalization insurance and Part B is supplementary medical insurance. An individual receives Part A hospital insurance automatically upon qualifying for Medicare. Part A is financed by employer and employee contributions from wages earned during a person's working years

(FICA taxes). Part B medical insurance is strictly voluntary and is financed by the federal government and by monthly premiums from those who enroll. The government pays about 2/3 of the actual premium cost, making Part B coverage a very attractive benefit. Individuals can arrange to have the premium deducted from their monthly Social Security check.[9]

The attainment of optometric recognition under Medicare in 1987 was a major milestone in optometric history. From its inception in 1966, only ophthalmologists could receive Medicare payment for covered services, even though optometrists were qualified to perform many of the same services. Between 1966 and 1986, optometrists lost a significant portion of their older patient population to ophthalmologists. Since many eye diseases are age-related, many of these Medicare patients could receive covered eye care from ophthalmologists, but not from optometrists. The American Optometric Association (AOA) made Medicare inclusion its top legislative priority. A partial victory was achieved in 1981 when optometrists were allowed to provide care for aphakic patients only. In 1986, the AOA was successful in having the Medicare law amended to allow optometrists full recognition and reimbursement for covered services.

For eye care, Medicare Part B is strictly a medical plan covering medically necessary services for the diagnosis and treatment of eye disease and injury. Routine eye care for refractive conditions is specifically excluded. Even when a medical eye diagnosis is made, Medicare will not cover the refractive portion of the examination. Refraction is considered a "noncovered service" for which the patient is responsible for paying.[12,13]

Part B of Medicare, which applies to optometric services, currently has a $75 deductible each calendar year. After the deductible has been paid, Medicare pays 80% of the approved charges for covered services. The patient must pay the annual deductible, the 20% coinsurance for covered services, and all fees for noncovered services, such as refraction (Table 84–3).

Medicare reimbursement is based on a retrospective fee analysis system known as the "customary, prevailing, and reasonable" (CPR) system. The CPR system is similar to the Blue Cross/Blue Shield UCR system discussed previously. The Medicare approved (or reasonable) charge is the lowest of the physician's "customary" charge, the "prevailing" community charge, or the submitted charge. The customary charge is the usual charge for a given service by a physician. If the customary charge for a service varies, the median (50th percentile) is used as the customary charge. The locality prevailing charge is the 75th percentile of the customary fees charged by all physicians of the same speciality in a given area for the procedure. Just as with Blue Shield UCR plans, the fees charged by all physicians or optometrists in a given area influence the Medicare reimbursement for that area. The prevailing charge for each service is recalculated each year, but annual increases are limited by the Medicare Economic Index to an amount that reflects the inflation rate.[11,14]

One should note that the Medicare customary charge has a

Table 84-3
Reimbursement Under Medicare

Medicare Pays:	Patient Pays:

80% of approved charges:
  Medically-necessary services
    (must have medical diagnosis)
  Spectacles and contact lenses
    following cataract surgery
	Annual deductible
	20% of approved charges
	All noncovered services:
	  Refraction, if performed
	  Routine eye examinations (no medical diagnosis)
	  Spectacles and contact lenses (phakic eye correction)
	  "Deluxe" frame charges, tints, coatings, and other lens
	    options (following cataract surgery)

different meaning than the Blue Cross/Blue Shield customary charge discussed in the previous section. The customary charge under Medicare is analogous to the Blue Cross/Blue Shield usual charge, and the Medicare prevailing charge is similar to the Blue Cross/Blue Shield customary charge. A comparison of reimbursement terminology is presented in Table 84-4.

The federal government contracts with commercial insurance companies or Blue Cross/Blue Shield organizations to administer the Medicare program throughout the United States. These carriers receive and process local Medicare claims and are given substantial autonomy in interpreting rules and regulations. As a result, there are regional differences in coding and processing Medicare claims.

Eyeglasses and contact lenses are also excluded (noncovered) services unless the patient has had cataract surgery. Medicare will cover spectacles and contact lenses only for aphakic or pseudophakic patients. If a patient is unilaterally aphakic (or pseudophakic), only the lens for the involved eye is covered. (A spectacle frame is still covered in a unilateral case.) For eligible patients, Medicare covers a basic frame and lenses. Options such as "deluxe" frames, tints, antireflection or scratch-resistant coatings, and photochromic lenses are excluded as well.

Each doctor must choose to either participate and accept Medicare assignment as full payment, or not to participate (Fig. 84-3). Nonparticipating physicians charge patients their usual fees, and submit an unassigned claim allowing the patient to receive the Medicare reimbursement. Nonparticipating physicians also have the option to accept Medicare assignment on a case-by-case basis. In an effort to reduce Medicare expenditures, the government recently imposed a "maximum allowable actual charge" (MAAC) on nonparticipating physicians. If a nonparticipating physician's fees exceed his or her MAAC on a Medicare patient, that physician will be forced to refund the balance to the patient and possibly be subject to penalties. By using MAACs, differential fee increases, and other mechanisms, the government is trying to convince all physicians to become participating providers for Medicare. In 1990,

44% of all physicians (MD and DO) are participating Medicare providers. Optometry and ophthalmology have approximately equal participation rates of 54% and 56%, respectively.[15]

Over half of Medicare recipients purchase private insurance policies to supplement Medicare benefits. Such "Medigap" insurance covers the 20% coinsurance not paid by Medicare, and some policies provide full or partial coverage for the deductible. If a Medicare beneficiary retains their pre-Medicare insurance, this coverage coordinates with Medicare and becomes secondary insurance. Like Medicare supplement plans, secondary insurance pays the coinsurance and sometimes the deductible. In many cases, Medicare carriers can automatically forward the claim directly to the supplementary or secondary company, saving both the practitioner and patient time and effort.

In response to rapidly escalating Medicare expenditures for Part B physician services, government policymakers have been seeking alternatives to the current method of physician payment. The CPR method has been criticized as being inflationary, inequitable, complex, and distorted. Beginning in 1992, a new Medicare fee schedule will be implemented that is based upon a Resource-Based Relative Value Scale (RBRVS). Unlike existing fee schedules that are based on actual physician charges, the RBRVS uses "physician resource inputs" to determine relative values for services and procedures. These input factors include (1) the work involved for services or procedures, including the time and intensity involved before, during, and after the service; (2) practice costs (including malpractice premiums); and (3) the opportunity cost of postgraduate training required to become a qualified specialist.[16,17]

The development of RBRVS did not include data for optometrists or other nonphysician "limited license" professionals. At the time of this writing, it is not known whether optometric Medicare reimbursement will be governed by the same formula used for ophthalmology. Once the new Medicare system is fully implemented, it is likely that other third-party payers (both governmental and nongovernmental) will adopt similar reimbursement schedules.

Table 84-4
Comparison of Reimbursement Terminology: Blue Shield vs Medicare

Description	Blue Shield		Medicare Part B	
	Term	Percentile	Term	Percentile
Charges by individual doctor	Usual	75th	Customary	50th
Charges by all doctors of same specialty and in same area	Customary	90th	Prevailing	75th

(Adapted from Cooper MG, Cooper DE. The medical assistant. New York: McGraw-Hill Book Co., 1986)

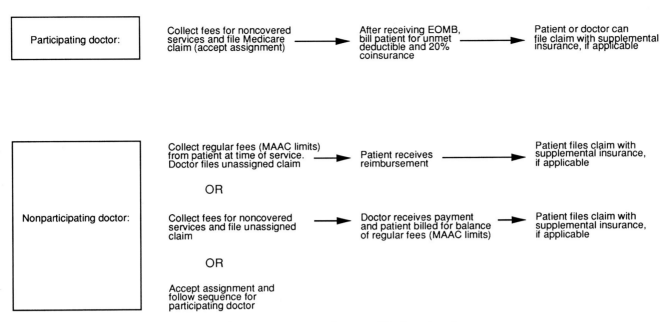

FIGURE 84–3. Flow chart for Medicare reimbursement. EOMB, explanation of Medicare benefits.

Medicaid

Medicaid is a medical assistance program for certain low-income individuals and families. The program is financed jointly by federal and state funds, with the federal contribution roughly related to each state's per capita income. Each state administers its own program within general guidelines specified by the federal government. Eligibility criteria and certain optional services vary widely among individual states. Arizona is currently the only state that does not have a Medicaid program.

In general, medical assistance is available to those receiving public assistance (welfare) payments such as Supplemental Security Income or Aid to Families with Dependent Children. Some states extend Medicaid eligibility to the "medically needy," meaning those who cannot pay their medical expenses, but are otherwise self-sufficient. In 1987 the Medicaid program covered nearly 23 million people and paid 45 billion dollars in benefits.[8]

Mandatory services provided by each state include inpatient and outpatient hospital services; laboratory and x-ray services; physician services; skilled nursing home services; home health services; family-planning services; and early and periodic screening, diagnosis, and treatment (EPSDT) for children under 21. Optional services offered by some states include prescription medications, dental care, and routine vision care, among others.[8]

Although routine vision care for adults is an optional service, vision care for children under aged 21 is mandated under the EPSDT program.[18] Under this program, each state must provide diagnostic services for physical and mental defects, health care treatments, and "other measures to correct or ameliorate defects and chronic conditions discovered."[19] Within the EPSDT program, however, each state again varies in the depth and frequency of vision and eye services provided. If a Medicaid recipient requires medical (nonroutine) eye care services, prior authorization is often necessary before the services or procedures are performed.

According to federal requirements, patients must present their Medicaid identification card at every visit to a provider's office. The Medicaid cards are issued monthly and prove eligibility for benefits for that month. If a patient cannot produce a current card, they are personally responsible for paying the bill. Physicians must agree to accept Medicaid reimbursement as full payment, realizing the Medicaid payment will be substantially less than their actual charges.[11]

Many elderly patients have coverage with both Medicaid and Medicare. If a medical diagnosis is made, the claim should be filed with Medicare first. The Medicare carrier will automatically forward the claim to the Medicaid agency. Medicaid, in this situation, serves as secondary insurance and pays the Medicare deductible and coinsurance (see previous section on Medicare). After receiving remittance notices from Medicare and Medicaid, the practitioner can file the refraction charge (a noncovered charge under Medicare) with Medicaid for reimbursement. If the examination results in a refractive diagnosis (routine examination), the claim can be filed directly with the Medicaid agency. Because of variation between state programs, the specific procedures for filing claims should be obtained from the state Medicaid agency.

Workers' Compensation

Workers' Compensation is insurance covering medical expenses and disability benefits for individuals with employment-related injuries or illnesses. All employers with more than a specified number of employees (according to state law) are required to have this insurance with the carrier of their choice. A special claim form is designed by each state, and claims are filed with the insurance company.

Before an injured employee sees a physician, the employer must authorize treatment. The patient may present a written report of the injury with authorization or the employer may telephone the physician before the visit. If no employer notification is received, the physician must determine if the problem was work-related. If so, the bills are sent to the employer's insurance company and not to the patient or the patient's insurance. (This is the reason all insurance claim forms ask if the patient's problem is work-related). The physician is required to send an initial report to the employer and subsequent reports as long as treatment or follow-up continues.[3,11]

Each state establishes the fee schedule for medical services and physicians are paid by the employer's insurance carrier. There may be special procedure codes required by the state in Workers'

Compensation cases. Specific information can be obtained from each state's Director of Workers' Compensation.

Alternative Delivery Systems

Because of rapidly escalating health care costs, the nation's health care system is in a state of transition. The federal government, insurance companies, hospitals, and large employers are all trying to control spiraling costs by imposing tighter controls on the utilization and delivery of health care services.

The traditional system for most Americans is based upon freedom-of-choice and fee-for-service. When an individual wishes to see a physician, he or she may see any physician they want, and that physician charges a fee for services rendered. If the patient has traditional indemnity insurance, a claim is filed, and the insurance company pays the bill. It is obvious that the traditional system simply rewards physicians for providing services: the more services performed, the greater the financial reward. It is also clear that the health care delivery system (physicians and hospitals) is entirely separate from the bill-paying system (insurance companies).[20]

Alternative delivery systems such as HMOs and PPOs are designed to control costs by integrating the delivery and the financing of health care within a single organization. Common cost-containment mechanisms include limiting the choice of providers, using reduced fee schedules or capitation payments, restricting hospital use and referrals to specialists, and strict utilization and peer review processes.

The growth of alternative delivery systems (also called *managed care plans*) has been quite remarkable. Between 1971 and 1987, the number of HMOs increased from 33 to 653, and the number of subscribers grew from 3.6 million to 30 million.[8] By the year 2000, over 50% of the United States population may be enrolled in an HMO. The Blue Cross/Blue Shield Association predicted that 85% of their 72 million enrollees will be in managed care programs by 1990.[21]

The implication for all health care providers is clear: participate in managed care plans with all their restrictions and reduced reimbursement, or potentially lose access to an ever-increasing patient population. Physicians, optometrists, and dentists may be salaried employees of free-standing staff-model HMOs or contract with the more popular individual practice association (IPA) HMOs. With the IPA arrangement, the doctor sees HMO patients in his or her own office, along with regular (non-HMO) patients. Although IPAs are certainly favored by private practitioners, they still greatly restrict practitioner autonomy. The majority make use of the "gate-keeper" concept, by which each patient has direct access to a personal physician who is responsible for coordinating all aspects of the patient's health care. The patient's gate-keeper is usually a primary care physician such as an internist or family practitioner. This individual decides whether the patient is admitted to a hospital, has advanced diagnostic or laboratory testing performed, or sees a specialist for care.[3]

Many IPAs allow free patient access to participating optometrists for routine eye care, such as a comprehensive eye examination and eyeglasses every 2 years. For nonroutine or medical eye care, the optometrist must seek approval from the patient's gate-keeper physician before providing the care. The gate-keeper may approve or deny the request, in which case the HMO will not reimburse the optometrist for the services (Fig. 84–4). In some plans, optometrists are limited to providing routine vision care only, whereas medical and surgical eye care is performed by ophthalmologists. In others, optometrists as well as ophthalmologists can provide medical eye care with approval by the patient's primary physician. In all cases, the patient must choose a physician on the HMO provider panel for eye care. Panel physicians are paid using either discounted fee schedules or capitation.

The use of capitation, for which the provider receives a fixed monthly payment (or "prepayment") for each HMO enrollee, places physicians at financial risk if services are overutilized. An optometrist might receive a certain capitation payment each month to cover a routine eye examination and ophthalmic materials for each HMO patient. The capitation payment is made to the optometrist regardless of whether the HMO patients actually use (or "consume") the vision care. If the overall utilization of optometric care is low or if the optometrist has been "efficient" in providing services, the unused capitation is the optometrist's

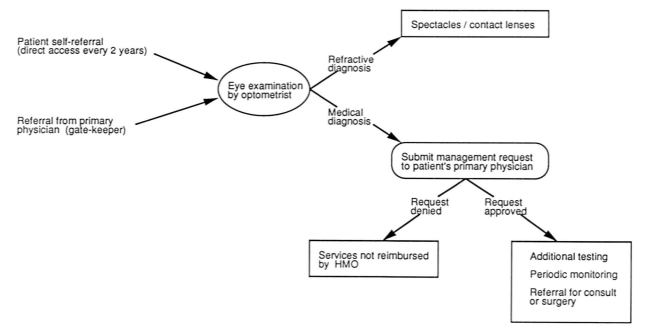

FIGURE 84–4. Example of eye care delivery in IPA-mode HMO illustrating patient access and role of "gate-keeper" in medical management.

profit. On the other hand, if utilization was higher than expected or if the optometrist provided more frequent or more costly services than were covered by the capitation, the optometrist loses money. The capitation system, therefore, uses financial incentives to limit utilization of services.

The PPOs are managed provider networks that offer a compromise between traditional indemnity plans and capitated HMOs. Unlike HMOs, enrollees in a PPO are not limited exclusively to panel providers. A PPO member may see a nonpanel physician if desired, but must pay a higher copayment or percentage than that required for a panel physician. Panel physicians are reimbursed by discounted fee schedules, avoiding the economic risk of capitation. Individuals covered by a PPO thus have a financial incentive to use the "preferred" panel physicians, but still retain the freedom to see nonpanel physicians. Panel physicians hope that gaining access to the PPO subscribers will offset the discounted fees for these patients. Like HMOs, PPOs have strict utilization review and quality control mechanisms to control costs and delivery of services.[3]

The various economic, political, demographic, and social forces currently in effect are leading to mergers and consolidation within the health insurance industry. Nearly all the major health insurers have been acquiring HMOs and PPOs or developing their own. It appears that the large insurance companies, national hospital chains, and regional and national HMOs will be controlling the future managed care environment. These "Super-Meds" will offer employers a menu of managed health insurance products that include HMO, PPO, and indemnity plans. Employers will be able to offer employees several health insurance options, while doing business with a single firm. The advent of the "triple-option" plan is encouraging for most practitioners, since private fee-for-service care is not precluded.[3,22]

PRACTICAL ASPECTS OF HEALTH INSURANCE CLAIMS

Despite the diversity among various insurance plans, there are some basic guidelines that will ensure efficient processing of insurance cases in practice.

1. All staff members, assistants, and technicians should understand the difference between medical plans and vision plans so they can properly educate patients and answer questions.
2. The office brochure or other patient information materials should clearly state the office policy on insurance, which plans are accepted and filed by the office, and the patients' responsibility for unassigned claims. For example, an office may accept Medicare and Medicaid, but not accept private health plans. Patients covered by private plans should understand before the examination that they must pay for all services rendered. It is their responsibility to obtain and complete a claim form and submit the claim to their carrier. Many offices complete and file the claim form as a courtesy service on unassigned claims. Patients should also understand that even if their insurance is accepted by the office, they may still be required to pay for deductibles, copayments, or noncovered services.
3. When a new patient calls for an appointment, the receptionist should inquire about medical and vision insurance. The patient should be instructed to bring any insurance identification cards to the examination. Upon a patient's arrival at the office, the receptionist should request to see the insurance card(s) to obtain the necessary information. Most offices also obtain insurance information on the patient information or registration form. This form can also state the office policy on insurance and accepted methods of payment.
4. Standardized insurance coding is necessary for all medical claims. Diagnostic and therapeutic procedure codes are found in Current Procedural Terminology (CPT) published each year by the American Medical Association. Diagnosis codes (devised by the World Health Organization) are obtained from the International Classification of Diseases (ICD) published by the Health Care Financing Administration. Medicare codes for ophthalmic materials are given in the HCFA Common Procedures Coding System (HCPCS). The American Optometric Association has compiled the most common CPT, ICD, and HCPCS codes pertaining to optometry in the Codes for Optometry manual.
5. Nearly all medical and optometric offices use a fee slip that itemizes the professional services and the corresponding CPT and ICD codes. Such a fee slip (also known as a "superbill") serves several important purposes. First, it minimizes or eliminates insurance paperwork on unassigned claims. All the necessary information required by the doctor should be present on the fee slip. The patient simply attaches the fee slip to the claim form, completes the demographic and policy information at the top of the claim form, and submits the claim to the insurance company. Second, the fee slip provides information to the receptionist or insurance clerk for assignment-accepted claims. The ICD and CPT codes will still be necessary for the staff member to complete the claim form or to enter information into the computer, Third, the fee slip serves as the patient's receipt, regardless of insurance status. Most are three-part carbonless forms of which one copy is submitted to the insurance company, one remains in the patient record, and one is the patient's receipt. Finally, the fee slip is an excellent internal marketing device that educates patients on the services and scope of optometric practice.[4]
6. All medical insurance carriers accept claims filed on the standard Medicare form (HCFA-1500). If a patient does not have their insurance company's specific form, the Medicare form can be used. Many optometric computer software programs are designed to complete continuous-feed Medicare forms.
7. As mentioned earlier, the diagnosis determines whether the eye examination and related procedures are covered by a given insurance plan. The corollary is that the clinician must make a diagnosis on each patient to determine appropriate insurance applicability. A patient may have both a medical eye diagnosis and a refractive diagnosis. If this patient has medical insurance, only the medical diagnosis should be listed on the fee slip or claim form. Any mention of a refractive diagnosis will likely cause immediate rejection of the claim, since claims processors automatically reject certain diagnoses and procedures that are exclusions from the policy (even if the other diagnoses are acceptable). This "shoot first and ask questions later" philosophy prevents insurance companies from paying a claim if there is any risk of a filing error.
8. Specific information on coding and filing health insurance claims is available from the Third-Party Committee of each state optometric association. In addition, local Medicare carriers, Medicaid agencies, and Blue Cross/Blue Shield offices have provider-relations personnel to assist in preparing and processing claims for these programs.

SUMMARY

Today's optometrist must understand and interact with the insurance system, in addition to providing excellent clinical care. The extent of private health insurance and the predicted decline of fee-for-service income mandate a working knowledge of the insurance process. Helping patients obtain their insurance benefit for optometric care is a valuable and much-appreciated service, given the high cost of coverage.

Optometric services are generally covered by medical plans or vision plans, depending upon the diagnosis. When a medical eye diagnosis is made, examinations and other medically necessary procedures are covered by medical insurance. Routine examinations for refractive conditions are covered by vision plans. Some insurance plans, such as HMOs, provide both types of eye care coverage.

Optometry's involvement with the insurance industry has greatly expanded in recent years commensurate with the expanding scope of practice. With the growth of managed care and triple-option plans, optometry's participation must increase to ensure our role as the primary provider of eye care in the future.

REFERENCES

1. Bartlett JD. Some predictions of optometrys' future. J Am Optom Assoc 1987;58:82–83.
2. Spivey BE, Gamble L. Providing ophthalmic services in a contracting environment. Ophthalmology 1987;94:296–297.
3. Farber L, ed. Encyclopedia of practice and financial management. Oradell, NJ: Medical Economics Books, 1988:247–271, 622–626.
4. Gordon A, Crooks CT. Optometric services and private health insurance. J Am Optom Assoc 1988;59:62–70.
5. Raffel MW. The US health system. New York: John Wiley & Sons, 1984:300–305.
6. Wilson FA, Neuhauser D. Health services in the United States. Cambridge: Ballinger Publishing, 1982:99–136.
7. Shulman AN. Health economics and financing. In: Newcomb RD, Jolley JL, eds. Public health and community optometry. Springfield: Charles C Thomas, 1980:229–252.
8. Health Insurance Association of America. Source book of health insurance data 1989. Washington, DC: Health Insurance Association of America, 1989.
9. Fordney MT, Follis JJ. Administrative medical assisting. New York: John Wiley & Sons, 1982:346–362.
10. Soroka M. Vision care and health insurance coverage. J Am Optom Assoc 1986;57:440–445.
11. Cooper MG, Cooper DE. The medical assistant. New York: McGraw-Hill Book Co., 1986:208–211, 276–303.
12. Crooks CT. Medicare reimbursement for optometry. South J Optom 1988;6(3):41–42.
13. Freeman D. Getting involved in Medicare: how to do it. Optom Manage September 1988:29–37.
14. Paxton HT. Medicare made relatively simple. Med Econ June 6, 1988: 164–174.
15. American Medical News. September 7, 1990, p. 3.
16. Hsiao WC, Braun P, Becker ER, et al. The resource-based relative value scale. JAMA 1987;258:799–802.
17. Hsiao WC, Braun P, Becker E, et al. A national study of resource-based relative value scales for physician services: final report, Department of Health Policy and Management, Harvard School of Public Health, September 27, 1988. HCFA contract no. 17-C-98795/1-03.
18. Jolley JL. Third-party payment programs. In: Newcomb RD, Jolley JL, eds. Public health and community optometry. Springfield: Charles C Thomas, 1980:253–280.
19. Spiegel A, Podair S, eds. Medicaid: lessons for national health insurance. Rockville: Aspen, 1975:8.
20. Mayer TR, Mayer GG. The health insurance alternative. New York: Perigee, 1984:29–41.
21. Hibbs JS. Contracting with managed health care plans in the present health care environment. Am J Ophthalmol 1987;103:321–327.
22. Goran M. The managed care environment. Ophthalmology 1987;94: 298–300.

Index

Page numbers in italics indicate figures; page numbers followed by a "t" indicate tables.